# Handbook of Dystonia

*Compliments of*

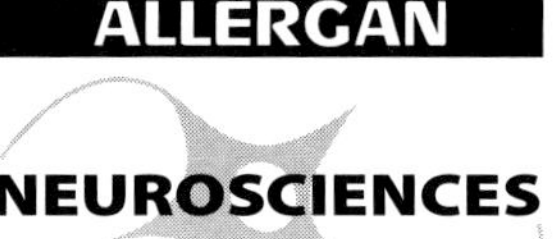

**NEUROLOGICAL DISEASE AND THERAPY**

1. Handbook of Parkinson's Disease, *edited by William C. Koller*
2. Medical Therapy of Acute Stroke, *edited by Mark Fisher*
3. Familial Alzheimer's Disease: Molecular Genetics and Clinical Perspectives, *edited by Gary D. Miner, Ralph W. Richter, John P. Blass, Jimmie L. Valentine, and Linda A. Winters-Miner*
4. Alzheimer's Disease: Treatment and Long-Term Management, *edited by Jeffrey L. Cummings and Bruce L. Miller*
5. Therapy of Parkinson's Disease, *edited by William C. Koller and George Paulson*
6. Handbook of Sleep Disorders, *edited by Michael J. Thorpy*
7. Epilepsy and Sudden Death, *edited by Claire M. Lathers and Paul L. Schraeder*
8. Handbook of Multiple Sclerosis, *edited by Stuart D. Cook*
9. Memory Disorders: Research and Clinical Practice, *edited by Takehiko Yanagihara and Ronald C. Petersen*
10. The Medical Treatment of Epilepsy, *edited by Stanley R. Resor, Jr., and Henn Kutt*
11. Cognitive Disorders: Pathophysiology and Treatment, *edited by Leon J. Thal, Walter H. Moos, and Elkan R. Gamzu*
12. Handbook of Amyotrophic Lateral Sclerosis, *edited by Richard Alan Smith*
13. Handbook of Parkinson's Disease: Second Edition, Revised and Expanded, *edited by William C. Koller*
14. Handbook of Pediatric Epilepsy, *edited by Jerome V. Murphy and Fereydoun Dehkharghani*
15. Handbook of Tourette's Syndrome and Related Tic and Behavioral Disorders, *edited by Roger Kurlan*
16. Handbook of Cerebellar Diseases, *edited by Richard Lechtenberg*
17. Handbook of Cerebrovascular Diseases, *edited by Harold P. Adams, Jr.*
18. Parkinsonian Syndromes, *edited by Matthew B. Stern and William C. Koller*
19. Handbook of Head and Spine Trauma, *edited by Jonathan Greenberg*
20. Brain Tumors: A Comprehensive Text, *edited by Robert A. Morantz and John W. Walsh*
21. Monoamine Oxidase Inhibitors in Neurological Diseases, *edited by Abraham Lieberman, C. Warren Olanow, Moussa B. H. Youdim, and Keith Tipton*
22. Handbook of Dementing Illnesses, *edited by John C. Morris*
23. Handbook of Myasthenia Gravis and Myasthenic Syndromes, *edited by Robert P. Lisak*
24. Handbook of Neurorehabilitation, *edited by David C. Good and James R. Couch, Jr.*
25. Therapy with Botulinum Toxin, *edited by Joseph Jankovic and Mark Hallett*
26. Principles of Neurotoxicology, *edited by Louis W. Chang*
27. Handbook of Neurovirology, *edited by Robert R. McKendall and William G. Stroop*
28. Handbook of Neuro-Urology, *edited by David N. Rushton*
29. Handbook of Neuroepidemiology, *edited by Philip B. Gorelick and Milton Alter*
30. Handbook of Tremor Disorders, *edited by Leslie J. Findley and William C. Koller*
31. Neuro-Ophthalmological Disorders: Diagnostic Work-Up and Management, *edited by Ronald J. Tusa and Steven A. Newman*
32. Handbook of Olfaction and Gustation, *edited by Richard L. Doty*
33. Handbook of Neurological Speech and Language Disorders, *edited by Howard S. Kirshner*
34. Therapy of Parkinson's Disease: Second Edition, Revised and Expanded, *edited by William C. Koller and George Paulson*
35. Evaluation and Management of Gait Disorders, *edited by Barney S. Spivack*
36. Handbook of Neurotoxicology, *edited by Louis W. Chang and Robert S. Dyer*
37. Neurological Complications of Cancer, *edited by Ronald G. Wiley*

38. Handbook of Autonomic Nervous System Dysfunction, *edited by Amos D. Korczyn*
39. Handbook of Dystonia, *edited by Joseph King Ching Tsui and Donald B. Calne*
40. Etiology of Parkinson's Disease, *edited by Jonas H. Ellenberg, William C. Koller and J. William Langston*
41. Practical Neurology of the Elderly, *edited by Jacob I. Sage and Margery H. Mark*
42. Handbook of Muscle Disease, *edited by Russell J. M. Lane*
43. Handbook of Multiple Sclerosis: Second Edition, Revised and Expanded, *edited by Stuart D. Cook*
44. Central Nervous System Infectious Diseases and Therapy, *edited by Karen L. Roos*
45. Subarachnoid Hemorrhage: Clinical Management, *edited by Takehiko Yanagihara, David G. Piepgras, and John L. D. Atkinson*
46. Neurology Practice Guidelines, *edited by Richard Lechtenberg and Henry S. Schutta*
47. Spinal Cord Diseases: Diagnosis and Treatment, *edited by Gordon L. Engler, Jonathan Cole, and W. Louis Merton*
48. Management of Acute Stroke, *edited by Ashfaq Shuaib and Larry B. Goldstein*
49. Sleep Disorders and Neurological Disease, *edited by Antonio Culebras*
50. Handbook of Ataxia Disorders, *edited by Thomas Klockgether*
51. The Autonomic Nervous System in Health and Disease, *David S. Goldstein*
52. Axonal Regeneration in the Central Nervous System, *edited by Nicholas A. Ingoglia and Marion Murray*
53. Handbook of Multiple Sclerosis: Third Edition, *edited by Stuart D. Cook*
54. Long-Term Effects of Stroke, *edited by Julien Bogousslavsky*
55. Handbook of the Autonomic Nervous System in Health and Disease, *edited by C. Liana Bolis, Julio Licinio, and Stefano Govoni*
56. Dopamine Receptors and Transporters: Function, Imaging, and Clinical Implication, Second Edition, *edited by Anita Sidhu, Marc Laruelle, and Philippe Vernier*
57. Handbook of Olfaction and Gustation: Second Edition, Revised and Expanded, *edited by Richard L. Doty*
58. Handbook of Stereotactic and Functional Neurosurgery, *edited by Michael Schulder*
59. Handbook of Parkinson's Disease: Third Edition, *edited by Rajesh Pahwa, Kelly E. Lyons, and William C. Koller*
60. Clinical Neurovirology, *edited by Avindra Nath and Joseph R. Berger*
61. Neuromuscular Junction Disorders: Diagnosis and Treatment, *Matthew N. Meriggioli, James F. Howard, Jr., and C. Michel Harper*
62. Drug-Induced Movement Disorders, *edited by Kapil D. Sethi*
63. Therapy of Parkinson's Disease: Third Edition, Revised and Expanded, *edited by Rajesh Pahwa, Kelly E. Lyons, and William C. Koller*
64. Epilepsy: Scientific Foundations of Clinical Practice, *edited by Jong M. Rho, Raman Sankar, and José E. Cavazos*
65. Handbook of Tourette's Syndrome and Related Tic and Behavioral Disorders: Second Edition, *edited by Roger Kurlan*
66. Handbook of Cerebrovascular Diseases: Second Edition, Revised and Expanded, *edited by Harold P. Adams, Jr.*
67. Emerging Neurological Infections, *edited by Christopher Power and Richard T. Johnson*
68. Treatment of Pediatric Neurologic Disorders, *edited by Harvey S. Singer, Eric H. Kossoff, Adam L. Hartman, and Thomas O. Crawford*

69. Synaptic Plasticity : Basic Mechanisms to Clinical Applications, *edited by Michel Baudry, Xiaoning Bi, and Steven S. Schreiber*
70. Handbook of Essential Tremor and Other Tremor Disorders, *edited by Kelly E. Lyons and Rajesh Pahwa*
71. Handbook of Peripheral Neuropathy, *edited by Mark B. Bromberg and A. Gordon Smith*
72. Carotid Artery Stenosis: Current and Emerging Treatments, *edited by Seemant Chaturvedi and Peter M. Rothwell*
73. Gait Disorders: Evaluation and Management, *edited by Jeffrey M. Hausdorff and Neil B. Alexander*
74. Surgical Management of Movement Disorders (HBK), *edited by Gordon H. Baltuch and Matthew B. Stern*
75. Neurogenetics: Scientific and Clinical Advances, *edited by David R. Lynch*
76. Epilepsy Surgery: Principles and Controversies, *edited by John W. Miller and Daniel L. Silbergeld*
77. Clinician's Guide To Sleep Disorders, *edited by Nathaniel F. Watson and Bradley Vaughn*
78. Amyotrophic Lateral Sclerosis, *edited by Hiroshi Mitsumoto, Serge Przedborski and Paul H. Gordon*
79. Duchenne Muscular Dystrophy: Advances in Therapeutics, *edited by Jeffrey S. Chamberlain and Thomas A. Rando*
80. Handbook of Multiple Sclerosis, Fourth Edition, *edited by Stuart D. Cook*
81. Brain Embolism, *edited by Louis R. Caplan and Warren J. Manning*
82. Handbook of Secondary Dementias, *edited by Roger Kurlan*
83. Parkinson's Disease: Genetics and Pathogenesis, *edited by Ted M. Dawson*
84. Migraine, *Russell Lane and Paul Davies*
85. Migraine and Other Headache Disorders, *edited by Richard B. Lipton and Marcelo Bigal*
86. Restless Legs Syndrome: Diagnosis and Treatment, *edited by William G. Ondo*
87. Handbook of Dementing Illnesses, Second Edition, *edited by John C. Morris, James E. Galvin, and David M. Holtzman*
88. Acute Stroke: Bench to Bedside, *edited by Anish Bhardwaj, Nabil J. Alkayed, Jeffrey R. Kirsch, and Richard J. Traystman*
89. Brain Tumors: Practical Guide to Diagnosis and Treatment, *edited by Joachim M. Baehring and Joseph M. Piepmeier*
90. Handbook of Dystonia, *edited by Mark A. Stacy*

# Handbook of Dystonia

edited by

Mark A. Stacy
*Movement Disorders Center*
*Duke University Medical Center*
*Durham, North Carolina, U.S.A.*

informa
healthcare

New York London

Informa Healthcare USA, Inc.
270 Madison Avenue
New York, NY 10016


Printed in the United States of America on acid-free paper
10 9 8 7 6 5 4 3 2 1

International Standard Book Number-10: 0-8493-7612-2 (Hardcover)
International Standard Book Number-13: 978-0-8493-7612-2 (Hardcover)



**Visit the Informa Web site at**
**www.informa.com**

**and the Informa Healthcare Web site at**
**www.informahealthcare.com**

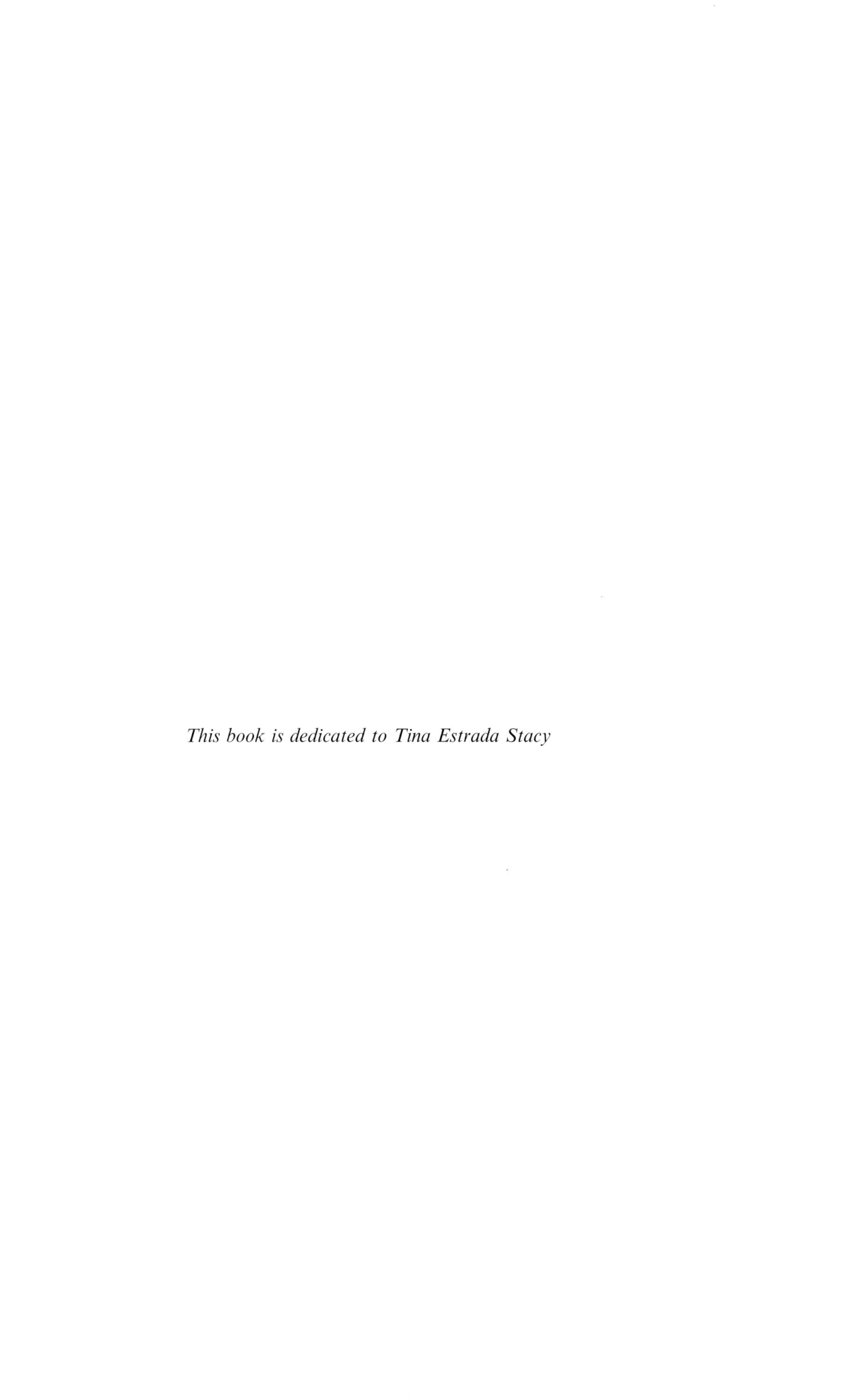

*This book is dedicated to Tina Estrada Stacy*

# Preface

Dystonia is a neurological condition that first was described as "dystonia muscularum deformans" nearly a century ago. Today, we know that dystonia is a movement disorder, typically characterized by an abnormal posture that is caused by a sustained muscle contraction. Given that the recognition of dystonia as a distinct diagnostic category did not occur until the 1970s, it is not surprising that an early, population-based prevalence study estimated that dystonia only affects approximately 24 per million people. However, with the development of botulinum toxin and an increased interest in this disorder, the prevalence of dystonia now is estimated to be nearly 100 times higher, potentially affecting 220 per million people worldwide.

While directed medical treatment began in the 1970s with the application of anticholinergic therapy, treatment of focal dystonia with botulinum toxin has led to a significant increase in the global recognition and research into this condition. Research conducted over the past 40 years has dramatically improved our understanding of dystonia. We now better understand its epidemiology, genetic risk factors, neurophysiology, and neuropathology. These advances have also improved and expanded treatment, not only with four marketed formulations of botulinum toxin, but also with phenol injection, baclofen pump therapy, and deep brain stimulation. These advances have dramatically improved the quality of life of patients affected with this disorder and have led to novel ideas for the investigation and treatment of other neurological disorders.

This volume was written to allow readers to quickly review the most current information regarding the pathogenesis and treatment of dystonia. The purpose of this book is to summarize the known information regarding this disorder and to present practical clinical assessment and treatment approaches.

The Handbook of Dystonia is organized in three basic sections: Epidemiology and Pathogenesis; Signs and Symptoms; and Treatment Options. After a well-rounded introduction, epidemiology and genetic factors are reviewed; these chapters are then followed by discussion regarding neuroanatomy, neurophysiology, neuropathology, and neuroimaging. Clinical descriptions for the idiopathic dystonias are grouped into generalized, cranial, cervical, limb and doparesponsive dystonia, with additional emphasis on other task-specific dystonias, such as musician's and sports-related dystonia. Secondary causes of dystonia are reviewed, with additional chapters on drug-induced and psychogenic presentations. In addition, because of the increasing emphasis on nonmotor symptoms in all areas of movement disorders, a chapter is devoted to this topic.

Treatment of dystonia is divided into four basic categories: medical treatment, botulinum toxin injections, phenol or neurolytic therapy, and surgical intervention. Given the relative importance of botulinum toxin in the treatment of dystonic disorders, three chapters are devoted to this topic. The surgical procedures for dystonia are divided into selective denervation for cervical dystonia and deep brain stimulation for generalized and other types of dystonia.

I would like to thank the contributors to this volume who have participated in bench and clinical research in dystonic disorders and have provided excellent summaries of these topics. I would also like to thank Informa Healthcare, specifically Susan B. Lee, Rick Werdann, Dana Bigelow, and Jinnie Kim, for their support and encouragement in preparing this book.

*Mark A. Stacy, MD*

# Contents

# Contributors

**Charles H. Adler** Department of Neurology, Mayo Clinic, Scottsdale, Arizona, U.S.A.

**Carlos A. Arce** Department of Neurosurgery, University of Florida HSC, Jacksonville, Florida, U.S.A.

**Richard L. Barbano** Department of Neurology, University of Rochester, Rochester, New York, U.S.A.

**Roongroj Bhidayasiri** Division of Neurology, Chulalongkorn University Hospital, Bangkok, Thailand, and Department of Neurology, David Geffen School of Medicine at UCLA, Los Angeles, California, U.S.A.

**Andrew Blitzer** New York Center for Voice and Swallowing Disorders, Head and Neck Surgical Group, St. Luke's Roosevelt Medical Center, New York, New York, U.S.A.

**Xandra O. Breakefield** Departments of Neurology and Radiology, Massachusetts General Hospital, Charlestown, Massachusetts, and Harvard Medical School, Boston, U.S.A.

**Nicole Calakos** Departments of Medicine/Neurology and Neurobiology, Center for Translational Neuroscience, Duke University, Durham, North Carolina, U.S.A.

**Francisco Cardoso** Department of Internal Medicine, Movement Disorders Clinic, Neurology Service, The Federal University of Minas Gerais, Brazil

**Arif Dalvi** Department of Neurology, University of Chicago, Chicago, Illinois, U.S.A.

**Khashayar Dashtipour** Department of Neurology, Loma Linda University, Loma Linda, California, U.S.A.

**Giovanni Defazio** Department of Neurological and Psychiatric Sciences, University of Bari, Bari, Italy

**Stewart A. Factor** Department of Neurology, Emory University School of Medicine, Wesley Woods Health Center, Atlanta, Georgia, U.S.A.

**Steven J. Frucht** The Neurological Institute, Columbia University Medical Center, New York, New York, U.S.A.

**Joanne Green** Department of Neurology, Emory University School of Medicine, Wesley Woods Health Center, Atlanta, Georgia, U.S.A.

**Mark Hallett** Human Motor Control Section, National Institute of Neurological Disorders and Stroke, National Institutes of Health, Bethesda, Maryland, U.S.A.

**Joseph Jankovic** Department of Neurology, Parkinson's Disease Center and Movement Disorders Clinic, Baylor College of Medicine, Houston, Texas, U.S.A.

**Barbara I. Karp** National Institute of Neurological Disorders and Stroke, National Institutes of Health, Bethesda, Maryland, U.S.A.

**Christine Klein** Department of Neurology, University of Luebeck, Luebeck, Germany

**Anthony E. Lang** Movement Disorders Unit, Toronto Western Hospital, and University of Toronto, Ontario, Canada

**Mark Lew** Department of Neurology, University of Southern California, Los Angeles, California, U.S.A.

**Steven E. Lo** The Neurological Institute, Columbia University Medical Center, New York, New York, U.S.A.

**Kelly E. Lyons** Department of Neurology, University of Kansas Medical Center, Kansas City, Kansas, U.S.A.

**William J. Marks, Jr.** Department of Neurology, University of California, San Francisco, California, U.S.A.

**Kevin StP. McNaught** Department of Neurology, Mount Sinai School of Medicine, New York, New York, U.S.A.

**Tanya K. Meyer** Department of Otorhinolaryngology, Head and Neck Surgery, University of Maryland Medical Center, Baltimore, Maryland, U.S.A.

**Jonathan W. Mink** Departments of Neurology, Pediatrics, Anatomy and Neurobiology, and Brain and Cognitive Sciences, University of Rochester, Rochester, New York, U.S.A.

**Nobuyoshi Nishiyama** Department of Laboratory of Chemical Pharmacology, Graduate School of Pharmaceutical Sciences, The University of Tokyo, Tokyo, Japan

**Yoshiko Nomura** Segawa Neurological Clinic for Children, Tokyo, Japan

**William G. Ondo** Department of Neurology, Baylor College of Medicine, Houston, Texas, U.S.A.

**Laurie J. Ozelius** Department of Molecular Genetics, Albert Einstein College of Medicine, Bronx, New York, U.S.A.

**Rajesh Pahwa** Department of Neurology, University of Kansas Medical Center, Kansas City, Kansas, U.S.A.

**Daniel P. Perl** Department of Pathology, Mount Sinai School of Medicine, New York, New York, U.S.A.

**Johan Samanta** Banner Good Samaritan Medical Center, Phoenix, and Department of Neurology, University of Arizona College of Medicine, Tucson, Arizona, U.S.A.

**Pankaj Satija** Department of Neurology, Baylor College of Medicine, Houston, Texas, U.S.A.

**Anette Schrag** University Department of Clinical Neurosciences, Royal Free and University College Medical School, London, U.K.

**Lauren C. Seeberger** Colorado Neurological Institute Movement Disorders Center, Englewood, and Department of Neurology, University of Colorado Health Sciences Center, Denver, Colorado, U.S.A.

**Masaya Segawa** Segawa Neurological Clinic for Children, Tokyo, Japan

**Joohi Shahed** Department of Neurology, Parkinson's Disease Center and Movement Disorders Clinic, Baylor College of Medicine, Houston, Texas, U.S.A.

**Holly A. Shill** Movement Disorder Section, Barrow Neurological Institute, Phoenix, Arizona, U.S.A.

**Mark A. Stacy** Department of Medicine/Neurology, and Movement Disorders Center, Duke University Medical Center, Durham, North Carolina, U.S.A.

**A. J. Stoessl** Pacific Parkinson's Research Centre, University of British Columbia, Vancouver, British Columbia, Canada

**Daniel Tarsy** Department of Neurology, Beth Israel Deaconess Medical Center, Harvard Medical School, Boston, Massachusetts, U.S.A.

**A. R. Troiano** Pacific Parkinson's Research Centre, University of British Columbia, Vancouver, British Columbia, Canada

**Ruth H. Walker** Department of Neurology, James J. Peters Veterans Affairs Medical Center, Bronx, and Mount Sinai School of Medicine, New York, New York, U.S.A.

# 1
# Introduction to Dystonia

**Joohi Shahed and Joseph Jankovic**
*Department of Neurology, Parkinson's Disease Center and Movement Disorders Clinic, Baylor College of Medicine, Houston, Texas, U.S.A.*

Although Hermann Oppenheim is usually credited with the introduction of the term "dystonia" in his landmark work published in 1911 (1), he was not the first to describe the abnormal postures and sustained muscle contractions that characterized this hyperkinetic movement disorder. In the 1830s, writer's cramp was recognized amongst members of the British Civil Service (2). In 1887, Horatio Wood, Chairman of Neurology at the University of Pennsylvania, the first Department of Neurology in the United States, described facial (blepharospasm) and oromandibular dystonia (3). In 1888, William Gowers (4) described dystonic postures in hands and feet, which he called "tetanoid chorea," in two siblings who were later diagnosed with Wilson's disease, a disorder that had not yet been named. In 1897, Barraquer Roviralta (5) described the generalized dystonia phenotype, but termed it "athetosis."

Since that time, the dystonic syndrome has been referred to by a variety of names, including "tonic cramps," (6) "torsion neurosis," (7) "progressive torsion spasm," and "dystonia lenticularis" (8). Schwalbe recognized the familial nature of dystonic disorders with his description of Jewish siblings in 1908 (6). He gave one of the most thorough descriptions of the disorder, and is therefore credited with "discovery" of dystonia. However, in his treatise "Tonic Cramps with Hysterical Symptoms," he highlighted the possible psychiatric overlay to these symptoms, sparking a controversy that influenced subsequent interpretations of the pathophysiology of dystonic disorders.

In 1911, in addition to the classical work by Oppenheim (1), two other landmark articles were published: one by Ziehen (7) and the other by Flatau and Sterling (9). Oppenheim (1) simultaneously named the syndrome "dystonia musculorum deformans" and "dysbasia lordotica progressiva." His classic description includes the characteristic "dromedary" gait. He termed the disorder "dystonia" to emphasize the seeming co-occurrence of increased and decreased tone in different parts of the body. The term "musculorum" incorporates Oppenheim's notion that dystonic postures were due to muscle abnormalities. The second term, on the other hand, emphasized the progressive nature of the symptoms while also recognizing the unusual twisted postures of the trunk and abnormal gait. Ziehen (7) recognized that dystonic movements seemed to increase with action and during emotional excitement, and argued for an organic cause of the symptoms.

After 1911, the term "dystonia" became the most widely accepted terminology for the disorder, and for a brief period, was referred to as "Oppenheim–Ziehen" disease. The term "dystonia musculorum deformans" coined by Oppenheim was criticized by Flatau and Sterling (9) because fluctuating muscle tone was not necessarily a characteristic of the disorder; the term "musculorum" incorrectly implied that the involuntary movement was due to a muscle disorder, and not all patients became deformed. They highlighted the genetic nature of the disorder and suggested the term "progressive torsion spasm."

Focal forms of dystonia were recognized before generalized dystonia, although they were often attributed to various occupations. Ramazzini (10), considered the father of occupational medicine, referred to symptoms consistent with writer's cramp in his 1713 treatise, "De Morbis Artificum Diatriba" or "Diseases of Workers." Duchenne also offered a description in 1855 (11), and Solly first termed the disorder "scrivener's palsy" in 1864 (2). Various other occupational cramping disorders were also described during the 18th and 19th centuries. In 1893, Gowers (12) described the clinical features and drew a pictorial representation of a 44-year-old man that was intended to depict spasmodic torticollis. However, in the drawing, the patient's right arm also appeared involved, as evidenced by its unusual posture and an open button, suggesting a more generalized dystonia. Subsequently, a vivid description of torticollis with photographs was published in 1896 by Thompson, referred to "wry neck" (13).

In 1929 Wimmer (14) referred to dystonia as a "syndrome" rather than a specific disease entity, thus acknowledging that the phenomenon is seen in various neurologic conditions including Wilson's disease, postencephalitic cases, and in instances of perinatal brain damage. He also recognized dystonic features in patients with Parkinson's disease and Huntington's chorea. Herz (15) later described the first large series of dystonia cases, comprised of 15 personal patients and a review of 100 from the literature in 1944. He documented the abnormal movements on film, analyzed them frame by frame, and so was able to characterize the sustained muscular contractions and flow of abnormal movements from one body part to another. Thus emerged a more precise explanation of the phenomenology of dystonia, and the disease "idiopathic torsion dystonia" as a distinct clinical entity.

Subsequent years in the history of dystonia were marked by efforts in elucidating its etiology. Despite early suspicion of the probable role of the basal ganglia in producing the abnormal movements, clinicopathologic correlations for this belief were lacking. In the 1930s (16) and again in the 1960s (17), published reports identified no specific neuropathologic changes in brains of patients with dystonia. Previous authors, including Oppenheim and Herz, had argued against a genetic influence for the development of dystonia. The aforementioned controversy surrounding psychogenic aspects of the disorder also hampered further scientific investigations. The phenomenon of a classic "geste antogoniste" fueled nonorganic theories. Later, recognition of dystonic features following the influenza/encephalitis epidemic of the 1920s strongly suggested that dystonia stemmed from an organic cause, but also led to confusion in the differentiation between primary and secondary forms of dystonia (18).

In the 1970s, after several authors reviewed familial cases of dystonia, the prevailing view was that in Jewish families inheritance was autosomal recessive, while non-Jewish forms were transmitted in an autosomal dominant fashion (18). Zeman and Dyken, however, performed detailed analyses of large families with dystonic disorders, and were the first to recognize that there were variable degrees of symptom severity in members of the same family, what they termed "formes frustes" of dystonia (17) more recently, the relative risk of spread of symptoms in patients with focal-onset primary dsytonias has been described (18).

The term "torsion dystonia" has been used in the literature, but because the term "torsion," which denotes "twisting," is not always part of dystonia (e.g., blepharospasm and oromandibular dystonia), this term seems redundant. Hence, the simple term "dystonia" is currently preferred when referring to the hyperkinetic movement disorder. In 1984, the Scientific Advisory Board of the Dystonia Medical Research Foundation proposed a formal definition of dystonia as "a syndrome of sustained muscle contractions, frequently causing twisting and repetitive movements, or abnormal postures" (19). This definition has since been further modified: "dystonia is a neurological disorder dominated by involuntary, sustained or spasmodic, repetitive, and patterned contractions of muscles, frequently causing twisting and other abnormal movements or postures." The term "patterned" refers to the repeated involvement of the same group of muscles, a feature that helps to differentiate dystonia from other hyperkinetic movement disorders. Dystonia has been also classified based on age at onset (early or late), parts of the body affected (focal, segmental, multifocal, or generalized), and etiology (primary or secondary) (20).

In the last two decades, there has been an explosion of knowledge about the pathophysiology and pathogenesis of dystonia. In 1985, two series of patients with hemidystonia (21,22) drew attention to the notion that lesions in the basal ganglia, particularly the putamen, can lead to such symptoms. The role of the basal ganglia in the pathophysiology of dystonia was later confirmed by several physiological and functional imaging studies (23,24). It is now thought that with focal forms of dystonia, genetic predisposition plays a significant role, either by rendering a decrease of inhibition, an increase of plasticity or an impairment in sensory function (25). Since the availability of new molecular techniques, several families with dystonia have been investigated. In 1989, the gene locus for idiopathic torsion dystonia (*DYT1*) was mapped to chromosome 9q in one North American family (20). Subsequently, a three base-pair (GAG) deletion was identified in the fifth exon of the *DYT1* (*TOR1A*) gene at the 9q34 locus, which codes for a novel 332 amino acid adenosine triphosphate-binding protein, termed torsinA (26,27). The mutation results in the loss of a pair of glutamic acid residues.

This important discovery not only enabled DNA testing for the abnormal *DYT1* (*TOR1A*) gene, but it also launched many fruitful research efforts into the cellular mechanisms of this inherited form of dystonia. TorsinA has now been localized to the nuclear envelope in studies using tissue cultures (28). Pathologic studies using brains of patients with *DYT1* dystonia have also demonstrated torsinA-positive perinuclear inclusion bodies within the midbrain reticular formation and periaqueductal gray of the pedunculopontine nucleus, cuneiform nucleus, and griseum centrale mesencephali, which also stain positively for ubiquitin and the nuclear envelope protein lamin A/C (29). Tau- and ubiquitin-immunoreactive aggregates were also noted in these inclusions as well as in the substantia nigra pars compacta and locus coeruleus, supporting the notion that *DYT1* dystonia is another neurodegenerative disorder associated with impaired protein handling, particularly in the brainstem nuclei. Interestingly, torsinA is also present in Lewy bodies, the pathological hallmark of Parkinson's disease, a finding that may provide insight into the frequent overlap of dystonia and parkinsonian disorders (30). Adding to this possible association is the common occurrence of joint or skeletal deformities in PD and parkinsonian disorders, which are most likely dystonic in origin (31).

Since the initial discovery of *DYT1* mutation, 14 other dystonic disorders have been given DYT designations and have been localized to specific chromosomes, though complete information on gene products and their functions are as yet unavailable. All except for *DYT2* (autosomal recessive) (32) and *DYT3* (Lubag, or X-linked dystonia-parkinsonism, autosomal recessive) (33) are autosomal dominant conditions. We now have a much greater pathophysiologic understanding of distinct dystonic disorders such as dopa-responsive dystonia (*DYT5* or Segawa disease, related to mutations in guanosine triphosphate cyclohydrolase I) (34,35) and myoclonus dystonia (*DYT11*, from mutations in the epsilon sarcoglycan gene) (36,37). Several susceptibility genes for dystonia have also been identified, such as the D5 dopamine receptor gene for familial blepharospasm (38) and familial cervical dystonia (39).

Along with advances in the understanding of the pathophysiology and genetics of dystonia have come developments in its treatment. Although surgical procedures for movement disorders have been in use for several decades, their use was limited due to an unacceptably high complication rate. The first surgeries in the 1940s and 1950s by Meyers (40) were ablative, and involved various subcortical structures. However, as microsurgical and recording techniques were not yet developed, there was a great deal of difficulty in ascertaining that the appropriate anatomic target had been reached. Two major sites emerged: the thalamus and the globus pallidus interna (GPi). In 1976, Cooper (41) published a 20-year follow-up report on over 200 patients treated with thalamotomy, noting that 70% of his patients experienced marked or moderate improvement in abnormal postures. Even at this early stage in the development of surgical techniques for dystonia, it was recognized that patients with genetic forms improved to a greater degree than those with secondary forms. Severe dysarthria from bilateral destructive lesions in the thalamus was a frequent complication, and attention soon turned to lesioning the GPi for control of dystonic symptoms. The first procedures were described in the 1950s in the anterodorsal region of the GPi, and were used to treat a variety of conditions including Parkinson's disease, dystonia, and other bradykinetic disorders (42). Over the years, the target was gradually moved to the posteroventral region of the GPi, with improved results. The modern pallidotomy, described by Laitenen et al. in 1992 (43), targets pallidal projections to the thalamus, seems to be much more effective in controlling dystonia, and does not carry the same risk of dysarthria. However, the uncertainty of outcome in a subpopulation of patients, namely progressive dystonia, despite an initial improvement, has also led to some hesitancy in pursuing this type of surgical procedure.

Over the past decade, deep brain stimulation, particularly targeting the GPi, has taken precedence over ablative procedures in the management of dystonia as well as other movement disorders (44,45). The adjustable and even reversible effects of stimulation offer the opportunity to tailor the stimulation parameters according to the needs of each patient. However, most reports continue to find that patients with genetic rather than secondary forms of dystonia have a more robust response to such procedures.

The most important development in the treatment of dystonic disorders has been the introduction of botulinum toxin injections. The first accurate medical description of botulism ("sausage poison") was reported in the early 1800s (46). Seven immunologically distinct botulinum toxins are now known, but only type A and B are in clinical use. In 1989, the U.S. Food and Drug Administration approved the original batch of botulinum toxin type A (produced in 1979) for use in patients with strabismus, blepharospasm, and facial nerve disorders such as hemifacial spasm. Neurologic applications for the toxin, including cervical and other forms

**Table 1** Milestones in the History of Dystonia

| Year | Author | Description |
|---|---|---|
| 1713 | Ramazzini (48) | Description of probable writer's cramp |
| 1804 | Solly (49) | "Scrivener's palsy" first named and described |
| 1800s | Kerner (50) | "Sausage poison" is a biologic toxin; motor and autonomic effects first noted |
| 1830s | From Pearce (2), 2005 | Writer's cramp described among British Civil Service |
| 1887 | Wood (3) | Facial and oromandibular dystonia |
| 1888 | Gowers (4) | "Tetanoid chorea"—two siblings who were later diagnosed with Wilson's disease |
| 1893 | Gowers (4) | Picture of torticollis, but patient most likely has generalized dystonia |
| 1895 | VanErmengem (51) | Bacillus botulinus first isolated from bodies of victims of food poisoning |
| 1896 | Thompson (13) | "Wry neck," photographs of cervical dystonia published |
| 1897 | Barraquer Roviralta (5) | "Athetosis" used to describe generalized dystonia |
| 1901 | Destarac (52) | "Torticolis spasmodique"—a 17-year-old girl with torticollis, tortipelvis, writer's cramp, and foot cramps; improved by sensory tricks, exacerbated with motor activity |
| 1903 | Leszynsky (53) | Hysterical spasms and gait |
| 1908 | Hunt (8) | "Myoclonia of the trunk," "tic spasms," hysterical |
| 1908 | Schwalbe (8) | Hereditary "tonic crampus" syndrome, maladie des tics—rapid movements; recognized the familial nature of dystonia in Jewish siblings (Lewin family); used scopolamine |
| 1911 | Ziehen (7) | "Torsion neurosis"—did not believe it to be hysterical; observed that "convulsive movements increased during voluntary movement" and during emotional excitement |
| 1911 | Oppenheim (1) | "Dystonia musculorum deformans" and "dysbasia lordotica progressiva"; "monkey" or "dromedary" gait first described along with "mobile spasms," sustained posturing, fluctuating muscle tone, rapid movement resembling tremor, chorea, and athetosis |
| 1911 | Flatau and Sterling (9) | "Progressive torsion spasm,"—noted hereditary, repetitive pattern, "jerky"; Jewish patients of high intelligence; objected to the term "deformans" because not all patients become disfigured and objected to the term "musculorum" because it implied a muscle condition |
| 1912 | Fraenkel (54) | Rapid, twisting, sustained movement, tortipelvis |
| 1912 | Wilson (8) | "Hepatolenticular degeneration"—"clonic" or "tic-like" spasms, "choreiform and athetoid" movements |
| 1916 | Hunt (55) | Slow, twisting or clonic, rhythmic movements |
| 1919 | Mendel (8) | "Torsion dystonia"—review of literature; 33 patients; "a morbid disease entity" |
| 1919 | Burke (56) | Botulinum toxin strains A and B identified |
| 1920 | Taylor (57) | "Dystonia lenticularis," postural ("myostatic") and kinetic forms of dystonia |

*(Continued)*

**Table 1** Milestones in the History of Dystonia (*Continued*)

| Year | Author | Description |
|---|---|---|
| 1920s | | Postencephalitic dystonia led to recognition of secondary forms |
| 1926 | Davidenkow (8) | "Myoclonic dystonia"—rapid "tic-like" movements |
| 1929 | Wimmer (14) | Dystonia is "not a disease but only a syndrome"—seen in Wilson's disease, postencephalitic cases, and perinatal brain damage |
| 1942 | Meyers (39) | Ablative surgical procedures used for dystonia |
| 1944 | Herz (15) | Idiopathic dystonia as a disease entity—15 personal cases and 105 from the literature; "slow, long-sustained, turning movements"; alternating "myorhythmia" or "very rapid, tic-like twitchings" |
| 1958 | Cooper (8) | Thalamotomy described for dystonia |
| 1959 | Zeman (58) | Autosomal dominant inheritance |
| 1960 | Zeman (59) | Formes frustes of dystonia |
| 1962 | Denny–Brown (60) | "Fixed or relatively fixed attitude" |
| 1967 | Zeman and Dyken (17) | No specific neuropathology in dystonia brains |
| 1976 | Cooper (40) | 20-year follow-up report on more than 200 patients with thalamotomy; genetic forms of dystonia improved the most |
| 1976 | Marsden (61) | Blepharospasm is a form of focal dystonia |
| 1983 | Fahn (62) | High dosage anticholinergic therapy relieves dystonia |
| 1983 | Jankovic and Patel (63) | Blepharospasm-oromandibular dystonia secondary to rostral brainstem-diencephalic lesion |
| 1984 | DMRF (64) | First formal definition of dystonia |
| 1985 | Scott et al. (65) | Botulinum toxin for blepharospasm |
| 1985 | Marsden et al. (21), Pettigrew and Jankovic (20) | Dystonia due to basal ganglia lesions |
| 1989 | Ozelius et al. (66) | Autosomal dominant dystonia linked to chromosome 9q32–34 (*DYT1*) |
| 1989 | | Botulinum toxin type A approved by the U.S. Food and Drug Administration |
| 1992 | Laitenen et al. (42) | Ablative procedures to pallidal projections to the thalamus are more effective than thalamotomy, with fewer side effects |
| 1994 | Ichinose et al. (67) | Mutations in the guanosine triphosphate-cyclohydrolase I on chromosome 14q22.1–22.2 identified as cause of autosomal dominant dopa-responsive-dystonia (DRD, Segawa disease) |
| 1995 | Ludecke (68) | Mutation in the tyrosine hydroxylaze gene on chromosome 11p15.5 causes autosomal recessive form of DRD |
| 1997 | Ozelius et al. (26) | Dystonia gene (*DYT1*) encodes torsinA, an adenosine triphosphate-binding protein |
| 2000 | | Botulinum toxin type A and Type B approved by the FDA for the treatment of cervical dystonia. |
| 2000 | | Pallidal deep brain stimulation demonstrated effective for dystonia |
| 2001 | Zimprich et al. (36) | Epsilon sarcoglycan gene mutation causes myoclonus-dystonia (*DYT11*) |

*Source*: Modified from Ref. 8.

of dystonia, soon followed. Since that time, the formulation was changed, resulting in less antigenicity. Numerous other medical indications for the toxin have been realized (47). Both medical and surgical treatments of dystonia have modified the natural history of dystonic disorders in that contractures, frequently seen in the past in untreated patients before such options were available, are now rarely observed. Furthermore, both patients with focal and generalized forms of dystonia are now able to reach their full potential and experience meaningful improvement in their quality of life.

The primary objective of this review has been to provide an introduction and historical perspective on dystonia and highlight some of the advances in our understanding of this neurological disorder (Table 1). Review of the diagnosis, appropriate investigations, and treatment options for various dystonic disorders is now available (69,70).

As a result of the advances in our medical and scientific knowledge about dystonia and dystonic disorders and available effective therapies, there is greater awareness of this hyperkinetic movement disorder among physicians and the general public. However, more work is needed to further our understanding of the pathogenesis of this complex disorder on a molecular level, and to develop more therapies targeted at cellular and biochemical changes that are continuously being elucidated through research endeavors. In this regard, the advances in lentiviral-mediated RNA interference therapy targeted against mutant torsinA are quite promising (71).

## REFERENCES


1. Oppenheim H. Über eine eigenartige Krampfkrankheit des kindlichen und jugendlichen Alters (Dysbasia lordotica progressiva, Dystonia musculorum deformans). Neurologisches Zentralblatt, Leipzig 1911; 30:1090–1107.
2. Pearce JM. A note on scrivener's palsy. J Neurol Neurosurg Psych 2005; 76:513.
3. Wood HC. Nervous Diseases and Their Diagnostics. Philadelphia: Lippincott, 1887.
4. Gowers WR. Gowers WR, ed. A Manual of Diseases of the Nervous System. Philadelphia: P. Blakiston, 1888:1375.
5. Barraquer Roviralta L. Contribución al estudio de la atetosis. Gac Med Catalana 1897; 20:385–391.
6. Schwalbe MW. Eine eigentumliche tonische krampfform mit hysterischen Symptomen. Inaugural Dissertation, Berlin, 1907.
7. Ziehen GT. Ein Fall von tonischer Torsionsneurose. Demonstrationen im Psychiatrischen Verein zu Berlin. Neurologisches Zentralblatt, Leipzig 1911; 30:109–110.
8. Jankovic J, Fahn S. Dystonic disorders. In: Jankovic J, Tolosa E, eds. Parkinson's Disease and Movement Disorders. 4th ed. Philadelphia: Lippincott Williams & Wilkins, 2002:331–357.
9. Flatau E, Sterling W. Progressiver Torsionsspasmus bei Kindern. Z Gesamte Neurol Psychiatr 1911; 7:586–612.
10. Ramazzini B. Diseases of Workers. In: Translated from De Morbis Artificum of 1713 by Wilmer Cave Wright. New York: Haffner, 1964.
11. Duchenne GBA. In: Poore GV, ed. Selections from the clinical works. London: New Sydenham Society; 1883, 399–409 from De L'electralisation localisée. 3rd ed. Paris: JB Baillière, 1855:1021–1034.
12. Gowers WR. A Manual of Diseases of the Nervous System. 2nd ed. Philadelphia: Blakiston, 1893:709–711.
13. Thompson JH. A Wry-Necked Family. Lancet 1896; ii:24.
14. Wimmer A. Le spasme de torsion. Rev Neurol 1929; 36:904–915.
15. Herz E. Dystonia. Arch Neurol Psych 1944; 51:305–355.

16. Goetz CG, Chmura TA, Lanska DJ. History of dystonia: Part 4 of the MDS-sponsored history of movement disorders exhibit, Barcelona, June, 2000. Mov Disord 2001; 16: 339–345.
17. Zeman W, Dyken P. Dystonia musculorum deformans: clinical, genetic and pathoanatomical studies. Psychiatr Neurol Neurochir 1967; 70:77–121.
18. Weiss EM, Hershey I, Karimi M, et al. Relative risk of spread of symptoms among the focal onset primary dystonias. Mov Disord 2006; 21:1175–1181.
19. Grundmann K. Primary torsion dystonia. Arch Neurol 2005; 62:682–685.
20. Tarsy D, Simon DK. Dystonia N Engl J Med 2006; 24; 355(8): 818–829.
21. Marsden CD, Obeso JA, Zarranz JJ, et al. The anatomical basis of symptomatic hemidystonia. Brain 1985; 108:463–483.
22. Pettigrew LC, Jankovic J. Hemidystonia: A report of 22 patients and a review of the literature. J Neurol Neurosurg Psychiatr 1985; 48:650–657.
23. Hallett M. Disorder of movement preparation in dystonia. Brain 2000; 123:1765–1766.
24. Eidelberg D, Moeller JR, Ishikawa T, et al. The metabolic topography of idiopathic torsion dystonia. Brain 1995; 118:1473–1484.
25. Hallett M. Pathophysiology of writer's cramp. Hum Mov Sci 2006; 19:[E pub ahead of print].
26. Ozelius LJ, Hewett JW, Page CE, et al. The early onset torsion dystonia gene (DYT1) encodes an ATP-binding protein. Nat Genet 1997; 17:40–48.
27. Breakfield XO, Kamm C, Hanson PI. TorsinA: movement at many levels. Neuron 2001; 31:9–12.
28. Naismith TV, Heuser JE, Breakefield XO, et al. TorsinA in the nuclear envelope. Proc Natl Acad Sci USA 2004; 101:7612–7617.
29. McNaught KS, Kapustin A, Jackson T, et al. Brainstem pathology in DYT1 primary torsion dystonia. Ann Neurol 2004; 56:540–547.
30. Jankovic J, Tintner R. Dystonia and Parkinsonism. Parkinsonism Relat Disord 2001; 8:109–121.
31. Ashour R, Jankovic J. Joint and skeletal deformities in Parkinson's disease, multiple system atrophy, and progressive supranuclear palsy. Mov Disord 2006; 28: [E pub ahead of print].
32. Khan NL, Wood NW, Bhatia KP. Autosomal recessive, DYT2-like primary torsion dystonia: a new family. Neurology 2003; 61:1801–1803.
33. Nolte D, Niemann S, Muller U. Specific sequence changes in multiple transcript system DYT3 are associated with X-linked dystonia parkinsonism. Proc Natl Acad Sci USA 2003; 100:10347–10352.
34. Segawa M, Nomura Y, Nishiyama N. Autosomal dominant guanosine triphosphate cyclohydrolase I deficiency (Segawa disease). Ann Neurol 2003; 54(suppl 6):S32–S45.
35. Chaila EC, McCabe DJ, Delanty N, Costello DJ, Murphy RP. Broadening the phenotype of childhood-onset dopa-responsive dystonia. Arch Neurol 2006; 63:1185–1188.
36. Zimprich A, Grabowski M, Asmus F, et al. Mutations in the gene encoding epsilon-sarcoglycan cause myoclonus-dystonia syndrome. Nat Genet 2001; 29:66–69.
37. Gerrits MC, Foncke EM, de Haan R, et al. Phenotype-genotype correlation in Dutch patients with myoclonus-dystonia. Neurology 2006; 66: 759-761.
38. Misbahuddin A, Placzek MR, Chaudhuri KR, et al. A polymorphism in the dopamine receptor DRD5 is associated with blepharospasm. Neurology 2002; 58:124–126.
39. Placzek MR, Misbahuddin A, Chaudhuri KR, et al Cervical dystonia is associated with a polymorphism in the dopamine (D5) receptor gene. J Neurol Neurosurg Psychiatr 2001; 71:262–264.
40. Meyers R. The present state of neurosurgical procedures directed against the extrapyramidal diseases. NY State J Med 1942; 42:317–325.
41. Cooper IS. 20-year follow-up study of the neurosurgical treatment of dystonia musculorum deformans. Adv Neurol 1976; 14:423–452.

42. Ford B. Pallidotomy for generalized dystonia. In: Fahn S, Hallet M, DeLong MR, eds. Dystonia 4: Advances in Neurology. Vol. 94. Philadelphia: Lippincott Williams & Wilkins, 2004:287–300.
43. Laitenen LV, Bergenheim AT, Hariz MI. Leksell's posteroventral pallidotomy in the treatment of Parkinson's disease. J Neurosurg 1992; 76:53–61.
44. Vidailhet M, Vercueil L, Houeto JL, et al, French Stimulation du Pallidum Interne dans la Dystonie (SPIDY) Study Group. Bilateral deep-brain stimulation of the globus pallidus in primary generalized dystonia. N Engl J Med 2005; 352:459–467.
45. Diamond A, Jankovic J. The effect of deep brain stimulation on quality of life in movement disorders. J Neurol Neurosurg Psychiatr 2005; 76:1188–1193.
46. Erbguth FJ. Historical notes on botulism, clostridium botulinum, botulinum toxin, and the idea of the therapeutic use of the toxin. Mov Disord 2004; 19(suppl 8):S2–S6.
47. Jankovic J. Botulinum toxin in clinical practice. J Neurol Neurosurg Psychiatr 2004; 75:951–957.
48. Ramazzini B. Diseases of Workers. Translated from De Morbis Artificum of 1713 by Wilmer Cave Wright. New York: Haffner, 1964.
49. Solly S. Pages of Samuel Solly; King's College London College Archives. Pearce JMS, 2004.
50. Kerner J. Neue Beobachtungen über die in Württemberg so häufig vorfallenden tödlichen Vergiftungen durch den Genuss geraücherter Würster. Tübingen: Osiander; 1820.
51. VanErmengem EP. Übereinen neuen anaeroben Bacillus und seine Beziehung zum Botulismus. Z Hyg Ingektionskrankh 1897: 26:1–56 (English version: Van Ermengem EP. A new anaerobic bacillus and its relation to bottlism. Rev Infect Dis 1979; 1:701–719.
52. Destarac T. Torticolis spasmodique et spasms fonctionnels. Rev Neurol 1901; 9:591–597.
53. Schwalbe W. Eine eigentümliche tonische Krampffotm mit hysterischen Symptomen: Medicin and Chirurgie. Berlin, Germany: Universitäts-Buchdruckerei G. Schade; 1908.
54. Wilson SAK. Progressive lenticular degeneration: a familial nervous disease associated with cirrhosis of the liver. Brain 1912; 34:295–509.
55. Mendel K. Torsionsdystonie (Dystonia musculorum deformans, Torsionsspasmus). Monatsschr Psychiatr Neurol 1919; 46:309–361.
56. Burke GS. The occurrence of Bacillus botulinus in nature. J Bacterial 1919; 4:541–553.
57. Jankovic J, Fahn S. Dystonic Disorders. In: Parkinson's Disease & Movement Disorders, 4th Ed. Jankovic J, Tolosa E, Eds. Philadelphia: Lippincott Williams & Wilkins, 2002: 331–357.
58. Jankovic J, Fahn S. Dystonic Disorders. In: Parkinson's Disease & Movement Disorders, 4th Ed. Jankovic J, Tolosa E, Eds. Philadelphia: Lippincott Williams & Wilkins, 2002: 331–357.
59. Cooper IS, Bravo G. Chemopallidectomy and chemothalamectomy. J Neurosurg 1958; 15(3):244–250.
60. Zeman W, Kaelbling R, Pasamanick B, Jenkins JT. Idiopathic dystonia musculorum deformans. I. The hereditary pattern. Am J Hum Genet 1959; 11(2 Part 1):188–202.
61. Zeman W, Kaelbling R, Pasamanick B. Idiopathic dystonia musculorum deformans. II. The formes frustes. Neurology 1960; 10:1068–1075.
62. Denny-Brown D. The basal ganglia and their relation to disorders of monkey: a PHAL study of subcortical projections. J Comp Neurol movement, London: Oxford University Press, 1962.
63. Marsden CD. Blepharospasm-oromandibular dystonia syndrome (Brueghel's syndrone). A variant of adult-onset torsion dystonia? J Neurol Neurosurg Psychiatry 1976; 39(12): 1204–1209.
64. Fahn S. High-dosage anticholinergic therapy in dystonia. Adv Neurol 1983; 37:177–188.
65. Jankovic J. Patel SC. Blepharospasm associated with brainstem lesions. Neurology 1983; 33(9):1237–1240.
66. Fahn S. Concept and classification of dystonia. Adv Neurol 1988; 50:1–8.

67. Scott AB. Kennedy RA, Stubbs HA. Botulinum A toxin injection as a treatment for blepharospasm. Arch Ophthalmol 1985; 103(3):347–350.
68. Ichinose H, Ohye T, Takahashi E, et al. Hereditary progressive dystonia with marked diurnal fluctuation caused by mutations in the GTP cyclohydrolase I gene. Nature Genet 1994; 8: 236–242.
69. Albanese A, Barnes MP, et al. A systematic review on the diagnosis and treatment of primary (idiopathic) dystonia and dystonia plus syndromes: report of an EFNS/MDS-ES Task Force. Eur J Neurol 2006; 13:433–444.
70. Geyer HL, Bressman SB. The diagnosis of dystonia. Lancet Neurol 2006; 5:780–790.
71. Ludecke B. Dworniczak B, Bartholome K. A point mutation in the tyrosine hydroxylase gene associated with Segawa's syndrome. Hum Genet 1995; 95(1):123–125.

# 2
# Epidemiology of Primary and Secondary Dystonia

**Giovanni Defazio**
*Department of Neurological and Psychiatric Sciences, University of Bari, Bari, Italy*

## INTRODUCTION

During the last decade, dystonia has been increasingly recognized. However, the body of work concerning the epidemiology of this condition is not extensive. In the past, barriers to epidemiologic study have included perceptions that dystonia is rare and associated with relatively low morbidity. In addition, the absence of validated diagnostic markers for dystonia has limited the careful classification of subjects with this hyperkinetic movement disorder. A further difficulty has arisen because dystonia is a heterogeneous condition that is classified according to the age of onset (early- and late-onset dystonia), body distribution (focal, segmental, multifocal, generalized, and hemidystonia), and etiology (primary and secondary dystonia) (1). Lastly, the evolution of numerous molecular and clinical subtyping systems has lead to some variation in neurologist attitudes in the recognition and treatment of dystonia (2).

## EPIDEMIOLOGY OF PRIMARY DYSTONIA

Traditionally, primary dystonia refers to a condition in which neurological findings are limited to the sustained involuntary posture, and no exogenous cause, associated degenerative disorder, or dramatic response to levodopa to suggest dopa-responsive dystonia may be found (1). Primary dystonia includes early-onset dystonia (presenting before 20 years) with onset in a limb and a tendency to generalize; and late-onset dystonia (presenting after 20 years) that most commonly manifests in focal (blepharospasm, oromandibular dystonia, cervical dystonia, laryngeal dystonia, and upper limb dystonia) or segmental forms (1,3).

### Prevalence and Incidence

Of the 14 studies of the prevalence of primary dystonia published as full papers in peer-reviewed journals or as chapter in books (4–18), six assessed both early- and

**Table 1** Range of Prevalence Rates Per Million on Early-Onset and Late-Onset Primary Dystonia According to Study Design

| Study design | References | Early-onset primary dystonia | Late-onset primary dystonia |
|---|---|---|---|
| Service-based studies | (5,6,8,10–14) | 3–50 | 61–254 |
| Record linkage system-based studies | (4,9,15) | 24–40 | 295–430 |
| Population-based studies | (7,16,17) | 50 | 30–7320 |

late-onset primary dystonia (4–7,10,15), two focused on early-onset primary dystonia alone (8,9), and six dealt with late-onset primary dystonia alone (11–14,16,17). Prevalence estimates ranged between 3 and 50 cases per million for early-onset dystonia, and between 30 and 7320 cases per million for late-onset dystonia (Table 1).

This substantial variability probably reflects differences in study design that influence validity, or differences in the characteristics of study populations (size, age, and ethnicity) that influence comparability.

Most studies were based on treatment settings (service-based studies) or record linkage systems. Because such studies fail to capture subjects not seeking medical advice or those incorrectly diagnosed with other disorders, resulting estimates tend to be in the lower to the middle range of variability (Table 1). In fact, careful family- and population-studies suggest that the percentage of underdiagnosis within primary dystonia may be as high as one- to two-thirds of the affected subjects (15,17,19–22).

Service-based and record linkage system–based studies differed from one another regarding additional factors related to study design, including case-finding procedures, method of case examination, and diagnostic criteria. These factors may impact on the variability of prevalence estimates. Thus, identifying the best results may provide information on the rate of patients with primary dystonia seeking medical advice and treatment. The methodologically more robust service-based/record linkage studies on early-onset dystonia were those that referred to specific diagnostic criteria, set no age-at-onset limits, and included affected relatives as valid cases. By these studies, the prevalence of patients with primary early-onset dystonia seeking medical attention ranged from 24 per million in Israel (9), to 40 per million in Northern England (15), and 50 per million in the Ashkenazi Jews of New York (Table 2) (8). The methodologically more-robust service-based/record linkage studies on late-onset dystonia recruited cases from both neurological and nonneurological services, provided diagnostic criteria, and included all forms of late-onset

**Table 2** Prevalence Rates Per Million (Crude Estimates) from Methodologically More Robust Service-Based/Record Linkage Studies on Early-Onset Primary Dystonia. Data Were Taken from the Original Report or Calculated According to Available Information

| First author, reference number, nation, years of observation | Population sample | Number of cases, prevalence estimate (95% confidence interval) |
|---|---|---|
| Zilber (9), Israel, 1949–1959 | 455,169 | 11, 24 (12–43) |
| Risch (8), USA (New York), 1990 | 1,466,800 | 73, 50 (39–63) |
| Butler (15), Northern England, 1993–2002 | 101,766 | 440 (11–101) |

dystonia. These surveys were conducted in Japan (6), Norway (13), Serbia (14), and Northern England (15). The crude prevalence of patients with primary late-onset dystonia seeking medical attention ranged from 101 to 430 per million in distinct populations (Table 2). This variability may arise from differences in access to the health system across countries, differences in ethnicity, or both.

Only a few prevalence studies have been population-based. Methodological efforts to reduce ascertainment error are improved with population-based protocols. Accordingly, two population studies provide the highest available estimates, China (7) on early-onset dystonia (50 per million; 95% confidence interval, 10–150) and Northern Italy (17) on late-onset dystonia (7320 per million; 95% confidence interval, 3190–15640). Noteworthily, the first was a crude estimate, while the latter was an age-specific prevalence rate. Nonetheless, even these population-based studies suffered from errors in data collection and neither report may be considered as a "gold standard" for population estimates of dystonia prevalence. The door-to-door study performed in China (7) screened for a number of neurological disorders and lacked a systematic approach to diagnosing dystonia. This may well have biased the resulting prevalence estimates. The Northern Italy survey (17) was performed by movement disorders experts who examined study subjects referring to specific diagnostic criteria. However, the study was based on a small population sample (707 individuals). Therefore, its point prevalence rate (7520 per million in the over 50s) might have been overestimated because of a chance-cluster of cases.

In general, the available prevalence studies on primary dystonia are limited by errors in data collection. The lack of valid studies means that the number of existing cases of primary dystonia in the population is difficult to estimate, and few inferences can be drawn about geographical differences in the prevalence of the condition. To provide more precise estimates, service-based studies may be adjusted for the likely fraction of underdiagnosis/misdiagnosis in a given area (Tables 2 and 3).

However, only a few studies provided this information. Based on the cases identified in the New York survey, considering a percentage of underdiagnosis or misdiagnosis as high as 50% in the study area, Risch et al. (8) estimated the true prevalence of primary early-onset dystonia among the Ashkenazim of the New York area to be 111 per million. The Northern England survey (15) considered that 20% to 30% of the local dystonia population still remained undetected, which yielded a possible crude prevalence of primary late-onset dystonia of about 600 per million. Finally, it has been suggested that the lower limit of the 95% confidence interval

**Table 3** Prevalence Rates Per Million (Crude Estimates) from Methodologically More Robust Service-Based/Record Linkage Studies, Studies on Late-Onset Primary Dystonia. Data Were Taken from the Original Report or Calculated According to Available Information

| First author, reference number, nation, years of observation | Population sample | Number of cases, prevalence estimate (95% confidence interval) |
|---|---|---|
| Matsumoto (6), Japan, 2000 | 1,459,130 | 146, 101 (84.5–118) |
| Dung Le (13), Norway, 1999–2002 | 508,726 | 129, 254 (212–301) |
| Pekmezovic (14), Serbia, 2001 | 1,602,226 | 165, 136 (116–159) |
| Butler (15), Northern England, 1993–2002 | 101,766 | 43, 430 (306–569) |

(approximately 3000 per million) of the estimate provided by the population survey performed in Northern Italy (17) may reflect the prevalence of late-onset dystonia in the Italian population aged 50 or more (23). Certainly, the foregoing considerations lack sound statistical support. Nevertheless, they suggest that primary dystonia is probably much more prevalent than previously thought.

The incidence of primary dystonia has been examined to date only in the study conducted by Nutt et al. (4) based on the Rochester epidemiology project. The resulting crude estimates found early-onset dystonia occurring in two per million persons per year, and late-onset primary dystonia in 24 per million persons per year. These estimates are considered to be low secondary to case ascertainment based on review of medical charts rather than on subject examination. The information is further limited by a change in the coding of patients, that the case-finding period was between the years 1950 and 1982, and late-onset focal dystonia was not recognized as a neurological disease until 1976 (24).

## Risk Factors and Etiology

Risk factors for primary dystonia include age, sex, and ethnicity. A number of studies have reported an age-associated rise in the prevalence of late-onset dystonia (6,10–14), and when rates are adjusted by gender, the expression of dystonia appears higher in women (11–14). Although it is not known whether increasing age in female gender plays a role in gene expression, a recent meta-analysis of 83 clinical series (25) suggests a caudal to rostral shift of site of onset of late-onset dystonia with increasing age. In this review, dystonic symptoms appeared in the upper limb and neck earlier than in the face. Interestingly, focal dystonias in the craniocervical area are more common in women and occupational limb cramps in men, while no clear gender difference is observed for early-onset generalized dystonia (15). Ethnicity as a risk factor is clearly supported by two prevalence studies. In Israel (9) early-onset dystonia was most common in Jews of Eastern European or Ashkenazi ancestry, with prevalence estimates being approximately 44 per million (and 24 per million overall). In Norway (13) the prevalence of late-onset dystonia was higher in subjects of European descent (283 per million) than among first-generation immigrants of Asian and African descent (34 per million).

Several studies have demonstrated unequivocally that primary dystonia can aggregate in families (19,21,26,27), and family history of dystonia is considered the most important of the known risk factors for primary dystonia. Although the presence of more than one affected member in the same family nucleus may be because of chance or because of shared environmental factors, a genetic contribution seems highly likely. To date, one gene (*DYT1*) and three disease-associated loci (*DYT6*, *DYT7*, and *DYT13*) have been identified (28). The *DYT1* gene is associated with a significant proportion of cases with early-onset generalized dystonia, but has more recently been linked to a family with late-onset limb dystonia. Most recently, it has been suggested that the haplotype of the *DYT1* gene can contribute to disease-risk for apparently sporadic primary dystonia (29).

The *DYT6* locus was mapped in two families with a form of childhood-onset and adult-onset cranial cervical dystonia (28). The *DYT7* locus localizes to the 30 cM region on chromosome 18 between D18S1153 and 18pter. This locus has been mapped in a large German family with predominantly adult-onset cervical dystonia (CD) (28). The *DYT13* locus was identified in an Italian family phenotypically heterogeneous for age of onset and affected body parts (28). It is worth noting that these associations have not be replicated in many other late-onset dystonia families, suggesting other yet unmapped loci (30,31).

In these primary dystonia families, the pattern of transmission is compatible with an autosomal dominant inheritance trait having about 40% to 60% penetrance for early-onset dystonia (32) and 20% penetrance for late-onset dystonia (33). This transmission pattern, the existence of intrafamilial differences in age of onset and disease severity (34), and the imperfect concordance of the clinical characteristics shown by identical twins with primary dystonia (35,36), suggest that environmental factors may contribute to the incomplete penetrance. However, only a few environmental factors have been assessed using epidemiological techniques.

An earlier case-control study of subjects with early-onset dystonia failed to demonstrate an association between history of abnormal birth, neonatal disorders, autoimmune diseases, and toxic exposure (37). More recently, Saunders et al. have postulated that childhood illnesses developing at age six or earlier may precipitate dystonia among *DYT1* carriers, thus suggesting the existence of a vulnerability window (38). A large Italian case-control study of late-onset dystonia subjects found no association with occupational hazards, wine drinking, life events, and age-related medical diseases such as diabetes mellitus and arterial hypertension (39). A number of controlled studies support local tissue injury as a trigger for topographically related focal dystonia, such as diseases of the anterior segment of the eye (blepharitis, kerato-conjunctivitis, dry eye) and blepharospasm (39,40), neck trauma and cervical dystonia (39), upper respiratory tract infection, and laryngeal dystonia (41). Furthermore, age of disease onset and the onset of blepharospasm was also suggested as a window of vulnerability for subjects developing blepharospasm (40).

Minor injuries associated with repetitive movements or postures of a certain body part have been also proposed as risk factors for focal dystonia. Focal hand, tongue, or embouchure dystonia in musicians represent possible repetitive injuries leading to occupational cramps. In an effort to replicate this paradigm, monkeys were trained to manipulate a vibrating joystick for long periods of time. Eventually the animals lost the ability to correctly accomplish these tasks for the delivery of a food pellet, and demonstrated motor control impairments suggestive of dystonia (42). To date, no controlled study specifically assessed activities at work associated with repetitive motor actions or changes in sensory stimuli as risk factors for focal dystonia. Nevertheless, there is indirect evidence linking focal hand dystonia with working activities that require repetitive and accurate motor tasks. Altenmuller estimated the prevalence of focal hand dystonia among musicians to be as high as 0.5% in 10,000 performing German musicians (43), whereas the prevalence of the condition in the general population was considerably lower (see previous section). Two observations further support a role of activity at work for the development of task-specific focal-hand dystonia among musicians. First, patients often date the onset of dystonia to an increase in practice time, change in technique, or an attempt to take a challenging repertoire (43,44). Second, the hand that performs the more complex task is more likely to develop dystonia (43).

The concept of peripheral injury inducing focal dystonia fits with current knowledge on the neurophysiology of dystonia. Repetitive motor actions and peripheral injury or its consequences (painful symptoms, immobilization procedures, or both) might induce plastic reorganization of cortical and subcortical structures leading to the changes of motor excitability and representation maps of sensorimotor cortex seen in dystonia (45). However, the limited number of controlled studies, the widespread occurrence of injury, the paucity of reported cases of focal dystonia following such an event, and the retrospective assessment of injury do not exclude the possibility of a coincidental association (46).

### Comorbidity

In the last few years, several controlled studies have reported clinical manifestations other than dystonia in patients with primary dystonia. A longitudinal study showed that patients with blepharospasm are more prone to develop Parkinson's disease (PD) than age- and sex-matched control subjects (47). This observation agrees with a recently reported animal model suggesting a minor reduction of the dopaminergic transmission as a permissive factor in the development of blepharospasm (48). Another report demonstrated the higher frequency of blepharospasm among hemifacial spasm patients than among age- and sex-matched neurological controls (49). Coexistence of these cranial movement disorders may indicate overlapping neurophysiological changes in the blink reflex circuitry (50). Two case-control studies found a higher frequency of idiopathic scoliosis developing in middle or late childhood or at around puberty in cervical dystonia than in control patients (51,52). Prior scoliosis may induce compensatory involuntary postures of the neck or alter peripheral sensory input from the trunk, thus inducing central cortical/subcortical reorganization leading to involuntary contractions of cervical muscles. Finally, some authors have reviewed the association of psychiatric disorders as part of the spectrum of primary dystonia. Brooks et al. (53), found a significantly higher frequency of compulsive symptoms in patients with primary blepharospasm than in patients with hemifacial spasm despite the clinical similarity. A recent controlled study documented an increased risk for recurrent major depression in *DYT1* carriers (54). Psychiatric comorbidity might indicate a common pathophysiologic background for primary dystonia, obsessive compulsive disorder, and depression, possibly a disturbed function of striato-thalamo-cortical circuitry.

## EPIDEMIOLOGY OF SECONDARY DYSTONIA

Secondary dystonia includes inherited disorders (i.e., dopa-responsive-dystonia, X-linked dystonia-parkinsonism, alcohol responsive myoclonus-dystonia, and heredodegenerative diseases such as Wilson's disease and Huntington's disease), parkinsonian (i.e., multiple system atrophy, progressive supranuclear palsy, and corticobasal degeneration) and environmental or acquired causes (i.e., perinatal injury, drug abuse, and stroke) (1).

Current prevalence data are available for dopa-responsive dystonia (0.5 cases per million in both England and Japan) (55) and X-linked recessive dystonia parkinsonism (1 out of 4000 in males in the Panay province of Capiz) (56). Given the phenotypic variability of both conditions and the possibility of misdiagnosis, these figures are probably underestimated.

The frequency of dystonia in heredodegenerative diseases remains debated because estimates were based on a few small clinical series from specialized clinics. For example, in Wilson's disease, the frequency of dystonia varied from 37% in a Yugoslavian series (57), to 81% in Maroc (58), and 96% in Eastern India (59). Furthermore, capture of clinical information often varies with collection methods. In a series of Huntington's disease patients followed by Columbia University, the prevalence of dystonia of any severity was reported to be 95%, but only 16.7% of the patients had dystonia that was severe and constant (60).

People with PD, particularly in younger-onset patients, may frequently report limb dystonia with exercise or with the declining (wearing-off) effect of antiparkinson therapies. In addition, axial or limb dystonia may often be helpful in subclassifying parkinsonism syndromes. Asymmetric limb dystonia, particularly affecting one arm, may be a common manifestation of corticobasal ganglionic degeneration: in a large clinical series of 66 patients, 59% had dystonia (61). Cervical or unilateral limb dystonia was reported to occur in 46% of 24 untreated clinically probable multiple system atrophy patients; in this sample, levodopa-induced dyskinesias occurring in 12 out of 18 patients were almost exclusively dystonic affecting craniocervical musculature (62). Dystonic features, mainly cranial and limb dystonia, occurred in 46% of 83 patients with clinically diagnosed progressive supranuclear palsy (63). However, in contrast to these clinical reports, very few clinicopathologic observations on multiple system atrophy (6 out of 140) and progressive supranuclear palsy (15 out of 118) included convincing dystonic manifestations (64).

Among the acquired forms of secondary dystonia, illicit and prescribed drug use and stroke are prominent causes. Although the list of drugs that can induce acute dystonic reactions and tardive dystonia is quite long, dopamine receptor-blocking drugs or neuroleptic drugs are probably the most frequent cause of acute dystonia. Tardive dystonia mainly affecting the cranial cervical area was reported to occur in 4% to 13% of the patients on long-term neuroleptic treatment (65,66). The poststroke frequency of dystonia is difficult to estimate because most reports are of isolated cases or series of patients with a given type of anatomical lesion. In a recent report (67), 56 out of 1500 patients with stroke developed abnormal involuntary movements including dystonia (16 patients, 1%) up to one year after stroke. Patients with stroke-related dystonic postures were younger than patients with other movement disorders. Dystonia was most frequently related to lentiform nucleus lesions, being less frequently associated with lesions of the brainstem, spinal cord, and cerebellum.

## CONCLUSIONS

The number of existing cases of primary dystonia in the population is not precisely known, but the condition is probably much more frequent than reported. By the best available estimates, primary dystonia should be considered the third most frequent movement disorder after essential tremor and PD. The most likely etiologic scenario suggested by epidemiological data is that primary dystonias are products of a genetic background and an environmental insult. Clinical onset in childhood/adolescence is not associated with birth or neonatal disorders. Likewise, clinical onset in the adult life is not associated to age-related medical conditions such as diabetes and arterial hypertension. Early viral childhood illnesses might favor the development of early onset generalized dystonia in *DYT1* carriers. Local injury may be a trigger for topographically related focal dystonia. Possibly, some environmental factors could closely interact with age to trigger dystonia. There is evidence suggesting that the spectrum of the disease might include other neurological (PD), psychiatric (obsessive compulsive disorder and depression), and orthopedic (idiopathic scoliosis) manifestations. Thus, the traditional view that the clinical features of primary dystonias are relatively restricted should no longer be accepted. Comorbidity might be a reflection of the genetic abnormality, indicating the substrate on which the dystonia develops, or a reflection of the developed dystonia on the background substrate.

The frequency of secondary dystonias is extremely difficult to estimate because methods of ascertainment are inconsistent and many cases are so rare as to make any true epidemiological estimation inaccurate with current data.

## REFERENCES


1. Fahn S, Bressman SB, Marsden CD. Classification of Dystonia. In: Fahn S, Marsden CD, DeLong MR, eds. Dystonia 3. Advances in Neurology. Vol. 78. Philadelphia: Lippincott-Raven, 1998:1–10.
2. Logroscino G, Livrea P, Anaclerio D, et al. Agreement among neurologists on the clinical diagnosis of dystonia at different body sites. J Neurol Neurosurg Psychiatr 2003; 74:348–350.
3. Defazio G, Berardelli A, Abbruzzese G, et al. Risk factors for the spread of primary adult onset blepharospasm: a multicentre investigation of the Italian Movement Disorders Study Group. J Neurol, Neurosurg Psychiat 1999; 67:613–619.
4. Nutt JG, Muenter MD, Aronson A, et al. Epidemiology of focal and generalized dystonia in Rochester, Minnesota. Mov Disord 1988; 3:188–194.
5. Castelon Konkiewitz E, Trender-Gerhard I, Kamm C, et al. Service-based survey of dystonia in Munich. Neuroepidemiology 2002; 21:202–206.
6. Matsumoto S, Nishimura M, Shibasaki H, Kaji R. Epidemiology of primary dystonias in Japan: comparison with western countries. Mov Disord 2003; 18:1196–1198.
7. Li S, Schoenberg B, Wang CC, et al. A prevalence survey of Parkinson's diseases and other movement disorders in the People's Republic of China. Arch Neurol 1985; 42:655–657.
8. Risch N, de Leon D, Ozelius L, et al. Genetic analysis of idiopathic torsion dystonia in Ashkenazi Jews and their recent descent from a small founder population. Nat Gen 1995; 9:152–159.
9. Zilber N, Korkzyn AD, Kahana E, et al. Inheritance of idiopathic torsion dystonia among Jews. J Med Gen 1984; 21:13–20.
10. Nakashima K, Kusumi M, Inoue Y, Takahashi K. Prevalence of focal dystonias in the western area of Tottori prefecture in Japan. Mov Disord 1995; 10:440–443.
11. The ESDE (Epidemiological Study of Dystonia in Europe) Collaborative Group. A prevalence study of primary dystonia in eight European countries. J Neurol 2000; 247:787–792.
12. Defazio G, Livrea P, De Salvia R, et al. Prevalence of primary blepharospasm in a community of Puglia region, Southern Italy. Neurology 2001; 56:1579–1581.
13. Dung Le K, Niulsen B, Dietrichs E. Prevalence of primary focal and segmental dystonia in Oslo. Neurology 2003; 61:1294–1296.
14. Pekmezovic T, Ivanovic N, Svetel M, et al. Prevalence of primary late-onset focal dystonia in the Belgrade population. Mov Disord 2003; 18:1389–1392.
15. Butler AG, Duffey PO, Hawthorne MR, Barnes MP. An epidemiologic survey of dystonia within the entire population of Northeast England over the past nine years. In: Fahn S, Hallett MK, DeLong MR, eds. Dystonia 4. Advances in Neurology. Vol. 94. Philadelphia: Lippincott, Williams and Wilkins, 2004:95–99.
16. Kandil M, Tohgamy SA, Fattah MA, et al. Prevalence of chorea, dystonia and athetosis in Assiut, Egypt: a clinical and epidemiological study. Neuroepidemiology 1994; 13:202–210.
17. Muller J, Kiechl S, Wenning GK, et al. The prevalence of primary dystonia in the general community. Neurology 2002; 59:941–943.
18. Fahn S. Concept and classification of dystonia. In: S Fahn, CD Marsden, DB Calne, eds. Advances in Neurology. Vol. 50. New York: Raven Press, 1988:1–8.
19. Waddy HM, Fletcher NA, Harding AE, Marsden CD. A genetic study of idiopathic focal dystonia. Ann Neurol 1991; 29:320–324.
20. Martino D, Aniello MS, Masi G, et al. Validity of family history data on primary adult-onset dystonia. Arch Neurol. 2004; 61:1569–1573.

21. Leube B, Kessler KR, Goecke T, et al. Frequency of familial inheritance among 488 index patients with idiopathic focal dystonia and clinical variability in a large family. Mov Disord 1997; 12:1000–1006.
22. Butler AG, Duffey PO, Hawthorne MR, Barnes MP. The socioeconomic implications of dystonia. In: Fahn S, Marsden CD, DeLong MR, eds. Dystonia 3. Advances in Neurology. Vol. 78. Philadelphia: Lippincott-Raven, 1998:349–358.
23. Defazio G, Abbruzzese G, Livrea P, Berardelli A. The epidemiology of primary dystonia. Lancet Neurol 2004; 3:673–678.
24. Marsden CD. The problem of adult-onset idiopathic torsion dystonia and other isolated dyskinesias in adult life (including blepharospasm, oromandibular dystonia, dystonic writer's cramp, and torticollis or axial dystonia). In: Eldridge R, Fahn S, eds. Advances in Neurology. Vol. 14. New York: Raven Press, 1976:1–10.
25. O'Riordan S, Raymond D, Lynch T, et al. Age at onset as a factor in determining the phenotype of primary torsion dystonia. Neurology 2004; 26(63):1423–1426.
26. Defazio G, Livrea P, Guanti G, et al. Genetic contribution to idiopathic adult-onset blepharospasm and cranial cervical dystonia. Eur Neurol 1993; 33:345–350.
27. Stojanovic M, Cvetkovic D, Kostic VS. A genetic study of idiopathic focal dystonias. J Neurol 1995; 242:508–510.
28. De Cavalho Aguiar PM, Ozelius LJ. Classification and genetics of dystonia. Lancet Neurol 2002; 1:316–325.
29. Clarimon J, Asgeirsonn H, Singleton A, et al. Torsin A haplotype predispose to idiopathic dystonia. Ann Neurol 2005; 57:765–767.
30. Brancati F, Defazio G, Caputo V, et al. Novel Italian family supports clinical and genetic heterogeneity of primary adult-onset torsion dystonia. Mov Disord 2002:392–397.
31. Defazio G, Brancati F, Valente EM, et al. Familial blepharospasm is inherited as an autosomal dominant trait and relates to a novel unassigned gene. Mov Disord 2003; 18:207–212.
32. Kramer PL, Heiman GA, Gasser T, et al. The DYT1 gene on 9q34 is responsible for most cases of early limb-onset idiopathic torsion dystonia in non-Jews. Am J Hum Genet 1994; 55:468–475.
33. Defazio G, Martino D, Aniello MS, et al. A family study on primary blepharospasm. J Neurol Neurosurg Psychiatry 2006; 77:252–254.
34. Fletcher NA, Harding AE, Marsden CD. Intrafamilial correlation in idiopathic torsion dystonia. Mov Disord 1991; 6:310–314.
35. Eldridge R, Ince SE, Chernow B, Milstien S, Lake CR. Dystonia in 61-year-old identical twins: observations over 45 years. Ann Neurol 1984; 16:356–358.
36. Wunderlich S, Reiners K, Gasser T, Naumann M. Cervical dystonia in monozygotic twins: case report and review of the literature. Mov Disord 2001; 16:714–718.
37. Fletcher NA, Harding AE, Marsden CD. A case-control study of idiopathic torsion dystonia. Mov Disord 1991; 6:304–309.
38. Saunders Pullman R, Shriberg J, Shanker V, Bressman SB. Penetrance and expression of dystonia genes. In: Fahn S, Hallett MK, DeLong MR, eds. Dystonia 4. Advances in Neurology. Vol. 94. Philadelphia: Lippincott, Williams and Wilkins, 2004:121–125.
39. Defazio G, Berardelli A, Abbruzzese G, et al. Possible risk factors for primary adult-onset distonia, a case-control investigation by the Italian Movement Disorders Study Group. J Neurol Neurosurg Psychiat 1998; 64:25–32.
40. Martino D, Defazio G, Alessio G, et al. Relationship between eye symptoms and blepharospasm: A multicenter case-control study. Mov Disord 2005:9. (Epub ahead of print).
41. Schweinfurth JM, Billante M, Courey MS. Risk factors and demographics in patients with spasmodic dysphonia. Laryngoscope 2002; 112:220–223.
42. Byl N, Merzenich MM, Jenkins WM. A primate genesis model of focal distonia and repetitive strain injury: I. Learning-induced dedifferentiation of the representation of the hand in the primary somatosensory cortex in adult monkeys. Neurology 1996; 47: 508–520.

43. Frucht SJ. Focal task specific distonia in musicians. In: Fahn S, Hallett MK, DeLong MR, eds. Dystonia 4. Advances in Neurology. Vol. 94. Philadelphia: Lippincott, Williams and Wilkins, 2004:225–230.
44. Frucht SJ, Fahn S, Greene PE, et al. The natural history of embouchure dystonia. Mov Disord 2001; 16:899–906.
45. Quartarone A, Bagnato s, Rizzo V, et al. Abnormal associative plasticità of the human motor cortex in writer's cramp. Brain 2003; 126:2586–2596.
46. Weiner WJ. Can peripheral trauma induce dystonia? No! Mov Disord 2001; 16:13–22.
47. Micheli F, Scorticati MC, Folgar S, Gatto E. Development of Parkinson's disease in patients with blepharospasm. Mov Disord 2004; 19:1069–1072.
48. Schicatano EJ, Basso MA, Evinger C. Animal models explains the origin of the cranial dystonia benign essential blepharospas. J Physiol 1997; 77:2842–2846.
49. Tan EK, Chan LL, Koh KK. Coexistent blepharospasm and hemifacial spasm: overlapping pathophysiologic mechanism? J Neurol Neurosurg Psychiatr 2004; 75:494–496.
50. Pavesi G, Cattaneo L, Chierici E, et al. Trigemino-facial inhibitory reflexes in idiopathic hemifacial spasm. Mov Disord 2003; 18:587–92.
51. Duane DD. Frequency of scoliosis in cervical dystonia patients and their relatives. Mov Disord 1998; 13(Suppl 2):99.
52. Defazio G, Abbruzzese G, Girlanda P, et al. Primary cervical distonia and scoliosis. A multicenter case-control study. Neurology 2003; 60:1012–1015.
53. Broocks A, Thiel A, Angerstein D, Dressler D. Higher prevalence of obsessive-compulsive symptoms in patients with blepharospasm than in patients with hemifacial spasm. Am J Psychiatry 1998; 155:555–557.
54. Heiman GA, Ottman R, Saunders-Pullman RJ, Ozelius LJ, Risch NJ, Bressman SB. Increased risk for recurrent major depression in DYT1 dystonia mutation carriers. Neurology 2004; 63:631–637.
55. Nygaard TG. Dopa-responsive dystonia: delineation of the clinical syndrome and clues to pathogenesis. Adv Neurol 1993; 60:577–585.
56. Kupke KG et al. X-linked recessive torsion dystonia in the Philippines. Am J Med Genet 1990; 36:237–242.
57. Svetel M, Kozic D, Stefanova E, Semnic R, Dragasevic N, Kostic VS. Dystonia in Wilson's disease. Mov Disord 2001; 16:719–723.
58. Bono W, Moutie O, Benomar A, et al. Wilson's disease. Clinical presentation, treatment and evolution in 21 cases. Rev Med Interne 2002; 23:419–431.
59. Sinha S, Jha DK, Sinha KK. Wilson's disease in Eastern India. J Assoc Physicians India 2001; 49:881–884.
60. Louis ED, Lee P, Quinn L, Marder K. Dystonia in Huntington's disease: prevalence and clinical characteristics. J Neurol Neurosurg Psychiat 2002; 72:300–303.
61. Vanez Z, Jankivic J. Dystonia in corticobasal degeneration. Mov Disord 2001; 16:252–257.
62. Boesch SM, Wenning GK, Ransmayr G, Poewe W. Dystonia in multiple system atrophy. J Neurol Neurosurg Psychiat 2002; 72:300–303.
63. Barclay CL, Lang AE. Dystonia in progressive supranuclear palsy. J Neurol Neurosurg Psychiatr 1997; 62:352–356.
64. Rivest J, Quinn N, Marsden CD. Dystonia. Dystonia in Parkinson's disease, multiple system atrophy, and progressive supranuclear palsy. Neurology 1990; 40:1571–1578.
65. van Harten PN, Matroos GE, Hock HW, Kahn RS. The prevalence of tardive dystonia, tardive dyskinesia, Parkinsonism and akathisia. The Curacao Extrapyramidal Syndromes Study: I. Schizophr Res 1996; 19:195–203.
66. Raja M. Tardive dystonia. Prevalence, risk factors, and comparison with tardive dyskinesia in a population of 200 acute psychiatric inpatients. Eur Arch Psychiatry Clin Neurosci 1995; 245:145–151.
67. Alarcon F, Zijlmans JC, Duenas G, Cevallos N. Post-stroke movement disorders: report of 56 patients. J Neurol Neurosurg Psychiat 2004; 75(11):1568–1574.

# 3
# Genetic Evaluation in Primary Dystonia

**Christine Klein**
*Department of Neurology, University of Luebeck, Luebeck, Germany*

**Laurie J. Ozelius**
*Department of Molecular Genetics, Albert Einstein College of Medicine, Bronx, New York, U.S.A.*

**Xandra O. Breakefield**
*Departments of Neurology and Radiology, Massachusetts General Hospital, Charlestown, Massachusetts, and Harvard Medical School, Boston, U.S.A.*

## INTRODUCTION

### Definition and Classifications

Inherited dystonias are a clinically and genetically heterogeneous group of movement disorders. Despite this variability, there is considerable overlap between different forms of dystonia, as they all share the common features of involuntary twisting and repetitive movements resulting in abnormal postures (1). More recently, efforts have been made to clarify the terminology of the dystonias, but confusing definitions remain. The term "dystonia" itself conveys three different meanings: first, a physical sign; second, a syndrome of sustained muscle contractions; third, the disease "idiopathic (or primary) dystonia" (2). The latter term "idiopathic dystonia" or "primary dystonia" usually refers to the genetic forms of dystonia that clinically manifests as dystonia and sometimes tremor (3).

Several classification schemes have been used to categorize the various forms of dystonia, and are useful when trying to establish the diagnosis of a specific (genetic) form of dystonia. The simplest classification of dystonia distinguishes primary and secondary forms. Recent studies indicate a prevalence of 1.8% of adults aged 50 to 89 years with primary or secondary dystonia (4). In the primary forms, dystonia is the only sign of the disease (with the exception of tremor), and the cause is either unknown or genetic. In the secondary forms, dystonia is usually only one of several disease manifestations and the cause may be genetic or due to other insults (e.g., lesions, trauma, drugs/toxins, and metabolic disorders). Uncertainties exist about how to categorize the dystonia-plus group that is considered a special subtype associated with other types of movement disorders, but not secondary to them. The traditional clinical categorization of the dystonias is based on age at onset, site of onset, distribution of symptoms (focal, segmental, multifocal, and generalized), and disease progression. Early onset dystonia often starts in a limb, tends to generalize, and frequently has a genetic origin, whereas adult onset dystonia usually spares the lower extremities, frequently involves cervical or cranial muscles, has a tendency to remain focal, and appears to be sporadic in most cases (5–7).

Genetic features used for classification purposes include mode of inheritance and molecular genetic data, such as linkage to a known gene locus or identification of a specific genetic defect (Table 1). In the past decade, monogenic defects have been found to underlie many forms of primary dystonia and dystonia-plus syndromes. These monogenic forms of dystonia have been "classified" according to the gene loci involved. However, this list of "DYTs" cannot be considered a classification in the true sense of the word. Rather, it represents an assortment of clinically and genetically heterogeneous disorders, which names the monogenic dystonia genes responsible in chronologic order based on their first appearance in the literature. Although some of these forms can be recognized clinically by a characteristic phenotype, considerable phenotypic overlap exists between several of the genetically defined forms. The list of DYT loci will continue to lengthen as additional genes are implicated in various forms of primary dystonia.

## Clinical and Genetic Heterogeneity of the Dystonias

The clinical and genetic heterogeneity of the dystonias often complicates diagnosis. First, phenotypic heterogeneity may lead to clinical misclassification. For example, carriers of the same GAG deletion in the *DYT1* gene may be unaffected or may present with mild writer's cramp, severe generalized dystonia or a jerky type of dystonic tremor reminiscent of myoclonus-dystonia (M-D) (8). Second, genetic heterogeneity exists in cases with virtually identical movement disorders, e.g., M-D, can be caused by defects in different genes [e.g., *DYT11* and *DYT15* (9)]. Third, phenotypically different manifestations of the underlying defect may appear in the same patient over time. For example, four members of a family with genetically proven SCA17 presented first with a purely dystonic syndrome, which was followed later by ataxia and other signs consistent with spinocerebellar ataxia (unpublished observation) (10). Patients with early onset Parkinson's disease, e.g., caused by mutations in the *Parkin* gene, frequently manifest first with dystonia (11).

## Evaluation of a Patient for Possible Genetic Dystonia

The majority of patients with primary dystonia suffer from focal dystonias that have been shown to be monogenic only in rare, single families (12–14). Most primary focal dystonia is believed to be multifactorial in etiology, with recent association studies implicating genes for torsinA and B (see DYT section). From a genetic testing point of view, it is, therefore, important to recognize possible features of dystonia pointing toward a monogenic form. In addition to an early age of onset, several other lines of evidence may indicate a genetic etiology, including a positive family history, a specific clinical picture [for example, dystonia with diurnal variation that worsens after exercise suggesting dopa-responsive dystonia (DRD)], and a specific ethnic background (for example, *DYT1* dystonia is more common among Ashkenazi Jews). It has to be stressed, however, that a genetic etiology should be suspected also in patients with a negative family history. Nonpaternity, adoption, small family size, reduced penetrance, variable expressivity, and de novo mutations may all account for a "pseudo"-negative family history in the presence of a monogenic dystonia.

**Table 1** Monogenic Forms of Dystonia (*DYT1–15*)

| Designation | Dystonia type | Mode of inheritance | Gene locus | Gene product | Genetic testing |
|---|---|---|---|---|---|
| *DYT1* | Early-onset generalized torsion dystonia (TD) | Autosomal dominant | 9q | TorsinA | Commercially available |
| *DYT2* | Autosomal recessive TD | Autosomal recessive | Unknown | Unknown | Unavailable |
| *DYT3* | X-linked dystonia Parkinsonism, "lubag" | X-chromosomal recessive | Xq | Disease-specific changes in DYT3 region | Available in select research laboratories |
| *DYT4* | "Non-DYT1" TD; whispering dysphonia | Autosomal dominant | Unknown | Unknown | Unavailable |
| *DYT5* | Dopa-responsive dystonia; Segawa syndrome | Autosomal dominant | 14q | GTP-cyclohydrolase I | Commercially available |
| | | Autosomal recessive | 11p | Tyrosine hydroxylase | Available in select research laboratories |
| *DYT6* | Adolescent-onset TD of mixed type | Autosomal dominant | 8p | Unknown | Unavailable |
| *DYT7* | Adult-onset focal TD | Autosomal dominant | 18p | Unknown | Unavailable |
| *DYT8* | Paroxysmal nonkinesigenic dyskinesia | Autosomal dominant | 2q | Myofibrillogenesis regulator 1 | Available in select research laboratories |
| *DYT9* | Paroxysmal choreoathetosis with episodic ataxia and spasticity | Autosomal dominant | 1p | Unknown | Unavailable |
| *DYT10* | Paroxysmal kinesigenic choreoathetosis | Autosomal dominant | 16p-q | Unknown | Unavailable |
| *DYT11* | Myoclonus-dystonia | Autosomal dominant | 7q | Epsilon-sarcoglycan | Commercially available |
| *DYT12* | Rapid-onset dystonia-parkinsonism | Autosomal dominant | 19q | $Na^+/K^+$ ATPase alpha 3 | Available in select research laboratories |
| *DYT13* | Multifocal/segmental dystonia | Autosomal dominant | 1p | Unknown | Unavailable |
| *DYT14* | Dopa-responsive dystonia | Autosomal dominant | 14q | Unknown | Unavailable |
| *DYT15* | Myoclonus-dystonia | Autosomal dominant | 18p | Unknown | Unavailable |

An accurate description of the dystonia phenotype is the second step when evaluating a patient for a monogenic form of dystonia. Important diagnostic hints can also be derived from the disease course (Fig. 1). For example, a sudden-onset dystonia disorder over a range of ages is compatible with rapid-onset dystonia-parkinsonism (*DYT12*). Many dystonias can be triggered or exacerbated by nonspecific factors, such as stress, fatigue, action or/and certain postures. However, more specific triggers may indicate a specific type of dystonia. For instance, alcohol, caffeine, sudden or prolonged movements, and exercise may each precipitate paroxysmal dystonias/dyskinesias (*DYT8* and *DYT10*). Response to treatment may also aid in the confirmation of a diagnosis, as a "therapeutic" response to alcohol is characteristic of M-D (*DYT11* and *DYT15*), and improvement with l-dopa supports a diagnosis of DRD (*DYT5*).

## Genetic Testing for Monogenic Dystonias

With the exception of *DYT1*, genetic testing guidelines for dystonia are still being formulated (15), and several important points need to be considered in evaluating the informativeness of testing (Table 2). These include the primary indication; mutation frequency; concerns regarding the implications of symptomatic, presymptomatic, and prenatal testing; availability and feasibility of specific dystonia gene screening; prognosis of the type of dystonia being diagnosed; therapeutic management decisions, and patient confidentiality concerns.

Several dystonia-associated genes contain a large number of exons [e.g., epsilon-sarcoglycan (*SGCE*) with 11 exons and $Na^+/K^+$ATPase alpha 3 (*ATP1A3*) with 23 exons], and gene dosage alterations (heterozygous deletions of whole exons or of the entire gene) have been found in cases, such as for the guanosine triphosphate cyclohydrolase I gene (*GCHI*) and the *SGCE* gene (16–18). Therefore, with the exception of testing for the recurrent GAG deletion in the *DYT1* gene (19), the mutational analysis of dystonia genes is technically demanding, labor-intense, and expensive. Importantly, a negative result does not fully exclude a mutation in the gene being tested, as introns and promoter regions are not usually sequenced and variations in those sequences are hard to interpret; gene dosage assays to test for whole exon deletions are not routinely performed, and the sensitivity and specificity of many of the methods used are less than 100%.

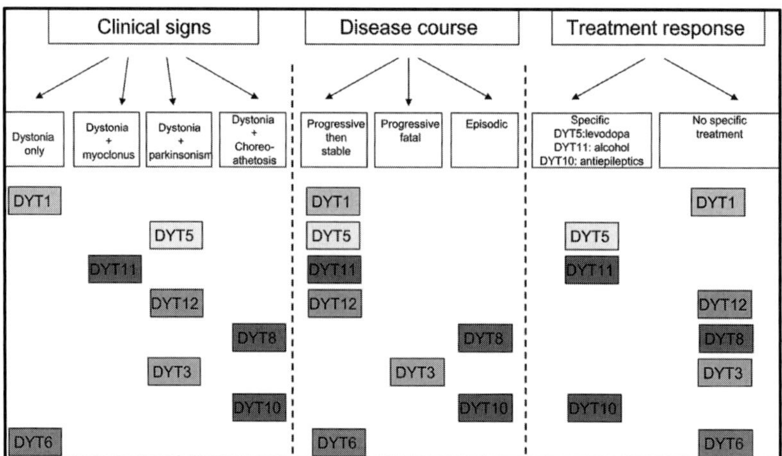


**Figure 1** Clinical classification of DYT dystonias.

**Table 2** Characteristics of DYT Syndromes

| | *DYT1* | *DYT5* | *DYT11* | *DYT12* | *DYT8* | *DYT3* | *DYT10* | *DYT6* |
|---|---|---|---|---|---|---|---|---|
| Clinical features | Dystonia with or without dystonic tremor | Dystonia with or without Parkinsonian features (sometimes atypical presentations) | Myoclonus with or without dystonia (rarely dystonia only) | Dystonia and parkinsonism | Paroxysmal dyskinesia, including choreoathetosis and dystonia | Dystonia and parkinsonism | Paroxysmal dyskinesia, including choreo-athetosis and dystonia | Dystonia, in particular cranial |
| Disease course | Frequently progresses with a caudorostral gradient, later often stabilizes | Diurnal variability of symptoms; often slowly progressive, especially if untreated | Often slowly progressive until young adulthood, then stable, rarely (partial) remission | Sudden onset; progresses with a rostrocaudal gradient, later often stabilizes | Attacks precipitated by alcohol, chocolate, fatigue, etc. often (partial) remission over time | Progressive dystonia-parkinsonism usually of adult onset | Attacks precipitated by sudden movement | Stabilizes after initial progression |
| Response to therapy | Variable response to anticholinergics; good response to deep brain stimulation | Excellent response to L-dopa | Often excellent response to alcohol | No specific treatment | No specific treatment | No specific treatment (L-dopa trial) | Antiepileptics | No specific treatment |
| Ethnic origin | Worldwide but more frequent in Ashkenazi Jews | Worldwide | Worldwide | Worldwide | Worldwide | Exclusively in Filipinos | Worldwide | Exclusively in Mennonites |

(*Continued*)

**Table 2** Characteristics of DYT Syndromes (*Continued*)

| | *DYT1* | *DYT5* | *DYT11* | *DYT12* | *DYT8* | *DYT3* | *DYT10* | *DYT6* |
|---|---|---|---|---|---|---|---|---|
| Genetic testing | GAG deletion in the DYT1 gene | Various mutations in the GCHI gene, including exon deletions | Various mutations in the SGCE gene, including exon deletions | Missense mutations in the Na/K ATPase alpha-3 gene | Missense mutations in the MR-1 gene | Disease-associated changes in the DYT3 gene | Linkage only | Linkage only |
| Availability of genetic test | Commercially available; technically simple; relatively inexpensive | Commercially available but not for exon deletions; relatively expensive | Commercially available but not for exon deletions; relatively expensive | In select research laboratories only | In select research laboratories only | In select research laboratories only | In select research laboratories only | In select research laboratories only |
| Genetic counseling | Reduced penetrance; variable expressivity | Reduced penetrance especially in men; variable expressivity | Disease usually transmitted through father due to maternal imprinting | Reduced penetrance; variable expressivity | Reduced penetrance; variable expressivity | Almost exclusively affects males; progressive and eventually fatal disorder | Reduced penetrance; variable expressivity | Reduced penetrance; variable expressivity |

*Note*: This table lists all DYT dystonias with known genes or gene loci that have been described in several families and implicated in genetic testing (in the order of occurrence in the manuscript). DYT7, 9, 13, 14, and 15 have each been described in a single family only. DYT2 and DYT4 dystonia have not yet been linked to a chromosomal location.
*Abbreviations*: GCHI, GTP cyclohydrolase I gene; MR-1, myofibrillogenesis regulator 1; SGCE, epsilon-sarcoglycan.

Genetic testing has become commercially available for several forms of dystonia, including *DYT1* (early onset torsion dystonia with a common mutation in the *TOR1A* gene), *DYT5a* (DRD with mutations in the *GCHI* gene), and *DYT11* (M-D with mutations in the *SGCE* gene). Mutations in the other known dystonia genes for *DYT3*, *DYT5b* [tyrosine hydroxylase (*TH*)], *DYT8* [myofibrillogenesis regulator 1 (*MR-1*)], and *DYT12* (*ATP1A3*) are currently only being analyzed in select research laboratories.

Genetic testing for monogenic dystonias, when available, can provide a powerful tool to identify at-risk individuals based on their mutational status. These advances are paralleled by the development of novel neuroimaging modalities and other techniques used to identify preclinical changes, such as abnormalities on positron emission tomography (PET) or magnetic resonance imaging (MRI) associated with *DYT1* carrier status (20–22). These subtle changes in brain metabolism and structure, and in motor sequence learning seen in unaffected *DYT1* carriers, for example, highlight the issue of where exactly to draw the line in designating an individual as "affected." More generally speaking, reduced penetrance and variable expressivity are important features of hereditary dystonias that need to be considered when it comes to genetic counseling of a dystonia patient. These issues will be specifically addressed for each of the monogenic dystonia forms discussed below.

## Monogenic Forms of Dystonia: *DYT1–15*

Currently, at least 15 different types of dystonia can be distinguished genetically, and are designated *DYT1-15* (Table 1). Six of these 15 dystonias are considered primary (*DYT1, DYT2, DYT4, DYT6, DYT7*, and *DYT13*), with the remainder classified as dystonia-plus syndromes. With the exception of three rare forms (*DYT2, DYT3*, and *DYT5b*), all of them follow an autosomal dominant pattern of transmission with reduced penetrance, and in at least one case (DYT11) with maternal imprinting. Genes have been identified for six of these monogenic dystonias (*DYT1, DYT3, DYT5, DYT8, DYT11*, and *DYT12*), and the chromosomal location is known for another seven forms (*DYT6, DYT7, DYT9, DYT10, DYT13, DYT14*, and *DYT15*). The known DYT gene products cover a broad range of functions including an endoplasmic reticulum (ER) chaperone protein (*DYT1*), transcription factor (*DYT3*), ion channel pump energizer (*DYT12*), putative detoxifying enzyme (*DYT8*), enzymes critical to dopamine synthesis (*DYT5*), and an interactive protein between the cell membrane and cytoskeleton (*DYT11*). Clearly, it is especially important for clinical neurologists to identity families with multiple members affected with these rarer forms and work with geneticists to define the clinical spectrum of the dystonia and identify the disease gene to provide insights into molecular etiology. Because most of the hereditary dystonias have reduced penetrance and no apparent neuronal degeneration, there is hope that understanding of the etiology can be used to reduce penetrance further and inform possible therapeutic interventions. This chapter is organized to provide information on the DYT dystonias in order of their prevalence.

# *DYT1* DYSTONIA (DYSTONIA MUSCULORUM DEFORMANS, OPPENHEIM'S DYSTONIA, AND EARLY ONSET GENERALIZED DYSTONIA)

Early-onset, generalized dystonia, caused by a mutation in the *TOR1A* gene, is the most common and severe of the hereditary dystonias, with an estimated frequency in the Ashkenazi Jewish population of at least 1 out of 9000 and a 5- to 10-fold lower frequency in non-Jewish populations (23,24). Symptoms, including sustained muscle contractions and abnormal posturing, typically begin in childhood (mean age 13 years, range 1–28 years) with twisting of an arm or leg, and progression to involve other limbs and torso, but usually not the face and neck (15,25). There is a tendency for symptoms to move up the body, and later onset cases to be less severe. Most cases are caused by a specific mutation, a three base pair (bp) deletion (GAG) in the coding region of the *TOR1A* gene. While this mutation accounts for about 60% of cases in the non-Jewish population, because of a founder effect, it comprises about 90% of cases in the Ashkenazi Jewish (15,19,26).

*DYT1* dystonia is inherited in an autosomal dominant manner with reduced penetrance (only about 30% of mutant gene carriers are affected) and variable expressivity with respect to age and site of onset and progression (27). If symptoms do not occur prior to 28 years of age in carriers, they usually remain unaffected for the rest of their life. Symptoms can be as mild as writer's cramp (28). Unaffected carriers have been shown to have a delay in motor sequence learning (20), as well as altered metabolic activity and anatomic pathways in certain brain regions as determined by PET and MRI, respectively (21,29). Recent studies also indicate an increase of depressive disorder in both affected and unaffected carriers (30). Collectively these findings suggest possible, developmental abnormalities in neuronal circuitry in *DYT1* mutation carriers. Factors contributing to penetrance have not been identified, but are presumed to involve coinheritance of other polymorphisms in functionally related loci or environmental insults. Although some have suggested that drug exposure (31), peripheral injury (31), viral infection (32), or polymorphisms at the *TOR1A* locus (Ozelius et al., unpublished data) may increase susceptibility, these hypotheses have not been proven.

The GAG deletion in *TOR1A* has occurred de novo in many ethnic populations, with a relatively high frequency, possibly due to repeated sequence in that region of the gene (33). Only a few other sequence variations in the coding region have been described, including an 18-bp deletion described in a family with M-D, which also carried a mutation in the *DYT11* gene (11,34) and a 4-bp deletion in an apparently normal individual, who was not examined neurologically (8). Several polymorphisms have been identified including a single-bp substitution in which an aspartic acid codon (allele frequency 88%) is replaced by a histidine codon (allele frequency 12%) (11). Interestingly, the frequency of the histidine codon is much reduced (allele frequency 4%) in affected *DYT1* carriers as compared to the normal population, suggesting it may have a role in penetrance (Ozelius, unpublished data). Several other polymorphisms have been described, which do not affect coding sequences of the *DYT1* gene, but which define a haplotype in the Icelandic population, which is strongly associated with apparently sporadic, late onset focal dystonia, suggesting a possible role for the *TOR1A* gene or the neighboring homologous *TOR1B* gene in these cases (35).

An understanding of the function of the protein, torsinA, encoded in *TOR1A* may provide some insight into the etiology of early onset torsion dystonia. TorsinA and its four homologues, torsinB, torp2, and torp3, are members of the superfamily of ATPases associated with a variety of activities ($AAA^{+}$) (26,36,37), which have many different functions including protein processing and degradation, organelle biogenesis, intracellular trafficking, and vesicle recycling (38,39). TorsinA is expressed throughout the body and at high levels in specific neuronal populations in the adult human brain, including in the substantia nigra, thalamus, and cerebellum (40–42). Interestingly, in the rodent and human brain highest levels of expression occur in the early postnatal period (43–45) and homozygous knockout mice for torsinA die at birth (46,47). This suggests that torsinA is needed in development of the nervous system, as well as for functional activity throughout life.

The function of torsinA is not yet delineated. Most of the protein appears to be located in the lumen of the ER and expression of the GAG-deleted cDNA (resulting in loss of a glutamic acid residue in the carboxy terminal region) leads to formation of whorled, membrane inclusions derived from the ER and abnormalities in the nuclear envelope (48–51). TorsinA-positive inclusions have been noted in the midbrain of *DYT1* patients (52), although no loss of neurons has been found in any brain regions (41,52–54). Different studies suggest involvement of torsinA in cytoskeletal dynamics, which may be important in neurite extension during development (55), in processing of proteins through the secretory pathway (56), and in degradation of mutant proteins (57,58).

Genetic testing for the GAG deletion in early onset dystonia is widely available, relatively inexpensive, and clearly indicated for any non-DRD case with onset in childhood (less than 26 years and without other medical symptoms), especially if the affected individual is of Ashkenazi Jewish descent or has other affected family members. Using age of onset of 26 as a criterion results in 100% sensitivity with acceptable specificities ranging from 43% (in non-Jews) to 63% (in Ashkenazi Jews) however, if criteria are set more narrowly to include only those with early limb onset specificity improves (70–80%), but sensitivity drops (94–96%) (15). Guidelines and advice on testing are available (15,19). However, there are a number of atypical dystonia cases where the GAG deletion has also been demonstrated including late onset after exposure to haloperidol with severe bulbar involvement (31), late onset manifesting as tremor (31), clonic dystonia and generalized dystonia with developmental delay (8), writer's cramp (13,28), stiff-person syndrome in a child (59), onset in cervical regions (15), onset at 64 or 73 years of age (19,60), and unilateral myoclonic dystonia (61). It is clear then that the *DYT1* GAG deletion can manifest, albeit rarely, in atypical ways and, at the same time, that a substantial fraction of classic early onset generalized dystonia, especially in the non-Jewish population, is not caused by this mutation. Other loci associated with adolescent-onset generalized dystonia, but with more prominent cranial and cervical involvement include *DYT6* in the Mennonite population (62) and *DYT13* in an Italian family (14). In addition to helping with differential diagnosis, information as to the presence of the GAG deletion can be used to advise other family members and may have a therapeutic correlate, as affected mutation carriers appear to respond well to deep brain stimulation (63,64). It is critical that genetic testing for *DYT1* be accompanied by counseling due to variable penetrance and expressivity of the *DYT1* mutation, the lack of a nonintrusive therapy, and the otherwise normal health and intelligence of mutation carriers.

## *DYT5* DYSTONIA (DOPA-RESPONSIVE DYSTONIA; SEGAWA SYNDROME)

DRD is characterized by childhood onset of dystonia, diurnal fluctuation of symptoms, and a dramatic response to L-dopa therapy. Later in the course of the disease, parkinsonian features may occur (65,66) and may, in rare cases, be the only sign of the condition (67). In addition, a variety of atypical presentations of DRD have been described that include for example, onset in the first week of life, generalized hypotonia, and proximal weakness (68,69) or psychiatric abnormalities (70,71). While a rare autosomal recessive form of DRD (*DYT5b*) is associated with mutations in the

*TH* gene, the more frequent form of DRD (*DYT5a*) is dominantly inherited and usually caused by mutations in the *GCHI* gene. *GCHI* encodes the enzyme GTPCH that catalyzes the first step in the biosynthesis of tetrahydrobiopterin (cofactor for *TH*) as a homodecamer (72). DRD patients have abnormally low levels of GTPCH activity due to a dominant-negative effect of the mutated allele, leading to dopamine depletion and explaining the remarkable therapeutic effect of L-dopa administration. However, *GCHI* mutations have only been identified in 40% to 60% of clinically typical DRD patients (73). Recently, heterozygous exon deletions in *GCHI* have been demonstrated (16,74,75) that were not detectable by conventional screening methods, suggesting that heterozygous exon deletions may account for at least 10% of the "mutation-negative" cases. Genetic heterogeneity is suggested by the report of a single family with autosomal dominant DRD that appears to map to a region on chromosome 14q13 located outside the *GCH1* gene region, which has been designated *DYT14* (76). This condition is associated with severely hypomelanized dopaminergic neurons in the substantia nigra and locus ceruleus, but no Lewy bodies (76).

Other autosomal recessive dystonia-plus syndromes, which have DRD as a component have mutations in other genes involved in biopterin and dopamine synthesis, including those encoding 6-pyruvoyl-tetrahydropterin synthase, sepiapterin reductase deficiency, dihydropterine reductase, and aromatic L-amino acid decarboxylase (77). In one family a haploinsufficiency of sepiapterin reductase also underlies a typical DRD phenotype (78).

Mutation carriers show a high degree of both inter- and intrafamilial phenotypic variability and reduced penetrance. Interestingly, penetrance is lower among men than women. The underlying mechanisms affecting penetrance are not yet resolved, but the ratio between wild-type transcript/protein and mutated transcript/protein seems to play a critical role as indicated in two small families with DRD and mutations in *GCHI* (79,80).

In most cases, the diagnosis of DRD can be established clinically (including a positive L-dopa response) and may be supported by the results of cerebrospinal fluid analysis showing decreased catecholamine metabolites and a phenylalanine-loading test with elevated phenylalanine/tyrosine levels (81). Genetic testing for *GCHI* mutations is commercially available, but does not include routine testing for heterozygous exon deletions. The latter accounts for a considerable number of "mutation-negative" cases, but is currently performed only in select research laboratories. *GCHI* mutations are spread across the entire gene (six exons) with most families having "private" mutations. [For a listing of known mutations see www.bh4.org/biomdb.summary.html (82)] Mutation-negative, clinically typical cases should ideally be tested for exon deletions. Overall, genetic analysis of the *GCHI* gene is relatively labor-intense and expensive. As the diagnosis can usually be made on clinical grounds and the detection of a mutation does not affect treatment or prognosis of the condition, genetic testing should be limited to patients and families with a special need for genetic counseling, to cases posing diagnostic difficulties or to the research setting. Important counseling issues, such as reduced penetrance and variable expressivity, cannot currently be predicted in individual cases even within families.

## *DYT11* (AND *DYT15*) MYOCLONUS-DYSTONIA

M-D is a movement disorder characterized by a combination of rapid, brief muscle contractions, and/or sustained twisting and repetitive movements that result in abnormal postures. Symptom onset is usually in childhood or early adolescence (13,83–88). The disease is inherited as an autosomal dominant trait with reduced penetrance (87,89). Loss-of-function mutations in the *SGCE* gene on chromosome 7q21 have been implicated in numerous families with *DYT11* M-D (9,17,18,34,86, 88,90–98). *DYT15* M-D, which has been described in a single family only, is phenotypically similar to *DYT11* M-D with an yet unidentified gene on chromosome 18p (99).

Various terms have been used to describe M-D in the literature, including myoclonic dystonia, inherited M-D syndrome, alcohol-responsive myoclonic dystonia, hereditary essential myoclonus, and *DYT11* and *DYT15* dystonia. Several articles address the issues underlying this terminology debate (83,100–102).

The myoclonic jerks typical of M-D are brief, lightning-like movements most often affecting the neck, trunk, and upper limbs with legs affected less prominently. Myoclonus is usually the presenting symptom. In most affected individuals, the myoclonic jerks show a dramatic lessening in response to alcohol (83,89,103). However, the alleviation of symptoms following alcohol ingestion varies among and between families (85,104). Approximately half of affected individuals have focal or segmental dystonia that presents as cervical dystonia and/or writer's cramp (34,86). In contrast to primary torsion dystonia (15), involvement of lower limbs is rare and usually does not occur at onset. In addition, the dystonia does not tend to worsen or generalize in the course of the disease. Rarely, dystonia is the only manifestation. Seizures have been reported in two families with M-D, but the significance of this finding is still unclear (93,105).

The most prominent nonmotor features have been psychiatric disease reported in some (103,106,107), but not all (108) families. Reported psychiatric problems include depression, anxiety, and obsessive-compulsive disorder (OCD) (107,109); depression, personality disorders, and addiction (106); and panic attacks (110). However, a systematic study of psychiatric illness was neither performed in most of these M-D families, nor did these features segregate with the M-D mutation. Saunders-Pullman et al. (109) did study psychiatric features in detail in three families linked to chromosome 7q and found an association between OCD and M-D. In agreement with these results, OCD was detected in combination with M-D in several other 7q-linked families (91,96).

Reduced penetrance on maternal transmission of the disease allele has been observed, suggesting maternal genomic imprinting of the *SGCE* gene (90). This suggestion is consistent with data showing that the murine *SGCE* gene is primarily transcribed from the paternal allele and is, therefore, maternally imprinted (110). Furthermore, using polymorphic markers and heterozygous *SGCE* knockout mice exclusive expression of the paternal allele was found in mouse brains (111). Two studies demonstrated paternal transmission of the *SGCE* mutant allele in affected individuals (92,112), as well as DNA methylation differences, supporting maternal imprinting of the human gene. It is speculated that because *SGCE* is maternally imprinted, the vast majority of affected individuals inherit their disease gene from their fathers and that the disease is caused by loss of function of this protein. However, up to 5% of cases inherit their mutated allele from their mothers (87,90,112) and presumably also express the wild-type allele from their fathers. In these instances, the phenotype may be milder. The reason for reversal of the maternal imprint in these cases is not known.

*SGCE*, a single transmembrane glycoprotein, is a member of a gene family that also includes alpha, beta, gamma, delta, and zeta sarcoglycans. The gene comprises 12 exons with exon 10 being differentially spliced and absent from most transcripts (113).

Two recent papers have identified other alternative splice variants in mouse brain that affect the C-terminal end of the encoded protein (114,115). The function of this *SGCE* protein is still largely unknown. The other members of the sarcoglycan family encode transmembrane components of the dystrophin-glycoprotein complex that links the cytoskeleton to the extracellular matrix. Mutations in the genes encoding these other sarcoglycans, which are mainly expressed in muscle, cause autosomal recessive limb-girdle muscular dystrophies (116). *SGCE* appears to be functionally similar to alpha-sarcoglycan in skeletal muscle (117) and is widely expressed in many tissues of the body (113,118) including various regions of the brain during both development and adulthood (90,115,119,120). In rodents, levels of *SCGE* are highest in the brain around birth (119) and in adults highest expression is found in the hippocampus, cortex, olfactory bulb, Purkinje cell layer of the cerebellum, and monoaminergic neurons in the midbrain (119,120). The function of *SGCE* in the brain is presently unknown.

All types of mutations have been reported in the *SGCE* gene including nonsense, missense, deletions, and insertions leading to frame shifts and splicing errors (9,17,34,86,88,90–98). Most of the mutations described to date have been localized in exons two to seven, implicating this region of the gene as important for function. Four nonsense mutations, R97X, W100X, R102X (all in exon three), and R372X (in exon nine), as well as two small deletions (in exons four and seven) have been found in more than one proband and appear to be recurrent mutations (86,88,90, 94,97,121). There is one confirmed de novo mutation (97) and several reported cases of "pseudo-negative" family history due to maternal imprinting, where the mutation was subsequently identified in the fathers (9,92,97). A recent report using quantitative polymerase chain reaction (PCR) indicates that exonic deletions in *SGCE* can also cause M-D (18).

Although the *SGCE* gene appears to represent the major locus for M-D, simplex and familial cases without identifiable *SGCE* mutations have been reported (88,94,97,98,121–123), suggesting locus heterogeneity. A large Canadian family with clinically typical M-D without a mutation in the *SGCE* gene has been linked to markers in a 16.5 cM region on chromosome 18p (locus DYT15) (99). Two other families also show possible linkage to this chromosome region (98). The overall contribution of this locus to M-D cannot be determined until the gene is identified. An additional family with a missense change in the D2 receptor (106) was subsequently found to have a mutation in *SGCE* (75), making the role of the D2 receptor mutation in this condition unclear.

Genetic testing for *SGCE* mutations is available, but the recent identification of exonic deletions complicates assessment. Based on the literature and excluding the exonic deletions, the mutation detection rate among familial cases of M-D is close to 50% (9,34,86,88,90–98), but the mutation detection rate among individuals with no family history is only about 12% to 13% (86,88,94,97,98,120,122,123). However, the two-exonic deletion families were previously screened for *SGCE* mutations and found to be "mutation-negative" (18), thus, the overall mutation rate in *SGCE* will be higher when deletion screening is included. Genotype-phenotype studies do not show any difference in phenotype associated with the different types of mutations in *SGCE* although the two families with the exonic deletions had a majority of members with a generalized distribution of myoclonus (18). In addition, there are no clear genotype–phenotype differences seen between *SGCE* mutation positive and negative cases, but from current studies, a positive family history and paternal inheritance are good indicators for identifying *SGCE* mutations and should be considered when trying to determine which M-D patients to test. Although the rate of mutation detection is low in cases without a family history, the identification of de novo mutations and the complication of maternal imprinting that leads to "pseudo-negative" family history both suggest that a negative family history should not preclude genetic testing in phenotypically typical cases. Importantly, in this specific type of dystonia, penetrance can be predicted in above 90% of the mutation carriers due to paternal expression/maternal imprinting of the mutated gene and should be considered upon counseling of an M-D patient and family members.

## OTHER HEREDITARY DYSTONIAS

Other clinically distinct forms of hereditary dystonia have been described which are rarer, including ones for which gene lesions have now been identified, *DYT8* (paroxysmal nonkinesigenic dyskinesia PNKD), *DYT12* (rapid onset dystonia–parkinsonism), and *DYT3* (X-linked dystonia–parkinsonism, lubag). Others have been linked to chromosomal locations without gene identification to date, including *DYT6* (adolescent-onset torsion dystonia of mixed phenotype), *DYT7* (adult-onset focal dystonia), *DYT9* (paroxysmal choreoathetosis with episodic ataxia and spasticity), *DYT10* (paroxysmal kinesigenic choreoathetosis), *DYT13* (multifocal/segmental dystonia), *DYT14* (DRD), and *DYT15* (M-D). Still others have not yet been linked to a chromosomal region, including *DYT2* (autosomal recessive, early-onset torsion dystonia) and *DYT4* (whispering dysphonia). We can anticipate that this list of dystonia genes will continue to increase slowly as neurologists and geneticists expand their efforts to identify, collect, and analyze families with rare forms of dystonia.

### *DYT12* Dystonia (Rapid Onset Dystonia-Parkinsonism)

*DYT12* dystonia (rapid onset dystonia-parkinsonism), first described by Dobyns et al. (124), is distinguished by sudden onset, which can be within hours to weeks, typically in adolescence or young adulthood (but as late as 55 years), in response to physical or mental stress, with persistence of symptoms throughout life. It is inherited in an autosomal dominant manner with reduced penetrance. Symptoms include dystonic spasms predominantly in the upper limbs, orofacial dystonia, dysarthria and dysphagia, and slowness of movement, sometimes along with symptoms of parkinsonism, including bradykinesia, rigidity, and postural instability (7,125). Other less common symptoms include depression, intermittent hemidystonia, paroxysmal dystonia, and seizures (126–128). Stressful events precipitating onset include fever, prolonged exercise, childbirth, and even giving oral presentations (124,125,128). Although some individuals show reduced levels of the dopamine metabolite, homovanillic acid in the CSF (129), there is no evidence for a decrease in the density of dopaminergic terminals (129) or clinical response to L-dopa treatment. A single affected brain has been analyzed to date with no evidence of neurodegeneration (128).

Four families have been found in which the disease phenotype links to chromosome 19q13 (130,131), while another family with more cranial-cervical involvement does not link to this region (8). Recently six different missense mutations were identified in the gene, *ATP1A3* on chromosome 19q13 (23 exons), which encodes the alpha 3 subunit of NaK ATPase (132). This is a subunit of a sodium pump responsible for maintenance of ionic gradients across cell membranes. The mutations are predicted to result in loss of activity or instability of the protein. Interestingly, mutations in the alpha-2 subunit of the $Na^+/K^+$ATPase have been implicated in familial hemiplegic migraine and infantile convulsions (133,134). Genetic testing for mutations in the *ATP1A3* locus is implicated in patients with abrupt onset of dystonia with features of parkinsonism over a few minutes to 30 days, with a rostral-caudal (face > arm > leg) gradient of symptoms and no response to dopaminergic medication (125).

### *DYT8* (Paroxysmal Dystonia/Dyskinesia)

This episodic form of dystonia was originally described by Mount and Reback (135). Movement abnormalities may manifest shortly after birth or in childhood or adolescence and can be precipitated with alcohol, caffeine, exercise, hunger, and fatigue (136). Symptoms include unilateral or bilateral dystonic and choreatic dyskinesias, lasting from minutes to hours with a frequency of 20 per day to twice per year (137). Many patients describe an aura preceding attacks and may experience attacks of variable severity. They lack a good response to antiepileptic drugs, and seizures are uncommon in patients with PNKD. Often, there is a decrease in attack frequency over time. Inheritance is autosomal dominant with reduced penetrance. Linkage analysis determined the *DYT8* gene to be localized to chromosome 2q33-q35 (138–140), but phenotypically similar families, which are not linked to this locus, have also been described (141). Mutations in the *MR-1* gene (10 exons) have now been identified in individuals from 13 families with this syndrome (142–145), however, only two single bp mutations have been identified and each results in the substitution of valine for alanine (at amino acid position 7 or 9). The function of MR-1 is not known, but it is homologous to glyoxalase hydroxyacylglutathione hydrolase, known to detoxify methylglyoxal, a compound in alcohol, cola, tea, and coffee, and a by-product of oxidative stress (146). This gene has several isoforms, one of which is specifically expressed in neurons and throughout many regions of the brain including the substantia nigra, red nucleus, cerebral cortex, and Purkinje cells and granule cells in cerebellum (142).

Genetic testing for PNKD should be considered in patients with paroxysmal dystonia/dyskinesia that presents with these clinical symptoms especially in cases with identified trigger for attacks and longer duration of attacks (30 minutes to two hours). PNKD can be differentiated on clinical grounds from paroxysmal kinesigenic choreoathetosis (PKC and *DYT10*) in which the attacks are shorter, more frequent, and triggered by sudden movement. Similarly, PNKD can be clinically differentiated from the rare paroxysmal exercise-induced dystonia that is precipitated by prolonged movement. At this time it may be justified to limit genetic testing for PNKD to the two recurrent mutations in the *MR-1* gene (145).

### *DYT3* (X-Linked Dystonia-Parkinonism, LUBAG)

This is the only DYT dystonia that is considered secondary and is described here only because it has been grouped under the DYT dystonias. X-linked recessive dystonia-parkinsonism is a neurodegenerative condition with a high incidence in males descending from the island of Panay in the Philippines (referred to in the local diatech as "lubag")due to a founder mutation, first described in 1976 (147,148). The age of onset is usually between 12 to 52 years starting with focal dystonia occurring in different regions of the body. Dystonic symptoms progress to become segmental or generalize over about six years with parkinsonian symptoms presenting later in the disease in about half of the patients. Penetrance is complete by 50 years of age.

A few Filipino women with the disease have been described, apparently due to homozygosity at the X-linked locus. A similar disorder has also been described in Caucasians, but it is not clear whether it is due to mutations in the *DYT3* gene (149,150). Neuroimaging shows atrophy of the caudate and putamen with neuroanatomically confirmed neuronal loss and astrocytosis, and severe depletion of striatosomes in these brain regions (151–153). The *DYT3* locus was initially mapped to Xq (154,155) with further definition to Xq13.1 (156). A number of disease-specific changes were identified in a 300 kb region including a deletion in an exon of a novel transcript and single bp changes in transcripts for the TATA-box binding protein-associated factor 1, a putative tumor suppressor (ING2), and a homologue of cytokine-inducible SH2 protein 4 (156). Genetic testing is implicated by dystonic symptoms that onset in adolescence or later years in males of Filipino extraction and can be carried out by PCR amplification of microsatellite markers in linkage disequilibrium with the founder mutation (157).

## OTHER DYT GENES

### *DYT2*

Less is known about the other *DYT* loci and they will be discussed here in numerical order. *DYT2* represents an autosomal recessive locus for dystonia that was first reported in three consanguineous Spanish gypsy families (158). Two of these families had a phenotype resembling *DYT1* dystonia with a mean age of onset of $15.0 \pm 6.6$ years, with dystonia starting in the feet, followed by rapid generalization in all affected children. The third family had primarily oromandibular dystonia and torticollis. Two recent reports of consanguineous families having children with generalized dystonia (159,160) add credence to this locus. To date, no genetic linkage studies or homozygosity mapping have been performed in any of these families.

### *DYT4*

This currently refers to a syndrome in an Australian family with whispering dysphonia and other dystonic symptoms ranging from focal to generalized dystonia, with some members manifesting psychiatric symptoms (161,162). It is an autosomal dominant trait with reduced penetrance, but linkage to a chromosomal location has not been established.

### *DYT6* (Adolescent Onset with Mixed Phenotype)

This has features of focal and generalized primary dystonia and was identified in three Mennonite families, who are related by a common ancestor dating to the mid-1700s (Saunders-Pullman R, Raymond D, Kramer P, et al. Unpublished data) (62). It is inherited in an autosomal dominant manner with penetrance estimated at 50%. Some phenotypic features overlap *DYT1* dystonia, but the onset is later in *DYT6* (mean 19 years; range 5–38 years) and there is more prominent cranial involvement, especially in muscles of the lung, larynx and face, with dysphonia being a predominant feature. $^{18}$F-Fluorodeoxyglucose PET imaging of regional glucose metabolism showed that affected individuals have bilateral hypermetabolism in the presupplementary motor area and parietal association cortices, as well as hypometabolism in the putamen and temporal cortex (21). The responsible locus has been mapped to the chromosome a 23 cM region spanning the centromere of chromosome 8 (Saunders-Pullman R, Raymond D, Kramer P, et al. Unpublished data.)

### *DYT7* (Adult Onset, Focal)

Adult-onset focal dystonia accounts for about 90% of all cases of dystonia with a prevalence estimated at 30 out of 100,000 of the general population (24,163). Late-onset primary torsion dystonia is probably more complex genetically than the early onset forms and the role of genes in the etiology of the various adult clinical subtypes is still under study. Genetic studies to determine the mode of inheritance using segregation analyses conclude that focal dystonia is inherited as an autosomal dominant trait with reduced penetrance of about 12% to 15% (164–166). Although the overall risk to first-degree relatives is 9.5% to 12% and the penetrance of the disease is low, several large multiplex (more penetrant) families have been described (12,167,168), including three multiplex families with musician's dystonia in the index patients and focal task-specific dystonia in other family members (169).

One form, *DYT7*, has been described in a single family from northwest Germany (12). In this family, symptoms usually affect a single body part—primarily the neck—causing cervical dystonia (torticollis), with eyes (blepharospasm), larynx (spasmodic dysphonia), and hands (postural tremor) affected in a few cases, and with a very low tendency to generalize. The mean age of onset is 43 years (range 28–70 years). The disease is inherited as an autosomal dominant trait with low penetrance. *DYT7* dystonia is linked to 18p and no neuropathology has been found. The 18p region is also implicated in other dystonias as patients with an 18p deletion can also exhibit dystonic symptoms (170,171) and one form of familial M-D (*DYT15*) is also linked in this region (99). Other families with a similar phenotype of adult onset torticollis/focal dystonia have been excluded from this locus (140,172–174) supporting locus heterogeneity.

### *DYT9* (Familial Paroxysmal Dyskinesia)

This is a complex paroxysmal phenotype manifesting episodic involuntary dystonic posture of limbs, dysarthria, paresthesias, and double vision, as well as, in some cases, paroxysmal choreoathetosis, spasticity, episodic ataxia, spastic paraplegia, and dyskinesia. A single family has been described (175) with autosomal dominant inheritance and onset at 2 to 15 years. Episodes usually last about 20 minutes and can occur anywhere from twice per day to twice per year. Symptoms are triggered by physical exercise, emotional stress, fatigue, and alcohol. The gene has been linked to chromosome 1p21-p13.3.

### *DYT10* (Paroxysmal Kinesigenic Dystonia/Dyskinesia, PKC)

This is the most frequent of the paroxysmal dyskinesias. It can be distinguished from *DYT8*, as in *DYT10* the onset is later, attacks are precipitated by sudden movements or startle (kinesigenic), of very short duration (seconds to minutes), very frequent (up to 100 times per day), and responsive to anticonvulsant therapy with no loss of consciousness or pain during attack (136,176–178). Symptoms can be precipitated by alcohol, caffeine, exercise, emotional stress, fatigue, or chocolate. It is inherited in an autosomal dominant manner with reduced penetrance. Linkage in eight Japanese families has been established to 16p11.2-q12.1 (179), a region that overlaps loci implicated in infantile convulsions, paroxysmal choreoathetosis, and rolandic epilepsy suggesting these might be allelic disorders (180,181).

### *DYT13* (Multifocal/Segmental Dystonia)

This syndrome has been described in a single large family from Italy with some similarities to *DYT6* dystonia. It is characterized by juvenile or early adult onset (mean 16 years, range 5–40 years), with the majority of cases showing segmental dystonia with prominent cranial cervical involvement, a mild course, slow progression, and only occasional generalization (14,182). It is inherited as an autosomal dominant syndrome with a penetrance of about 60%. The locus has been mapped to chromosome 1p36.1-p36.32 (in the same region as *PARK7*).

In addition to these numbered DYT genes, there are several other new forms of dystonia emerging, which are distinguished by their phenotype and lack of linkage to known loci, including autosomal dominant blepharospasm with adult onset in two families (183); early-onset generalized dystonia with mild parkinsonian signs (184); typical early-onset generalized dystonia accompanied by cervical dystonia or writer's cramp beginning at age 30 (172), and adult-onset cranio-cervical torsion dystonia (141).

## REFERENCES

1. Fahn S, Bressman SB, Marsden CD. Classification of dystonia. Adv Neurol 1998; 78:1–13.
2. Quinn NP. Parkinsonism and dystonia, pseudo-parkinsonism and pseudodystonia. Adv Neurol 1993; 60:540–543.
3. Bressman SB. Dystonia genotypes, phenotypes, and classification. Adv Neurol 2004; 94:101–107.
4. Wenning GK, Kiechl S, Seppi K, et al. Prevalence of movement disorders in men and women aged 50–89 years (Bruneck Study cohort): a population-based study. Lancet Neurol 2005; 4:815–820.
5. Klein C, Breakefield XO, Ozelius LJ. Genetics of primary dystonia. Semin Neurol 1999; 19:271–280.
6. Klein C, Ozelius LJ. Movement disorders: classifications. J Inherit Metab Dis 2002; 28:425–439.
7. Klein C. Movement disorders: classifications. J Inherit Metab Dis 2005; 28:425–439.
8. Kabakci K, Hedrich K, Leung J-C, et al. Mutations in DYT1: extension of the phenotypic and mutational spectrum. Neurology 2004; 62:395–400.
9. Kock N, Kasten M, Schule B, et al. Clinical and genetic features of myoclonus-dystonia in 3 cases: a video presentation. Mov Disord 2004; 19:231–234.
10. Hagenah JM, Zuhlke C, Hellenbroich Y, et al. Focal dystonia as a presenting sign of spinocerebellar ataxia 17. Mov Disord 2004; 19:217–220.
11. Leung J, Klein C, Friedman J, et al. Novel mutation in the TOR1A (DYT1) gene in atypical, early onset dystonia and polymorphisms in dystonia and early onset parkinsonism. Neurogenetics 2001; 3:133–143.
12. Leube B, Rudnicki D, Ratzlaff T, et al. Idiopathic torsion dystonia: assignment of a gene to chromosome 18p in a German family with adult onset, autosomal dominant inheritance and purely focal distribution. Hum Mol Genet 1996; 5:1673–1677.
13. Gasser T, Windgassen K, Bereznai B, et al. Phenotypic expression of the DYT1 mutant: a family with writer's cramp of juvenile onset. Ann Neurol 1998; 44:126–128.
14. Valente EM, Bentivoglio AR, Cassetta E, et al. DYT13, a novel primary torsion dystonia locus, maps to chromosome 1p36.13—36.32 in an Italian family with cranial-cervical or upper limb onset. Ann Neurol 2001; 49:362–366.
15. Bressman SB, Sabatti C, Raymond D, et al. The DYT1 phenotype and guidelines for diagnostic testing. Neurology 2000; 54:1746–1752.
16. Hagenah J, Saunders-Pullman R, Hedrich K, et al. High mutation rate in dopa-responsive dystonia: detection with comprehensive GCHI screening. Neurology 2005; 64:908–911.

17. DeBerardinis RJ, Conforto D, Russell K, et al. Myoclonus in a patient with a deletion of the epsilon-sarcoglycan locus on chromosome 7q21. Am J Med Genet 2003; 121A:31–36.
18. Asmus F, Salih F, Hjermind LE, et al. Myoclonus-dystonia due to genomic deletions in the epsilon-sarcoglycan gene. Ann Neurol 2005; 58:792–797.
19. Klein C, Friedman J, Bressman S, et al. Genetic testing for early-onset torsion dystonia (DYT1): Introduction of a simple screening method, experiences from testing of a large patient cohort, and ethical aspects. Genet Test 1999; 3:323–328.
20. Ghilardi MR, Carbon M, Silvestri G, et al. Impaired sequence learning in carriers of the DYT1 dystonia mutation. Ann Neurol 2003; 54:102–109.
21. Carbon M, Kingsley PB, Su S, et al. Microstructural white matter changes in carriers of the DYT1 gene mutation. Ann Neurol 2004; 56:283–286.
22. Asanuma K, Ma Y, Okulski J, et al. Decreased striatal D2 receptor binding in non-manifesting carriers of the DYT1 dystonia mutation. Neurology 2005; 64:347–349.
23. Risch N, de Leon D, Ozelius LJ, et al. Genetic analysis of idiopathic torsion dystonia in Ashkenazi Jews and their recent descent from a small founder population. Nat Genet 1995; 9:152–159.
24. Nutt JG, Muenter MD, Aronson A, et al. Epidemiology of focal and generalized dystonia in Rochester, Minnesota. Mov Disord 1988; 3:188–194.
25. Bressman SB, de Leon MS, Kramer PL, et al. Dystonia in Ashkenazi Jews: clinical characterization of a founder mutation. Ann Neurol 1994; 36:771–777.
26. Ozelius LJ, Hewett J, Page C, et al. The early-onset torsion dystonia gene (DYT1) encodes an ATP-binding protein. Nat Genet 1997; 17:40–48.
27. Risch NJ, Bressman SB, de Leon D, et al. Segregation analysis of idiopathic torsion dystonia in Ashkenazi Jews suggests autosomal dominant inheritance. Am J Hum Genet 1990; 46:533–538.
28. Kamm C, Naumann M, Mueller J, et al. The DYT1 GAG deletion is infrequent in sporadic and familial writer' s cramp. Mov Disord 2000; 15:1238–1241.
29. Eidelberg D, Moeller JR, Antonini A, et al. Functional brain networks in DYT1 dystonia. Ann Neurol 1998; 44:299–300.
30. Heiman GA, Ottman R, Saunders-Pullman RJ, et al. Increased risk for recurrent major depression in DYT1 dystonia mutation carriers. Neurology 2004; 63:631–637.
31. Edwards M, Huang Y-Z, Wood NW, et al. Different patterns of electrophysiological deficits in manifesting and non-manifesting carriers of the DYT1 gene mutation. Brain 2003; 126:2074–2080.
32. Saunders-Pullman R, Shriberg J, Shanker V, et al. Penetrance and expression of dystonia genes. Adv Neurol 2004; 94:121–125.
33. Klein C, Brin MF, de Leon D, et al. *De novo* mutations (GAG deletion) in the DYT1 gene in two non-Jewish patients with early-onset dystonia. Hum Mol Genet 1998; 7:1133–1136.
34. Klein C, Liu L, Doheny D, et al. Epsilon-sarcoglycan mutations found in combination with other dystonia gene mutations. Ann Neurol 2002; 52:675–679.
35. Clarimon J, Asgeirsson H, Singleton A, et al. TorsinA haplotype predisposes to idiopathic dystonia. Ann Neurol 2005; 57:765–767.
36. Neuwald AF, Aravind L, Spouge JL, et al. AAA+: a class of chaperone-like ATPases associated with the assembly, operation, and disassembly of protein complexes. Genome Res 1999; 9:27–43.
37. Lupas A, Flanagan JM, Tamura T, et al. Self-compartmentalization proteases. Trends Biochem Sci 1997; 22:399–404.
38. Hanson PI, Whiteheart SW. AAA+ proteins: have engine, will work. Nat Rev Mol Cell Biol 2005; 6:519–529.
39. Vale RD. AAA proteins: Lords of the ring. J Cell Biol 2000; 150:F13–F19.
40. Augood SJ, Keller-McGandy CE, Siriani A, et al. Distribution and ultrastructural localization of torsinA immunoreactivity in the human brain. Brain Res 2003; 986:12–21.
41. Rostasy K, Augood SJ, Hewett JW, et al. TorsinA protein and neuropathology in early onset generalized dystonia with GAG deletion. Neurobiol Dis 2003; 12:11–24.

42. Shashidharan P, Kramer BC, Walker R, et al. Immunohistochemical localization and distribution of torsinA in normal human and rat brain. Brain Res 2000; 853:197–206.
43. Xiao J, Gong S, Zhao Y, et al. Developmental expression of rat torsinA transcript and protein. Brain Res Dev Brain Res 2004; 152:47–60.
44. Siegert S, Bahn E, Kramer M, et al. TorsinA expression is detectable in human infants as young as four weeks old. Brain Res Dev Brain Res 2005; 157:19–26.
45. Vasudevan A, Breakefield XO, Bhide PG. TorsinA and torsinB expression in the developing mouse brain. Mol Brain Res: 2006;1073–1074: 139–145.
46. Goodchild RE, Kim CE, Dauer WT. Loss of the dystonia-associated protein torsinA selectively disrupts the neuronal nuclear envelope. Neuron 2005; 48:923–932.
47. Dang M, Yokoi F, Li Y. Motor deficits and hyperactivity in DYT1 knockdown mice. Mol Brain Res 2005; 196:452–463.
48. Hewett J, Gonzalez-Agosti C, Slater D, et al. Mutant torsinA, responsible for early onset torsion dystonia, forms membrane inclusions in cultured neural cells. Hum Mol Genet 2000; 22:1403–1413.
49. Kustedjo K, Bracey MH, Cravatt BF. TorsinA and its torsion dystonia-associated mutant forms are lumenal glycoproteins that exhibit distinct subcellular localizations. J Biol Chem 2000; 275:27933–27939.
50. Naismith TV, Heuser JE, Breakefield XO, et al. TorsinA in the nuclear envelope. Proc Natl Acad Sci USA 2004; 101:7612–7617.
51. Goodchild RE, Dauer WT. The AAA+ protein torsinA interacts with a conserved domain present in LAP1 and a novel ER protein. Cell Biol 2005; 168:855–862.
52. McNaught KS, Kapustin A, Jackson T, et al. Brainstem pathology in DYT1 primary torsion dystonia. Ann Neurol 2004; 56:540–547.
53. Hedreen JC, Zweig RM, DeLong MR, et al. Primary dystonias: a review of the pathology and suggestions for new directions of study. Adv Neurol 1988; 50:123–132.
54. Walker RH, Brin MF, Sandu D, et al. TorsinA immunoreactivity in brains of patients with DYT1 and non-DYT1 dystonia. Neurology 2002; 58:120–124.
55. Hewett J, Zeng J, Bragg DC, Breakefield XO. Dystonia-causing mutant form of torsinA inhibits cell adhesion and neurite extension through interference with cytoskeletal dynamics. Neurobiol Dis 2006; 22:98–111.
56. Torres GE, Sweeney AL, Beaulieu JM, et al. Effect of torsinA on membrane proteins reveals a loss of function and a dominant negative phenotype of the dystonia-associated {Delta}E-torsinA mutant. Proc Natl Acad Sci USA 2004; 101:15650–15655.
57. McLean PJ, Kawamata H, Shariff S, et al. TorsinA and heat shock proteins act as molecular chaperones: suppression of alpha-synuclein aggregation. J Neurochem 2002; 83:846–854.
58. Cao S, Gelwix CC, Caldwell KA, et al. Torsin-mediated protection from cellular stress in the dopaminergic neurons of *Caenorhabditis elegans*. J Neurosci 2005; 25:3801–3812.
59. Wong VCN, Lam C-W, Fung WC. Stiff child syndrome with mutation of DYT1 gene. Neurology 2005; 65:1465–1466.
60. Opal P, Tintner R, Jankovic J, et al. Intrafamilial phenotypic variability of the DYT1 dystonia: from asymptomatic TOR1A gene carrier status to dystonic storm. Mov Disord 2002; 17:339–345.
61. Gatto EM, Pardal MM, Micheli FE. Unusual phenotypic expression of the DYT1 mutation. Parkinsonism Relat Disord 2003; 9:277–279.
62. Almasy L, Bressman SB, de Leon D, et al. Idiopathic torsion dystonia linked to chromosome 8 in two Mennonite families. Ann Neurol 1997; 42:670–673.
63. Toda H, Hamani C, Lozano A. Deep brain stimulation in the treatment of dyskinesia and dystonia. Neurosurg Focus 2004; 17:E2 Rev.
64. Coubes P, Cif L, El Fertit H, et al. Electrical stimulation of the globus pallidus internus in patients with primary generalized dystonia: long-term results. J Neurosurg 2004; 101:189–194.
65. Segawa M, Hosaka A, Miyagawa F, et al. Hereditary progressive dystonia with marked diurnal fluctuation. Adv Neurol 1976; 14:215–233.

66. Blau N, Bonafe L, Thony B. Tetrahydrobiopterin deficiencies without hyperphenylalaninemia: diagnosis and genetics of dopa-responsive dystonia and sepiapterin reductase deficiency. Mol Genet Metab 2001; 74:172–185.
67. Grimes DA, Barclay CL, Duff J, et al. Phenocopies in a large GCH1 mutation positive family with dopa responsive dystonia: confusing the picture? J Neurol Neurosurg Psychiatry 2002; 72:801–804.
68. Bandmann O, Valente EM, Holmans P, et al. Dopa-responsive dystonia: a clinical and molecular genetic study. Ann Neurol 1998; 44:649–656.
69. Kong CK, Ko CH, Tong SF, et al. Atypical presentation of dopa-responsive dystonia: generalized hypotonia and proximal weakness. Neurology 2001; 57:1121–1124.
70. Hahn H, Trant MR, Brownstein MJ, et al. Neurologic and psychiatric manifestations in a family with a mutation in exon 2 of the guanosine triphosphate-cyclohydrolase gene. Arch Neurol 2001; 58:749–755.
71. Van Hove JLK, Steyaert J, Matthijs G, et al. Expanded motor and psychiatric phenotype in autosomal dominant Segawa syndrome due to GTP cyclohydrolase deficiency. J Neurol Neurosurg Psychiatry 2006; 77:18–23.
72. Nar H, Huber R, Auerbach G, et al. Active site topology and reaction mechanism of GTP cyclohydrolase I. Proc Natl Acad Sci USA 1995; 92:12120–12125.
73. Nygaard TG, Wooten GF. Dopa-responsive dystonia: some pieces of the puzzle are still missing. Neurology 1998; 50:853–855.
74. Furukawa Y, Guttman M, Sparagana SP, et al. Dopa-responsive dystonia due to a large deletion in the GTP cyclohydrolase I gene. Ann Neurol 2000; 47:517–520.
75. Klein C, Hedrich K, Kabakci K, et al. Exon deletions in the GCHI gene in two of four Turkish families with dopa-responsive dystonia. Neurology 2002; 59:1783–1786.
76. Grotzsch H, Pizzolato GP, Ghika J, et al. Neuropathology of a case of dopa-responsive dystonia associated with a new genetic locus, DYT14. Neurology 2002; 58:1839–1842.
77. Friedman J, Standaert DG. Neurogenetics of dystonia and paroxysmal dyskinesias. In: Lynch DR, ed. Neurogenetics: Scientific and Clinical Advances. Marcel Dekker, New York 2005:403–426.
78. Steinberger D, Blau N, Goriuonov D, et al. Heterozygous mutation in 5'-untranslated region of sepiapterin reductase gene (SPR) in a patient with dopa-responsive dystonia. Neurogenetics 2004; 5:187–190.
79. Hirano M, Tamaru Y, Ito H, et al. Mutant GTPcyclohydrolaseI mRNA levels contribute to dopa-responsive dystonia onset. Ann Neurol 1996; 40:796–798.
80. Hirano M, Imaiso Y, Ueno S. Differential splicing of the GTP cyclohydrolase I RNA in dopa-responsive dystonia. Biochem Biophys Res Commun 1997; 234:316–319.
81. Saunders-Pullman R, Blau N, Hyland K, et al. Phenylalanine loading as a diagnostic test for DRD: interpreting the utility of the test. Mol Genet Metab 2004; 83:207–212.
82. www.bh4.org/biomdb.summary.html.
83. Quinn NP. Essential myoclonus and myoclonic dystonia. Mov Disord 1996; 11:119–124.
84. Klein C, Gurvich N, Sena-Esteves M, et al. Evaluation of the role of the D2 dopamine receptor in myoclonus dystonia. Ann Neurol 2000; 47:369–373.
85. Vidailhet M, Tassin J, Durif F, et al. A major locus for several phenotypes of myoclonus-dystonia on chromosome 7q. Neurology 2001; 56:1213–1216.
86. Asmus F, Zimprich A, Tezenas Du Montcel S, et al. Myoclonus-dystonia syndrome: epsilon-sarcoglycan mutations and phenotype. Ann Neurol 2002; 52:489–492.
87. Klein C. Myoclonus and myoclonus-dystonias. In: Pulst S, ed. Genetics of Movement Disorders. San Diego: Academic Press, 2003:449–469.
88. Valente EM, Edwards MJ, Mir P, et al. The epsilon-sarcoglycan gene in myoclonic syndromes. Neurology 2005; 64:737–739.
89. Mahooudji M, Pikielny RT. Hereditary essential myoclonus. Brain 1967; 90:669–674.
90. Zimprich A, Grabowski M, Asmus F, et al. Mutations in the gene encoding epsilon-sarcoglycan cause myoclonus-dystonia syndrome. Nat Genet 2001; 29:66–69.

91. Doheny DO, Brin MF, Morrison CE, et al. Phenotypic features of myoclonus-dystonia in three kindreds. Neurology 2002; 59:1187–1196.
92. Muller B, Hedrich K, Kock N, et al. Evidence that paternal expression of the epsilon-sarcoglycan gene accounts for reduced penetrance in myoclonus-dystonia. Am J Hum Genet 2002; 71:1303–1311.
93. Foncke EM, Klein C, Koelman JH, et al. Hereditary myoclonus-dystonia associated with epilepsy. Neurology 2003; 60:1988–1990.
94. Han F, Lang AE, Racacho L, et al. Mutations in the epsilon-sarcoglycan gene found to be uncommon in seven myoclonus-dystonia families. Neurology 2003; 61:244–246.
95. Hjermind LE, Werdelin LM, Eiberg H, et al. A novel mutation in the epsilon-sarcoglycan gene causing myoclonus-dystonia syndrome. Neurology 2003; 60:1536–1539.
96. Marechal L, Raux G, Dumanchin C, et al. Severe myoclonus-dystonia syndrome associated with a novel epsilon-sarcoglycan gene truncating mutation. Am J Med Genet 2003; 119B:114–117.
97. Hedrich K, Meyer EM, Schule B, et al. Myoclonus-dystonia: detection of novel, recurrent, and de novo SGCE mutations. Neurology 2004; 62:1229–1231.
98. Schule B, Kock N, Svetel M, et al. Genetic heterogeneity in ten families with myoclonus-dystonia. J Neurol Neurosurg Psychiatry 2004; 75:1181–1185.
99. Grimes DA, Han F, Lang AE, et al. A novel locus for inherited myoclonus-dystonia on 18p11. Neurology 2002; 59:1182–1186.
100. Quinn NP, Rothwell JC, Thompson PD, et al. Hereditary myoclonic dystonia, hereditary torsion dystonia and hereditary essential myoclonus: an area of confusion. Adv Neurol 1988; 50:391–401.
101. Lang AE. Essential myoclonus and myoclonic dystonia. Mov Disord 1997; 12:127.
102. Saunders-Pullman R, Ozelius L, Bressman SB. Inherited myoclonus-dystonia. Adv Neurol 2002; 89:185–191.
103. Kyllerman M, Forsgren L, Sanner G, et al. Alcohol-responsive myoclonic dystonia in a large family: Dominant inheritance and phenotypic variation. Mov Disord 1990; 5: 270–279.
104. Klein C, Schilling K, Saunders-Pullman RJ, et al. A major locus for myoclonus-dystonia maps to chromosome 7q in eight families. Am J Hum Genet 2000; 67:1314–1319.
105. O'Riordan S, Ozelius LJ, de Carvalho Aguiar P, et al. Inherited myoclonus-dystonia and epilepsy: further evidence of an association? Mov Disord 2004; 19:1456–1459.
106. Klein C, Brin MF, Kramer P, et al. Association of a missense change in the D2 dopamine receptor with myoclonus dystonia. Proc Natl Acad Sci USA 1999; 27:5173–5176.
107. Nygaard TG, Raymond D, Chen C, et al. Localization of a gene for myoclonus-dystonia to chromosome 7q21-q31. Ann Neurol 1999; 46:794–798.
108. Asmus F, Zimprich A, Naumann M, et al. Inherited myoclonus-dystonia syndrome: narrowing the 7q21-q31 locus in German families. Ann Neurol 2001; 49:121–124.
109. Saunders-Pullman R, Shriberg J, Heiman G, et al. Myoclonus dystonia: possible association with obsessive-compulsive disorder and alcohol dependence. Neurology 2002; 58:242–245.
110. Scheidtmann K, Muller F, Hartmann E, et al. Familial myoclonus-dystonia syndrome associated with panic attacks. Nervenarzt 2000; 71:839–842.
111. Piras G, El Kharroubi A, Kozlov S, et al. Zac1 (Lot1), a potential tumor suppressor gene, and the gene for epsilon-sarcoglycan are maternally imprinted genes: identification by a subtractive screen of novel uniparental fibroblast lines. Mol Cell Biol 2000; 20:3308–3315.
112. Grabowski M, Zimprich A, Lorenz-Depiereux B, et al. The epsilon-sarcoglycan gene (SGCE), mutated in myoclonus-dystonia syndrome, is maternally imprinted. Eur J Hum Genet 2003; 11:138–144.
113. McNally EM, Ly CT, Kunkel LM. Human epsilon-sarcoglycan is highly related to alpha-sarcoglycan (adhalin), the limb girdle muscular dystrophy 2D gene. FEBS Lett 1998; 422:27–32.

114. Yokoi F, Dang MT, Mitsui S, et al. Exclusive paternal expression and novel alternatively spliced variants of epsilon-sarcoglycan mRNA in mouse brain. FEBS Lett 2005; 579:4822–4828.
115. Nishiyama A, Endo T, Takeda S, et al. Identification and characterization of epsilon-sarcoglycans in the central nervous system. Brain Res Mol Brain Res 2004; 125:1–12.
116. Hack AA, Groh ME, McNally EM. Sarcoglycans in muscular dystrophy. Microsc Res Tech 2000; 48:167–180.
117. Liu LA, Engvall E. Sarcoglycan isoforms in skeletal muscle. J Biol Chem 1999; 274:38171–38176.
118. Ettinger AJ, Feng G, Sanes JR. Epsilon-sarcoglycan, a broadly expressed homologue of the gene mutated in limb-girdle muscular dystrophy 2D. J Biol Chem 1997; 272:32534–32538.
119. Xiao J, LeDoux MS. Cloning, developmental regulation and neural localization of rat epsilon-sarcoglycan. Brain Res Mol Brain Res 2003; 119:132–143.
120. Chan P, Gonzalez-Maeso J, Ruf F, et al. Epsilon-sarcoglycan immunoreactivity and mRNA expression in mouse brain. J Comp Neurol 2005; 482:50–73.
121. Tezenas du Montcel S, Clot F, Vidailhet M, et al. Epsilon sarcoglycan mutations and phenotype in French patients with myoclonic syndromes. J Med Genet 2005; 43:394–400.
122. Valente EM, Misbahuddin A, Brancati F, et al. Analysis of the epsilon-sarcoglycan gene in familial and sporadic myoclonus-dystonia: evidence for genetic heterogeneity. Mov Disord 2003; 18:1047–1051.
123. Grundmann K, Laubis-Herrmann U, Dressler D, et al. Lack of mutations in the epsilon-sarcoglycan gene in patients with different subtypes of primary dystonias. Mov Disord 2004; 19:1294–1297.
124. Dobyns WB, Ozelius LJ, Kramer PL, et al. Rapid-onset dystonia-parkinsonism. Neurology 1993; 43:2596–2602.
125. Brashear A, Farlow MR, Butler IJ, et al. Variable phenotype of rapid-onset dystonia–parkinsonism. Mov Disord 1996; 2:151–156.
126. Brashear A, de Leon D, Bressman S, et al. Rapid onset dystonia-parkinsonism: a report of a second family. Neurol 1997; 48:1066–1069.
127. Webb DW, Broderick A, Brashear A, et al. Rapid onset dystonia-parkinsonism in a 14-year-old girl. Europ J Paediatr Neurol 1999; 3:171–173.
128. Pittock SJ, Joyce CO, Keane V. Rapid onset dystonia-parkinsonism: a clinical and genetic analysis of a new kindred. Neurology 2000; 55:991–995.
129. Brashear A, Butler IJ, Hyland K, et al. Cerebrospinal fluid homovanillic acid levels in rapid-onset dystonia-parkinsonism. Ann Neurol 1998; 43:521–526.
130. Kramer PL, Mineta M, Klein C, et al. Rapid-onset dystonia parkinsonism: Linkage to chromosome 19q13. Ann Neurol 1999; 46:176–182.
131. Zaremba J, Mierzewska H, Lysiak Z, et al. Rapid-onset dystonia-parkinsonism: a fourth family consistent with linkage to chromosome 19q13. Mov Disord 2004; 19:1506–1510.
132. de Carvalho Aguiar P, Sweadner KJ, Penniston J, et al. Mutations in the $Na^+K^+$-ATPase 3 gene ATP1A3 are associated with rapid onset dystonia parkinsonism. Neuron 2004; 43:169–175.
133. De Fusco M, Marconi R, Silvestri L, et al. Haploinsufficiency of ATP1A2 encoding the $Na^+/K^+$ pump alpha2 subunit associated with familial hemiplegic migraine type 2. Nat Genet 2003; 33:192–196.
134. Vanmolkot KR, Kors EE, Hottenga JJ, et al. Novel mutations in the $Na^+$, $K^+$-ATPase pump gene ATP1A2 associated with familial hemiplegic migraine and benign familial infantile convulsions. Ann Neurol 2003; 54:360–366.
135. Mount L, Reback S. Familial paroxysmal choreoathetosis preliminary report on an mitheric undescribed clinical syndrome. Arch Neurol Psychiatry 1940; 44:841–847.
136. Fahn S. Concept and classification of dystonia. Adv Neurol 1988; 50:1–8.
137. Demirkiran M, Jankovic J. Paroxysmal dyskinesias: clinical features and classification. Ann Neurol 1995; 38:571–579.

138. Fouad GT, Servidei S, Durcan S, et al. A gene for familial paroxysmal dyskinesia (FPD1) maps to chromosome 2q. Am J Hum Genet 1996; 59:135–139.
139. Fink JK, Rainier S, Wilkowski J, et al. Paroxysmal dystonic choreoathetosis: Tight linkage to chromosome 2q. Am J Hum Genet 1996; 59:140–145.
140. Raskind WH, Bolin T, Wolff J, et al. Further localization of a gene for paroxysmal dystonic choreoathetosis to a 5-cM region on chromosome 2q34. Hum Genet 1998; 102:93–97.
141. Munchau A, Valente EM, Davis MB, et al. A Yorkshire family with adult-onset cranio-cervical primary torsion dystonia. Mov Disord 2000; 15:954–959.
142. Lee HY, Xu Y, Huang Y, et al. The gene for paroxysmal non-kinesigenic dyskinesia encodes an enzyme in a stress response pathway. Hum Mol Genet 2004; 13:3161–3170.
143. Rainier S, Thomas D, Tokarz D, et al. Myofibrillogenesis regulator 1 gene mutations cause paroxysmal dystonic choreoathetosis. Arch Neurol 2004; 61:1025–1029.
144. Chen DH, Matsushita M, Rainier S, et al. Presence of alanine-to-valine substitutions in myofibrillogenesis regulator 1 in paroxysmal nonkinesigenic dyskinesia: confirmation in 2 kindreds. Arch Neurol 2005; 62:597–600.
145. Djarmali A, Svetel M, Momcilovic D, et al. Significance of recurrent mutations in the myofibrillogenesis regulator 1 gene. Arch Neurol 2005; 62:1641.
146. Thornalley PJ. The glyoxalase system in health and disease. Mol Aspects Med 1993; 14:287–371.
147. Lee LV, Pascasio FM, Fuentes FD, et al. Torsion dystonia in Panay, Philippines. Adv Neurol 1976; 14:137–151.
148. Evidente VG, Nolte D, Niemann S, et al. Phenotypic and molecular analyses of X-linked dystonia-parkinsonism ("lubag") in women. Arch Neurol 2004; 61:1956–1959.
149. Factor SA, Barron KD. Mosaic pattern of gliosis in the neostriatum of a North American man with craniocervical dystonia and parkinsonism. Mov Disord 1997; 12:783–789.
150. Gibb WR, Kilford L, Marsden CD. Severe generalised dystonia associated with a mosaic pattern of striatal gliosis. Mov Disord 1992; 7:217–223.
151. Waters CH, Faust PL, Powers J, et al. Neuropathology of lubag (X-linked dystonia parkinsonism). Mov Disord 1993; 8:387–390.
152. Lee LV, Munoz EL, Tan KT, et al. Sex linked recessive dystonia parkinsonism of Panay, Philippines (XDP). Mol Pathol 2001; 54:362–368.
153. Goto S, Lee LV, Munoz EL, et al. Functional anatomy of the basal ganglia in X-linked recessive dystonia-parkinsonism. Ann Neurol 2005; 58:7–17.
154. Kupke KG, Lee LV, Mueller U. Assigment of the X-linked torsion dystonia gene to Xq21 by linkage analysis. Neurology 1990; 40:1438–1442.
155. Wilhelmsen KD, Weeks DE, Nygaard TG, et al. Genetic mapping of "lubag" (X-linked Dystonia-Parkinsonism) is a Filipino kindred to the pericentromeric region of the X chromosomes. Ann Neurol 1991; 29:124–131.
156. Nolte D, Niemann S, Muller U. Specific sequence changes in multiple transcript system DYT3 are associated with X-linked dystonia parkinsonism. Proc Natl Acad Sci USA 2003; 100:10347–10352.
157. Plummer C, Bradfield J, Singleton AB, et al. First case report of X linked dystonia parkinsonism (XDP) or 'lubag' in Australia. J Clin Neurosci 2005; 12:946–947.
158. Gimenez-Roldan S, Delgado G, Marin M, et al. Hereditary torsion dystonia in gypsies. Adv Neurol 1988; 50:73–81.
159. Khan NL, Wood NW, Bhatia KP. Autosomal recessive, DYT2-like primary torsion dystonia: a new family. Neurology 2003; 61:1801–1803.
160. Moretti P, Hedera P, Wald J, et al. Autosomal recessive primary generalized dystonia in two siblings from a consanguineous family. Mov Disord 2005; 20:245–247.
161. Parker N. Hereditary whispering dysphonia. J Neurol Neurosurg Psychiatry 1985; 48:218–224.
162. Ahmad F, Davis MB, Waddy HM, et al. Evidence for locus heterogeneity in autosomal dominant torsion dystonia. Genomics 1993; 15:9–12.

163. ESDE Collaborative Group. A prevalence study of primary dystonia in eight European countries. J Neurol 2000; 247:787–792.
164. Defazio G, Livrea P, Guanti G, et al. Genetic contribution to idiopathic adult-onset blepharospasm and cranial-cervical dystonia. Eur Neurol 1993; 33:345–350.
165. Waddy HM, Fletcher NA, Harding AE, et al. A genetic study of idiopathic focal dystonias. Ann Neurol 1991; 29:320–324.
166. Leube B, Kessler KR, Goecke T, et al. Frequency of familial inheritance among 488 index patients with idiopathic focal dystonia and clinical variability in a large family. Mov Disord 1997; 12:1000–1006.
167. Uitti RJ, Maraganore DM. Adult onset familial cervical dystonia: report of a family including monozygotic twins. Mov Disord 1993; 8:489–494.
168. Bressman SB, Warner TT, Almasy L, et al. Exclusion of the DYT1 locus in familial torticollis. Ann Neurol 1996; 40:681–684.
169. Schmidt A, Jabusch HC, Altemmuller E, et al. Dominantly transmitted focal dystonia in families of patients with musician's cramp. Neurology. 2006; 67:691–693.
170. Klein C, Page CE, LeWitt P, et al. Genetic analysis of three patients with an 18p-syndrome and dystonia. Neurology 1999; 52:649–651.
171. Tezzon F, Zanoni T, Passarin MG, et al. Dystonia in a patient with deletion of 18p. Ital J Neurol Sci 1998; 19:90–93.
172. Klein C, Pramstaller PO, Claudio MD, et al. Clinical and genetic evaluation of a family with a mixed dystonia phenotype from South Tyrol. Ann Neurol 1998; 44:394–398.
173. Jarman PR, del Grosso N, Valente EM, et al. Primary torsion dystonia: the search for genes is not over. J Neurol Neurosurg Psychiatry 1999; 67:395–397.
174. Brancati F, Defazio G, Caputo V, et al. Novel Italian family supports clinical and genetic heterogeneity of primary adult-onset torsion dystonia. Mov Disord 2002; 17:392–397.
175. Auburger G, Ratzlaff T, Lunkes A, et al. A gene for autosomal dominant paroxysmal choreoathetosis/spasticity (CSE) maps to the vicinity of a potassium channel gene cluster on chromosome 1p, probably within 2 cM between D1S443 and D1S197. Genomics 1996; 31:90–94.
176. Kertesz A. Paroxysmal kinesigenic choreoathetosis. An entity within the paroxysmal choreoathetosis syndrome. Description of 10 cases, including 1 autopsied. Neurology 1967; 17:680–690.
177. Walker ES. Familial paroxysmal dystonic choreoathetosis: a neurologic disorder simulating psychiatric illness. Johns Hopkins Med J 1981; 148:108–113.
178. Bruno MK, Hallett M, Gwinn-Hardy K, et al. Clinical evaluation of idiopathic paroxysmal kinesigenic dyskinesia: new diagnostic criteria. Neurology 2004; 63:2280–2287.
179. Tomita H, Nagamitsu S, Wakui K, et al. Paroxysmal kinesigenic choreoathetosis locus maps to chromosome 16p11.2-q12.1. Am J Hum Genet 1999; 65:1688–1697.
180. Swoboda KJ, Soong BW, McKenna C, et al. Paroxysmal kinesigenic dyskinesia and infantile convulsions. Clinical and linkage studies. Neurology 2001; 57:S42–S48.
181. Caraballo R, Pavek S, Lemainque A, et al. Linkage of benign familial infantile convulsions to chromosome 16p12-q12 suggests allelism to the infantile convulsions and choreoathetosis syndrome. Am J Hum Genet 2001; 68:788–794.
182. Bentivoglio AR, Del Grosso N, Albanese A, et al. Non-DYT1 dystonia in a large Italian family. J Neurol Neurosurg Psychiatry 1997; 62:357–360.
183. Defazio G, Brancati F, Valente EM, et al. Familial blepharospasm is inherited as an autosomal dominant trait and relates to a novel unassigned gene. Mov Disord 2003; 18:207–212.
184. Fabbrini G, Brancati F, Vacca L, et al. A novel family with an unusual early-onset generalized dystonia. Mov Disord 2005; 20:81–86.

# 4
# Functional Anatomy of the Basal Ganglia

**Jonathan W. Mink**
*Departments of Neurology, Pediatrics, Anatomy and Neurobiology, and Brain and Cognitive Sciences, University of Rochester, Rochester, New York, U.S.A.*

## INTRODUCTION

The basal ganglia are thought to be the primary site of neuronal dysfunction in the majority of movement disorders. Although most forms of dystonia do not have clearly identified pathology, focal brain lesions that produce dystonia are most commonly located in the basal ganglia or thalamic target of the basal ganglia (1). Even in forms of dystonia where there is evidence for cerebral cortical abnormalities, basal ganglia abnormalities have also been identified (2,3). Indeed, some authors view cortical dysfunction in dystonia as a secondary consequence of basal ganglia dysfunction (4–6). Thus, knowledge of the organization and function of basal ganglia-thalamo-cortical circuits is important to understanding the underlying pathophysiology of dystonia.

The basal ganglia include the striatum (caudate, putamen, nucleus accumbens), the subthalamic nucleus (STN), the globus pallidus [internal segment, external segment, ventral pallidum (VP)], and the substantia nigra pars compacta (SNpc) and substantia nigra pars reticulata (SNpr) (Fig. 1). The striatum and STN receive the majority of inputs from outside of the basal ganglia. Most of those inputs come from cerebral cortex, but thalamic nuclei also provide strong inputs to striatum. The bulk of the outputs from the basal ganglia arise from the internal segment of the globus pallidus (GPi), VP, and SNpr. These outputs are inhibitory to the pedunculopontine area in the brainstem and to thalamic nuclei that in turn project to the frontal lobe.

## BASAL GANGLIA INPUTS

### Striatum

The striatum receives the bulk of extrinsic input to the basal ganglia. While the striatum receives excitatory input from virtually all of cerebral cortex (7), the ventral striatum (nucleus accumbens and rostroventral extensions of caudate and putamen) receive inputs from the hippocampus and amygdala (8). The glutamatergic cortical afferents terminate largely on the heads of the dendritic spines of medium spiny neurons in a generally topographic organization (9). It has been suggested that this topography provides the basis for a segregation of functionally different circuits in

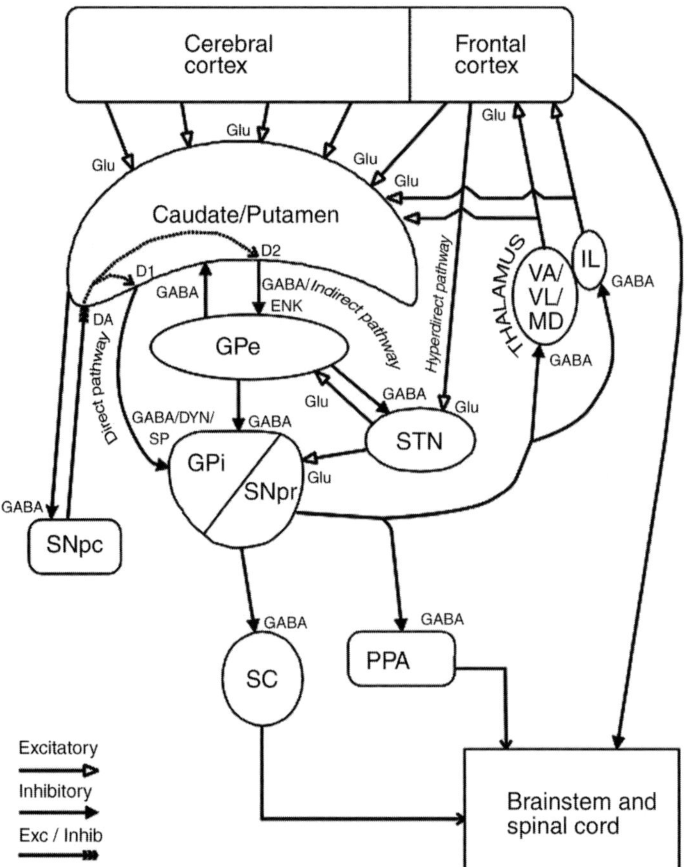


**Figure 1** Simplified schematic diagram of basal ganglia—thalamo-cortical circuitry. Excitatory connections are indicated by open arrows; inhibitory connections by filled arrows. The modulatory dopamine projection is indicated by a three-headed arrow. *Abbreviations*: DYN, dynorphin; ENK, enkephalin; GABA, γ-amino butyric acid, Glu, glutamate; GPe, globus pallidus pars externa; GPi, globus pallidus pars interna; IL, intralaminar thalamic nuclei; MD, mediodorsal nucleus, PPA, pedunculopontine area; SC, superior colliculus; SNpc, substantia nigra pars compacta; SNpr, substantia nigra pars reticulata; SP, substance P; STN, subthalamic nucleus; VA, ventral anterior nucleus; VL, ventral lateral nucleus.

the basal ganglia (10). Although the topography implies a certain degree of parallel organization, there is also evidence for convergence and divergence in the corticostriatal projection. The large dendritic fields of medium spiny neurons (11) allow them to receive input from adjacent projections, which arise from different areas of cortex. Inputs to striatum from several functionally related cortical areas overlap, and a single cortical area projects divergently to multiple striatal zones (12,13). Thus, there is a multiply convergent and divergent organization within a broader framework of functionally different parallel circuits. This organization provides an anatomical framework for the integration and transformation of cortical information in the striatum.

Medium spiny striatal neurons make up the great majority of the striatal neuron population. They project outside of the striatum and receive a number of inputs in addition to the important cortical enervation; these include (i) excitatory glutamatergic inputs from the thalamus; (ii) cholinergic input from striatal interneurons;

(iii) $\gamma$-amino-butyric acid (GABA), substance P, and enkephalin input from adjacent medium spiny striatal neurons; (iv) GABA input from small, parvalbumin positive, fast-spiking interneurons; (v) a large input from dopamine-containing neurons in the SNpc; (vi) a more sparse input from the serotonin-containing neurons in the dorsal and median raphe nuclei.

In recent years, there has been increasing recognition of the importance of the fast-spiking GABAergic striatal interneurons. These cells make up less than 2% of the striatal neuron population, but they exert powerful inhibition on medium spiny neurons. Like medium spiny neurons, they receive excitatory input from the cerebral cortex. They appear to play an important role in focusing the spatial pattern of medium spiny neuron activation (14).

The dopamine input to the striatum terminates largely on the shafts of the dendritic spines of medium spiny neurons where it is in a position to modulate transmission from the cerebral cortex to the striatum (15). The action of dopamine on striatal neurons depends on the type of dopamine receptor involved. Five types of G protein-coupled dopamine receptors have been described (D1–D5) (16). These have been grouped into two families based on their linkage to adenyl cyclase activity and response to agonists. The D1 family includes D1 and D5 receptors and the D2 family includes D2, D3, and D4 receptors. The conventional view has been that dopamine acts at D1 receptors to facilitate the activity of postsynaptic neurons and at D2 receptors to inhibit postsynaptic neurons (17). Indeed, this is a fundamental concept for currently popular models of basal ganglia pathophysiology (18,19). However, the physiologic effect of dopamine on striatal neurons is more complex. While activation of dopamine D1 receptors potentiates the effect of cortical input to striatal neurons in some states, it reduces the efficacy of cortical input in others (20). Activation of D2 receptors more consistently decreases the effect of cortical input to striatal neurons (21). Dopamine contributes to focusing the spatial and temporal patterns of striatal activity.

In addition to short-term facilitation or inhibition of striatal activity, there is evidence that dopamine can modulate corticostriatal transmission by mechanisms of long-term depression (LTD) and long-term potentiation (LTP). Through these mechanisms, dopamine strengthens or weakens the efficacy of corticostriatal synapses and can thus mediate reinforcement of specific discharge patterns. LTP and LTD are thought to be fundamental to many neural mechanisms of learning and may underlie the hypothesized role of the basal ganglia in habit learning (22). SNpc dopamine neurons fire in relation to behaviorally significant events and reward (23). These signals are likely to modify the responses of striatal neurons to inputs that occur in conjunction with the dopamine signal resulting in the reinforcement of motor and other behavior patterns. Striatal lesions or focal striatal dopamine depletion impairs the learning of new movement sequences (24), supporting a role for the basal ganglia in certain types of procedural learning.

Medium spiny striatal neurons contain the inhibitory neurotransmitter GABA and colocalized peptide neurotransmitters (25). Based on the type of neurotransmitters and the predominant type of dopamine receptor they contain, the medium spiny neurons can be divided into two populations. One population contains GABA, dynorphin, and substance P and primarily expresses D1 dopamine receptors. These neurons project to the basal ganglia output nuclei, GPi, and SNpr. The second population contains GABA and enkephalin and primarily expresses D2 dopamine receptors. These neurons project to the external segment of the globus pallidus (GPe) (18).

Although there are no apparent regional differences in the striatum based on cell type, an intricate internal organization has been revealed with special stains. When the striatum is stained for acetylcholinesterase (AChE), there is a patchy distribution of lightly staining regions within more heavily stained regions (26). The AChE-poor patches have been called "striosomes" and the AChE-rich areas have been called the extrastriosomal matrix. The matrix forms the bulk of the striatal volume and receives input from most areas of cerebral cortex. Within the matrix are clusters of neurons with similar inputs that have been termed "matrisomes." The bulk of the output from cells in the matrix is to both segments of the GP, VP, and to SNpr. The striosomes receive input from prefrontal cortex and send output to SNpc (27). Immunohistochemical techniques have demonstrated that many substances such as substance P, dynorphin, and enkephalin have a patchy distribution that may be partly or wholly in register with the striosomes. The striosome-matrix organization suggests a level of functional segregation within the striatum that may be important in understanding the variety of symptoms in Tourette's syndrome.

### Subthalamic Nucleus

The STN receives an excitatory, glutamatergic input from many areas of frontal lobes with especially large inputs from motor areas of cortex (28). The STN also receives an inhibitory GABA input from GPe. The output from the STN is glutamatergic and excitatory to the basal ganglia output nuclei, GPi, VP, and SNpr. STN also sends an excitatory projection back to GPe. There is a somatopic organization in STN (29) and a relative topographic separation of "motor" and "cognitive" inputs to STN.

## BASAL GANGLIA OUTPUTS

The primary basal ganglia output arises from GPi, a GPi-like component of VP, and SNpr. As described above, GPi and SNpr receive excitatory input from STN and inhibitory input from striatum. They also receive an inhibitory input from GPe. The dendritic fields of GPi, VP, and SNpr neurons span up to 1 mm diameter and thus have the potential to integrate a large number of converging inputs (30). The output from GPi, VP, and SNpr is inhibitory and uses GABA as its neurotransmitter. The primary output is directed to thalamic nuclei that project to the frontal lobes: the ventrolateral, ventroanterior, and mediodorsal nuclei. The thalamic targets of GPi, VP, and SNpr project, in turn, to frontal lobe, with the strongest output going to motor areas. Collaterals of the axons projecting to thalamus project to an area at the junction of the midbrain and pons near the pedunculopontine nucleus (31). Other output neurons (20%) project to intralaminar nuclei of the thalamus, to the lateral habenula, or to the superior colliculus (32).

The basal ganglia motor output has a somatotopic organization such that the body below the neck is largely represented in GPi and the head and eyes are largely represented in SNpr. The separate representation of different body parts is maintained throughout the basal ganglia. Within the representation of an individual body part, it also appears that there is segregation of outputs to different motor areas of cortex and that an individual GPi neuron sends output via thalamus to just one area of cortex (33). Thus, GPi neurons that project via thalamus to motor cortex are adjacent to, but separate from, those that project to premotor cortex or supplementary motor area. GPi neurons that project via thalamus to prefrontal cortex are also separate from those projecting to motor areas and from VP neurons projecting via thalamus to orbitofrontal cortex. The anatomic segregation of basal ganglia-thalamocortical outputs suggests functional segregation at the output level, but other anatomic evidence suggests interactions between circuits within the basal ganglia (see above) (34).

## INTRINSIC BASAL GANGLIA NUCLEI

The GPe, and the GPe-like part of VP may be viewed as intrinsic nuclei of the basal ganglia. Like GPi and SNpr, GPe receives an inhibitory projection from the striatum and an excitatory one from STN. Unlike GPi, the striatal projection to GPe contains GABA and enkephalin but not substance P (18). The output of GPe is quite different from the output of GPi. The output is GABAergic and inhibitory and the majority of the output projects to STN. The connections from striatum to GPe, from GPe to STN, and from STN to GPi form the "indirect" striatopallidal pathway to GPi (Fig. 1) (35). In addition, there is a monosynaptic GABAergic inhibitory output from GPe directly to GPi and to SNpr and a GABAergic projection back to striatum (36). Thus, GPe neurons are in a position to provide feedback inhibition to neurons in striatum and STN and feedforward inhibition to neurons in GPi and SNpr. This circuitry suggests that GPe may act to oppose, limit, or focus the effect of the striatal and STN projections to GPi and SNpr as well as focus activity in these output nuclei.

Dopamine input to the striatum arises from SNpc and the ventral tegmental area (VTA). SNpc projects to most of the striatum; VTA projects to the ventral striatum. The SNpc and VTA are made up of large dopamine-containing cells. SNpc receives input from the striatum, specifically from the striosomes. This input is GABAergic and inhibitory. The SNpc and VTA dopamine neurons project to caudate and putamen in a topographic manner (34), but with overlap. The nigral dopamine neurons receive inputs from one striatal circuit and project back to the same and to adjacent circuits. Thus, they appear to be in a position to modulate activity across functionally different circuits.

## FUNCTIONAL ORGANIZATION

Although the basal ganglia intrinsic circuitry is complex, the overall picture is of two primary pathways through the basal ganglia from cerebral cortex with the output directed via thalamus at the frontal lobes. These pathways consist of two disynaptic pathways from cortex to the basal ganglia output (Fig. 1). In addition, there are several multisynaptic pathways involving GPe. The two disynaptic pathways are from cortex through (i) striatum (the direct pathway) and (ii) STN (the hyperdirect pathway) to the basal ganglia outputs. These pathways have important anatomical and functional differences. First, the cortical input to STN comes only from frontal lobe whereas the input to striatum arises from virtually all areas of cerebral cortex. Second, the output from STN is excitatory, whereas the output from striatum is inhibitory. Third, the excitatory route through STN is faster than the inhibitory route through striatum (37). Finally, the STN projection to GPi is divergent and the striatal projection is more focused (38). Thus, the two disynaptic pathways from cerebral cortex to the basal ganglia output nuclei, GPi and SNpr, provide fast,

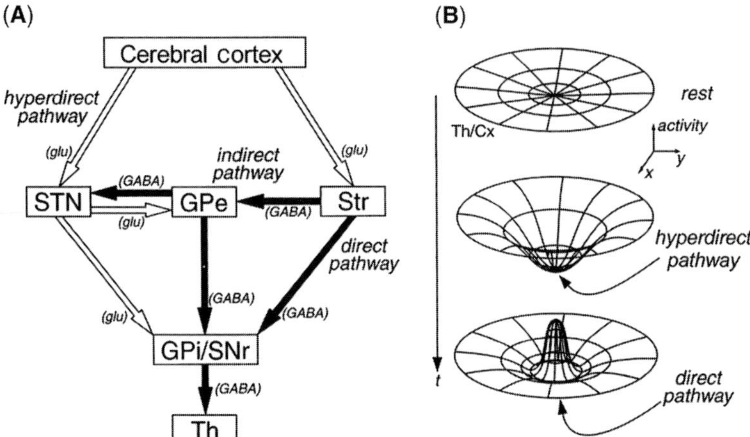


**Figure 2** (**A**) A schematic diagram of the hyperdirect cortico-subthalamo-pallidal, direct cortico-striato-pallidal, and indirect cortico-striato-GPe-subthalamo-GPi pathways. White and black arrows represent excitatory glutamatergic and inhibitory GABAergic projections, respectively. (**B**) A schematic diagram explaining the activity change over time (t) in the Th/Cx projection following the sequential inputs through the hyperdirect cortico-subthalamo-pallidal (*middle*) and direct cortico-striato-pallidal (*bottom*) pathways. *Abbreviations*: GPe, globus pallidus pars externa; GPi, globus pallidus pars interna; SNr, substantia nigra pars reticulata; STN, subthalamic nucleus; Str, striatum; Th, thalamus; glu, glutamatergic; GABA, γ-amino butyric acid; Th/Cx, thalamocortical. *Source*: From Ref. 37.

widespread, divergent excitation through STN and slower, focused, inhibition through striatum. This organization provides an anatomical basis for focused inhibition and surround excitation of neurons in GPi and SNpr (Fig. 2). Because the output of GPi and SNpr is inhibitory, this would result in focused facilitation and surround inhibition of basal ganglia thalamocortical targets.

## FOCUSED FACILITATION AND SURROUND INHIBITION OF COMPETING MOTOR PATTERNS

A functional representation of normal basal ganglia motor function based on anatomical, physiological, and lesion studies has been postulated (28,39). In this scheme, the tonically active inhibitory output of the basal ganglia acts as a "brake" on motor pattern generators (MPGs) in the cerebral cortex (via the thalamus) and brainstem. When a movement is initiated by a particular MPG, basal ganglia output neurons projecting to competing MPGs increase their firing rate, thereby increasing inhibition and applying a "brake" on those generators. Other basal ganglia output neurons projecting to the generators involved in the desired movement decrease their discharge, thereby removing tonic inhibition and releasing the brake from the desired motor patterns. Thus, the intended movement is enabled and competing movements are prevented from interfering with the desired one.

The anatomical arrangement of STN and striatal inputs to GPi and SNpr form the basis for a functional center-surround organization as shown in Figure 3. When a voluntary movement is initiated by cortical mechanisms, a separate signal is sent to STN, exciting it. STN projects in a widespread pattern and excites GPi.

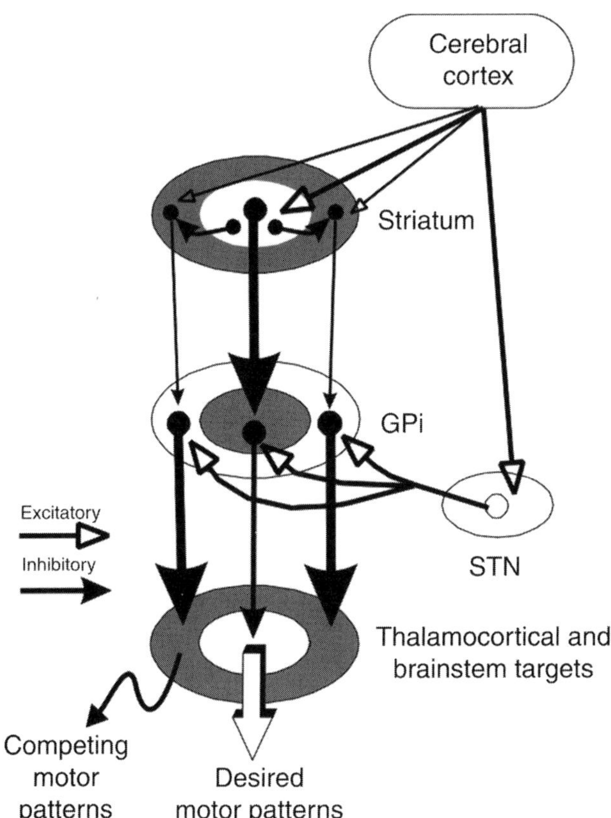


**Figure 3** Schematic of normal functional organization of the basal ganglia output. Excitatory projections are indicated with open arrows; inhibitory projections are indicated with filled arrows. Relative magnitude of activity is represented by line thickness. *Abbreviations:* STN, subthalamic nucleus; GPi, globus pallidus pars interna. *Source:* From Ref. 40.

The increased GPi activity causes inhibition of thalamocortical motor mechanisms. In parallel to the pathway through STN, signals are sent from all areas of cerebral cortex to striatum. The cortical inputs are transformed by the striatal integrative circuitry to a focused, context-dependent output that inhibits specific neurons in GPi. The inhibitory striatal input to GPi is slower, but more powerful, than the excitatory STN input. The resulting focally decreased activity in GPi selectively disinhibits the desired thalamocortical MPGs. Indirect pathways from striatum to GPi (striatum→GPe→GPi and striatum→GPe→STN→GPi) (Fig. 1) result in further focusing of the output. The net result of basal ganglia activity during a voluntary movement is the inhibition ("braking") of competing motor patterns and focused facilitation (releasing the "brake") from the selected voluntary movement pattern generators.

This scheme provides a framework for understanding both the pathophysiology of parkinsonism (28,41) and involuntary movements (28,39). Different involuntary movements such as parkinsonism, chorea, dystonia, or tics result from different abnormalities in the basal ganglia circuits. Loss of dopamine input to the striatum results in a loss of normal pauses of GPi discharge during voluntary movement. Hence, there is excessive inhibition of MPGs and ultimately bradykinesia (41). Furthermore, loss of dopamine results in abnormal synchrony of GPi neuronal discharge and loss of the normal spatial and temporal focus of GPi activity (41–43). Broad lesions of GPi or SNpr disinhibit both desired and unwanted motor patterns leading to inappropriate activation of competing motor patterns, but normal generation of the wanted movement. Thus, lesions of GPi cause dystonia with cocontraction of multiple muscle groups and difficulty turning off unwanted motor patterns, but do not affect movement initiation (44). Lesions of SNpr cause unwanted saccadic eye movements that interfere with the ability to maintain visual fixation, but do not impair the initiation of voluntary saccades (45). Lesions of putamen may cause dystonia due to the loss of focused inhibition in GPi (39). Lesions of STN produce continuous involuntary movements of the contralateral limbs (hemiballism or hemichorea) (39). Despite the involuntary movements, voluntary movements can still be performed. Although structural lesions of putamen, GPi, SNpr, or STN produce certain types of unwanted movements or behaviors, they do not produce tics. Tics are more likely to arise from abnormal activity patterns, most likely in the striatum (39).

## RELATIONSHIP OF BASAL GANGLIA ORGANIZATION TO DYSTONIA

Relatively little is known about basal ganglia neuronal activity in dystonia, but knowledge is increasing with the growing use of neurosurgical treatment for dystonia. There appears to be reduced tonic firing of GPi neurons accompanied by abnormal temporal discharge patterns in some individuals with dystonia (4), but there may be a confounding effect of anesthesia (46). The size of somatosensory receptive fields in GPi neurons is increased in patients with dystonia. These data have been used to support the idea that dystonia is associated with increased activity in the "direct" pathway from striatum to GPi, leading to excessive inhibition of GPi and excessive disinhibition of motor cortical areas. This would be reflected as enhanced facilitation and possibly expansion of the "center" of the present center–surround model (Fig. 3). An alternative scheme, based on reduced dopamine D2 receptor binding in striatum in dystonic monkeys and in people with dystonia, is that abnormal activity in the "indirect" pathway influencing activity in the STN–GPi projection is the basis for decreased GPi discharge in dystonia (47). In the present model, this would be seen as reduced activity in the inhibitory "surround" (Fig. 4).

The fact that pallidotomy and deep brain stimulation of GPi are effective treatments for dystonia creates some problems for the hypothesis that decreased GPi discharge alone is the fundamental basis for dystonia (4). To account for this, it has been proposed that an abnormal temporal pattern of the GPi output could be the basis for dystonia. However, abnormal temporal (bursting) patterns have been described in Parkinson's disease, chorea/hemiballism, and dystonia (4,48), and it is not clear whether there are critical differences in those patterns that explain the unique characteristics of the different movement disorders. It is possible that dystonia results from incomplete suppression of competing motor patterns due to insufficient surround inhibition of competing MPGs (Fig. 4) (47). This deficient surround inhibition may also lead to expansion of the facilitatory center, which would lead to "overflow" contraction of adjacent muscles. Decreased efficacy of the surround with or without expansion of the center causes inappropriate disinhibition of unwanted muscle activity.

The scheme presented here differs in emphasis from the now classic model of basal ganglia circuitry that emphasizes opposing direct and indirect pathways from striatum to GPi/SNpr (18,19). These models have contributed substantially to

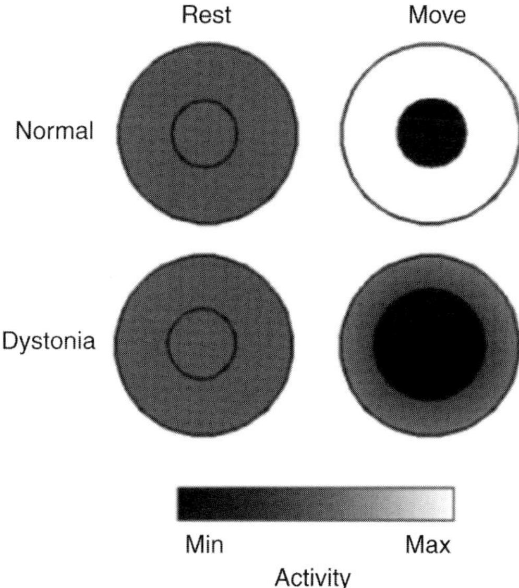


**Figure 4** Schematic representation of hypothetical changes in globus pallidus pars interna activity associated with parkinsonism and dystonia. In dystonia, there is little change at rest, but volitional movement is associated with a broadening of the facilitatory center and reduced activity of the inhibitory surround. Conventions as described for Figure 3.

advances in basal ganglia research over the past 15 years. If the success of a model is measured by the amount of research it stimulates, these schemes have been extraordinarily successful. In simple terms, these models proposed that hypokinetic movement disorders (e.g., parkinsonism) are distinguished from hyperkinetic movement disorders (e.g., chorea, dystonia, tics) based on the magnitude of basal ganglia output. Both clinical and basic research findings have required revision of the classic model (4,28,39,46,49). New emphasis on (i) the importance of timing cortical input to the STN and the timing of STN input to GPi/SNpr (28,37), (ii) the temporal-spatial organization of activity patterns in the different basal ganglia nuclei (28,39), and (iii) the importance of spike train patterns (4,42) reflect our improved understanding of basal ganglia function and dysfunction.

## SUMMARY

Basal ganglia circuitry is rich with complexity, but some simple organizational principles can aid understanding of normal and abnormal function. The hypothesis of selective facilitation and surround inhibition by the basal ganglia is perhaps most relevant for understanding brain mechanisms of dystonia (50). Increased understanding of these mechanisms and of the effect of disordered patterns of neuron discharge in basal ganglia circuits has the potential to increase the efficacy of current treatments and may point the direction to new brain-based interventions.

## ACKNOWLEDGMENTS

Supported by NIH R01NS39821 and R21NS40086.

## REFERENCES


1. Marsden CD, Obeso JA, Zarranz JJ, et al. The anatomical basis of symptomatic hemidystonia. Brain 1985; 108:463–483.
2. Feiwell RJ, Black KJ, McGee-Minnich LA, et al. Diminished regional cerebral blood flow response to vibration in patients with blepharospasm. Neurology 1999; 52:291–297.
3. Perlmutter JS, Stambuk MK, Markham J, et al. Decreased [18F]spiperone binding in putamen in idiopathic focal dystonia. J Neurosci 1997; 17(2):843–850.
4. Vitek JL. Pathophysiology of dystonia: a neuronal model. Mov Disord 2002; 17:S49–S62.
5. Hallett M. The neurophysiology of dystonia. Arch Neurol 1998; 55(5):601–603.
6. Berardelli A, Rothwell JC, Hallett M, et al. The pathophysiology of primary dystonia. Brain 1998; 121:1195–1212.
7. Kemp JM, Powell TPS. The corticostriate projection in the monkey. Brain 1970; 93:525–546.
8. Fudge J, Kunishio K, Walsh C, et al. Amygdaloid projections to ventromedial striatal subterritories in the primate. Neuroscience 2002; 110:257–275.
9. Cherubini E, Herrling PL, Lanfumey L, et al. Excitatory amino acids in synaptic excitation of rat striatal neurones in vitro. J Physiol 1988; 400:677–690.
10. Alexander GE, DeLong MR, Strick PL. Parallel organization of functionally segregated circuits linking basal ganglia and cortex. Annu Rev Neurosci 1986; 9:357–381.
11. Wilson CJ, Groves PM. Fine structure and synaptic connections of the common spiny neuron of the rat neostriatum: a study employing intracellular injection of horseradish peroxidase. J Comp Neurol 1980; 194:599–614.
12. Selemon LD, Goldman-Rakic PS. Longitudinal topography and interdigitation of corticostriatal projections in the rhesus monkey. J Neurosci 1985; 5:776–794.
13. Flaherty AW, Graybiel AM. Corticostriatal transformations in the primate somatosensory system. Projections from phsyiologically mapped body-part representations. J Neurophysiol 1991; 66(4):1249–1263.
14. Mallet N, Le Moine C, Charpier S, et al. Feedforward inhibition of projection neurons by fast-spiking gaba interneurons in the rat striatum in vivo. J Neurosci 2005; 25(15): 3857–3869.
15. Bouyer JJ, Park DH, Joh TH, et al. Chemical and structural analysis of the relation between cortical inputs and tyrosine hydroxylase-containing terminals in rat neostriatum. Brain Res 1984; 302:267–275.
16. Sibley DR, Monsma FJ. Molecular biology of dopamine receptors. Trends Pharmacol Sci 1992; 13:61–69.
17. Gerfen CR, Engber TM, Mahan LC, et al. $D_1$ and $D_2$ dopamine receptor-regulated gene expression of striatonigral and striatopallidal neurons. Science 1990; 250:1429–1432.
18. Albin RL, Young AB, Penney JB. The functional anatomy of basal ganglia disorders. Trends Neurosci 1989; 12:366–375.
19. DeLong MR. Primate models of movement disorders of basal ganglia origin. Trends Neurosci 1990; 13:281–285.
20. Hernandez-Lopez S, Bargas J, Surmeier DJ, et al. D1 receptor activation enhances evoked discharge in neostriatal medium spiny neurons by modulating an L-type Ca2+ conductance. J Neurosci 1997; 17(9):3334–3342.
21. Nicola S, Surmeier J, Malenka R. Dopaminergic modulation of neuronal excitability in the striatum and nucleus accumbens. Annu Rev Neurosci 2000; 23:185–215.
22. Jog M, Kubota Y, Connolly C, et al. Building neural representations of habits. Science 1999; 286:1745–1749.
23. Schultz W, Romo R, Ljungberg T, et al. Reward-related signals carried by dopamine neurons. In: Houk JC, Davis JL, Beiser DG, eds. Models of Information Processing in the Basal Ganglia. Cambridge: MIT Press, 1995:233–249.
24. Matsumoto N, Hanakawa T, Maki S, et al. Role of nigrostriatal dopamine system in learning to perform sequential motor tasks in a predictive manner. J Neurophysiol 1999; 82:978–998.

25. Penny GR, Afsharpour S, Kitai ST. The glutamate decarboxylase-, leucine enkephalin-, methionine enkephalin- and substance P-immunoreactive neurons in the neostriatum of the rat and cat: evidence for partial population overlap. Neuroscience 1986; 17:1011–1045.
26. Graybiel AM, Aosaki T, Flaherty AW, et al. The basal ganglia and adaptive motor control. Science 1994; 265:1826–1831.
27. Gerfen CR. The neostriatal mosaic: multiple levels of compartmental organization in the basal ganglia. Annu Rev Neurosci 1992; 15:285–320.
28. Mink JW. The basal ganglia: focused selection and inhibition of competing motor programs. Prog Neurobiol 1996; 50:381–425.
29. Nambu A, Takada M, Inase M, et al. Dual somatotopical representations in the primate subthalamic nucleus: evidence for ordered but reversed body-map transformations from the primary motor cortex and the supplementary motor area. J Neurosci 1996; 16(8):2671–2683.
30. Percheron G, Yelnik J, Francois C. A Golgi analysis of the primate globus pallidus. III. Spatial organization of the striato-pallidal complex. J Comp Neurol 1984; 227:214–227.
31. Parent A. Extrinsic connections of the basal ganglia. Trends Neurosci 1990; 13(7): 254–258.
32. Francois C, Percheron G, Yelnik J, et al. A topographic study of the course of nigral axons and of the distribution of pallidal axonal endings in the centre median-parafascicular complex of macaques. Brain Res 1988; 473:181–186.
33. Hoover JE, Strick PL. Multiple output channels in the basal ganglia. Science 1993; 259:819–821.
34. Haber SN, Fudge JL, McFarland NR. Striatonigrostriatal pathways in primates form an ascending spiral from the shell to the dorsolateral striatum. J Neurosci 2000; 20: 2369–2382.
35. Alexander GE, Crutcher MD. Functional architecture of basal ganglia circuits: neural substrates of parallel processing. Trends Neurosci 1990; 13(7):266–271.
36. Bolam JP, Hanley JJ, Booth PA, et al. Synaptic organisation of the basal ganglia. J Anat 2000; 196:527–542.
37. Nambu A, Tokuno H, Hamada I, et al. Excitatory cortical inputs to pallidal neurons via the subthalamic nucleus in the monkey. J Neurophysiol 2000; 84:289–300.
38. Parent A, Hazrati LN. Anatomical aspects of information processing in primate basal ganglia. Trends Neurosci 1993; 16(3):111–116.
39. Mink J. The basal ganglia and involuntary movements: impaired inhibition of competing motor patterns. Arch Neurol 2003; 60:1365–1368.
40. Mink JW. Basal ganglia dysfunction in Tourette's syndrome: a new hypothesis. Pediatr Neurol 2001; 25:190–198.
41. Boraud T, Bezard E, Bioulac B, et al. From single extracellular unit recording in experimental and human parkinsonism to the development of a functional concept of the role played by the basal ganglia in motor control. Prog Neurobiol 2002; 66:265–283.
42. Raz A, Vaadia E, Bergman H. Firing patterns and correlations of spontaneous discharge of pallidal neurons in the normal and the tremulous 1-methyl-4-phenyl-1,2,3,6-tetrahydropyridine vervet model of parkinsonism. J Neurosci 2000; 20:8559–8571.
43. Tremblay L, Filion M, Bedard PJ. Responses of pallidal neurons to striatal stimulation in monkeys with MPTP-induce parkinsonism. Brain Res 1989; 498:17–33.
44. Mink JW, Thach WT. Basal ganglia motor control. III. Pallidal ablation: normal reaction time, muscle cocontraction, and slow movement. J Neurophysiol 1991; 65:330–351.
45. Hikosaka O, Wurtz RH. Modification of saccadic eye movements by GABA-related substances. II. Effects of muscimol in monkey substantia nigra pars reticulata. J Neurophysiol 1985; 53(1):292–308.
46. Hutchison WD, Lang AE, Dostrovsky JO, et al. Pallidal neuronal activity: implications for models of dystonia. Ann Neurol 2003; 53:480–488.
47. Perlmutter JS, Tempel LW, Black KJ, et al. MPTP induces dystonia and parkinsonism. Clues to the pathophysiology of dystonia. Neurology 1997; 49:1432–1438.

48. Wichmann T, DeLong MR. Functional and pathophysiological models of the basal ganglia. Curr Opin Neurobiol 1996; 6:751–758.
49. Hutchison WD, Dostrovsky JO, Walters JR, et al. Neuronal oscillations in the basal ganglia and movement disorders: evidence from whole animal and human recordings. J Neurosci 2004; 24:9240–9243.
50. Hallett M. Dystonia: abnormal movements result from loss of inhibition. Adv Neurol 2004; 94:1–9.

# 5
# Physiology of Primary Dystonia

**Holly A. Shill**
*Movement Disorder Section, Barrow Neurological Institute, Phoenix, Arizona, U.S.A.*

**Mark Hallett**
*Human Motor Control Section, National Institute of Neurological Disorders and Stroke, National Institutes of Health, Bethesda, Maryland, U.S.A.*

## INTRODUCTION

This chapter will review the pathophysiology of primary dystonia. Primary generalized dystonia of children may differ from the focal dystonias of adults, and it is important to keep in mind that most physiology has been done with focal dystonia. Anatomical pathology is usually described as normal, but in fact there is very little information. Recently, signs of neural degeneration have been found in the brainstem in patients with primary generalized dystonia (1). Anatomical speculation largely comes from secondary dystonia, and many abnormalities have been found in these pathways. We will focus mainly on neurophysiological investigation with electromyography (EMG), electroencephalography (EEG), and transcranial magnetic stimulation (TMS). Another chapter will cover neuroimaging findings of dystonia.

It is likely that, similar to most disorders, dystonia is a resultant of a genetic background and an environmental influence. Three lines of physiological abnormalities have been found in dystonia, and they might represent the physiological consequence of the genetic disorder.

## LOSS OF INHIBITION

Clinically, dystonia is characterized by sustained, tonic contractions, abnormal postures and, less commonly, superimposed tremor and myoclonic jerking. The basic physiological mechanism behind these movements can be attributed to a loss of inhibition at many levels of the neuraxis. This loss of inhibition can be most easily evaluated physiologically with electromyography. The characteristic finding is that of unwanted, sustained contractions in the agonist muscle, overflow of activity into unwanted muscles, and antagonist cocontraction, all of which contribute to the abnormal posture. EMG bursts in dystonia often last seconds. Even when myoclonic contractions are present, these seem to be prolonged, lasting 100 to 300 msec (which helps to differentiate them from myoclonus of cortical origin). A detailed EMG study performed in patients with hand cramps of various types found cocontracting agonist and antagonist bursts with unusually prolonged activity in the muscles studied (2). The EMG findings are thought to reflect loss of inhibition necessary for suppressing unwanted muscle activity, as well as turning off muscle activity when appropriate. This supposition is supported by findings with reflex studies and with TMS.

Reciprocal inhibition is the physiological process of inhibition of the antagonist muscle during agonist action. One aspect of reciprocal inhibition is a spinal suppression of antagonist muscles mediated through the agonist Ia afferent. This reflex is abnormal in patients with dystonia (3,4) and may be partly responsible for the abnormal cocontraction of the antagonist muscle. In patients with blepharospasm, the blink reflex recovery curve (the blink response to paired stimuli with progressively increasing interstimulus intervals) has been studied and is abnormal (5,6). These types of reflex studies support loss of inhibition at the spinal and brainstem levels, respectively.

TMS is a physiological tool used to assess integrity of central motor pathways. With direct stimulation of the motor cortex, a motor-evoked potential (MEP) is generated in the target muscle (most commonly the hand muscles are used since the cortical hand area is easily accessed noninvasively over the scalp). Combined with a test pulse to produce an MEP, a second, conditioning, pulse can be given just before at either subthreshold (not sufficient to generate an MEP) or suprathreshold levels. At short interstimulus intervals (less than 5 msec), there is inhibition of the MEP with a subthreshold conditioning pulse; this is called short intracortical inhibition (SICI). At interstimulus intervals (ISIs) between 8 and 30 msec, there is facilitation of the MEP. A suprathreshold prepulse with an ISI longer than 50 msec produces inhibition again, called long intracortical inhibition (LICI). Additionally, when a single pulse is given during ongoing EMG activity, there is inhibition called the silent period (SP). The first part of the SP is likely Renshaw-cell–mediated inhibition at the spinal level. However, the latter part of the SP is cortical. SICI is largely mediated by GABA-A (7). LICI and SP are both likely mediated by GABA-B (8,9).

SICI is reduced in patients with dystonia (Fig. 1) (10). This being seen in both motor cortices in patients with unilateral writer's cramp suggests that it is a primary defect in dystonia. LICI and the SP are abnormal only on the affected side in writer's cramp (11,12). Taken together, this suggests that the SICI abnormality may be primary, perhaps resulting from genetic malfunction, and that the LICI and SP abnormality may develop with symptomatic expression.

Surround inhibition is a concept that has been recently investigated in dystonia. Sensory surround inhibition is well understood and accepted (13). Its role in the motor system is less well understood; however, basal ganglia are thought to have a primary role in the selection of motor programs from among a set of differing motor programs (14). A motor command is given by the cortex, and this is further refined by the basal ganglia in response to the spatial constraints of the task. Given that dystonia is characterized by overflow of muscle activity, it is logical that a failure of basal ganglia surround inhibition may be at play. Surround inhibition in the motor system has been demonstrated clinically using TMS. Significant surround inhibition has been shown in muscles of the contralateral limb during finger movement (15) and in the ipsilateral limb for a muscle not involved in the task (16). With these techniques, defective surround inhibition has been demonstrated in focal hand dystonia (17,18).

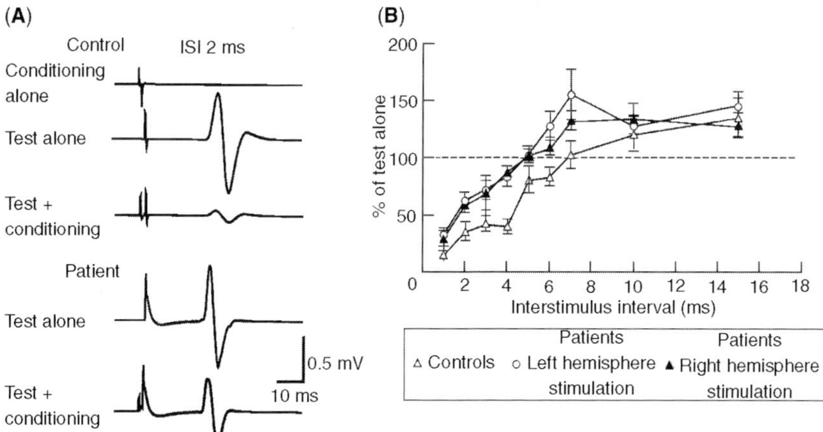


**Figure 1** Corticocortical inhibition in healthy controls and patients with focal hand dystonia. (**A**) Raw data from an individual control subject (*top 3 traces*) and a patient with writer's cramp (*bottom 2 traces*). These data were obtained after L-hemispheric stimulation, with responses recorded in the relaxed right first dorsal interosseous muscle. In the control subject, there is clear suppression of the response when a conditioning pulse is given 2 msec before the test response, whereas in the patient, there is less suppression. (**B**) Data obtained across all interstimulus intervals in both patient and controls (stimulation of both right and left hemisphere). *Source*: From Ref. 10.

Globus pallidus interna lesioning or stimulation leads to significant improvements in patients with primary dystonia (19). Recordings of the globus pallidus interna (Gpi) neurons during pallidal surgery for dystonia have led to some confusion. Reduction in the tonic neuronal firing is often found, although changes are also seen in the temporal pattern (with more irregularity seen in the discharges) (20). This is hard to reconcile with the fact that lesioning reduces the degree of dystonia. This suggests that the firing pattern itself may be more important that the background discharge rate. Further evidence for the center surround theory should also be found in direct recording in humans with dystonia.

## SENSORY CHANGES

Involvement of the sensory system in dystonia has been suspected for years given the frequent presence of the sensory trick in patients with cervical dystonia in particular. Basic sensory modalities have generally been thought to be normal in patients with dystonia. However, more careful evaluations have shown loss of spatial and temporal discrimination in the hands of patients with focal hand dystonia (21,22). Mapping of the cortical sensory representation of the hand in dystonia shows disruption of the orderly arrangement of the homunculus (Fig. 2) (23), and is present in both hands in patients with unilateral writer's cramp (24). Brain mapping of the globus pallidus and thalamus during surgery for dystonia support enlargement of the sensory receptive fields in these areas (20). Sensory spatial discrimination has been used to identify subclinical abnormality in relatives of patients with focal dystonia (25).

The effect of a sensory stimulus on motor performance (sensorimotor integration) has also been studied and is abnormal in dystonia. This can be studied by

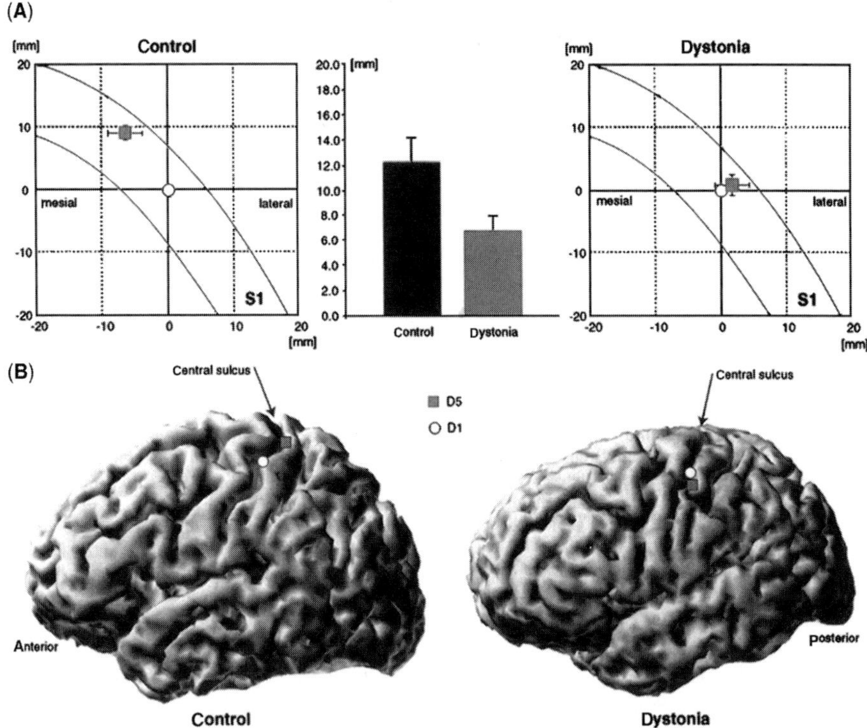


**Figure 2** Schematic of the left paracentral gyrus (somatosensory cortex) for six controls (*left*) and six patients with hand dystonia (*right*) showing the localization for the primary cortical somatosensory evoked potential (N20) in the coronal plane for digits 1 (D1) and 5 (D5). The bar graph in the middle displays the distance in mm between D1 and D5 in the coronal plane. This distance is reduced in patients with focal hand dystonia. The 3-D reconstruction of the brain shows the localization in the cortex of the N20 for D1 and D5 for controls (*left*) and patients (*right*). The normal cortical homuncular arrangement of fingers is degraded in patients with dystonia. *Source*: From Ref. 23.

using the somatosensory-evoked potential (SSEP) in a paradigm called sensorimotor gating, where a stimulus to the median nerve is given before and during movement, and the cortical SSEP is evaluated. In patients with dystonia, the premovement gating of the SSEP before voluntary movement is abnormal compared with controls, supporting abnormal sensorimotor integration (26). Additionally, a sensory stimulus about 100 to 200 msec prior to a TMS pulse usually produces inhibition of the MEP; however, in dystonia, this same stimulus produces facilitation (27). Vibration of the hand can trigger dystonic hand movements in patient with writer's cramp and this can be blocked by local weak lidocaine that should influence just the gamma motoneurons (28), suggesting a primary abnormality in processing of spindle sensory afferents. Finally, lack of sensory surround inhibition has been demonstrated using a combination of median and ulnar SSEPs. In patients with dystonia, the combination potential of the double simultaneous stimulation was higher that that for controls, despite normal responses to the individual stimuli, supporting lack of surround inhibition (29).

Taken together, the abnormalities found in the sensory system support abnormalities in sensory processing and lack of sensory inhibition. Relating this to the motor system changes supports a widespread deficit in inhibitory processes, more specifically in surround inhibition, of both the motor and sensory systems. Clinically, the sensory trick may work by "focusing" the sensory response in order to appropriately inhibit the surrounding, unwanted motor programs.

## PLASTICITY

The third aspect of dystonia that appears important is abnormal plasticity of the nervous system. Clinically, patients with focal dystonia do not develop the abnormal movement until adulthood and often, in response to some type of repetitive use or injury to the effected body part. Writer's cramp is often seen in accountants; a musician's dystonia is specific to the body part used. Even the "yips" of golfing may be a task-specific dystonia (30). These clinical observations suggest that it takes some maladaptive response of the central nervous system to develop dystonia, and this suggests that deranged plasticity might be responsible.

There is growing support for abnormal plasticity. One animal model that mimics dystonia is created by training monkeys to repetitively hold a manipulandum for long periods of time (31). They eventually develop a motor control disorder reminiscent of dystonia and show somatosensory cortex abnormalities that may be similar to those seen with human dystonia. A model of long-term potentiation using TMS demonstrates that patients with dystonia have an abnormal physiological response to ongoing associative sensory stimulation with increasing corticospinal excitability and reduced intracortical inhibition compared to controls (32). Another study shows that the homeostatic function of plasticity may be lost in patients with dystonia (33). These studies would indicate that some of the changes seen in chronic dystonia may occur as secondary changes. On the other hand, loss of inhibition will lead to increased plasticity; so the inhibitory dysfunction may be primary.

## CONCLUSIONS

In summary, primary dystonia is accompanied by many changes at all levels of the neuroaxis with a recurring theme of dysfunction and lack of inhibition of the motor and sensory pathways. How this relates to the abnormal plasticity is not well understood. Teasing out what comes first is certainly challenging, and this will help decipher what the genetic abnormality produces. Uncovering these relationships will not only lead to a better understanding of the primary mechanisms behind focal and generalized primary dystonia, but also will give suggestions about possible rehabilitation strategies.

## REFERENCES


1. McNaught KS, Kapustin A, Jackson T, et al. Brainstem pathology in DYT1 primary torsion dystonia. Ann Neurol 2004; 56(4):540–547.
2. Cohen LG, Hallett M. Hand cramps: clinical features and electromyographic patterns in a focal dystonia. Neurology 1988; 38(7):1005–1012.
3. Nakashima K, Rothwell JC, Day BL, et al. Reciprocal inhibition between forearm muscles in patients with writer's cramp and other occupational cramps, symptomatic hemidystonia and hemiparesis due to stroke. Brain 1989; 112(Pt 3):681–697.

4. Panizza M, Lelli S, Nilsson J, et al. H-reflex recovery curve and reciprocal inhibition of H-reflex in different kinds of dystonia. Neurology 1990; 40(5):824–828.
5. Berardelli A, Rothwell JC, Day BL, et al. Pathophysiology of blepharospasm and oromandibular dystonia. Brain 1985; 108(Pt 3):593–608.
6. Eekhof JL, Aramideh M, Bour LJ, et al. Blink reflex recovery curves in blepharospasm, torticollis spasmodica, and hemifacial spasm. Muscle Nerve 1996; 19(1):10–15.
7. Di Lazzaro V, Oliviero A, Meglio M, et al. Direct demonstration of the effect of lorazepam on the excitability of the human motor cortex. Clin Neurophysiol 2000; 111(5): 794–799.
8. Werhahn KJ, Kunesch E, Noachtar S, et al. Differential effects on motorcortical inhibition induced by blockade of GABA uptake in humans. J Physiol 1999; 517(Pt 2): 591–597.
9. Siebner HR, Dressnandt J, Auer C, et al. Continuous intrathecal baclofen infusions induced a marked increase of the transcranially evoked silent period in a patient with generalized dystonia. Muscle Nerve 1998; 21(9):1209–1212.
10. Ridding MC, Sheean G, Rothwell JC, et al. Changes in the balance between motor cortical excitation and inhibition in focal, task specific dystonia. J Neurol Neurosurg Psychiatry 1995; 59(5):493–498.
11. Chen R, Wassermann EM, Canos M, et al. Impaired inhibition in writer's cramp during voluntary muscle activation. Neurology 1997; 49(4):1054–1059.
12. Filipovic SR, Ljubisavljevic M, Svetel M, et al. Impairment of cortical inhibition in writer's cramp as revealed by changes in electromyographic silent period after transcranial magnetic stimulation. Neurosci Lett 1997; 222(3):167–170.
13. Angelucci A, Levitt JB, Lund JS. Anatomical origins of the classical receptive field and modulatory surround field of single neurons in macaque visual cortical area V1. Prog Brain Res 2002; 136:373–388.
14. Mink JW. The basal ganglia: focused selection and inhibition of competing motor programs. Prog Neurobiol 1996; 50(4):381–425.
15. Sohn YH, Jung HY, Kaelin-Lang A, et al. Excitability of the ipsilateral motor cortex during phasic voluntary hand movement. Exp Brain Res 2003; 148(2):176–185.
16. Sohn YH, Hallett M. Surround inhibition in human motor system. Exp Brain Res 2004; 158(4):397–404.
17. Sohn YH, Hallett M. Disturbed surround inhibition in focal hand dystonia. Ann Neurol 2004; 56(4):595–599.
18. Stinear CM, Byblow WD. Impaired modulation of intracortical inhibition in focal hand dystonia. Cereb Cortex 2004; 14(5):555–561.
19. Vidailhet M, Vercueil L, Houeto JL, et al. Bilateral deep-brain stimulation of the globus pallidus in primary generalized dystonia. N Engl J Med 2005; 352(5):459–467.
20. Vitek JL, Chockkan V, Zhang JY, et al. Neuronal activity in the basal ganglia in patients with generalized dystonia and hemiballismus. Ann Neurol 1999; 46(1):22–35.
21. Molloy FM, Carr TD, Zeuner KE, et al. Abnormalities of spatial discrimination in focal and generalized dystonia. Brain 2003; 126(Pt 10):2175–2182.
22. Bara-Jimenez W, Shelton P, Sanger TD, et al. Sensory discrimination capabilities in patients with focal hand dystonia. Ann Neurol 2000; 47(3):377–380.
23. Bara-Jimenez W, Catalan MJ, Hallett M, et al. Abnormal somatosensory homunculus in dystonia of the hand. Ann Neurol 1998; 44(5):828–831.
24. Meunier S, Garnero L, Ducorps A, et al. Human brain mapping in dystonia reveals both endophenotypic traits and adaptive reorganization. Ann Neurol 2001; 50(4):521–527.
25. O'Dwyer JP, O'Riordan S, Saunders-Pullman R, et al. Sensory abnormalities in unaffected relatives in familial adult-onset dystonia. Neurology 2005; 65(6):938–940.
26. Murase N, Kaji R, Shimazu H, et al. Abnormal premovement gating of somatosensory input in writer's cramp. Brain 2000; 123(Pt 9):1813–1829.
27. Abbruzzese G, Marchese R, Buccolieri A, et al. Abnormalities of sensorimotor integration in focal dystonia: a transcranial magnetic stimulation study. Brain 2001; 124(Pt 3):537–545.

28. Kaji R, Rothwell JC, Katayama M, et al. Tonic vibration reflex and muscle afferent block in writer's cramp. Ann Neurol 1995; 38(2):155–162.
29. Tinazzi M, Priori A, Bertolasi L, et al. Abnormal central integration of a dual somatosensory input in dystonia. Evidence for sensory overflow. Brain 2000; 123(Pt 1):42–50.
30. Adler CH, Crews D, Hentz JG, et al. Abnormal co-contraction in yips-affected but not unaffected golfers: evidence for focal dystonia. Neurology 2005; 64(10):1813–1814.
31. Byl NN, Merzenich MM, Jenkins WM. A primate genesis model of focal dystonia and repetitive strain injury: I. Learning-induced dedifferentiation of the representation of the hand in the primary somatosensory cortex in adult monkeys. Neurology 1996; 47(2):508–520.
32. Quartarone A, Bagnato S, Rizzo V, et al. Abnormal associative plasticity of the human motor cortex in writer's cramp. Brain 2003; 126(Pt 12):2586–2596.
33. Quartarone A, Rizzo V, Bagnato S, et al. Homeostatic-like plasticity of the primary motor hand area is impaired in focal hand dystonia. Brain 2005; 128(Pt 8):1943–1950.

# 6
# Pathology of the Dystonias

**Ruth H. Walker**
*Department of Neurology, James J. Peters Veterans Affairs Medical Center, Bronx, and Mount Sinai School of Medicine, New York, New York, U.S.A.*

**Kevin StP. McNaught**
*Department of Neurology, Mount Sinai School of Medicine, New York, New York, U.S.A.*

**Daniel P. Perl**
*Department of Pathology, Mount Sinai School of Medicine, New York, New York, U.S.A.*

## INTRODUCTION

Relatively little is known about the neuropathology of the primary dystonias because of the very limited availability of post mortem tissue (Table 1). Additional factors are that only a small number of genes responsible for these disorders have been identified, and many of the primary dystonias and dystonia-plus syndromes such as DYT4, DYT6, DYT7, DYT13, and DYT15 have been identified by linkage only, and in some cases, not even that. In general, neuroimaging studies indicate that any structural changes are minor, and that the pathophysiology of dystonia is more likely related to functional changes rather than specific neurodegeneration.

A number of reports of neuropathology of single cases and small series are available from the premolecular era, but in the absence of genetic identification, it is challenging to interpret these observations. Accordingly, we limit this review to conditions in which the genetic identity is known. The paroxysmal dyskinesias (DYT8, DYT9, and DYT10) are not discussed here.

The secondary dystonias represent a large and diverse group of disease entities in which dystonia may be seen as an accompanying clinical feature. In some examples, dystonia represents a relatively constant feature while in others it is seen in only some cases with the disorder. With many of these conditions, the distribution of the pathologic changes is widespread, which makes it difficult to determine what specific areas of involvement have led to the dystonic symptomatology. Here, we will discuss those disease entities where dystonia is seen with reasonable regularity and for which consistent neuropathologic changes have been described in the literature. However, it should be pointed out for almost all the examples of the secondary dystonias, cliniconeuropathologic correlation to the dystonic aspects of the disorder is lacking.

**Table 1** Pathology of Primary Dystonia

| Disease | Dystonia | Other clinical conditions | Caudate | Putamen | GPe | GPi | STN | SNr | SNc | Thalamus | Cerebellum | Other |
|---|---|---|---|---|---|---|---|---|---|---|---|---|
| DYT1 | +++ | – | – | – | – | – | – | – | – | – | – | PPN inclusions |
| DYT3 (Lubag) (1–3) | ++ | Parkinsonism | +++ Striosomes (GABAergic neurons) | +++ Striosomes (GABAergic neurons) | + | – | – | – | + | – | ++ | – |
| DYT5, DYT14 (dopa-responsive dystonia; AR or AD) (4,5) | +++ | Parkinsonism | – | – | – | – | – | – | +++ | – | – | – |
| DYT11 (myoclonus dystonia) (one case–obligate carrier) | ++ | Myoclonus | – | – | – | – | – | – | – | – | – | – |
| DYT12 (rapid-onset dystonia-parkinsonism; one case) | +++ | Parkinsonism | – | – | – | – | – | – | – | – | – | – |

*Note*: The severity of involvement is indicated from mild (+) to severe (+++).
*Abbreviations*: AR, autosomal recessive; AD, autosomal dominant; GPe, globus pallidus external segment; GPi, globus pallidus internal segment; PPN, pedunculopontine nucleus; STN, subthalamic nucleus; SNc, substantia nigra pars compacta; SNr, substantia nigra pars reticulata.

## PATHOLOGY OF PRIMARY DYSTONIA; DYT1 DYSTONIA

The pathological basis of DYT1 dystonia (dystonia musculorum deformans, Oppenheim's disease) has eluded investigators since the illness was first described. Only a few neuropathological studies have been reported, and the findings of these are inconsistent. This has been limited, in part, by the absence of genetic identification and testing for the dystonias. One patient with dystonia musculorum deformans, presumed to have the *DYT1* mutation, who died at the age of 29, was found to have mild neuronal loss with neurofibrillary tangles (NFTs) in the locus coeruleus (LC) and infrequent NFTs in the substantia nigra pars compacta (SNc), pedunculopontine nucleus (PPN), and dorsal raphe nucleus (19). More recently, in a case confirmed to carry the *DYT1* mutation, no evidence of pathological change was seen in selected regions, nor were there abnormalities on using an antibody to torsinA (20). However, minor changes have been reported in the SNc of four patients with DYT1 dystonia. Although these brains exhibited an increase in size and decrease in spacing of dopaminergic neurons, no evidence of protein aggregation, inclusion body formation, or neuronal death was noted (21).

### Brainstem Pathology in DYT1 Dystonia

Novel antibodies to ubiquitin-protein conjugates (UPC) are highly sensitive to ubiquitin and α-synuclein in detecting protein aggregates in neurodegenerative disorders such as Parkinson's disease (PD) and dementia with Lewy bodies (22). Using UPC antibodies, inclusion bodies in the midbrain reticular formation and periaqueductal gray (PAG) have been demonstrated in four patients with DYT1 dystonia (Fig. 1) (23). These inclusions were spherical and found at perinuclear sites in cells of the PPN, cuneiform nucleus (CN), and griseum centrale mesencephali. The inclusions stained intensely for UPC and the nuclear envelope protein lamin A/C (Fig. 2), but staining was less intense and less frequent for ubiquitin, torsinA, and the endoplasmic reticulum marker protein disulphide isomerase (Fig. 2). The inclusion bodies were not labeled using antibodies to several other proteins including α-synuclein and were present in cholinergic and other neurons, but not in glia (23). Inclusion bodies were located in proximity to or directly associated with the nucleus and often appeared compressed, contorted, and abnormal (Fig. 2). This finding is consistent with cell culture studies showing that mutations in torsinA cause the protein to accumulate in the nuclear envelope and to form perinuclear inclusions (24–27). It has also been shown that the nuclear envelope of neurons is abnormal in torsinA null and homozygous disease mutant "knock-in" mice (28).

In addition, the presence of protein aggregates in the neuromelanin-pigmented neurons of the SNc and LC in DYT1 dystonia has also been noted (23). These protein aggregates were immunoreactive for tau and ubiquitin, but not torsinA, and were reminiscent of the NFTs previously reported in the patient with dystonia musculorum deformans (19).

### Brainstem Pathology in DYT1 Transgenic Mice

Consistent with protein accumulation in the brains of patients with DYT1 dystonia, these changes have also been reported as protein aggregates and perinuclear inclusion bodies in the brainstem of transgenic mice expressing mutant torsinA (29,30). These protein aggregates and inclusion bodies were immunoreactive for

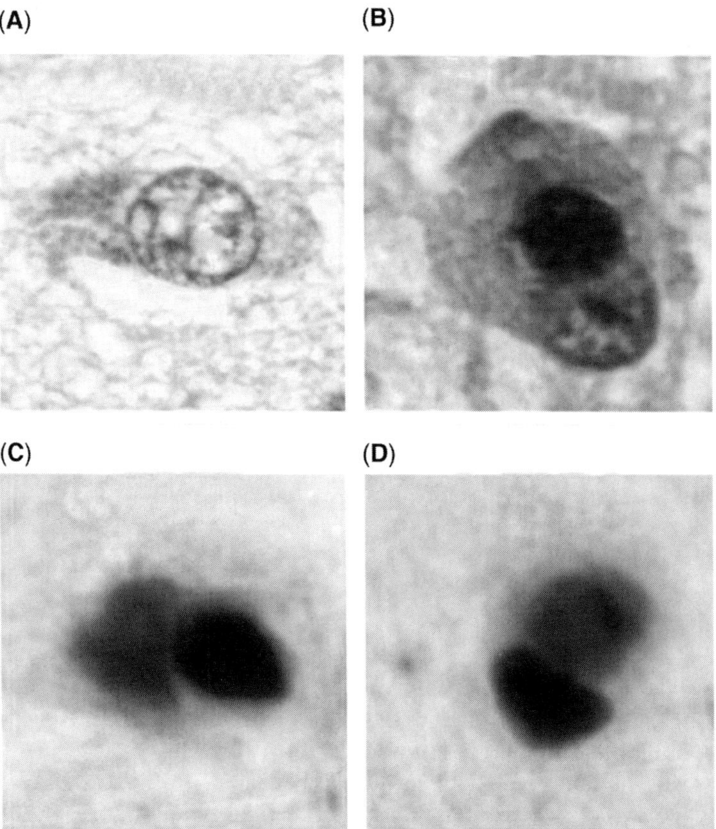


**Figure 1** (*See color insert*) Intracellular inclusion bodies in DYT1 dystonia. In the brainstems of patients with DYT1 dystonia and controls, antibodies to ubiquitinated proteins (**A**, **B**, **C**) and ubiquitin (**D**), show low intracellular staining in controls (**A**), and intensely stained inclusion bodies in DYT1 dystonia (**B**, **C**, **D**). The chromogen is 3,3-diaminobenzidine (brown) and nuclei are counterstained with hematoxylin (blue). *Source*: Modified from Ref. 23 with permission.

ubiquitin, torsinA, and lamin A/C and were localized to cells in the pontine and mesencephalic brainstem and in the PAG.

## Conclusion

The finding of protein aggregates and inclusion bodies in brainstem nuclei of patients with DYT1 dystonia, and similar pathological changes in DYT1 transgenic mice, suggests that protein accumulation is likely a direct result of the mutation in torsinA. It is notable that these pathologic findings are found in the PPN and CN, which play important roles in motor function through extensive efferent and afferent connections with the basal ganglia, thalamus, cerebral cortex, and spinal cord (31–35). Indeed, the PPN and CN constitute the so-called mesencephalic locomotor region (MLR), which is thought to regulate muscle tone and rhythmic limb movements during locomotion (31–34,36). The PAG is also thought to be functionally associated with the MLR (33). Thus, it is reasonable to hypothesize that mutant torsinA-induced neuronal dysfunction or degeneration in these brainstem nuclei underlies the pathophysiology of DYT1 and perhaps other forms of dystonia.

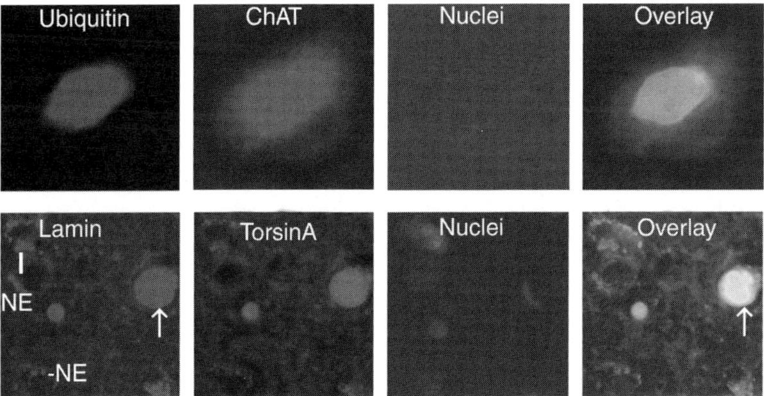


**Figure 2** (*See color insert*) Perinuclear inclusions in DYT1 dystonia. Top row; inclusion bodies contain ubiquitin (red, Alexa Fluor 594) and are present in cholinergic neurons stained for cholineacetyl transferase (ChAT; green, Alexa Fluor 488). Bottom row; inclusion bodies also contain the nuclear envelope (NE) marker lamin A/C (red) and torsinA (green). Cell nuclei stained with blue (bisbenzimide, Hoechst 3358). *Source*: Modified from Ref. 23 with permission.

## PATHOLOGY OF DYSTONIA-PLUS SYNDROMES AND SECONDARY DYSTONIA

### Introduction

Of the inherited dystonia-plus syndromes, DYT11 (myoclonus-dystonia)(RHW, personal observations) and rapid-onset dystonia-parkinsonism (DYT12) (37) do not show evidence of neurodegeneration on neuroimaging or in the limited neuropathological studies available in the literature (Table 1). Dopa-responsive dystonia (DRD; DYT5 and DYT14) does not show frank neuronal loss, however, there are distinct neuropathological findings. Neurodegeneration is found in DYT3 (Lubag).

The commonly accepted model of basal ganglia function (Fig. 3A) (39,40) only partially explains the clinical generation of movement disorders, and in fact may be least suitable to explaining the phenomenology of dystonia. A more complex model has been proposed with the detailed report of the neuropathology of Lubag (Filipino dystonia-parkinsonism; DYT3) (1) and may provide a better explanation.

Dystonia may be caused by anatomic lesions in a variety of locations, although the basal ganglia are typically involved. Of the various nuclei of the basal ganglia, the most commonly affected sites appear to be the caudate nucleus and putamen, however, it appears that lesions involving almost any of the nuclei may cause dystonia (Tables 2–4).

When dystonia is caused by a structural lesion of the putamen, the model would predict that neurons of the indirect pathway are preferentially damaged, as decreased function of the first connection of the indirect pathway is postulated (as opposed to increased activity in the striato-GPi direct pathway)(Fig. 3B). While in most causes of dystonia, there is no neuropathological evidence to support this model, the exception to this is Lubag (DYT3), where recent neuropathological evidence (1) suggests a mechanism by which increased activity of the direct pathway may occur. In addition, the currently accepted model does not explain why both

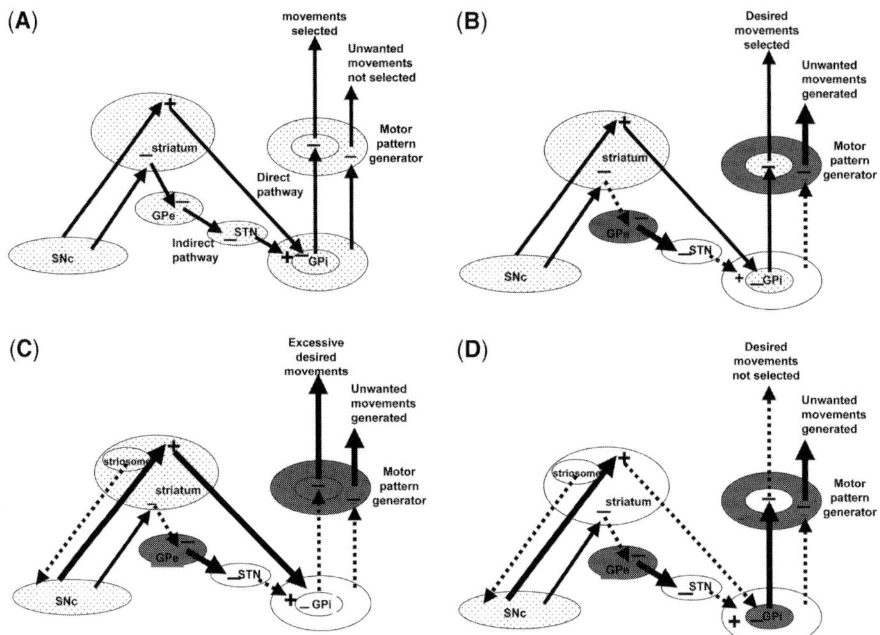


**Figure 3** Model of basal ganglia circuitry in dystonia. (**A**) During normal function of the basal ganglia, the direct pathway from the striatum inhibits neurons of the GPi, disinhibiting the motor pattern generator, consisting of the motor thalamic nuclei and their projections to the cortex. The neurons which select the motor program are represented as being surrounded by a network, controlled by the indirect pathway, which reduces the generation of unwanted movements. (**B**) In dystonia, there is decreased surround inhibition via the indirect pathway, with loss of inhibition of unselected movements. (**C**) Incorporating the "third-pathway" (38), as has been postulated from the neuropathology of Lubag (DYT3) (1), preferential loss of striosomal neurons projecting to the SNc results in increased dopaminergic input to the striatum, thus is the cause of the increased output via the direct pathway and the decreased output via the indirect pathway. (**D**) In the parkinsonian stage of this disorder, loss of the remaining neurons in the matrix results in damage to the direct pathway, and hence increased output from the GPi/STN, as is seen in Parkinson's disease.

pallidotomy and deep brain stimulation should reduce the symptoms of dystonia, although current thinking suggests that abnormal neuronal firing pattern, rather than absolute firing rate, is the critical factor. The role of the brainstem structures in which neuronal pathology is found in DYT1 is unclear, but may implicate impaired downstream processing of motor signals.

## Caudate Nucleus/Putamen

The caudate nucleus and putamen are frequently involved when the clinical presentation is of dystonia. However, they are also often affected in disorders in which the predominant movement disorder is chorea, such as Huntington's disease (HD). In HD, as in a number of other neurodegenerative disorders affecting the basal ganglia, a variety of movement disorders including tics, dystonia, chorea, myoclonus, and parkinsonism may be observed. At present it is unclear what the difference is at the neuropathological level between patients with different clinical phenotypes.

**Table 2** Pathology of Secondary Dystonia; Autosomal Dominant Inheritance

| Disease | Dystonia | Other clinical conditions | Caudate | Putamen | GPe | GPi | STN | SNr | SNc | Thalamus | Cerebellum | Other |
|---|---|---|---|---|---|---|---|---|---|---|---|---|
| Huntington's disease | + | Chorea, parkinsonism, dementia | +++ | +++ | ++ | + | + | ++ | ++ | + | + | NIIBs in neocortex |
| Huntington's disease-like 2 (6,7) | ++ | Chorea, parkinsonism, dementia | +++ | +++ | + | + | + | + | ++ | + | – | NIIBs in neocortex |
| Spinocerebellar ataxia III | + | Ataxia | – | – | – | – | – | – | + | – | Dentate +++ | NIIBs in affected areas; atrophy of dorsal and lateral spinal tracts |
| Spinocerebellar ataxia 17 | + | Ataxia | ++ | ++ | – | – | – | – | – | + | Purkinje +++ | NIIBs in affected areas |
| Dentatorubro-pallidoluysian atrophy | + | Ataxia, chorea, myoclonus, dementia | – | – | +++ | ++ | ++ | – | – | – | Dentate ++ | NIIBs in dentate, pons |
| Neuroferritinopathy (8) | ++ | Chorea, parkinsonism | – | + | +++ | +++ | – | – | – | – | ++ | White matter, neuroaxonal spheroids |

*Note*: The severity of involvement is indicated from mild (+) to severe (+++).
*Abbreviations*: GPe, globus pallidus external segment; GPi, globus pallidus internal segment; NIIB, neuronal intranuclear inclusion bodies; STN, subthalamic nucleus; SNc, substantia nigra pars compacta; SNr, substantia nigra pars reticulata.

**Table 3** Pathology of Secondary Dystonia; Autosomal Recessive Inheritance

| Disease | Dystonia | Other clinical conditions | Caudate | Putamen | GPe | GPi | STN | SNr | SNc | Thalamus | Cerebellum | Other |
|---|---|---|---|---|---|---|---|---|---|---|---|---|
| Wilson's disease | + | Chorea, psychiatric symptoms, coarse tremor, liver disease | + | +++ | ++ | ++ | + | – | – | – | Dentate + | Alzheimer type II astrocytes in cortex |
| Pantothenate kinase–associated neurodegeneration | ++ | Chorea, dementia, retinal pigmentation | – | – | + | +++ | | ++ | – | – | – | Iron deposition, neuroaxonal spheroids, GCIs, LBs in brainstem |
| Chorea-acanthocytosis (9–12) | ++ | Chorea, parkinsonism, dementia, peripheral neuropathy and myopathy | +++ | +++ | ++ | ++ | – | – | + | + | – | Axonal neuropathy |
| Aceruloplasminemia | ++ | Diabetes, retinal degeneration, ataxia, dementia | +++ | +++ | ++ | ++ | – | ++ | ++ | +++ | Purkinje, dentate ++ | Iron deposition in astrocytes |
| Friedreich's ataxia | + | Ataxia, peripheral neuropathy, (spasticity) | – | – | – | – | – | – | + | + | Dentate +++ | Corticospinal, dorsal/lateral spinal tracts |
| Ataxia–telangiectasia | + | Ataxia, chorea, oculomotor apraxia | – | – | – | – | – | – | + | – | Cortex, Purkinje, granule +++ | Telangiectasiae in conjunctivae, skin, meninges, brain |

| | | | | | | | | | | | | |
|---|---|---|---|---|---|---|---|---|---|---|---|---|
| $GM_1$ gangliosidosis | + | Parkinsonism | ++ | ++ | + | + | – | – | – | – | Purkinje+ | $GM_1$ ganglioside throughout brain, PAS+ |
| $GM_2$ gangliosidosis | + | Variable | + | + | – | – | + | + | + | + | ++ | $GM_2$ ganglioside throughout brain, PAS+ |
| Niemann-Pick type C | + | Vertical gaze palsy | ++ | ++ | ++ | ++ | – | – | – | + | Dentate, cortex ++ | Sphingolipid accumulation in cortex |
| Neuronal ceroid lipofuscinosis | + | Variable, often retinal involvement | ++ | ++ | ++ | ++ | ++ | ++ | ++ | ++ | ++ | Granular inclusions PAS+ |
| Metachromatic leukodystrophy | + | Quadriparesis, spasticity, ataxia | + | + | + | + | + | + | + | + | + | Demyelination; sulphatide in neurons |
| Homocystinuria | + | Vascular disease, ectopia lentis | – | – | – | – | – | – | – | – | – | Vascular occlusion and infarction |
| Hartnup disease | + | Variable; skin and GI symptoms | – | – | – | – | – | – | – | ++ | Cortex | Cortical atrophy; demyelination |
| Glutaric aciduria | ++ | Episodes of ketoacidosis, fever | ++ | ++ | – | – | – | – | – | – | Cortical atrophy | – |
| Neuronal intranuclear inclusion disease (13) | + | Variable | – | – | – | – | – | + | +++ | – | Purkinje ++ | Eosinophilic NIIBs in brain and anterior horn cells |

*Note*: The severity of involvement is indicated from mild (+) to severe (+++).

*Abbreviations*: GCI, glial cytoplasmic inclusions; GI, gastrointestinal; GPe, globus pallidus external segment; GPi, globus pallidus internal segment; LB, Lewy body; NIIB, neuronal intranuclear inclusion bodies; PAS, periodic acid Schiff; STN, subthalamic nucleus; SNc, substantia nigra pars compacta; SNr, substantia nigra pars reticulata.

**Table 4** Pathology of Secondary Dystonia; Other (X-Linked or Mixed Inheritance, Mitochondrial, Sporadic)

| Disease | Dystonia | Other clinical | Caudate | Putamen | GPe | GPi | STN | SNr | SNc | Thalamus | Cerebellum | Other |
|---|---|---|---|---|---|---|---|---|---|---|---|---|
| Lesch–Nyhan | + | Chorea, self-mutilation | + | + | + | + | + | + | + | + | + | Nonspecific necrotic changes throughout brain |
| McLeod syndrome (12,14,15) | ++ | Chorea, parkinsonism, dementia, peripheral neuropathy and myopathy | +++ | +++ | ++ | ++ | – | – | – | – | – | Peripheral neuropathy and myopathy |
| Fahr's disease (Autosomal dominant, mitochon-drial, or other) | ++ | Chorea, parkinsonism, dementia | +++ | +++ | ++ | ++ | – | – | – | + | +++dentate, white matter | Calcium in blood vessel walls |
| Leigh's syndrome | ++ | Chorea, dementia, | + | + | – | – | – | ++ | ++ | – | ++dentate, inf. olive | Periaqueductal grey |
| Mohr–Tranebjaerg disease | +++ | Deafness ± | +++ | +++ | +++ | +++ | – | – | – | – | – | |
| Parkinson's disease | + | Parkinsonism | – | – | – | – | – | – | +++ | + | + | LBs in many brainstem/midbrain regions, and cortex |
| Progressive supranuclear palsy | ++ | Parkinsonism, supranuclear gaze palsy | – | – | ++ | ++ | ++ | ++ | +++ | ++ | + | Midbrain +++ tau+ NFTs |

| | | | | | | | | | | | | |
|---|---|---|---|---|---|---|---|---|---|---|---|---|
| Multiple system atrophy | + | Parkinsonism, autonomic/ cerebellar dysfunction | ++ | ++ | – | – | – | – | ++ | – | ++ (cerebellar subtype) | GCIs; locus coeruleus; inferomediolateral columns (Shy-Drager) |
| Corticobasal degeneration | ++ | Parkinsonism | ++ | ++ | + | + | + | + | ++ | + | +/– | Asymmetric cortical atrophy, ballooned neurons, tau+ |
| Primary pallidal degeneration (16) | ++ | Bradykinesia | – | – | ++ | ++ | – | – | – | – | – | |
| Pallidoluysian atrophy (17) | +– | Dysarthria, gait disorder, vertical gaze palsy | – | – | +++ | – | +++ | – | – | – | – | |
| Creutzfeldt–Jakob disease | ++ | Chorea, dementia, myoclonus (progression over months) | ++ | ++ | – | – | – | – | – | ++ | ++ | Cortex; spongiform degeneration in affected regions (variable) |
| Alzheimer's disease | + | Dementia, rigidity, myoclonus | – | – | – | – | – | – | – | – | + | Cortical atrophy, plaques, NFTs; degeneration of nucleus basalis of Meynert |
| Neuronal intermediate filament inclusion disease (18) | + | Variable | +++ | ++ | ++ | ++ | ++ | ++ | ++ | +++ | – | Frontal/temporal cortex; neurofilament+ inclusions |

*Note*: The severity of involvement is indicated from mild (+) to severe (+++).
*Abbreviations*: GCI, glial cytoplasmic inclusions; GPe, globus pallidus external segment; GPi, globus pallidus internal segment; LB, Lewy body; NFT, neurofibrillary tangle; NIIB, neuronal intranuclear inclusion bodies; STN, subthalamic nucleus; SNc, substantia nigra pars compacta; SNr, substantia nigra pars reticulata.

Many of the disorders described below have pathology extending into the external and internal segments of the globus pallidus (GP). This is especially true of structural lesions causing dystonia (41), such as infarction, arteriovenous malformation, tumor, or hemorrhage. The clinical results from such a lesion may be quite variable and involve a variety of neurological and psychiatric symptoms (42). However, it is apparent that lesions limited to the putamen may also result in pure dystonia without apparent psychiatric symptoms (43).

*Lubag*

Analysis of the neuropathology of Lubag (DYT3) has generated provocative results, potentially shedding light upon the mechanism of dystonia (1). Parkinsonian cases of Lubag were compared with cases in which dystonia was the major clinical presentation. In dystonic cases, there was a predominant loss of striatal projection neurons in striosomes and patchy loss in the surrounding matrix (38). The authors postulate that the loss of the GABAergic inhibitory striosomal projection to the SNc results in increased nigrostriatal activity, thus causing increased activity of the neurons of the direct pathway via excitatory dopamine D1 receptors (Fig. 3C). This would result in increased inhibition, and hence decreased activity of the GPi, in accordance with the predictions of the traditional model in dystonia. As the disease progresses, striatal neuronal loss becomes more widespread, and loss of the striato-GPi neurons of the direct pathway, which were previously hyperactive, results in parkinsonism (Fig. 3D).

Additional studies of the neuropathology of Lubag reported verify caudate/putamen involvement and also suggest moderate cerebellar Purkinje cell loss and mild fibrillary gliosis without neuronal loss of the GP and SN (2,44).

*Huntington's Disease*

HD is the most common neurodegenerative disorder primarily affecting the caudate/putamen and may produce dystonia as part of a clinical phenotype of a mixed movement disorder. Because of its relatively high incidence, it has been possible to study the neuropathology in detail at different disease stages. The juvenile form, known as the Westphal variant, with age of onset younger than 20, is characterized by a parkinsonian presentation, often with marked dystonia. In adult-onset HD, as the disease advances, chorea often gives way to more parkinsonian and dystonic features, with severe bradykinesia or akinesia, rigidity, and postural impairment (45,46). Initially, striatal neurons projecting to the GPe, comprising the indirect pathway, are affected (47). It is postulated that this corresponds to the initial appearance of chorea, progressing to parkinsonism as the direct pathway is affected. The pathophysiology of dystonia in HD is not well understood. Involvement of the striatum is said to be more severe in the juvenile form than in those with midlife onset, even though the duration of disease from onset to death may be equivalent. The subtype of striatal neurons preferentially affected in this parkinsonian phenotype has not been specifically reported. However, the juvenile form may respond to both l-dopa (48) and dopamine agonists (49), suggesting that the deficit is of presynaptic nigral dopaminergic neurons, rather than postsynaptic striatal neurons. Although degeneration of striatal medium spiny neurons is well documented as the primary neuropathologic abnormality, loss of neurons from the SN, both pars compacta and pars reticulata, has also been described (50,51). Ubiquitin- and huntingtin-immunoreactive intranuclear inclusions are found in the cortex in both juvenile and adult forms of the illness.

*Huntington's Disease-like 2*

There are several other neurodegenerative disorders affecting the basal ganglia, in which the predominant movement disorder is chorea but dystonia is often a major feature, such as Huntington's disease-like 2 (HDL2) (6,52,53). Because neuropathological studies in these rare disorders are usually only available in cases that have succumbed to advanced disease, it is has not been possible to perform studies to determine if particular neuronal types are lost from the striatum or to correlate neuropathological findings with the clinical presentation.

In HDL2 the neuropathological findings in the small number of cases with advanced disease are very similar to those seen in HD, with marked atrophy and gliosis of the caudate-putamen, and to a lesser extent of the GP. Also strikingly similar to HD, there were numerous ubiquitin-immunoreactive neuronal intranuclear inclusions throughout the cortex, accompanied by moderate neuronal loss and gliosis (6,7).

*Neuroacanthocytosis Syndromes*

Post mortem findings in autosomal recessive chorea-acanthocytosis (54,55) reveal severe neuronal loss and gliosis of the caudate, putamen (9–11), and, to a lesser extent, the GP (10–12) and SN (12). There is occasional atrophy with gliosis of the thalamus (11), with involvement of the anterior nuclei and centromedian nucleus (10). Similar findings are seen in X-linked McLeod syndrome (54,55), with marked atrophy and gliosis of the caudate nucleus and putamen (12,14) and moderate gliosis and neuronal loss of the GP (15).

*Corticobasal Degeneration*

Corticobasal degeneration (CBD) is characterized by an asymmetric presentation of parkinsonism, dystonia, and cortical deficits, attributed to pathology of the basal ganglia and cortex. Limb dystonia may result in flexion contractures of the hand and arm. The leg tends to be extended at the knee and the foot plantar-flexed and inverted. The brain, upon gross examination, shows a variable degree of selective atrophy of the cerebral cortex, which is usually distinctly asymmetric. The frontal or parietal cortex is most commonly affected, although this feature may be quite subtle. The midbrain appears somewhat shrunken, the aqueduct of Sylvius is enlarged, and the SNc depigmented. Within the area of cortical atrophy, one sees severe neuronal loss with gliosis. Scattered in these areas are remaining ballooned neurons with a loss of Nissl substance and a rounded eosinophilic cytoplasm. In addition, in the caudate, putamen, and adjacent white matter, one sees numerous thread-like processes that stain with silver impregnation stains as well as antibodies directed against abnormally phosphorylated tau. Tau-positive inclusions are also noted in oligodendroglial cells, where they appear similar to those seen in cases of progressive supranuclear palsy (PSP). The nosologic distinction between these two entities is under discussion, with suggestions that they may be variants of the same disorder.

*Multiple System Atrophy*

Patients with multiple system atrophy (MSA) may present with a wide range of clinical features. Although 90% of MSA patients will show some degree of parkinsonian features, individuals with this disease are subclassified as Parkinson-predominant (MSA-P) or cerebellar-predominant (MSA-C) forms. Although dystonic symptoms are not frequent, they may be encountered in the parkinsonian subtype. Typically, the parkinsonism is midline with axial rigidity and falling, and cervical antecollis is often seen (56). Limb dystonia may also be present (56). A number of brain regions undergo neurodegeneration with neuronal loss, gliosis, and the presence of α-synuclein-immunoreactive glial cytoplasmic inclusions. These regions include the SN and LC, putamen, and subthalamic nucleus (STN). With cerebellar dysfunction there is loss of Purkinje cells and neurons of the inferior olivary nuclei. There is considerable variability in the extent of involvement in these various regions, and, at the present time, it is unclear which area of particular damage correlates with the presence of prominent dystonia in MSA patients. Iron deposition in the lateral rim of the putamen is a characteristic finding on magnetic resonance imaging (MRI), suggesting degeneration of medium spiny striatal neurons. The limited benefit to the parkinsonism from dopaminergic medications implies postsynaptic loss of dopamine receptors on striatal neurons projecting to the GPi, in addition to the loss of dopaminergic SNc neurons. It is not yet known if neuronal loss in the putamen follows a specific distribution in patients with dystonia, for example, affecting the neurons of the indirect rather than the direct pathway (Fig. 3B).

*Wilson's Disease*

Wilson's disease (WD) may present with a variety of abnormal movements including dystonia of face, neck, trunk, and limbs, although this is rarely the sole or presenting feature (57). The causative mutation is of the *ATP7B* gene, resulting in an inability to transport copper onto ceruloplasmin, with resultant copper accumulation in putamen (and to a much lesser extent, the caudate nucleus and the GP) and in extraneuronal sites including the liver and cornea (58–60). Copper deposition and cavitation is also seen in the GP. Alzheimer type II astrocytes, secondary to liver disease, are found in gray matter throughout the brain. Dystonia of the face, tongue, and pharynx may be seen and may result in dysarthria. The classical "risus sardonicus" of WD is caused by dystonia affecting the lower facial muscles. Hereditary whispering dysphonia (DYT4) is associated with WD (61), although the mechanism of pathophysiology and neuropathology are not known.

*Idiopathic Basal Ganglia Calcification*

Fahr's disease [idiopathic basal ganglia calcification (IBGC)] refers to a heterogeneous group of disorders in which there is deposition of calcium in the basal ganglia and other cerebral regions, particularly the deep cerebellar nuclei. The clinical picture may include dystonia, parkinsonism, chorea, ataxia, cognitive impairment, and behavioral changes. In one family, linkage to 14q was demonstrated (IBC1) (62), although the gene has not yet been identified. In several families with autosomal dominant inheritance, linkage to this locus has been excluded (63,64). In other families (65,66), the pattern of inheritance and additional clinical features suggest mitochondrial inheritance. Pathologically, abundant calcium deposition is found predominantly in the putamen, caudate nucleus, and dentate nucleus. Calcium is also found in the walls of blood vessels, although vascular disease is not a typical feature.

*$GM_1$ Gangliosidosis*

The late-onset, chronic form of $GM_1$ gangliosidosis (adult; type 3), caused by autosomal recessive inheritance of a deficiency of β-galactosidase, is slowly progressive and may present during childhood or as late as the fourth decade of life. This form involves only the CNS and does not affect the skeletal system. Dystonia is often marked, especially orofacial, and dysarthria and dysphagia may be severe. Features of parkinsonism are also reported (67–70). MRI frequently shows bilateral putamenal hyperintensities on T2 sequences (68,70), which are reflected by the neuropathologic findings. In the adult-onset cases, the extent of involvement tends to be more limited, with neuronal storage seen in caudate, putamen, and, to a lesser degree, the amygdala, GP, and Purkinje cells of the cerebellum (69). There is evidence of intraneuronal storage with swollen neuronal perikarya and accumulation in adjacent glial cells. Membranous cytoplasmic bodies are seen ultrastructurally in affected cells.

#### *$GM_2$ Gangliosidosis*

The late-onset forms of $GM_2$ gangliosidosis, due to autosomal recessive deficiency of hexosaminidase A, may occur in childhood, adolescence, or adulthood as either subacute or chronic forms. Dystonia and choreoathetosis have been reported in the subacute forms, along with dysarthria, speech loss, ataxia, spasticity, seizures, and behavioral changes (71–73). In general, cerebellar and corticospinal abnormalities tend to predominate over basal ganglia–related symptomatology. Storage material accumulates in the neurons and glia of the cortex and cerebellum. In some variants, the SN and the basal ganglia are mildly involved.

#### *Niemann–Pick Type C*

Niemann–Pick type C may present in childhood or even late into adulthood, with cerebellar signs, action tremor and myoclonus, seizures, and dysarthria. This autosomal recessive neurodegenerative disease is related to a failure of cholesterol trafficking in the endosomal–lysosomal pathway. Dystonia, particularly of the lower facial muscles, and choreoathetosis, may be present. As with $GM_2$ gangliosidosis, the presence of supranuclear gaze palsy, specifically loss of vertical gaze, may lead this disorder to resemble PSP (74,75). Typically, there is visceral storage of sphingomyelin primarily in macrophages ("sea-blue histiocytes"). The neuropathologic features tend to be rather variable, with some cases showing widespread neuronal storage and others a more localized involvement (generally in chronic progressive adult-onset cases). Neuronal cytoplasm is filled with sphingomyelin material. In patients with the chronic progressive form of the disease, NFTs, similar to those seen in Alzheimer's disease, are also noted.

#### *Neuronal Ceroid Lipofuscinosis*

Dystonia is occasionally seen in the various forms of neuronal ceroid lipofuscinosis, the different types of which are associated with mutations of a number of genes (*CLN1, CLN2, CLN3, CLN5, CLN6,* and *CLN8*) for various endosomal-lysosomal proteins (76). Accumulation of proteins results in the diagnostic autofluorescent material within neurons. The specific neuropathological findings vary with the different types. Dystonia has been reported rarely in the infantile form, along with an unusual phenotype of microcephaly and hypotonia, with atrophy of the caudate nuclei, due to mutation of *CLN2* (77). In the juvenile form (late-onset Batten disease; Spielmeyer–Vogt disease), usually due to mutations of *CLN3*, involvement of the extrapyramidal system is a late feature, with occasional dystonia (78), accompanied by intellectual decline, visual loss, and seizures (79). In the adult form, Kufs' disease, the cerebellum and brainstem are predominantly involved, and the striatum and thalamus can also be affected.

#### *Glutaric Aciduria Type I*

The striatum appears particularly vulnerable to accumulation of glutaric acid, in glutaric aciduria type I, due to autosomal recessive inheritance of deficiency of glutaryl-CoA dehydrogenase. Dystonic posturing, especially facial grimacing, appears during infancy and, occasionally, in later life. Degeneration primarily of the striatum is found on neuroimaging and on neuropathological examination.

#### *Lesch–Nyhan Syndrome*

Lesch–Nyhan syndrome is an X-linked disorder caused by mutation of hypoxanthine phosphoribosyl transferase, and presents at three to six months with psychomotor retardation and hypotonia. Subsequently, spasticity, dystonia, and choreoathetosis develop. A typical feature is self-mutilation, with biting of the hands and lips. The enzyme deficiency results in the accumulation of uric acid, as there is impaired phosphorylation of hypoxanthine and guanine.

#### *Mitochondrial Disorders*

Leigh's syndrome may be attributed to a number of different mutations of mitochondrial DNA and presents in early childhood, although adult-onset presentation has been reported (80). A variety of different neurological signs may be present, including acute encephalopathy, psychomotor retardation, hypotonia, spasticity, myopathy, dysarthria, seizures, dystonia, and chorea. An overlap with mitochondrial encephalopathy with lactic acidosis and stroke-like episodes (MELAS) may occur (81). Characteristically, lesions in the thalamus, caudate, putamen, midbrain, pons, and, variably, the GP, are seen on neuroimaging, corresponding neuropathologically with vascular proliferation, gliosis, neuronal loss, demyelination, and cystic cavitation of these structures (82). In Mohr–Tranebjaerg syndrome, initially described as X-linked dystonia and deafness, but subsequently determined to be due to a mitochondrial mutation (83,84), neuronal loss and gliosis of the caudate, putamen, and GP have been reported (85).

#### *Creutzfeldt–Jakob Disease*

Various movement disorders may be seen in Creutzfeldt–Jakob disease, typically myoclonus and chorea, but sometimes dystonia. Spongiform changes are found particularly in the cortex, caudate/putamen, thalamus, and cerebellum. Diagnostic immunoreactivity to the prion protein PrP is seen in various patterns, depending upon the genotypic variant.

#### *Neuronal Intermediate Filament Inclusion Disease*

Neuronal intermediate filament inclusion disease (NIFID) is a rare, apparently sporadic, disorder, in which the neuropathologic findings of intermediate neurofilament inclusions are widespread throughout the brain, affecting particularly the frontal and temporal lobes and the caudate nucleus. Clinically, symptoms develop in early-mid adulthood (18) and correspond to the distribution of the lesions.

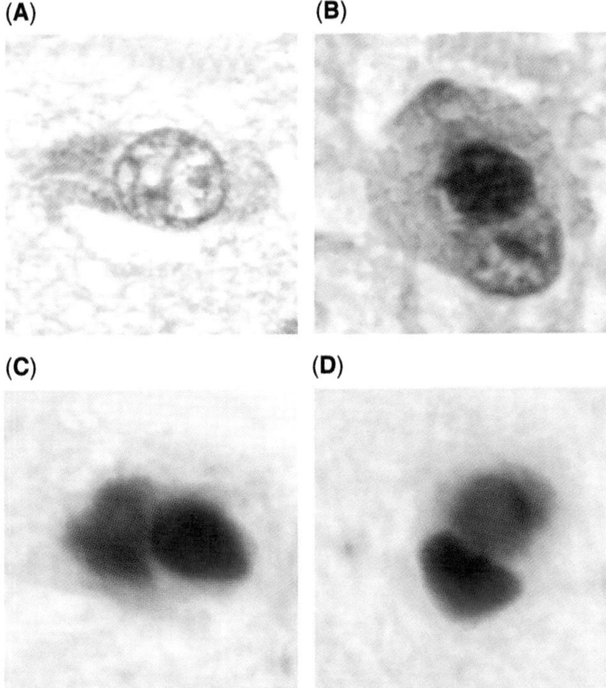


**Figure 6.1** Intracellular inclusion bodies in DYT1 dystonia. In the brainstems of patients with DYT1 dystonia and controls, antibodies to ubiquitinated proteins (**A**, **B**, **C**) and ubiquitin (**D**), show low intracellular staining in controls (**A**), and intensely stained inclusion bodies in DYT1 dystonia (**B**, **C**, **D**). The chromogen is 3,3-diaminobenzidine (*brown*) and nuclei are counterstained with hematoxylin (*blue*). (*See p. 68*)

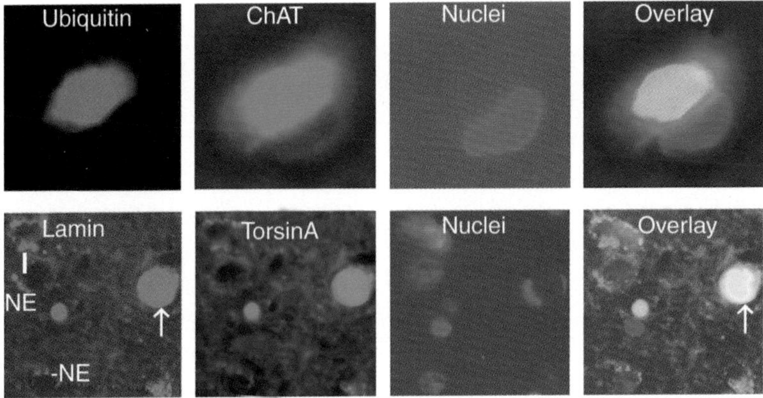


**Figure 6.2** Perinuclear inclusions in DYT1 dystonia. Top row; inclusion bodies contain ubiquitin (*red*, Alexa Fluor 594) and are present in cholinergic neurons stained for cholineacetyl transferase (ChAT; *green*, Alexa Fluor 488). Bottom row; inclusion bodies also contain the nuclear envelope (NE) marker lamin A/C (*red*) and torsinA (*green*). Cell nuclei stained with blue (bisbenzimide, Hoechst 3358). (*See p. 69*)

*Actin/Cofilin Aggregation*

In a single pair of identical twins afflicted by an unnamed developmental and neurodegenerative condition, with rapidly progressive generalized dystonia, spherical deposits containing actin and cofilin were found in the caudate/putamen. These structures were also found in the GP and the SN. There was no frank neuronal loss or gliosis. Rod-shaped structures of similar composition were seen in the neocortex and thalamus (86).

*Tardive Dystonia*

One of the forms of dystonia most commonly encountered in the clinic is tardive dystonia, due to chronic administration of the classical neuroleptic or dopamine receptor–blocking agents (DRBA). The pathophysiology of this condition and of the other tardive movement disorders is still unknown; however, the role of DRBA suggests involvement of the caudate and putamen. While acute neuroleptic-induced dystonic reactions are usually seen in younger patients, the appearance of tardive dystonia and dyskinesia (chorea) is seen more typically in older people with cognitive impairment (87). This increased vulnerability suggests that progressive neuronal loss because of factors such as normal aging, chronic psychiatric illness, cerebrovascular disease, or Alzheimer's disease, may play a role. There have been reports of normal brains on pathological examination (88) or of various findings that are likely to be nonspecific (89).

## GP-Pars Externa/GP-Pars Interna/Substantia Nigra Pars Reticulata

Lesions or neurodegenerative processes usually appear to involve both segments of the GP, internal and external, thus, they are considered here together. The neuronal constituents of these two nuclei are very similar, consisting predominantly of large GABAergic projection neurons. The main output target of the GPe is the GPi, thus the effects of damage to the external segment are likely to be masked by the effects of damage to the internal segment. The SNr is homologous to the GPi, consisting also of GABAergic neurons and with very similar afferent and efferent connections, thus, the pathology of either nucleus would have very similar effects upon the output of the basal ganglia.

Intraoperative electrophysiological recordings suggest that decreased neuronal activity of the GPi is found in dystonia (90,91). This correlates well with the direct/indirect pathway model (Fig. 3B and C) and the causation of dystonia by lesions in the nucleus. However, both high-frequency stimulation and lesions of the GPi have a therapeutic benefit in dystonia (92), thus, it is hypothesized that disruption of aberrant signal from the GPi in dystonia is of more clinical importance than the restoration of a normal signal.

*Progressive Supranuclear Palsy*

Several types of dystonia may be seen in the otherwise parkinsonian condition of PSP. Extension of the trunk and neck are characteristic, with retropulsion, and blepharospasm is a frequent feature. Although usually associated with a diagnosis of CBD, limb dystonia has been reported in neuropathologically–confirmed PSP (93,94). Dystonic dyskinesias are rare as side effects of l-dopa therapy in this condition but may occur (93,95). Patients with PSP show evidence of neurodegeneration in a number of brain regions including the thalamus, GP, STN, PAG, and SN. There is also a variable degree of involvement of the dentate nucleus of the cerebellum. The areas of neurodegeneration reveal neuronal loss and gliosis with NFT formation is some remaining neurons. In addition, in astrocytes and in particular, oligodendroglial cells in these regions, one encounters comma-shaped tau-immunoreactive inclusion bodies referred to as coiled bodies.

### *Primary Pallidal Degeneration*

Conditions in which neuropathological changes are limited to the GP are relatively rare; however, bradykinesia and dystonia have been reported in primary pallidal degeneration (16). In this small series, the onset was in adulthood, and the disease was distinct from PD in that there was no increase in muscle tone. Onset at younger age has also been reported, associated with marked rigidity and more choreiform and dystonic movements. Neuronal degeneration and gliosis was limited to neurons of the GP.

### *Dentatorubropallidoluysian Atrophy*

Dentatorubropallidoluysian atrophy (DRPLA) is a condition in which the neurodegenerative process affects the external segment of the GP more than the internal segment. DRPLA is caused by CAG repeat expansions in the gene coding for atrophin-1 and may present with dystonia, myoclonus, and chorea, in addition to dementia and ataxia. The model seems to be inaccurate in this example as a primary lesion in the GPe should result in parkinsonism, not dystonia. However, one explanation, consistent with the model, is that the neurodegeneration in the STN prevents the effects of GPe damage from being clinically manifest. Cases generally show evidence of severe neuronal loss in the GPe and the cerebellum (dentate nucleus) with prominent atrophy of the superior cerebellar peduncles. Less prominent neuronal loss is seen in the red nucleus, STN, caudate and putamen, thalamus, SN, and inferior olives. Atrophin-1–immunoreactive inclusions are seen in neuronal nuclei and more generally in neuronal cytoplasm.

### *Pallidoluysian Atrophy*

Isolated pallidoluysian atrophy has been reported, presenting in mid-adulthood with progressive generalized dystonia, bradykinesia, gait disorder, dysarthria, and supranuclear gaze paresis (17). Neuronal atrophy and gliosis involved only the GPe and the STN, supporting a mechanism of decreased GPi activity due to loss of excitatory STN input, as the cause of dystonia.

### *Neurodegeneration with Brain Iron Accumulation*

Several disorders are included under the classification of neurodegeneration with brain iron accumulation (NBIA), resulting in iron deposition in the GP. These include typical (and less commonly, atypical) pantothenate kinase–associated neurodegeneration, neuroferritinopathy, aceruloplasminemia, and Karak syndrome (96). High levels of iron deposition are reported in the GP and are likely to be due to disrupted iron metabolism (97,98).

Pantothenate kinase–associated neurodegeneration (PKAN) is caused by mutations of pantothenate kinase 2 (*PANK2*) (99) and presents with mixed features of orofacial and limb dystonia, choreoathetosis, cognitive impairment, and spasticity (100). The typical MRI "eye-of-the-tiger" pattern of iron deposition in the GP is highly suggestive of the diagnosis (100). The majority of clinically typical cases are due to mutations of *PANK2*, causing protein truncation. Pantothenate kinase catalyses the rate-limiting step in the synthesis of coenzyme A from vitamin B5 (pantothenate). The amount of active enzyme correlates with the disease phenotype, as typical patients have no active enzyme but atypical patients, in whom there may be a missense mutation of *PANK2*, may have some enzyme function (100). The distribution of the neurological lesions is thought to relate to the accumulation of iron and other neurotoxic substances and to local tissue demand for coenzyme-A (99). Iron deposition with marked pigmentation is found in both segments of the GP and the SNr, with neuronal loss and gliosis.

Neuroferritinopathy is caused by mutation of ferritin light chain and also results in iron deposition in the basal ganglia (8). Cystic changes affect predominantly the GP and the caudate/putamen to a lesser extent. Spherical inclusions containing iron and ferritin are found predominantly in the GP, but also in the forebrain and cerebellum. Neuroaxonal spheroids, immunoreactive for ubiquitin, tau, and neurofilament are found diffusely in the GP, putamen, and white matter (8). Unlike the other disorders (PKAN, aceruloplasminemia, etc.), most of which are inherited in an autosomal recessive fashion, this is an autosomal dominant disorder. The result is a variety of movement disorders including chorea, dystonia, and parkinsonism (101,102), with onset at age 40 to 55 years, and rarely cognitive impairment (103). Serum ferritin values tend to be below or at the lower end of the normal range.

## Substantia Nigra Pars Compacta

Disruption of dopaminergic function has long been believed to play a major role in dystonia, and this is now supported by a growing body of direct evidence (21,104–107).

The involvement of the SNc, with degeneration of dopaminergic neurons, in the production of dystonia is unclear in some of the disorders described here, in which neurodegeneration is widespread. In many of these diseases a variety of movement disorders may be seen, including parkinsonism in addition to dystonia. This makes it challenging to precisely determine the pathophysiological substrate for the generation of dystonia. One potential mechanism for the production of movement disorders may be imbalance in dopamine neurotransmission between the direct and indirect pathways or within striatal microcircuits.

### *Parkinson's Disease*

A frequent presentation of early PD is painful foot dystonia, which is also seen in later stages when l-dopa is wearing off. With more advanced disease, severe truncal dystonia may be seen, resulting in forward and/or lateral flexion of the spine (camptocormia) (108). Dystonia of the cervical, cranial, and upper limb muscles has also been reported in PD (109–112). Dystonia is often a component of l-dopa–induced dyskinesias (LIDs), a motor phenomenon typically associated with elevated plasma levels of this agent.

There is debate as to whether disease due to some of the mutations identified to date, such as of *parkin* and *PARK8,* can truly be called PD, as the pathologic hallmark, the Lewy body, is often (but not invariably) absent in these cases (113). Mutation of the *parkin* gene typically results in disease onset in early adulthood, often with prominent dystonia, sometimes exercise induced (114), as a presenting feature (114–117). The response to l-dopa is usually striking, and this feature, in combination with marked dystonia, may even suggest a diagnosis of DRD, thus neuropathological findings are important in making the correct diagnosis (118).

Dystonia does not appear to be as typical in disease caused by the other mutations identified to date, such as of *α-synuclein* (119), *UCH-L1* (120), *DJ-1* (121), *PINK1* (122), or localized to the *PARK8* locus (123), although these are rare (124), and a typical phenotype is not yet fully characterized.

#### *Dopa-Responsive Dystonia*

Dopamine deficiency in the absence of nigral neurodegeneration is seen in dopa-responsive dystonia (DRD; DYT5 and DYT14). Neuropathologically, there is decreased immunoreactivity for tyrosine hydroxylase (TH) in the SNc, but no signs of neuronal loss or Lewy bodies (4,5,125,126). Biochemically, dopamine levels are reduced in the SN and in the striatum. The genetic defects interfere with the production of cofactors or enzymes required for dopamine synthesis. The defects may occur at several different points in the biosynthetic pathway and include guanosine triphosphate cyclohydrolase-1 (GTP-CH1) deficiency (DYT5; autosomal dominant) (4) and TH (DYT5; autosomal recessive).

#### *Neuronal Intranuclear (Hyaline) Inclusion Disease*

Neuronal intranuclear (hyaline) inclusion disease is a genetically heterogeneous disorder diagnosed neuropathologically, with widespread intranuclear inclusions throughout the central, peripheral, and autonomic nervous system (13). The onset may be at any age, and those with young onset tend to have parkinsonism and dystonia, in addition to behavioral changes, corticospinal cerebellar signs, and seizures. Depigmentation of the SNc is often a major neuropathologic feature, and one case has been reported with l-dopa–responsive dystonia, with marked SNc neuronal loss in addition to more widespread lesions (127).

### Subthalamic Nucleus

The primary condition in which STN degeneration is associated with dystonia is DRPLA, however, the multinuclear nature of the pathology makes it difficult to associate lesions of this particular nucleus with specific symptoms. STN lesions are classically associated with hemiballismus, although bilateral STN lesions in PD, or with incorrect settings of STN deep brain stimulation electrodes, may result in severely dystonic speech. Certainly, STN underactivity will result in decreased GPi neuronal firing. As the STN projects predominantly to the GPi, it is possible that it is the pathology of this nucleus that plays a more significant role clinically.

### Thalamus

According to the basal ganglia model, the thalamus, or at least the motor nuclei, should be overactive in dystonia. This is concordant with the use of thalamotomy being used to treat generalized dystonia until the advent of deep brain stimulation in the 1990s. The precise localization of the lesions varied, but often involved the motor nuclei (ventroanterior and ventrolateral). A moderate to marked improvement is reported in approximately half of patients who underwent this procedure

(128–130). However, dysarthria from dystonic speech was often amongst the post-surgical complications of bilateral procedures (131).

Lesions of the thalamus have occasionally been reported as causing dystonia. When this does occur, the characteristics of the involuntary movements are typically different from those seen with other basal ganglia lesions. Vascular lesions affecting the posterior motor nuclei have been reported as causing contralateral dystonic posturing of the hand, with athetoid movements typical of cases presumed to be due to loss of sensory input ("pseudoathetosis"), and myoclonus (132). This was usually in the setting of contralateral hemiparesis and hemianaesthesia, and occasionally a rubral-type tremor.

## Cerebellum

The cerebellum is not typically invoked as a potential pathologic site for the cause of dystonia, however, there is some evidence for its involvement, for example from neuroimaging studies in humans (133). There is more evidence for the involvement of the cerebellum from animal models, for example the dystonic dt rat, in which the removal of the cerebellum results in marked reduction of dystonia (134,135).

### *Spinocerebellar Ataxias*

Dystonia may be seen in a number of the spinocerebellar ataxias (SCAs), particularly SCA III, (Machado–Joseph disease). However, in addition to cerebellar pathology, the SNc may also be involved, which may account for parkinsonian features, and possibly also dystonia.

A variety of movement disorders may be seen in SCA 17, including parkinsonism, dystonia, and chorea (136,137), in addition to the typical phenotype of ataxia, dementia and hyperreflexia. Neuropathologically, cerebellar Purkinje cells are affected, in addition to the caudate/putamen and cerebral cortex (138).

Dystonia may be seen in the autosomal recessive ataxias, particularly in the setting of spasticity. Again, the predominant neuropathogical abnormality is of the cerebellum.

In Friedreich's ataxia, the most common form of familial spinocerebellar degeneration, the characteristic symmetrical loss of myelin in the posterior columns and lateral corticospinal tracts are unlikely to account for the dystonia occasionally seen. In the cerebellum there is a loss of neurons in the dentate nucleus but the Purkinje cells remain intact. Abnormal iron metabolism is implicated in the neurodegenerative process.

The neuropathologic lesion in ataxia–telangiectasia involves the cerebellum with prominent degeneration of the cerebellar cortex, including loss of Purkinje cells and internal granule cells. Transneuronal degeneration of the inferior olivary nuclei is also encountered.

## White Matter

White matter disorders present with a variety of neurological symptoms, including dystonia. Metachromatic leukodystrophy, due to autosomal recessive inheritance of mutations of aryl sulphatase-A, typically presents with cognitive and psychiatric impairment, and occasionally generalized dystonia. The white matter is predominantly involved, but accumulated sulphatides are found in neurons throughout the brain.

Movement disorders are uncommon in disorders of amino acid metabolism, apart from glutaric aciduria type-I, but may be reported in homocystinuria. Neuroimaging demonstrates white matter lesions, corresponding neuropathologically with a vasculopathy. Hartnup disease is an autosomal recessive disorder related to mutations involving an apical membrane-situated amino acid transporter. This is thought to lead to a deficiency in neutral amino acid absorption. Because of the failure of tryptophan absorption, patients develop a pellagra-like syndrome with widespread nervous system impairment. In the few autopsied cases, diffuse cerebral atrophy with demyelination, cerebral cortical, and Purkinje cell loss have been described (139,140).

### Neocortex

Nuchal or truncal dystonia may be seen in Alzheimer's disease, typically in more advanced cases, and in the setting of generalized rigidity and spasticity. The precise relationship of the neuropathological findings to the development of movement disorders is not yet defined, but is likely secondary to cortical neurodegeneration. Drug-induced dystonia may be caused by DRBA, such as risperidone (141) and acetylcholinesterase inhibitors (142,143).

## CONCLUSIONS

It is clear that with more precise molecular characterization of the primary dystonias and the application of better tools to identify and localize proteinaceous accumulations, a neuropathologic picture is beginning to emerge. Additional cases, well characterized both clinically and molecularly, are required to better understand these disorders from a pathogenetic standpoint. With this the long sought-after goal of identifying a consistent recognizable pattern of neuropathologic involvement will be realized and the underlying pathophysiology of primary dystonia can be finally articulated. The situation with the secondary dystonias is more complex because it appears that many brain areas may be involved in such cases. Nevertheless, as a better understanding of the pathophysiology of dystonia is reached, hopefully this can begin to be applied to at least some these cases.

## REFERENCES

1. Goto S, Lee LV, Munoz EL, et al. Functional anatomy of the basal ganglia in X-linked recessive dystonia-parkinsonism. Ann Neurol 2005; 58(1):7–17.
2. Waters CH, Faust PL, Powers J, et al. Neuropathology of Lubag (X-Linked Dystonia Parkinsonism). Mov Disord 1993; 8:387–390.
3. Singleton A, Hague S, Hernandez D. X-linked recessive dystonia parkinsonism (XDP; Lubag; DYT3). Adv Neurol 2004; 94:139–142.
4. Ichinose H, Suzuki T, Inagaki H, et al. Molecular genetics of dopa-responsive dystonia. Biol Chem 1999; 380(12):1355–1364.
5. Grotzsch H, Pizzolato GP, Ghika J, et al. Neuropathology of a case of dopa-responsive dystonia associated with a new genetic locus, DYT14. Neurology 2002; 58(12):1839–1842.
6. Margolis RL, O'Hearn E, Rosenblatt A, et al. A disorder similar to Huntington's disease is associated with a novel CAG repeat expansion. Ann Neurol 2001; 50(6):373–380.
7. Walker RH, Morgello S, Davidoff-Feldman B, et al. Autosomal dominant chorea-acanthocytosis with polyglutamine-containing neuronal inclusions. Neurology 2002; 58(7):1031–1037.

8. Curtis AR, Fey C, Morris CM, et al. Mutation in the gene encoding ferritin light polypeptide causes dominant adult-onset basal ganglia disease. Nat Genet 2001; 28(4):350–354.
9. Arzberger T, Heinsen H, Buresch N, et al. The neuropathology of chorea-acanthocytosis: from stereology to an immunohistochemical detection of chorein. Mov Disord 2005; 20(12):1679.
10. Alonso ME, Teixeira F, Jimenez G, et al. Chorea-acanthocytosis: report of a family and neuropathological study of two cases. Can J Neurol Sci 1989; 16(4):426–431.
11. Vital A, Bouillot S, Burbaud P, et al. Chorea-acanthocytosis: neuropathology of brain and peripheral nerve. Clin Neuropathol 2002; 21(2):77–81.
12. Hardie RJ, Pullon HW, Harding AE, et al. Neuroacanthocytosis. A clinical, haematological and pathological study of 19 cases. Brain 1991; 114:13–49.
13. Takahashi-Fujigasaki J. Neuronal intranuclear hyaline inclusion disease. Neuropathology 2003; 23(4):351–359.
14. Brin MF, Hays A, Symmans WA, et al. Neuropathology of McLeod phenotype is like chorea-acanthocytosis (CA). Can J Neurol Sci 1993; 20(suppl 4):234.
15. Rinne JO, Daniel SE, Scaravilli F, et al. Nigral degeneration in neuroacanthocytosis. Neurology 1994; 44:1629–1632.
16. Aizawa H, Kwak S, Shimizu T, et al. A case of adult onset pure pallidal degeneration. I. Clinical manifestations and neuropathological observations. J Neurol Sci 1991; 102(1):76–82.
17. Wooten GF, Lopes MBS, Harris WO, et al. Pallidoluysian atrophy: dystonia and basal ganglia functional anatomy. Neurology 1993; 43:1764–1768.
18. Cairns NJ, Grossman M, Arnold SE, et al. Clinical and neuropathologic variation in neuronal intermediate filament inclusion disease. Neurology 2004; 63(8):1376–1384.
19. Zweig RM, Hedreen JC, Jankel WR, et al. Pathology in brainstem regions of individuals with primary dystonia. Neurology 1988; 38(5):702–706.
20. Walker RH, Brin MF, Sandu D, et al. TorsinA immunoreactivity in brains of patients with DYT1 and non-DYT1 dystonia. Neurology 2002; 58(1):120–124.
21. Rostasy K, Augood SJ, Hewett JW, et al. TorsinA protein and neuropathology in early onset generalized dystonia with GAG deletion. Neurobiol Dis 2003; 12(1):11–24.
22. McNaught KS, Shashidharan P, Perl DP, et al. Aggresome-related biogenesis of Lewy bodies. Eur J Neurosci 2002; 16(11):2136–2148.
23. McNaught KS, Kapustin A, Jackson T, et al. Brainstem pathology in DYT1 primary torsion dystonia. Ann Neurol 2004; 56(4):540–547.
24. Gonzalez-Alegre P, Paulson HL. Aberrant cellular behavior of mutant torsinA implicates nuclear envelope dysfunction in DYT1 dystonia. J Neurosci 2004; 24(11): 2593–2601.
25. Goodchild RE, Dauer WT. Mislocalization to the nuclear envelope: an effect of the dystonia-causing torsinA mutation. Proc Natl Acad Sci U S A 2004; 101(3):847–852.
26. Naismith TV, Heuser JE, Breakefield XO, et al. TorsinA in the nuclear envelope. Proc Natl Acad Sci U S A 2004; 101(20):7612–7617.
27. Bragg DC, Camp SM, Kaufman CA, et al. Perinuclear biogenesis of mutant torsin-A inclusions in cultured cells infected with tetracycline-regulated herpes simplex virus type 1 amplicon vectors. Neuroscience 2004; 125(3):651–661.
28. Goodchild RE, Kim CE, Dauer WT. Loss of the dystonia-associated protein torsina selectively disrupts the neuronal nuclear envelope. Neuron 2005; 48(6):923–932.
29. Dang MT, Yokoi F, McNaught KS, et al. Generation and characterization of Dyt1 DeltaGAG knock-in mouse as a model for early-onset dystonia. Exp Neurol 2005; 196(2):452–463.
30. Shashidharan P, Sandu D, Potla U, et al. Transgenic mouse model of early-onset DYT1 dystonia. Hum Mol Genet 2005; 14(1):125–133.
31. Takakusaki K, Oohinata-Sugimoto J, Saitoh K, et al. Role of basal ganglia-brainstem systems in the control of postural muscle tone and locomotion. Prog Brain Res 2004; 143:231–237.

32. Takakusaki K, Habaguchi T, Ohtinata-Sugimoto J, et al. Basal ganglia efferents to the brainstem centers controlling postural muscle tone and locomotion: a new concept for understanding motor disorders in basal ganglia dysfunction. Neuroscience 2003; 119(1):293–308.
33. Jordan LM. Initiation of locomotion in mammals. Ann N Y Acad Sci 1998; 860:83–93.
34. Pahapill PA, Lozano AM. The pedunculopontine nucleus and Parkinson's disease. Brain 2000; 123(Pt 9):1767–1783.
35. Mena-Segovia J, Bolam JP, Magill PJ. Pedunculopontine nucleus and basal ganglia: distant relatives or part of the same family? Trends Neurosci 2004; 27(10):585–588.
36. Skinner RD, Garcia-Rill E. The mesencephalic locomotor region (MLR) in the rat. Brain Res 1984; 323(2):385–389.
37. Pittock SJ, Joyce C, O'Keane V, et al. Rapid-onset dystonia-parkinsonism - A clinical and genetic analysis of a new kindred. Neurology 2000; 55(7):991–995.
38. Graybiel AM, Canales JJ, Capper-Loup C. Levodopa-induced dyskinesias and dopamine-dependent stereotypies: a new hypothesis. Trends Neurosci 2000; 23(10):S71–S77.
39. Albin RL, Young AB, Penney JB. The functional anatomy of basal ganglia disorders. TINS 1989; 12:366–375.
40. DeLong MR. Primate models of movement disorders of basal ganglia origin. Trends Neurosci 1990; 13:281–285.
41. Marsden CD, Obeso JA, Zarranz JJ, et al. The anatomical basis of symptomatic hemidystonia. Brain 1985; 108:463–483.
42. Bhatia KP, Marsden CD. The behavioural and motor consequences of focal lesions of the basal ganglia in man. Brain 1994; 117:859–876.
43. Walker RH, Purohit DP, Good PF, et al. Severe generalized dystonia due to primary putaminal degeneration: case report and review of the literature. Mov Disord 2002; 17(3):576–584.
44. Altrocchi PM, Forno LM. Spontaneous oral-facial dyskinesia: neuropathology of a case. Neurology 1983; 33(6):802–805.
45. Kremer B, Weber B, Hayden MR. New insights into the clinical features, pathogenesis and molecular genetics of Huntington disease. Brain Pathol 1992; 2(4):321–335.
46. Penney JB, Young AB, Shoulson I, et al. Huntington's disease in Venezuela: 7 years of follow-up on symptomatic and asymptomatic individuals. Mov Disord 1990; 5(2):93–99.
47. Reiner A, Albin RL, Anderson KD, et al. Differential loss of striatal projection neurons in Huntington disease. Proc Natl Acad Sci USA 1988; 85(15):5733–5737.
48. Low PA, Allsop JL. Huntington's chorea—the rigid form (Westphal variant) treated with l-DOPA: a case report. Proc Aust Assoc Neurol 1973; 10(0):45–46.
49. Bonelli RM, Niederwieser G, Diez J, et al. Pramipexole ameliorates neurologic and psychiatric symptoms in a Westphal variant of Huntington's disease. Clin Neuropharmacol 2002; 25(1):58–60.
50. Oyanagi K, Takeda S, Takahashi H, et al. A quantitative investigation of the substantia nigra in Huntington's disease. Ann Neurol 1989; 26(1):13–19.
51. Bugiani O, Tabaton M, Cammarata S. Huntington's disease: survival of large striatal neurons in the rigid variant. Ann Neurol 1984; 15(2):154–156.
52. Walker RH, Rasmussen A, Rudnicki D, et al. Huntington's Disease-like 2 can present as chorea-acanthocytosis. Neurology 2003; 61(7):1002–1004.
53. Walker RH, Jankovic J, O'Hearn E, et al. Phenotypic Features of Huntington Disease-like 2. Mov Disord 2003; 18(12):1527–1530.
54. Danek A, Walker RH. Neuroacanthocytosis. Curr Opin Neurol 2005; 18(4):386–392.
55. Rampoldi L, Danek A, Monaco AP. Clinical features and molecular bases of neuroacanthocytosis. J Mol Med 2002; 80(8):475–491.
56. Boesch SM, Wenning GK, Ransmayr G, et al. Dystonia in multiple system atrophy. J Neurol Neurosurg Psychiatry 2002; 72(3):300–303.
57. Risvoll H, Kerty E. To test or not? The value of diagnostic tests in cervical dystonia. Mov Disord 2001; 16(2):286–289.

58. Magalhaes AC, Caramelli P, Menezes JR, et al. Wilson's disease: MRI with clinical correlation. Neuroradiology 1994; 36(2):97–100.
59. Page RA, Davie CA, Macmanus D, et al. Clinical correlation of brain MRI and MRS abnormalities in patients with Wilson disease. Neurology 2004; 63(4):638–643.
60. Sener RN. Diffusion MR imaging changes associated with Wilson disease. AJNR Am J Neuroradiol 2003; 24(5):965–967.
61. Elwes R, Saunders M. Generalized dystonia, whispering dysphonia and Wilson's disease in members of the same family [letter]. J Neurol Neurosurg Psychiatry 1986; 49:107.
62. Geschwind DH, Loginov M, Stern JM. Identification of a locus on chromosome 14q for idiopathic basal ganglia calcification (Fahr disease). Am J Hum Genet 1999; 65(3): 764–772.
63. Brodaty H, Mitchell P, Luscombe G, et al. Familial idiopathic basal ganglia calcification (Fahr's disease) without neurological, cognitive and psychiatric symptoms is not linked to the IBGC1 locus on chromosome 14q. Hum Genet 2002; 110(1):8–14.
64. Oliveira JR, Spiteri E, Sobrido MJ, et al. Genetic heterogeneity in familial idiopathic basal ganglia calcification (Fahr disease). Neurology 2004; 63(11):2165–2167.
65. Younes-Mhenni S, Thobois S, Streichenberger N, et al. [Mitochondrial encephalomyopathy, lactic acidosis and stroke-like episodes (Melas) associated with a Fahr disease and cerebellar calcifications]. Rev Med Interne 2002; 23(12):1027–1029.
66. Reske-Nielsen E, Jensen PK, Hein-Sorensen O, et al. Calcification of the central nervous system in a new hereditary neurological syndrome. Acta Neuropathol (Berl) 1988; 75(6): 590–596.
67. Goldman JE, Katz D, Rapin I, et al. Chronic GM1 gangliosidosis presenting as dystonia: I. Clinical and pathological features. Ann Neurol 1981; 9:465–475.
68. Uyama E, Terasaki T, Watanabe S, et al. Type-3 GM1 gangliosidosis: characteristic MRI findings correlated with dystonia. Acta Neurol Scand 1992; 86:609–615.
69. Yoshida K, Ikeda S, Kawaguchi K, et al. Adult GM1 gangliosidosis: immunohistochemical and ultrastructural findings in an autopsy case. Neurology 1994; 44(12): 2376–2382.
70. Muthane U, Chickabasaviah Y, Kaneski C, et al. Clinical features of adult GM1 gangliosidosis: report of three Indian patients and review of 40 cases. Mov Disord 2004; 19(11):1334–1341.
71. Meek D, Wolfe LS, Andermann E, et al. Juvenile progressive dystonia: a new phenotype of GM2 gangliosidosis. Ann Neurol 1984; 15(4):348–352.
72. Nardocci N, Bertagnolio B, Rumi V, et al. Progressive dystonia symptomatic of juvenile GM2 gangliosidosis [see comments]. Mov Disord 1992; 7:64–67.
73. Hardie RJ, Young EP, Morgan-Hughes JA. Hexosaminidase A deficiency presenting as juvenile progressive dystonia [letter]. J Neurol Neurosurg Psychiatry 1988; 51(3):446–447.
74. Cardoso F, Camargos S. Juvenile parkinsonism: a heterogeneous entity. Eur J Neurol 2000; 7(5):467–471.
75. Coleman RJ, Robb SA, Lake BD, et al. The diverse neurological features of Niemann-Pick disease type C: a report of two cases. Mov Disord 1988; 3(4):295–299.
76. Mole SE. The genetic spectrum of human neuronal ceroid-lipofuscinoses. Brain Pathol 2004; 14(1):70–76.
77. Simonati A, Santorum E, Tessa A, et al. A CLN2 gene nonsense mutation is associated with severe caudate atrophy and dystonia in LINCL. Neuropediatrics 2000; 31(4): 199–201.
78. Boustany RM, Alroy J, Kolodny EH. Clinical classification of neuronal ceroid-lipofuscinosis subtypes. Am J Med Genet Suppl 1988; 5:47–58.
79. Aberg LE, Rinne JO, Rajantie I, et al. A favorable response to antiparkinsonian treatment in juvenile neuronal ceroid lipofuscinosis. Neurology 2001; 56(9):1236–1239.
80. Goldenberg PC, Steiner RD, Merkens LS, et al. Remarkable improvement in adult Leigh syndrome with partial cytochrome c oxidase deficiency. Neurology 2003; 60(5): 865–868.

81. Crimi M, Galbiati S, Moroni I, et al. A missense mutation in the mitochondrial ND5 gene associated with a Leigh-MELAS overlap syndrome. Neurology 2003; 60(1): 1857–1861.
82. Tanji K, Kunimatsu T, Vu TH, et al. Neuropathological features of mitochondrial disorders. Semin Cell Dev Biol 2001; 12(6):429–439.
83. Tranebjaerg L, Jensen PK, van Ghelue M, et al. Neuronal cell death in the visual cortex is a prominent feature of the X-linked recessive mitochondrial deafness-dystonia syndrome caused by mutations in the TIMM8a gene. Ophthalmic Genet 2001; 22(4): 207–223.
84. Swerdlow RH, Wooten GF. A novel deafness/dystonia peptide gene mutation that causes dystonia in female carriers of Mohr-Tranebjaerg syndrome. Ann Neurol 2001; 50(4):537–540.
85. Scribanu N, Kennedy C. Familial Syndrome With Dystonia, Neural Deafness, and Possible Intellectual Impairment: Clinical Course and Pathological Findings. New York: Raven Press, 1976:235–243.
86. Gearing M, Juncos JL, Procaccio V, et al. Aggregation of actin and cofilin in identical twins with juvenile-onset dystonia. Ann Neurol 2002; 52(4):465–476.
87. Smith JM, Oswald WT, Kucharski LT, et al. Tardive dyskinesia: age and sex differences in hospitalized schizophrenics. Psychopharmacology (Berl) 1978; 58(2):207–211.
88. Hunter R, Blackwood W, Smith MC, et al. Neuropathological findings in three cases of persistent dyskinesia following phenothiazine medication. J Neurol Sci 1968; 7(2): 263–273.
89. Christensen E, Moller JE, Faurbye A. Neuropathological investigation of 28 brains from patients with dyskinesia. Acta Psychiatr Scand 1970; 46(1):14–23.
90. Vitek JL, Chockkan V, Zhang JY, et al. Neuronal activity in the basal ganglia in patients with generalized dystonia and hemiballismus. Ann Neurol 1999; 46(1):22–35.
91. Silberstein P, Kuhn AA, Kupsch A, et al. Patterning of globus pallidus local field potentials differs between Parkinson's disease and dystonia. Brain 2003; 126:2597–2608.
92. Vidailhet M, Vercueil L, Houeto JL, et al. Bilateral deep-brain stimulation of the globus pallidus in primary generalized dystonia. N Engl J Med 2005; 352(5):459–467.
93. Barclay CL, Lang AE. Dystonia in progressive supranuclear palsy. J Neurol Neurosurg Psychiatry 1997; 62(4):352–356.
94. Oide T, Ohara S, Yazawa M, et al. Progressive supranuclear palsy with asymmetric tau pathology presenting with unilateral limb dystonia. Acta Neuropathol (Berl) 2002; 104(2):209–214.
95. Tan EK, Chan LL, Wong MC. Levodopa-induced oromandibular dystonia in progressive supranuclear palsy. Clin Neurol Neurosurg 2003; 105(2):132–134.
96. Mubaidin A, Roberts E, Hampshire D, et al. Karak syndrome: a novel degenerative disorder of the basal ganglia and cerebellum. J Med Genet 2003; 40(7):543–546.
97. Thomas M, Jankovic J. Neurodegenerative disease and iron storage in the brain. Curr Opin Neurol 2004; 17(4):437–442.
98. Rouault TA. Iron on the brain. Nat Genet 2001; 28(4):299–300.
99. Zhou B, Westaway SK, Levinson B, et al. A novel pantothenate kinase gene (*PANK2*) is defective in Hallervorden-Spatz syndrome. Nat Genet 2001; 28(4):345–349.
100. Hayflick SJ, Westaway SK, Levinson B, et al. Genetic, clinical, and radiographic delineation of Hallervorden-Spatz syndrome. N Engl J Med 2003; 348(1):33–40.
101. Crompton DE, Chinnery PF, Bates D, et al. Spectrum of movement disorders in neuroferritinopathy. Mov Disord 2004; 20(1):95–99.
102. Mir P, Edwards MJ, Curtis AR, et al. Adult-onset generalized dystonia due to a mutation in the neuroferritinopathy gene. Mov Disord 2004; 20(2):243–245.
103. Wills AJ, Sawle GV, Guilbert PR, et al. Palatal tremor and cognitive decline in neuroferritinopathy. J Neurol Neurosurg Psychiatry 2002; 73(1):91–92.
104. Playford ED, Fletcher NA, Sawle GV, et al. Striatal [F-18]dopa uptake in familial idiopathic dystonia. Brain 1993; 116:1191–1199.

105. Perlmutter JS, Stambuk MK, Markham J, et al. Decreased [18F]spiperone binding in putamen in dystonia. Adv Neurol 1998; 78:161–168.
106. Rinne JO, Iivanainen M, Metsahonkala L, et al. Striatal dopaminergic system in dopa-responsive dystonia: a multi-tracer PET study shows increased D2 receptors. J Neural Transm 2004; 111(1):59–67.
107. Augood SJ, Hollingsworth Z, Albers DS, et al. Dopamine transmission in DYT1 dystonia: a biochemical and autoradiographical study. Neurology 2002; 59(3):445–448.
108. Djaldetti R, Mosberg-Galili R, Sroka H, et al. Camptocormia (bent spine) in patients with Parkinson's disease—characterization and possible pathogenesis of an unusual phenomenon. Mov Disord 1999; 14(3):443–447.
109. Morrison PJ, Patterson VH. Cranial dystonia (Meige syndrome) in postencephalitic parkinsonism. Mov Disord 1992; 7(1):90–91.
110. LeWitt PA, Burns RS, Newman RP. Dystonia in untreated parkinsonism. Clin Neuropharm 1986; 9(3):293–297.
111. Poewe WH, Lees AJ, Stern GM. Dystonia in Parkinson's disease: clinical and pharmacological features. Ann Neurol 1988; 23(1):73–78.
112. Katchen M, Duvoisin RC. Parkinsonism following dystonia in three patients. Mov Disord 1986; 1(2):151–157.
113. Singleton A. What does PINK1 mean for Parkinson diseases? Neurology 2004; 63(8):1350–1351.
114. Khan NL, Graham E, Critchley P, et al. Parkin disease: a phenotypic study of a large case series. Brain 2003; 126(6):1279–1292.
115. Tan LC, Tanner CM, Chen R, et al. Marked variation in clinical presentation and age of onset in a family with a heterozygous parkin mutation. Mov Disord 2003; 18(7):758–763.
116. Lohmann E, Periquet M, Bonifati V, et al. How much phenotypic variation can be attributed to parkin genotype? Ann Neurol 2003; 54(2):176–185.
117. Quinn N, Critchley P, Marsden CD. Young onset Parkinson's disease. Mov Disord 1987; 2(2):73–91.
118. Tassin J, Durr A, Bonnet AM, et al. Levodopa-responsive dystonia. GTP cyclohydrolase I or parkin mutations? Brain 2000; 123 Pt 6:1112–1121.
119. Polymeropoulos MH, Lavedan C, Leroy E, et al. Mutation in the alpha-synuclein gene identified in families with Parkinson's disease. Science 1997; 276(5321):2045–2047.
120. Leroy E, Boyer R, Auburger G, et al. The ubiquitin pathway in Parkinson's disease. Nature 1998; 395(6701):451–452.
121. Bonifati V, Rizzu P, Squitieri F, et al. DJ-1(PARK7), a novel gene for autosomal recessive, early onset parkinsonism. Neurol Sci 2003; 24(3):159–160.
122. Valente EM, Abou-Sleiman PM, Caputo V, et al. Hereditary early-onset Parkinson's disease caused by mutations in PINK1. Science 2004; 304(5674):1158–1160.
123. Zimprich A, Muller-Myhsok B, Farrer M, et al. The PARK8 locus in autosomal dominant parkinsonism: confirmation of linkage and further delineation of the disease-containing interval. Am J Hum Genet 2004; 74(1):11–19.
124. Clark LN, Afridi S, Mejia-Santana H, et al. Analysis of an early-onset Parkinson's disease cohort for DJ-1 mutations. Mov Disord 2004; 19(7):796–800.
125. Rajput A, Kishore A, Snow B, et al. Dopa-responsive, nonprogressive juvenile parkinsonism: report of a case. Mov Disord 1997; 12(3):453–456.
126. Segawa M, Nishiyama N, Nomura Y. DOPA-responsive dystonic parkinsonism—pathophysiologic considerations. Adv Neurol 1999; 80:389–400.
127. Paviour DC, Revesz T, Holton JL, et al. Neuronal intranuclear inclusion disease: report on a case originally diagnosed as dopa-responsive dystonia with Lewy bodies. Mov Disord 2005; 20(10):1345–1349.
128. Cooper IS. 20-year followup study of the neurosurgical treatment of dystonia musculorum deformans. Adv Neurol 1976; 14:423–452.
129. Tasker RR, Doorly T, Yamashiro K. Thalamotomy in generalized dystonia. Adv Neurol 1988; 50:615–632.

130. Cardoso F, Jankovic J, Grossman RG, et al. Outcome after stereotactic thalamotomy for dystonia and hemiballismus. Neurosurgery 1995; 36(3):501–507.
131. Yamashiro K, Tasker RR. Stereotactic thalamotomy for dystonic patients. Stereotact Funct Neurosurg 1993; 60:81–85.
132. Lehericy S, Grand S, Pollak P, et al. Clinical characteristics and topography of lesions in movement disorders due to thalamic lesions. Neurology 2001; 57(6):1055–1066.
133. Asanuma K, Ma Y, Huang C, et al. The metabolic pathology of dopa-responsive dystonia. Ann Neurol 2005; 57(4):596–600.
134. Ledoux MS, Lorden JF. Abnormal cerebellar output in the genetically dystonic rat. Adv Neurol 1998; 78:63–78.
135. Ledoux MS, Lorden JF, Ervin JM. Cerebellectomy eliminates the motor syndrome of the genetically dystonic rat. Exp Neurol 1993; 120:302–310.
136. Stevanin G, Fujigasaki H, Lebre AS, et al. Huntington's disease-like phenotype due to trinucleotide repeat expansions in the TBP and JPH3 genes. Brain 2003; 126:1599–1603.
137. Zuhlke C, Gehlken U, Hellenbroich Y, et al. Phenotypical variability of expanded alleles in the TATA-binding protein gene. Reduced penetrance in SCA17? J Neurol 2003; 250(2):161–163.
138. Nakamura K, Jeong SY, Uchihara T, et al. SCA17, a novel autosomal dominant cerebellar ataxia caused by an expanded polyglutamine in TATA-binding protein. Hum Mol Genet 2001; 10(14):1441–1448.
139. Schmidtke K, Endres W, Roscher A, et al. Hartnup syndrome, progressive encephalopathy and allo-albuminaemia. A clinico-pathological case study. Eur J Pediatr 1992; 151(12): 899–903.
140. Tahmoush AJ, Alpers DH, Feigin RD, et al. Hartnup disease. Clinical, pathological, and biochemical observations. Arch Neurol 1976; 33(12):797–807.
141. Magnuson TM, Roccaforte WH, Wengel SP, et al. Medication-induced dystonias in nine patients with dementia. J Neuropsychiatry Clin Neurosci 2000; 12(2):219–225.
142. Miyaoka T, Seno H, Yamamori C, et al. Pisa syndrome due to a cholinesterase inhibitor (donepezil): a case report. J Clin Psychiatry 2001; 62(7):573–574.
143. Kwak YT, Han IW, Baik J, et al. Relation between cholinesterase inhibitor and Pisa syndrome. Lancet 2000; 355(9222):2222.

# 7

# Neuroimaging in Dystonia

**A. R. Troiano and A. J. Stoessl**
*Pacific Parkinson's Research Centre, University of British Columbia, Vancouver, British Columbia, Canada*

## INTRODUCTION

In the last decades, technological innovations have provided a deeper understanding of the mechanisms underlying neurological disorders. Magnetic resonance imaging (MRI) has evolved into functional magnetic resonance imaging (fMRI), with the ability to discern changes in cerebral function with good temporal resolution. Increases in spatial resolution of positron-emission tomography (PET) and single-photon emission computed tomography (SPECT), associated with the development of new radiotracers, have also allowed novel approaches to the study of disease. The impact of such advances is particularly pronounced in the fields of movement disorders (MDs) and epilepsy. The investigation of Parkinson's disease (PD) and dystonia has benefited substantially from this more widely available technology. In PD, functional imaging is useful in detecting dopaminergic cell loss and changes in cerebral metabolic rates during the performance of behavioral or motor tasks. As for the various forms of dystonia, imaging has corroborated what was suggested in clinical and pathological investigations: instead of a single pathologic focus, dystonia is the consequence of dysfunction in the cortico-subcortical networks of sensorimotor control, in which the basal ganglia represent only one of the players.

This chapter discusses the contributions of structural and functional imaging in studying dystonia of various etiologies. In keeping with other segments of this book, imaging challenges in dystonia will be approached from an etiologic basis.

## SECONDARY DYSTONIAS

Dystonia may be the presenting feature or a late accompanying symptom of a vast number of neurological disorders (Table 1). Age and mode of onset, family history, associated signs, and presentation are helpful clinical clues to distinguish idiopathic from secondary dystonia. Unless dystonia is restricted to the face or neck, virtually every patient with dystonia without a clear family history of MD will undergo structural imaging. This is indicated because dystonia is the most common MD following insults to the basal ganglia. Putamen and globus pallidus (GP) lesions are more

**Table 1** Structural Imaging Findings in Secondary Dystonia

| | |
|---|---|
| *Dystonia-plus syndrome* | |
| Progressive supranuclear palsy | Decreased midbrain area (1) |
| Multiple system atrophy—parkinsonism | Putaminal "slit," midbrain hyperintensity, MRS decreased NAA/Cr ratios (2), DWI increased putaminal diffusivity (3), MRI volumetry decreased striatal and brainstem volumes (4) |
| Corticobasal degeneration | Asymmetric posterior frontal and parietal atrophy |
| Dopa-responsive dystonia | Normal |
| Dystonia-myoclonus | Normal |
| *Heredodegenerative* | |
| X-linked | |
| Lubag | Striatal atrophy |
| Pelizaeus-Merzbacher disease | MRI "tigroid" hemispheric white matter lesions, MRS white matter high NAA/Cho, low Cho/Cr ratios (5) |
| Lesch-Nyhan syndrome | Caudate atrophy (6) |
| Autosomal dominant | |
| Huntington's disease | Caudate and putamen atrophy |
| Autosomal recessive | |
| Wilson's disease | Signal changes in basal ganglia (may improve with therapy) |
| Neurodegeneration with brain iron accumulation type 1, pantothenate kinase-associated neurodegeneration | Iron deposition in globus pallidus (eye-of-the-tiger sign, not always present) (7) |
| Acanthocytosis | Cortical atrophy, signal alteration, or atrophy on caudate and putamen |
| Ataxia-telangiectasia | Cerebellar atrophy |
| Unknown mode of inheritance | |
| Rett syndrome | Nonspecific cortical and white matter atrophy |
| Familial basal ganglia calcifications | Basal ganglia calcifications (particularly on CT scan) |
| *Metabolic disorders* | |
| Glutaric academia | Brain atrophy or hypoplasia, white matter changes, wide open opercula, and basal ganglia lesions (8) |
| Methylmalonic acidemia | Hyperintensity globus pallidus (9) |
| Homocystinuria | Nonspecific findings |
| Metachromatic leukodystrophy | "Tigroid," "leopard-skin" in deep white matter (10) |
| Ceroid lipofuscinosis | Cerebral and cerebellar atrophy, cortical thinning, and white matter changes (11) |
| Niemann-Pick type C | Cerebral atrophy, brainstem abnormalities |
| GM1 Gangliosidosis | Bilateral putaminal abnormalities |
| GM2 Gangliosidosis | Childhood onset: basal ganglia and thalamic abnormalities, thalamic hyperdensity (12), juvenile onset: cortical, white matter, and cerebellar atrophy (12–14) |
| *Mitochondrial disorders* | |
| Leigh's disease | Hyperintensities in basal ganglia (putamen), brainstem, and dentate nucleus |
| Leber's disease | White matter changes, possible association with multiple sclerosis–like presentation |

*Abbreviations*: Cho, choline; Cr, creatine; CT, computerized tomography; DWI, diffusion-weighted imaging; MRI, magnetic resonance imaging; MRS, magnetic resonance spectroscopy; NAA, *N*-acetylaspartate.

frequently associated with dystonia than caudate lesions. The latter lead more often to behavioral or cognitive, rather than motor disturbances (15). While lesions to the putamen are commonly unilateral, because the GP is susceptible to widespread injury due to hypoxia or exogenous intoxications, bilateral damage is common. Rarely, lacunar infarcts of the thalamus may lead to dystonia or myoclonic dystonia, with well-circumscribed lesions of the centromedian, sensory (16), ventral intermediate, and ventral caudal nuclei having been reported (17).

## Cerebrovascular Disease

Cerebrovascular disease of distinct etiologies may evolve into dystonia. Although *chorea* is the most prevalent dyskinesia after stroke (18), generalized dystonia or hemidystonia may develop from days to months after the vascular event. Typically, MRI will demonstrate lesions of the basal ganglia and thalamus, but brainstem and telencephalic lesions of frontal, temporal, occipital, and parietal lobes are also seen (18). Dystonic contraction of the upper limb is seen in the setting of parietal lobe stroke, particularly of the posterior division of the parietal branch of the Sylvian artery (19). A variable time interval between insult and onset of MD is also seen in hemidystonia. The lesions are usually of vascular origin, but small vascular tumors have also been described. Although vascular lesions are often suggested by the presence of risk factors for stroke or a history of craniocerebral trauma (including perinatal trauma) (20), in cases of childhood-onset progressive hemidystonia it is advisable to rule out primary antiphospholipid syndrome (21–26).

## Craniocerebral Trauma

Traumatic brain injury (TBI) is uncommonly followed by the appearance of dystonia. There is often a time lapse between the event and development of dystonia. This interval could be due to initial hemiplegia preventing the manifestation of dystonia or due to neuronal plasticity that may be more prominent in young individuals (27). While severe trauma is associated with extensive neuro-radiological findings, the effects of relatively minor head trauma remain unknown. With severe head trauma, imaging consistently identifies lesions in contralateral subcortical nuclei. Review of two large dystonia-related TBI studies totaling 19 subjects finds that lesions of the internal capsule were noted in 11 individuals and in every instance were associated with other striatal and pallidal lesions. Whenever putamen and caudate were considered in isolation, putaminal lesions were observed in eight individuals and caudate in four others. Lesions of the lentiform nucleus as a whole (putamen and GP) were present in four patients. Pallidal and thalamic lesions were observed in four individuals each. In addition to this topography, there was a vast array of telencephalic lesions, comprising fronto-temporal and occipital hypodensities and, on long-term follow-up, regional cerebral atrophy with dilated lateral ventricles and white matter changes (27,28).

## Dystonia-Plus Syndromes

The interpretation of MRI findings in dystonia-plus syndromes remains somewhat speculative, given that description of imaging findings by necessity cannot focus only on lesions associated with dystonic muscle contractions. While not typically used to confirm the diagnosis of progressive supranuclear palsy, MRI may demonstrate decreased midbrain area when compared to other forms of parkinsonism (1,29).

In multiple system atrophy (MSA), predominance of parkinsonian features correlates with a rim on the dorsolateral putamen detected on MRI, secondary to gliosis and local deposits of iron (30). Whether this striatal abnormality also correlates with dystonic cramping is not known. Pontine signal changes ("hot cross bun sign") are also seen in MSA, and are consistently more related to cerebellar disturbances (31).

Dystonia may be an early feature of Huntington's disease (HD), more so in early-onset rigid-akinetic forms. Internal shoulder rotation, fist clenching, and excessive knee flexion are its most common forms (32). In pregenetic testing times, computed tomography (CT) scan was regularly employed for the diagnosis of HD, showing bilateral atrophy of the caudate and putamen with an apparent increase of the lateral ventricles. More recently, magnetic resonance-based spectroscopy and voxel-based morphometry (VBM) allow the study of more specific disease-related alterations that could potentially be followed in the future, because new treatments emerge. In early HD, VBM showed a pattern of degeneration comparable to that of pathological studies, in which dorsal and caudal striatum are primarily affected (33).

Neurodegeneration with brain iron accumulation type 1 (NBIA1) is a rare autosomal recessive neurological disorder of variable age of onset, attributed to mutation of the pantothenate kinase 2 (*PANK2*) gene. Most individuals with childhood onset (typical NBIA1) display dystonia, and more commonly, choreathetosis, corticospinal tract signs, retinitis pigmentosa, optic atrophy, and cognitive impairment. Adult-onset (atypical NBIA1) cases predominantly manifest with parkinsonism. Virtually all individuals homozygous for the *PANK2* mutation demonstrate a pathognomonic MRI pattern, characterized by bilateral hypointensity of the GP with a central area of hyperintensity on T2-weighted images—classically termed the "eye-of-the-tiger" sign. However, this MRI finding may be present only early in the disease. A report of one child with progressive neurological decline demonstrated this MRI finding after four years of symptoms with a follow-up scan at 11 years showing only nonspecific pallidal changes (7).

Although the neurological form of Wilson's disease (WD) typically starts with dysarthria, tremor, and dysgraphia, 40% to 65% of patients develop dystonia in the course of disease, 50% of those displaying generalized dystonia (34,35). Similar to other secondary conditions, peripheral putaminal lesions on T2-weighted images correlate with the presence of dystonic movements, whereas parkinsonism is related to both striatal and nigral lesions (36). Functional imaging suggests a relationship between regional or global cerebral blood flow and disease severity (37,38). In Wilson's disease (WD) displaying parkinsonism or dystonia, there is evidence for presynaptic dopaminergic abnormalities, as shown with [$^{18}$F] dopa (39) and [$^{11}$C]-(+)-nomifensine, which binds to the dopamine transporter (DAT) (40). Interestingly, both MRI lesions and decreased binding to D2 receptors tend to improve with D-penicillamine or other chelation therapy (41,42).

## THE DOPAMINE SYSTEM IN DYSTONIA

Evidence linking impairment of the dopaminergic axis to symptoms of dystonia remains unclear, but may be a function of dynamic rather than slowly progressive changes. From a clinical perspective, the "off"-period dystonia in PD is quite likely associated with falling levels of synaptic nigrostriatal dopamine (DA), while acute drug-induced dystonia is seen in the setting of recent introduction of DA receptor blocking drugs. In addition, animals exposed to N-methyl-4-phenyl-1,2,3,6-tetrahydropyridine (MPTP) display dystonic symptoms as they evolved to more characteristic signs of parkinsonism (43). While dysfunction of the dopaminergic pathways is less convincing in the setting of primary dystonia, postmortem examination has demonstrated moderate depletion of DA in anterior striatal regions, but the overall change does not appear to be sufficient to cause dystonia (44,45). Given other reports of increased striatal levels of the DA metabolite 3,4-dihydroxyphenylacetic acid in the setting of lower DA levels, perhaps these findings suggest alterations in DA turnover, and relatively dynamic changes at nigrostriatal synapse (46).

Functional neurologic imaging has not provided clear insight into the role of DA turnover in dystonia. An early PET study demonstrating increased striatal $^{18}$F-dopa was the first to suggest increased DA turnover in primary dystonia. In this investigation, Otsuka and coworkers assessed eight subjects, three with generalized symptoms and five with segmental or focal signs. Surprisingly, even in individuals displaying asymmetric clinical findings, the increase in $^{18}$F-dopa uptake was not different between striatal sides (47). In addition, other investigations have reported normal or decreased $^{18}$F-dopa uptake in primary dystonia (24,48,49). Although it is difficult to resolve these data, it should be noted that the presence of reduced $^{18}$F-dopa uptake in individuals with hemidystonia should be viewed with caution, for in most instances there is an associated structural lesion of the contralateral striatum. Furthermore, regional pathologic alterations are associated with vascular changes that alter the uptake of ligand, but may not necessarily reflect neurotransmitter abnormalities.

Another means of measuring presynaptic DA function is to assess DAT availability. Despite inherent limitations, such as variations related to compensatory regulation or the effects of pharmacological intervention, the DAT can be studied using a variety of approaches. Although data concerning the role of the DAT in dystonia remain scarce, Naumann et al. report preservation of presynaptic function using $^{123}$I-β-CIT SPECT in patients with cervical dystonia (50). Given the recent discovery of reduced cell membrane expression of DAT associated with the *DYT1* mutation (51), the role of DA in generalized dystonia may be reemphasized.

## Dopa-Responsive Dystonia

Investigation of presynaptic dopaminergic integrity has been repeatedly targeted in individuals with dopa-responsive dystonia (DRD). The typical form of this disease is inherited as an autosomal dominant trait with loss of function of the guanosine triphosphate cyclohydrolase 1 (*GTPCH1*) gene, limiting the synthesis of DA. DRD may also present with parkinsonism in addition to dystonia, creating a diagnostic uncertainty between DRD and early-onset Parkinson's disease (EOPD) that is usually resolved with genetic testing (52). In such cases, diagnosis may be determined with functional imaging (Table 2). Although initial reports suggested decrease in striatal uptake of [$^{18}$F]-dopa (53,54), Snow et al. (55) demonstrated normal values. Given that *GTPCH1* mutations result in reduced activity of tyrosine hydroxylase, DA striatal uptake in DRD should not be affected (70), and the observation by Snow et al. is now accepted. In retrospect, the neurochemical substrate for DRD was thus predicted by PET studies prior to the identification of mutations in *GTPCH1*, and remains useful in evaluating subjects with variable symptoms of dystonia.

PET visualization of vesicular monoamine transporter (VMAT) (56) and DAT (56,57) confirms postmortem findings that presynaptic dopaminergic terminals are intact in DRD. Indeed, there is an increase in VMAT binding in untreated DRD, possibly reflecting the effects of profound depletion of intravesicular DA, and also explaining the prolonged response to levodopa in this condition, in contrast to

**Table 2** Functional Imaging in Primary Dystonia[a]

| | |
|---|---|
| Dopaminergic radioligands | |
| Primary generalized dystonia | |
| [$^{18}$F]-DOPA | Increased (47), normal (47,48), or decreased (24,49) |
| DAT | Normal (50) |
| Dopa-responsive dystonia | |
| Presynaptic | |
| [$^{18}$F]-DOPA | Decreased (53,54), normal (55) |
| VMAT2 | Elevated (56) |
| DAT | Normal (56–60) |
| Postsynaptic | |
| D1 receptors | Normal (57) |
| Pre/postsynaptic | |
| D2 receptors | Elevated (57,61,62) |
| Cerebral blood flow (CBF) and metabolism | |
| Dystonia-related pattern | Increased metabolism lentiform, pons, midbrain, lateral frontal cortex, and SMA (63,64) |
| Regional CBF | |
| Metabolic disruption of connectivity | Striatum ⟷ premotor cortex (65)<br>Thalamus ⟷ caudate/lentiform nucleus (64,66) |
| Sensorimotor cortex | Increased (67) or decreased (68) |
| Premotor area (at rest) | Increased (64,69) |
| Supplementary motor area | Increased (68) |

[a]Findings of presynaptic dopaminergic integrity are variable, although DAT is usually normal. Increases in D2 receptors in DRD may be due to decreased dopamine synthesis or use of [$^{11}$C]-raclopride as radioligand (see text). Studies of cerebral blood flow disclose metabolic changes in sensorimotor and frontal regions, as well as in the striatum and midbrain.

*Abbreviations*: DAT, dopamine transporter; SMA, supplementary motor area; VMAT2, vesicular monoamine transporter type 2.

PD, in which vesicular trapping of DA is impaired (56,71). Furthermore, unlike the PET findings in DRD, DAT binding is consistently decreased in EOPD. Most studies comparing DAT changes between DRD and EOPD employ SPECT (58–60). This offers a practical advantage, because neuro-PET scanners are usually restricted to research centers and SPECT is more widely available.

In addition to the limited synthesis of DA, D2-like receptors are upregulated in DRD (57,61,62). This cannot be attributed to DA deficiency alone, because the same increase is observed in asymptomatic gene carriers and in symptomatic individuals after prolonged treatment with levodopa (61). These findings suggest that *GTPCH1* gene mutations also lead to cellular changes postsynaptically, instead of a pure presynaptic deficiency of DA.

Although [$^{11}$C]-raclopride binding is susceptible to changes in the availability of endogenous DA, this would not be the case when higher affinity D2 ligands, such as [$^{18}$F]- or [$^{11}$C]-spiperone and [$^{18}$F]-benperidol are used. D1-like receptors are reportedly normal in DRD (57).

## IMAGING STUDIES IN *DYT1* DYSTONIA

Given the paucity of neuropathologic change in idiopathic torsion dystonia, functional neuro-imaging has an important role in determining disease pathogenesis.

While some changes in the dopaminergic axis have been postulated, the role and mechanisms for this pharmacologic alteration are more likely to occur is concert with molecular changes associated with torsinA activity. The *DYT1* gene, localized on chromosome 9q34, encodes torsinA, which is mostly found in the perinuclear envelope of neurons, particularly in the brainstem, cerebellum, and hippocampus (72,73). Molecular diagnosis has allowed the demonstration of neurophysiological evidence that nonmanifesting *DYT1* (*NMDYT*) carriers display abnormal inhibitory cortical mechanisms, but to a lesser extent than individuals manifesting dystonia (74,75). Recently, concurrent positron emission tomography with $H_2{}^{15}O$ demonstrated that, in order to perform the sequence memorization, gene carriers activated larger proportions of prefrontal cortex (right supplementary motor area and left ventral prefrontal cortex), occipital association cortex, and cerebellar hemisphere, while the posterior cingulate cortex was underactive (tasks executed with the right hand) (76). Perhaps these enhanced cortical activations reflect striatal alterations, given that altered supplementary motor area (SMA) pattern activation seems to be part of a more widespread set of network changes in *DYT1* carriers.

Diffusion tensor imaging is another tool, previously used to assess stroke and demyelinating disease, used to discern the spectrum of changes separately manifesting from *NMDYT* carriers (77,78). This image sequencing process, by measuring fractional anisotropy, an index of water diffusivity and organization of axons in parallel bundles of fibers (79), has demonstrated white matter changes underlying the sensorimotor cortex in carriers of torsinA mutations (80). While the subtle changes in myelin seen with *DYT1* may reflect changes underlying pathophysiology of dystonia, the link between DA metabolism and D2-like receptor expression have not been established. However, in vivo investigations suggest that pharmacological stimulation of D2 receptors decreases GP regional blood flow, thereby modulating cortical motor activity (81). Furthermore, speculation concerning the role of the indirect pathway is also relevant, given the decrease in striatal D2 receptor expression associated with the *DYT1* mutation (82–84).

In an effort to better assess the role of DA in *DYT1* dystonia, it is useful to review traditional PET analysis with complex statistical models [Scaled Subprofile Model (SSM)]. Applied to PD, this principle identifies a network composed of increased subcortical metabolism (pallidum, thalamus, and pons) and decreased cortical activation (SMA, lateral premotor, dorsolateral prefrontal cortex (DLPFC), and parietooccipital association cortices) (63,85). In contrast, dystonia features a relative overactivation of the SMA, as well as hypermetabolism of the lentiform nucleus (Fig. 1) (63), and suggests that increased SMA metabolism leads to the muscle co-contractions that characterize dystonia (86). In addition, a disparity of activation between the basal ganglia and thalamus is also noted, with pallidal metabolism uncoupled to thalamic activity (64,66). This lentiform-thalamic dissociation suggests that pallidal activity may be a preponderant factor in the physiopathology of dystonia, and may be a distant effect of mutant torsinA expression in the midbrain reticular formation and periaqueductal grey area, and reduced expression in the basal ganglia (73). Partial support for this concept is the observation of symptomatic benefit from deep brain stimulation (DBS) of the GP (87). Furthermore, regional cerebral blood flow PET has demonstrated that pallidal DBS ameliorates the frontal overactivity observed during performance of a joystick task (88). The abnormalities demonstrated by SSM are highly predictive of patients with symptomatic dystonia (89). This pattern may evolve with disease progression. Thus, *NMDYT* individuals demonstrate increased metabolic activity of the cerebellum, caudate, lentiform nuclei, and SMA

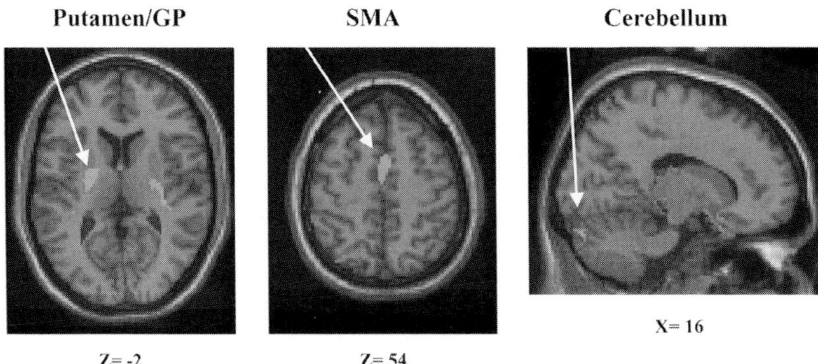


**Figure 1** Fluorodeoxyglucose positron-emission tomography of *DYT1* dystonia. With appropriate statistical models, functional imaging identifies a network of regions responsible for the manifestation of dystonia. Such network, referred to as torsion dystonia-related pattern, is composed of increased metabolism of the globus pallidus, putamen, supplementary motor area, and cerebellar hemisphere. *Abbreviations*: GP, globus pallidus; SMA, supplementary motor area. *Source*: From Ref. 63.

with decreased midbrain activation. Affected *DYT1* patients not only continue to exhibit increased metabolism of the cerebellum and to a lesser extent, cerebral hemispheres (SMA and lateral premotor cortex), but also show increased midbrain and thalamic activity.

## IMAGING STUDIES IN FOCAL DYSTONIA

Current imaging studies in *DYT1* dystonia do not suggest sensory cortex input to the metabolic network studied in dystonia. However, it is difficult to discount the role of sensory modulation in the presence of the *geste antagoniste* in some forms of focal dystonia, as well as the tendency for vibratory stimuli to induce dystonic posturing in writer's cramp (90). Imaging studies in studies of focal dystonia remain difficult to interpret, and disparate findings may be due, in part, to distinct study protocols, and continually improving imaging technology (65,67,68,91). Because writer's cramp is easy to produce in an fMRI protocol, this condition is ideal for this technology. Early fMRI study disclosed abnormal mechanisms of muscle relaxation in writer's cramp (92). Delmaire and colleagues postulated that changes in fluidity of muscle contraction and relaxation, while thought to be a basal ganglia function, may represent somatotopic misrepresentations of the cortex (93). Using fMRI during the performance of finger and toe movements on the affected side (without triggering dystonia), patients activated portions of the contralateral putamen when compared to normal controls.

The connections between frontal areas and basal ganglia, as part of the cortico-striato-pallidal-cortical loop, are a point of particular interest, because disrupted communication between structures could underlie the emergence of dystonia. Loss of normal coupling between thalamus and caudate/lentiform metabolism was reported in earlier studies (66) and replicated with more recent PET methods (64). A similar disconnection was shown in patients with writer's cramp, in which discrepant metabolic rates were noted between the striatum and premotor cortex and between contralateral premotor cortices (Fig. 2) (65).

In individuals scanned at rest, there is consistent premotor hypermetabolism (64,69). Findings are less clear when voluntary movement comes into play: during

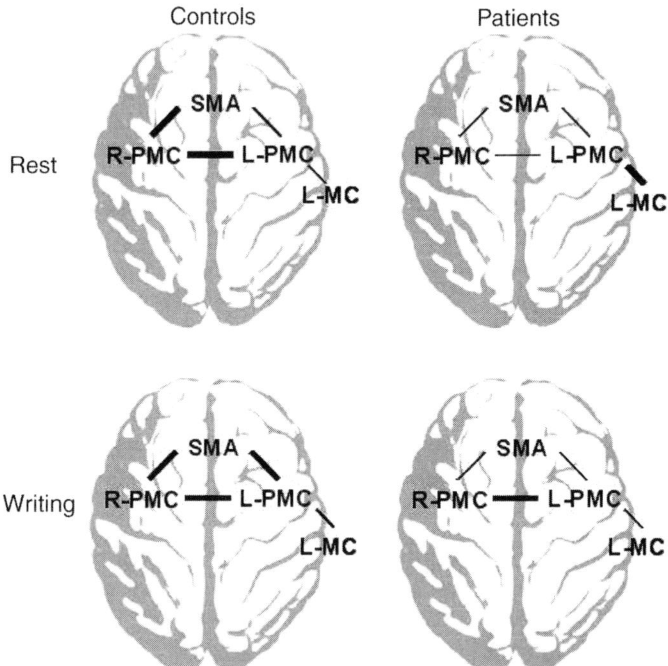


**Figure 2** Schematic representation of cortical activations obtained with rCBF positron-emission tomography at rest and during handwriting in individuals with writer's cramp and controls. At rest and during the writing task, the connections between frontal regions are decreased in patients, compared to controls. Thick lines represent statistically significant correlations. *Abbreviations*: PMC, premotor cortex; SMA, supplementary motor area; MC, motor cortex (L=left, R=right). *Source*: Adapted from Ref. 65.

dystonia-inducing tasks, metabolic activity in the premotor area may either decrease (65,67) or increase (94). Analogous increments are also observed during joystick manipulation (91). The failure of activation of premotor areas [as well as caudal SMA (68)] could potentially explain the slowness of movements observed in dystonia. While this literature remains controversial, elevated metabolism of some cortical areas is used to justify dystonia (91), while decreased activation is thought to explain bradykinesia, reflecting our limited understanding of motor control (64,68,95).

## CONCLUSION

Neuroimaging has become an indispensable part of the assessment and research of dystonia. In primary forms of the disease, functional imaging endorses prior hypotheses of disturbances of the DA system, constituted by pre- and postsynaptic alterations. This is also the case with DRD, in which D2 receptors are upregulated. Studies of cerebral blood flow and glucose consumption suggest that interconnected cortico-subcortical structures participate in the physiopathology of this condition. Whereas the basal ganglia display conspicuously increased metabolism, prefrontal, premotor, and sensorimotor areas present variable metabolic changes. This can be a result of disease mechanisms that differ between focal and generalized dystonia and distinct study methods. PET studies associated with sensory stimuli support the concept that dystonia is the result of impaired sensory and motor processing, rather than an exclusively motor disorder.

Interference with abnormal pallidal activity could underlie the clinical improvement following globus pallidus deep brain stimulation (GPi DBS) in selected patients. In secondary dystonia, structural imaging frequently identifies putaminal lesions. In addition, MRI virtually establishes the diagnosis in conditions such as NBIA1, supports clinical decision making in MSA and might help treatment follow-up in WD. Future developments might establish the role of functional and structural imaging in the differential diagnosis of dystonic disorders and treatment follow up.

## REFERENCES

1. Oba H, Yagishita A, Terada H, et al. New and reliable MRI diagnosis for progressive supranuclear palsy. Neurology 2005; 64:2050–2055.
2. Davie CA, Wenning GK, Barker GJ, et al. Differentiation of multiple system atrophy from idiopathic Parkinson's disease using proton magnetic resonance spectroscopy. Ann Neurol 1995; 37:204–210.
3. Seppi K, Schocke MF, Donnemiller E, et al. Comparison of diffusion-weighted imaging and [123I]IBZM-SPECT for the differentiation of patients with the Parkinson variant of multiple system atrophy from those with Parkinson's disease. Mov Disord 2004; 19:1438–1445.
4. Schulz JB, Skalej M, Wedekind D, et al. Magnetic resonance imaging-based volumetry differentiates idiopathic Parkinson's syndrome from multiple system atrophy and progressive supranuclear palsy. Ann Neurol 1999; 45:65–74.
5. Sener RN. Pelizaeus-Merzbacher disease: diffusion MR imaging and proton MR spectroscopy findings. J Neuroradiol 2004; 31:138–141.
6. Harris JC, Lee RR, Jinnah HA, et al. Craniocerebral magnetic resonance imaging measurement and findings in Lesch-Nyhan syndrome. Arch Neurol 1998; 55:547–553.
7. Baumeister FA, Auer DP, Hortnagel K, et al. The eye-of-the-tiger sign is not a reliable disease marker for Hallervorden-Spatz syndrome. Neuropediatrics 2005; 36:221–222.
8. Brismar J, Ozand PT. CT and MR of the brain in glutaric acidemia type I: a review of 59 published cases and a report of 5 new patients. AJNR Am J Neuroradiol 1995; 16:675–683.
9. Yesildag A, Ayata A, Baykal B, et al. Magnetic resonance imaging and diffusion-weighted imaging in methylmalonic acidemia. Acta Radiol 2005; 46:101–103.
10. Faerber EN, Melvin J, Smergel EM. MRI appearances of metachromatic leukodystrophy. Pediatr Radiol 1999; 29:669–672.
11. D'Incerti L. MRI in neuronal ceroid lipofuscinosis. Neurol Sci 2000; 21:S71–S73.
12. Caliskan M, Ozmen M, Beck M, et al. Thalamic hyperdensity—is it a diagnostic marker for Sandhoff disease? Brain Dev 1993; 15:387–388.
13. Grosso S, Farnetani MA, Berardi R, et al. GM2 gangliosidosis variant B1 neuroradiological findings. J Neurol 2003; 250:17–21.
14. Mugikura S, Takahashi S, Higano S, et al. MR findings in Tay-Sachs disease. J Comput Assist Tomogr 1996; 20:551–555.
15. Bhatia KP, Marsden CD. The behavioural and motor consequences of focal lesions of the basal ganglia in man. Brain 1994; 117(Pt 4):859–876.
16. Krystkowiak P, Martinat P, Defebvre L, et al. Dystonia after striatopallidal and thalamic stroke: clinicoradiological correlations and pathophysiological mechanisms. J Neurol Neurosurg Psychiatry 1998; 65:703–708.
17. Lehericy S, Grand S, Pollak P, et al. Clinical characteristics and topography of lesions in movement disorders due to thalamic lesions. Neurology 2001; 57:1055–1066.
18. Alarcon F, Zijlmans JC, Duenas G, et al. Post-stroke movement disorders: report of 56 patients. J Neurol Neurosurg Psychiatry 2004; 75:1568–1574.
19. Ghika J, Ghika-Schmid F, Bogousslasvky J. Parietal motor syndrome: a clinical description in 32 patients in the acute phase of pure parietal strokes studied prospectively. Clin Neurol Neurosurg 1998; 100:271–282.

20. Rondot P, Bathien N, Tempier P, et al. [Topography of secondary dystonia lesions]. Bull Acad Natl Med 2001; 185:103–104.
21. Akbostanci MC, Yigit A, Ulkatan S. Cavernous angioma presenting with hemidystonia. Clin Neurol Neurosurg 1998; 100:234–237.
22. Angelini L, Rumi V, Nardocci N, et al. Hemidystonia symptomatic of primary antiphospholipid syndrome in childhood. Mov Disord 1993; 8:383–386.
23. Gille M, Van den BP, Ghariani S, et al. Delayed-onset hemidystonia and chorea following contralateral infarction of the posterolateral thalamus. A case report. Acta Neurol Belg 1996; 96:307–311.
24. Leenders KL, Frackowiak RS, Quinn N, et al. Ipsilateral blepharospasm and contralateral hemidystonia and parkinsonism in a patient with a unilateral rostral brainstem-thalamic lesion: structural and functional abnormalities studied with CT, MRI, and PET scanning. Mov Disord 1986; 1:51–58.
25. Matsuda M, Hashimoto T, Shimizu Y, et al. Coexistence of hemidystonia and hemiballism in a diabetic patient with striatal hyperintensity on T1-weighted MRI. J Neurol 2001; 248:1096–1098.
26. Nardocci N, Zorzi G, Grisoli M, et al. Acquired hemidystonia in childhood: a clinical and neuroradiological study of thirteen patients. Pediatr Neurol 1996; 15:108–113.
27. Lee MS, Rinne JO, Ceballos-Baumann A, et al. Dystonia after head trauma. Neurology 1994; 44:1374–1378.
28. Krauss JK, Mohadjer M, Braus DF, et al. Dystonia following head trauma: a report of nine patients and review of the literature. Mov Disord 1992; 7:263–272.
29. Warmuth-Metz M, Naumann M, Csoti I, et al. Measurement of the midbrain diameter on routine magnetic resonance imaging: a simple and accurate method of differentiating between Parkinson disease and progressive supranuclear palsy. Arch Neurol 2001; 58:1076–1079.
30. Savoiardo M. Differential diagnosis of Parkinson's disease and atypical parkinsonian disorders by magnetic resonance imaging. Neurol Sci 2003; 24(Suppl 1):S35–S37.
31. Watanabe H, Saito Y, Terao S, et al. Progression and prognosis in multiple system atrophy: an analysis of 230 Japanese patients. Brain 2002; 125:1070–1083.
32. Louis ED, Lee P, Quinn L, et al. Dystonia in Huntington's disease: prevalence and clinical characteristics. Mov Disord 1999; 14:95–101.
33. Kassubek J, Juengling FD, Kioschies T, et al. Topography of cerebral atrophy in early Huntington's disease: a voxel based morphometric MRI study. J Neurol Neurosurg Psychiatry 2004; 75:213–220.
34. Starosta-Rubinstein S, Young AB, Kluin K, et al. Clinical assessment of 31 patients with Wilson's disease. Correlations with structural changes on magnetic resonance imaging. Arch Neurol 1987; 44:365–370.
35. Svetel M, Kozic D, Stefanova E, et al. Dystonia in Wilson's disease. Mov Disord 2001; 16:719–723.
36. Magalhaes AC, Caramelli P, Menezes JR, et al. Wilson's disease: MRI with clinical correlation. Neuroradiology 1994; 36:97–100.
37. Cordato DJ, Fulham MJ, Yiannikas C. Pretreatment and posttreatment positron emission tomographic scan imaging in a 20-year-old patient with Wilson's disease. Mov Disord 1998; 13:162–166.
38. Schlaug G, Hefter H, Engelbrecht V, et al. Neurological impairment and recovery in Wilson's disease: evidence from PET and MRI. J Neurol Sci 1996; 136:129–139.
39. Snow BJ, Bhatt M, Martin WR, et al. The nigrostriatal dopaminergic pathway in Wilson's disease studied with positron emission tomography. J Neurol Neurosurg Psychiatry 1991; 54:12–17.
40. Westermark K, Tedroff J, Thuomas KA, et al. Neurological Wilson's disease studied with magnetic resonance imaging and with positron emission tomography using dopaminergic markers. Mov Disord 1995; 10:596–603.
41. Schlaug G, Hefter H, Nebeling B, et al. Dopamine D2 receptor binding and cerebral glucose metabolism recover after D-penicillamine-therapy in Wilson's disease. J Neurol 1994; 241:577–584.

42. Schwarz J, Antonini A, Kraft E, et al. Treatment with D-penicillamine improves dopamine D2-receptor binding and T2-signal intensity in de novo Wilson's disease. Neurology 1994; 44:1079–1082.
43. Perlmutter JS, Tempel LW, Black KJ, et al. MPTP induces dystonia and parkinsonism. Clues to the pathophysiology of dystonia. Neurology 1997; 49:1432–1438.
44. Furukawa Y, Hornykiewicz O, Fahn S, et al. Striatal dopamine in early-onset primary torsion dystonia with the DYT1 mutation. Neurology 2000; 54:1193–1195.
45. Hornykiewicz O, Kish SJ, Becker LE, et al. Brain neurotransmitters in dystonia musculorum deformans. N Engl J Med 1986; 315:347–353.
46. Augood SJ, Hollingsworth Z, Albers DS, et al. Dopamine transmission in DYT1 dystonia: a biochemical and autoradiographical study. Neurology 2002; 59:445–448.
47. Otsuka M, Ichiya Y, Shima F, et al. Increased striatal 18F-dopa uptake and normal glucose metabolism in idiopathic dystonia syndrome. J Neurol Sci 1992; 111:195–199.
48. Playford ED, Fletcher NA, Sawle GV, et al. Striatal [18F]dopa uptake in familial idiopathic dystonia. Brain 1993; 116(Pt 5):1191–1199.
49. Leenders KL, Quinn N, Frackowiak RS, et al. Brain dopaminergic system studied in patients with dystonia using positron emission tomography. Adv Neurol 1988; 50:243–247.
50. Naumann M, Pirker W, Reiners K, et al. Imaging the pre- and postsynaptic side of striatal dopaminergic synapses in idiopathic cervical dystonia: a SPECT study using [123I] epidepride and [123I] beta-CIT. Mov Disord 1998; 13:319–323.
51. Torres GE, Sweeney AL, Beaulieu JM, et al. Effect of torsinA on membrane proteins reveals a loss of function and a dominant-negative phenotype of the dystonia-associated DeltaE-torsinA mutant. Proc Natl Acad Sci U S A 2004; 101:15650–15655.
52. Ichinose H, Ohye T, Takahashi E, et al. Hereditary progressive dystonia with marked diurnal fluctuation caused by mutations in the GTP cyclohydrolase I gene. Nat Genet 1994; 8:236–242.
53. Sawle GV, Leenders KL, Brooks DJ, et al. Dopa-responsive dystonia: [18F]dopa positron emission tomography. Ann Neurol 1991; 30:24–30.
54. Turjanski N, Bhatia K, Burn DJ, et al. Comparison of striatal 18F-dopa uptake in adult-onset dystonia-parkinsonism, Parkinson's disease, and dopa-responsive dystonia. Neurology 1993; 43:1563–1568.
55. Snow BJ, Nygaard TG, Takahashi H, et al. Positron emission tomographic studies of dopa-responsive dystonia and early-onset idiopathic parkinsonism. Ann Neurol 1993; 34:733–738.
56. Fuente-Fernandez R, Furtado S, Guttman M, et al. VMAT2 binding is elevated in dopa-responsive dystonia: visualizing empty vesicles by PET. Synapse 2003; 49:20–28.
57. Rinne JO, Iivanainen M, Metsahonkala L, et al. Striatal dopaminergic system in dopa-responsive dystonia: a multi-tracer PET study shows increased D2 receptors. J Neural Transm 2004; 111:59–67.
58. Jeon BS, Jeong JM, Park SS, et al. Dopamine transporter density measured by [123I] beta-CIT single-photon emission computed tomography is normal in dopa-responsive dystonia. Ann Neurol 1998; 43:792–800.
59. Naumann M, Pirker W, Reiners K, et al. [123I]beta-CIT single-photon emission tomography in DOPA-responsive dystonia. Mov Disord 1997; 12:448–451.
60. O'Sullivan JD, Costa DC, Gacinovic S, et al. SPECT imaging of the dopamine transporter in juvenile-onset dystonia. Neurology 2001; 56:266–267.
61. Kishore A, Nygaard TG, Fuente-Fernandez R, et al. Striatal D2 receptors in symptomatic and asymptomatic carriers of dopa-responsive dystonia measured with [11C]-raclopride and positron-emission tomography. Neurology 1998; 50:1028–1032.
62. Kunig G, Leenders KL, Antonini A, et al. D2 receptor binding in dopa-responsive dystonia. Ann Neurol 1998; 44:758–762.
63. Carbon M, Trost M, Ghilardi MF, et al. Abnormal brain networks in primary torsion dystonia. Adv Neurol 2004; 94:155–161.

64. Eidelberg D, Moeller JR, Ishikawa T, et al. The metabolic topography of idiopathic torsion dystonia. Brain 1995; 118(Pt 6):1473–1484.
65. Ibanez V, Sadato N, Karp B, et al. Deficient activation of the motor cortical network in patients with writer's cramp. Neurology 1999; 53:96–105.
66. Stoessl AJ, Martin WR, Clark C, et al. PET studies of cerebral glucose metabolism in idiopathic torticollis. Neurology 1986; 36:653–657.
67. Pujol J, Roset-Llobet J, Rosines-Cubells D, et al. Brain cortical activation during guitar-induced hand dystonia studied by functional MRI. Neuroimage 2000; 12:257–267.
68. Ceballos-Baumann AO, Passingham RE, Warner T, et al. Overactive prefrontal and underactive motor cortical areas in idiopathic dystonia. Ann Neurol 1995; 37:363–372.
69. Galardi G, Perani D, Grassi F, et al. Basal ganglia and thalamo-cortical hypermetabolism in patients with spasmodic torticollis. Acta Neurol Scand 1996; 94:172–176.
70. Furukawa Y, Nygaard TG, Gutlich M, et al. Striatal biopterin and tyrosine hydroxylase protein reduction in dopa-responsive dystonia. Neurology 1999; 53:1032–1041.
71. Fuente-Fernandez R, Schulzer M, Mak E, et al. Presynaptic mechanisms of motor fluctuations in Parkinson's disease: a probabilistic model. Brain 2004; 127:888–899.
72. Augood SJ, Penney JB Jr, Friberg IK, et al. Expression of the early-onset torsion dystonia gene (DYT1) in human brain. Ann Neurol 1998; 43:669–673.
73. McNaught KS, Kapustin A, Jackson T, et al. Brainstem pathology in DYT1 primary torsion dystonia. Ann Neurol 2004; 56:540–547.
74. Edwards MJ, Huang YZ, Wood NW, et al. Different patterns of electrophysiological deficits in manifesting and non-manifesting carriers of the DYT1 gene mutation. Brain 2003; 126:2074–2080.
75. Sharma N, Baxter MG, Petravicz J, et al. Impaired motor learning in mice expressing torsinA with the DYT1 dystonia mutation. J Neurosci 2005; 25:5351–5355.
76. Ghilardi MF, Carbon M, Silvestri G, et al. Impaired sequence learning in carriers of the DYT1 dystonia mutation. Ann Neurol 2003; 54:102–109.
77. Oppenheim C, Rodrigo S, Poupon C, et al. [Diffusion tensor MR imaging of the brain. Clinical applications.]. J Radiol 2004; 85:287–296.
78. Ramnani N, Behrens TE, Penny W, et al. New approaches for exploring anatomical and functional connectivity in the human brain. Biol Psychiatry 2004; 56:613–619.
79. Le Bihan D. Looking into the functional architecture of the brain with diffusion MRI. Nat Rev Neurosci 2003; 4:469–480.
80. Carbon M, Kingsley PB, Su S, et al. Microstructural white matter changes in carriers of the DYT1 gene mutation. Ann Neurol 2004; 56:283–286.
81. Black KJ, Gado MH, Perlmutter JS. PET measurement of dopamine D2 receptor-mediated changes in striatopallidal function. J Neurosci 1997; 17:3168–3177.
82. Asanuma K, Ma Y, Okulski J, et al. Decreased striatal D2 receptor binding in non-manifesting carriers of the DYT1 dystonia mutation. Neurology 2005; 64:347–349.
83. Perlmutter JS, Stambuk MK, Markham J, et al. Decreased [18F]spiperone binding in putamen in idiopathic focal dystonia. J Neurosci 1997; 17:843–850.
84. Nobrega JN, Richter A, Tozman N, et al. Quantitative autoradiography reveals regionally selective changes in dopamine D1 and D2 receptor binding in the genetically dystonic hamster. Neuroscience 1996; 71:927–937.
85. Eidelberg D, Moeller JR, Dhawan V, et al. The metabolic topography of parkinsonism. J Cereb Blood Flow Metab 1994; 14:783–801.
86. Trost M, Carbon M, Edwards C, et al. Primary dystonia: is abnormal functional brain architecture linked to genotype?. Ann Neurol 2002; 52:853–856.
87. Lozano AM, Abosch A. Pallidal stimulation for dystonia. Adv Neurol 2004; 94:301–308.
88. Detante O, Vercueil L, Thobois S, et al. Globus pallidus internus stimulation in primary generalized dystonia: a H215O PET study. Brain 2004; 127:1899–1908.
89. Eidelberg D, Moeller JR, Antonini A, et al. Functional brain networks in DYT1 dystonia. Ann Neurol 1998; 44:303–312.

90. Kaji R, Rothwell JC, Katayama M, et al. Tonic vibration reflex and muscle afferent block in writer's cramp. Ann Neurol 1995; 38:155–162.
91. Playford ED, Passingham RE, Marsden CD, et al. Increased activation of frontal areas during arm movement in idiopathic torsion dystonia. Mov Disord 1998; 13:309–318.
92. Oga T, Honda M, Toma K, et al. Abnormal cortical mechanisms of voluntary muscle relaxation in patients with writer's cramp: an fMRI study. Brain 2002; 125:895–903.
93. Delmaire C, Krainik A, Tezenas du MS, et al. Disorganized somatotopy in the putamen of patients with focal hand dystonia. Neurology 2005; 64:1391–1396.
94. Odergren T, Stone-Elander S, Ingvar M. Cerebral and cerebellar activation in correlation to the action-induced dystonia in writer's cramp. Mov Disord 1998; 13:497–508.
95. Karbe H, Holthoff VA, Rudolf J, et al. Positron emission tomography demonstrates frontal cortex and basal ganglia hypometabolism in dystonia. Neurology 1992; 42:1540–1544.

# 8
# Primary Generalized Dystonia

**Johan Samanta**
*Banner Good Samaritan Medical Center, Phoenix, and Department of Neurology, University of Arizona College of Medicine, Tucson, Arizona, U.S.A.*

## INTRODUCTION

Dystonia is a syndrome of sustained, repetitive, patterned muscle contractions producing twisting (e.g., torticollis) or squeezing (e.g., blepharospasm) movements or abnormal postures that may be present at rest, with changing posture, or when performing a specific motor activity. Severity and extent of involvement, however, can vary considerably from task-specific contractions of a single limb to continuous and generalized contraction of limb and axial muscles.

Oppenheim coined the term *Dystonia Musculorum Deformans* in 1911 to describe a group of children with abnormal postures and progressive disability (1). However, because dystonia is not a disorder of the muscle and does not always produce postural deformity, the shortened term is now preferred. Over the last 95 years, the classification of this disorder has evolved from one of primarily clinical characterization (e.g., focal, segmental, or generalized dystonia) to etiological characterization with molecular designations describing a number of alleles associated with these conditions (2). Increasingly, careful phenotypic analyses within specific kindreds have lead to the realization that a wide range of clinical presentations may exist within a specific genotype. Thus, the current use of two broad etiologic categories: primary (or idiopathic) and secondary (symptomatic).

Secondary dystonia (Chapter 16) can be associated with a number of disorders that are either acquired (e.g., neuroleptic-induced, postinfectious, cerebrovascular) or are part of an inherited disorder (e.g., Wilson's disease, Huntington's disease, and Hallervorden-Spatz). These secondary dystonias typically present with other abnormalities on examination beyond dystonia (e.g., ataxia, dementia, pathological reflexes, parkinsonism), and laboratory and imaging findings can be instrumental in making a diagnosis. Primary dystonia, however, should present with no other examination findings than the dystonia itself. A consistent pattern of abnormality on laboratory and imaging studies has not been described in primary dystonia. Thus, such studies are usually unremarkable.

It is the ongoing elucidation and characterization of the genetic basis of the childhood- and adult-onset primary dystonias that may provide the strongest clinical aid to diagnosis and, eventually, to more definitive treatments. The first of these genetic characterizations, DYT1, is an autosomal dominant disorder localized to chromosome 9q32–34. It is this population that represents the *Dystonia Musculorum Deformans* subjects originally described by Oppenheim and is now termed "idiopathic torsion dystonia" (ITD). Because the epidemiology (Chapter 2), genetics (Chapter 3), and pathophysiology (Chapters 5 and 6) of primary dystonia have already been covered in detail, this chapter will review clinical presentation and course, differential diagnosis, and approach to treatment, particularly as related to early-onset and generalized primary dystonia.

## CLINICAL PRESENTATION

The clinical range of primary dystonia is quite variable, and familial and population studies of allele carriers demonstrate a wide range of symptom involvement from generalized (affecting the entire body) to focal (confined to one body part). Focal dystonias can involve the head (cranial dystonia), neck (cervical dystonia), or limb. Cervical dystonia is the most common focal dystonia followed by blepharospasm, limb, and laryngeal dystonia. The most common form of limb dystonia is writer's cramp, a task-specific dystonia. While the presentation and course of a subject with primary dystonia is highly variable, it usually begins as a focal dystonia, and is present only with certain actions. However, symptoms may progress to involve the trunk, neck, face, and upper limbs, and may also become more persistently present, eventually persisting even at rest.

Age of onset appears to be closely linked to both likelihood and degree of progression in primary dystonia. There is a bimodal distribution in age of onset with modes at nine years (early- or childhood-onset) and 45 years of age (late- or adult-onset) with a nadir at 27 years (3). Adult-onset primary dystonia usually presents with cervical, cranial, or upper limb involvement and only about 20% to 30% progress to segmental involvement, with generalized dystonia being quite unusual. Adult onset of generalized dystonia is strongly suggestive of a secondary dystonia. Conversely, childhood-onset patients most often present with dystonia of a single limb with progression to segmental or generalized dystonia occurring in the great majority of patients (Table 1). The body region first affected is significant as well, with onset in the leg associated with earlier onset (approximately 8.5 years of age vs. 11 years), as well as greater likelihood of and more rapid progression to generalized

**Table 1** Presentation and Progression of Primary Dystonia by Age at Onset

| |
|---|
| Onset < age 13 |
| Presentation most often in limb (leg > arm) |
| Progression to generalized dystonia common |
| Often familial |
| Onset ages 13–20 |
| Presentation in arm > leg, but cervical and cranial onset common also |
| Most often remains focal or segmental, but generalized dystonia occurs |
| Onset > age 20 |
| Presentation most often with cervical or cranial dystonia, onset in leg is rare |
| Remains focal > segmental (~20%) > generalized (rare) |
| Typically sporadic |

dystonia than when onset is in the arm (4,5). While child- and adolescent-onset primary dystonia is more common in Jews of Ashkenazi ancestry, there does not appear to be significant difference in clinical presentation and course between Jewish and non-Jewish patients. It should be noted that exceptions to this pattern do exist and should be considered when evaluating any patient with dystonia. Leg dystonia in patients beyond 30 years of age should prompt a concern for idiopathic Parkinson's disease. In children, the development of leg dystonia, particularly in the presence of diurnal fluctuation of symptom severity, may represent the initial onset of dopa-responsive dystonia (DRD).

Primary dystonia in a limb (regardless of age at onset) often starts as a task-specific dystonia, occurring only when performing a specific motor activity (e.g., walking or writing). Progression may manifest as activation of the dystonia with less specific motor activities (e.g., walking and running, writing and typing) or with actions of other parts of the body and may eventually lead to persistent dystonic activity even while at rest. The presence of dystonia at rest, if left untreated, may lead to fixed postures and eventually to permanent contractures.

Progression may also occur as a spreading from focal involvement (e.g., a single limb) at onset to involvement of adjacent segments of the body and eventually more distally (generalized) dystonia. This may first present with involvement of muscles not normally used in the provoking task. This phenomenon, termed "overflow," may produce forearm pronation and wrist flexion in addition to lower-limb dystonia when walking, or elbow elevation and shoulder abduction in addition to exaggeration of grip and wrist flexion when writing. Lower limb dystonia of childhood-onset tends to spread to bilateral lower limb involvement followed by involvement of the trunk and eventually may include upper limb, cervical, and cranial dystonia as well. The rate of progression to generalized dystonia with onset in a leg is less than five years, compared to more than 11 years with arm-onset. Rarely, dystonia may progress to involve only the other ipsilateral limb, producing a hemidystonia. However, this is not typical in the setting of primary dystonia and the presence of hemidystonia is overwhelmingly associated with secondary rather than primary dystonia (6,7).

An important clinical feature of primary dystonia is that certain postures or "sensory tricks" (geste antagoniste) can transiently diminish or even completely relieve dystonic movements. Classically, gentle counter pressure to the neck or jaw may enable the patient with cervical dystonia to achieve and maintain a normal head position. While cervical dystonia is most commonly associated with benefit from sensory tricks, patients with other focal as well as generalized dystonia may successfully employ similar strategies. Another clinical feature often present in primary dystonia is tremor. Termed dystonic tremor, it is felt to arise from the patient's attempt (often unconsciously) to overcome the abnormal posture of their dystonia. Dystonic tremor is a focal, action-type tremor and tends to be irregular in both amplitude and rhythm. It is most pronounced when the patient actively works to resist the pulling of the dystonic muscle groups and may be silent when the patient permits the involved body part to assume its full dystonic posture (8). Dystonic tremor has been reported as the first and, sometimes, only manifestation of dystonia. Additionally, the presence of tremor resembling essential tremor has been reported in up to 20% of patients in some series, though linkage analysis has not supported a common genetic origin with essential tremor thus far (9,10). Rapid dystonic movements resembling myoclonus can occur in some patients as well. They are usually seen on voluntary muscle activation and tend to be superimposed on dystonic muscle spasms (11). Emotional stress and fatigue also tend to aggravate dystonia and associated

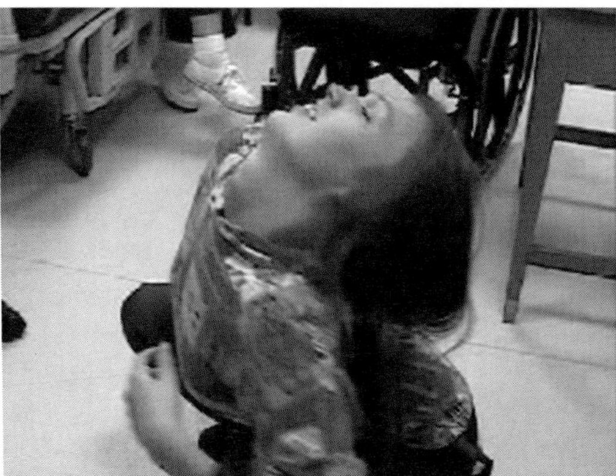

**Figure 1** Patient with generalized dystonia displaying "dromedary gait." *Source*: Photo courtesy Mark Stacy.

movements, while relaxation and rest tend to reduce the spasms. Dystonia resolves during deep sleep. With the exception of cervical dystonia and some presentations of posttraumatic dystonia (see below), pain is not common in primary dystonia. Similarly, patients with generalized dystonia and cervical involvement may report pain in that area only.

Gait, especially in early-onset dystonia, can be affected. Commonly, the leg swings forward abnormally with abduction at the hip and the lower leg and foot angled medially, nearly striking the opposite leg. However, other postures and gaits can be seen as well. When the axial muscles are involved, the patient may develop what has been termed "dromedary gait," with the trunk bent forward at the hips and the neck extended (Fig. 1). This pattern of posture and ambulation is in contrast to the cervical and axial hyperextension or opisthotonus seen in tardive dystonia. Over time, some patients with generalized dystonia may become unable to walk at all or only for a few steps before being overwhelmed by their dystonia.

Although primary dystonia is considered a chronic lifelong disorder, remissions do occur. Partial-to-complete remissions have been reported in up to 20% of adult-onset primary dystonia. Remissions are more common in cervical dystonia, tend to occur during the first two to three years from onset, and are transient, lasting from days to several years (12). Conversely, child-onset primary dystonia is only rarely associated with remission that is typically brief and partial (13).

## DIFFERENTIAL DIAGNOSIS

While the genetic basis of primary generalized dystonia has been well established, there is increasing evidence that many adult-onset focal dystonias are genetically based as well. Molecular descriptions of dystonic conditions have been reported with ITD (*DYT1*), focal dystonia (*DYT7*), mixed dystonia (*DYT6* and *DYT13*), DRD, myoclonic dystonia, rapid-onset dystonia parkinsonism, Fahr disease, Hallervorden-Spatz syndrome, X-linked dystonia parkinsonism, deafness-dystonia syndrome, mitochondrial dystonias, myoclonic dystonia, neuroacanthocytosis, and the paroxysmal dystonias/dyskinesias (14). Additionally, focal dystonias may emerge in families exhibiting generalized dystonia (15), and have also been related to the *DYT1* allele (16). While the gene test for the *DYT1* mutation remains the only one available for primary dystonia, genetic testing is currently available for several other dystonic syndromes.

Extrapyramidal syndromes such as Wilson's disease, Parkinson's disease, progressive supranuclear palsy, corticobasal ganglionic degeneration (CBGD), and multiple system atrophy may be associated with dystonia. While focal and segmental dystonia is seen most often in these disorders, axial and generalized involvement can occur as well. Lower limb dystonia can be the presenting symptom of idiopathic Parkinson's disease, especially in young-onset individuals. Writer's cramp, torticollis, oromandibular dystonia, and blepharospasm have been observed to precede the onset of Parkinson's as well. Patients with progressive supranuclear palsy often present with dystonic muscle contraction of the axial muscles as well as blepharospasm, and some patients with CBGD exhibit profound limb dystonia in addition to, and sometimes masking, symptoms of the "alien-limb" phenomenon. Tonic spasms of multiple sclerosis are typically transient attacks of the limbs, and can present as limb dystonia, hemidystonia, or even generalized dystonia. Other secondary causes of dystonia include exposure to dopamine (DA) receptor-blocking drugs (tardive dystonia), hypoxic encephalopathy (particularly in child-onset dystonia), head trauma, encephalitis, human immunodeficiency virus and other infections, peripheral or segmental nerve injury, reflex sympathetic dystrophy, inherited disorders (e.g., Wilson's disease), metabolic disorders, and other inborn errors of metabolism, mitochondrial disorders, and chromosomal abnormalities (Table 2).

Central nervous system lesions are well recognized as causes of dystonia. Chuang et al. (17) reviewed 190 cases of hemidystonia, and found the most common etiologies of hemidystonia to be stroke, trauma, and perinatal injury. In these subjects, the mean age of onset was 20 to 25.7 years, and the average latency from insult to dystonia was 2.8 to 4.1 years. Basal ganglia lesions were seen in almost 50% of the patients with the putamen most commonly involved. Cerebral infarction in the posterolateral thalamic nuclei may be associated with contralateral hand dystonia, and large lenticular or caudatocapsulolenticular lesions may give rise to foot dystonia (18). Other structural abnormalities associated with dystonia include cavernous angioma of the basal ganglia (19), subdural hematoma (20), left frontal meningioma (21), calcification of the head of the right caudate nucleus (22), and cervical cord lesion secondary to multiple sclerosis (23). Movement disorders after severe head injury have been reported in 13% to 66% of the patients (24). Generalized dystonia in children has been associated with head injury and can present as focal dystonia with progression to generalized dystonia over months to years (25). Basal ganglia and thalamic lesions are usually seen on brain imaging. Perinatal brain injury can result in a dystonic form of cerebral palsy (26).

Although peripheral trauma as a cause of dystonia remains controversial, it has been suggested that pain, prominent in nearly all reported cases of posttraumatic dystonia, may be a critical pathogenic factor (27). Increased blood flow in the basal ganglia is associated with painful thermal stimulation or capsaicin injection of the hand using Positron emission tomography analysis (28,29). Typically, dystonia after peripheral trauma presents as either focal or segmental dystonia.

Psychogenic dystonia should only be diagnosed by exclusion and after thorough consideration of all other possibilities. Clinical features suggestive of a psychogenic dystonia include give-way weakness, atypical sensory or pain complaints,

**Table 2** Differential Diagnosis of Dystonia

*Idiopathic (primary) dystonia*
- Sporadic (ITD)
- Inherited (hereditary torsion dystonia)
  - Autosomal dominant ITD (*DYT1*)
  - Autosomal dominant torsion dystonia of mixed phenotype (*DYT6*)
  - Autosomal dominant late onset focal dystonia (*DYT7*)
  - Segmental dystonia (*DYT13*)

*Secondary dystonia*
- Dystonia-plus syndromes
  - Myoclonic dystonia (not *DYT1* gene)
  - Dopa-responsive dystonia GTP cyclohydrolase I; 14Q22.1-q22.2gene defect
  - Autosomal recessive tyrosine hydroxylase deficiency
  - Rapid-onset dystonia—parkinsonism
  - Early-onset parkinsonism with dystonia
  - Paroxysmal dystonia—choreoathetosis
- Associated with neurodegenerative disorders
  - Sporadic
    - Parkinson's disease
    - Progressive supranuclear palsy
    - Multiple system atrophy
    - Corticobasal ganglionic degeneration
    - Multiple sclerosis
    - Central pontine myelinolysis
  - Inherited
    - Wilson's disease
    - Huntington's disease
    - Juvenile parkinsonism-dystonia
    - Progressive pallidal degeneration
    - Hallervorden-Spatz disease
    - Hypoprebetalipoproteinemia, acanthocytosis, retinitis pigmentosa, and pallidal degeneration (HARP syndrome)
    - Joseph's disease
    - Ataxia telangiectasia
    - Neuroacanthocytosis
    - Rett's syndrome (?)
    - Intraneuronal inclusion disease
    - Infantile bilateral striatal necrosis
    - Familial basal ganglia calcifications
    - Spinocerebellar degeneration
    - Olivopontocerebellar atrophy
    - Hereditary spastic paraplegia with dystonia
    - X-linked dystonia parkinsonism or Lubag (pericentromeric) deletion of 18q
- Associated with metabolic disorders
  - Amino acid disorders
    - Glutamic acidemia
    - Methylmalonic acidemia
    - Homocystenuria
    - Hartnup's disease
    - Tyrosinosis

(*Continued*)

**Table 2** Differential Diagnosis of Dystonia (*Continued*)

- Lipid disorders
  - Metachromatic leukodystrophy
  - Ceroid lipofuscinosis
  - Dystonic lipidosis ("sea blue" histiocytosis)
  - Gangliosidoses (GM1-, GM2-variants)
  - Hexosaminidase A and B deficiency
- Miscellaneous metabolic disorders
  - Wilson's disease
  - Mitochondrial encephalopathies (Leigh's disease, Leber's disease)
  - Lesch-Nyhan syndrome
  - Triosephosphate isomerase deficiency
  - Vitamin E deficiency
  - Biopterin deficiency

Due to a known specific cause

- Perinatal cerebral injury and kernicterus (athetoid cerebral palsy, delayed-onset dystonia)
- Infection (viral encephalitis, encephalitis lethargica, Reye's syndrome, subacute sclerosing panencephalitis, Jakob-Creutzfeld disease, AIDS)
- Other (tuberculosis, syphilis, acute infectious torticollis)
- Paraneoplastic brainstem encephalitis
- Cerebral, vascular, and ischemic injury
- Brain tumor
- Arteriovenous malformation
- Head trauma and brain surgery
- Peripheral trauma
- Toxins (Mn, CO, $CS_2$, methanol, disulfiram, wasp sting)
- Drugs (levodopa, bromocriptine, antipsychotic agents, metoclopramide, fenfluramine, flecainide, ergot agents, anticonvulsant agents, certain calcium channel blocking agents)

*Other hyperkinetic syndromes associated with dystonia*

- Tic disorders with dystonic tics
- Paroxysmal Dyskinesias
  - Paroxysmal kinesigenic choreoathetosis
  - Paroxysmal dystonic choreoathetosis
  - Intermediate paroxysmal dyskinesia
  - Benign infantile dyskinesia

*Psychogenic*

*Pseudodystonia*

- Atlanto-axial subluxation
- Syringomyelia
- Arnold-Chiari malformation
- Trochlear nerve palsy
- Vestibular torticollis
- Posterior fossa mass
- Soft tissue neck mass
- Congenital postural torticollis
- Congenital Klippel-Feil syndrome
- Isaac's syndrome
- Sandiffer's syndrome
- Satoyoshi syndrome
- Stiff-person syndrome

*Abbreviations*: ITD, idiopathic torsion dystonia; GTP, guanosine triposphate.

fixed postures, lack of modification of the movement disorder by action, and shifting areas of involvement (e.g., the dystonia moves from a leg to the opposite arm and then to the trunk).

## DIAGNOSTIC APPROACH

The diagnosis of primary dystonia should be considered in any patient presenting with an abnormal posture. Information concerning age at onset, initial and subsequent areas of involvement, course and progression, tremor or other movement disorders, possible birth injury, developmental milestones, and exposure to neuroleptic medications, as well as a family history of dystonia, parkinsonism, or other movement disorders should be reviewed. Because phenotypic expression of ITD is highly varied in this population, extreme care should be taken in recording family data with particular attention to consanguinity or Jewish ancestry. Clinically, in primary dystonia, the only neurological abnormality is the presence of dystonic postures and movements. Thus secondary dystonia must be considered when evidence of other neurological dysfunction (e.g., cognitive, cranial nerve, pyramidal, sensory, or cerebellar deficits) is present. Obtaining serum ceruloplasmin levels and slit-lamp testing should be considered in all patients under the age of 50. Blood sample for genetic assessment, storage diseases, and metabolic disorders should be evaluated individually. Presentation with lower limb dystonia and abnormal gait in a child or young adult should prompt consideration of DRD and a trial of levodopa. Levodopa, in this setting, is both therapeutic and diagnostic because DRD is typically dramatically responsive at low doses (50–200 mg/day). Imaging of the brain (magnetic resonance imaging or computed tomography scan) may be indicated in children and in adult-onset patients with a short history of limb dystonia or when other neurological symptoms are present in conjunction with dystonia.

## MANAGEMENT

The role of patient education and supportive care in primary dystonia should not be underestimated. Physical and occupational therapy play an important role in preventing contractures, maintaining independence, and developing coping strategies for existing limitations. Specialty braces can be used as a substitute for a sensory trick. Many patients report benefit with various relaxation techniques and biofeedback therapy.

Anticholinergic drugs can be effective in generalized dystonia, particularly in children. Fahn (30) found that 61% of children compared to just 38% of adults improved with high-dose anticholinergic therapy. Lack of tolerability due to anticholinergic side effects often limits the usefulness of these drugs, especially in adults. Slow titration may improve the likelihood of a patient reaching a therapeutic dose (approximately 30 mg/day for trihexyphenidyl). Patients with primary, segmental, and generalized dystonia beginning in childhood or adolescence should receive a trial of levodopa (with a dopa decarboxylase inhibitor) up to 1000 mg/day. DRD patients are typically well maintained on levodopa doses of 50 to 200 mg/day and unlike juvenile-onset Parkinson's patients, this group does not develop fluctuations (31). Dopamine-depleting drugs such as tetrabenazine and atypical antipsychotic drugs such as clozapine have been found useful in some patients with dystonia. These drugs are particularly useful in patients with tardive dystonia (32–34). In some patients with a component of tremor, beta-blocking agents may be useful (35). Baclofen or tizanidine are commonly used in treating symptoms of dystonia, and may be most appropriate in patients with a history of hypoxic or traumatic brain injury. Benzodiazepines, particularly if patients report sleep difficulty, are also useful. In one series of 190 patients, approximately one-third of patients experienced some benefit from medical therapy, which included anticholinergics, benzodiazepines, clonazepam, and diazepam (17).

Botulinum toxin injections are highly effective in the treatment of focal dystonia (36–41). Injection strategy is determined by a combination of functional observation, muscle palpation, and electrophysiolgic assessment. The sheer number of muscles involved limits the role of botulinum toxin injections in generalized dystonia. However, selective injection of muscles to reduce a particularly troublesome focal component can be considered (e.g., foot dystonia or retrocollis). A recent retrospective analysis of 235 patients receiving a total of 2616 injections with botulinum toxin—type A found continued benefit at five years (42). Interestingly, benefit was sustained in 100% of the lower-limb affected subjects and only 56% of the writer's cramp population. In this large series, 16.6% of the patients developed resistance over the course of 10 years' follow-up. Adverse effects developed in 27% of the patients at any one time, occurring in over 4.5% of injection sessions, but were significantly lower in the limb dystonia groups. Another retrospective study of 62 cervical dystonia patients found that while 82% of those patients had been employed prior to onset of symptoms, only 47% were still employed at initiation of treatment. Long-term treatment (ranging from 1.5–10 years) with botulinum toxin resulted in 67% of those on medical leave returning to work (43). Currently, two botulinum serotypes (type A or type B) are available for commercial usage.

Perineural injection with 3% phenol has been used for more than 20 years in the management of spasticity in children, and may occasionally be considered in patients with spastic dystonia of a limb (44). This intervention requires considerable time, and best results are seen with careful management of patient expectations, and identification of potential response with injection of lidocaine prior to injection of phenol (45). Duration of benefit for spasticity ranges from one month to more than two years, and injection in the upper extremities generally show greater benefit than lower extremity procedures. Side effects include chronic dysesthesia and permanent nerve palsy (46). Motor point stimulation is useful for localization, and, although mixed motor and sensory nerves may be injected, injection of pure motor nerves (such as the musculocutaneous nerve) is associated with less pain.

Intrathecal baclofen (ITB) may be of benefit in generalized dystonia especially when associated with cerebral palsy. Abright et al. (47) report benefit from ITB infusion in a large group of subjects ranging in age from 3 to 42 years. All participants carried the diagnosis of generalized dystonia refractory to oral medications, 71% also carried the diagnosis of cerebral palsy. In this series, improvement was reported in 80 of 86 subjects with bolus injections; subsequently 77 participants underwent intrathecal catheter implantation. Seventy-two of these subjects demonstrated benefit for a median follow-up up to 29 months. However, surgical complications such as cerebrospinal fluid leaks, infections, and catheter problems occurred in 29 subjects. Interestingly, these authors note a better response with the catheter placed above T-4, when compared to the benefit seen with placement below T-6. The benefit of ITB in primary generalized dystonia is not well established.

Stereotactic neurosurgical intervention should be considered in primary dystonia patients who have severe dystonia and have not achieved adequate symptomatic

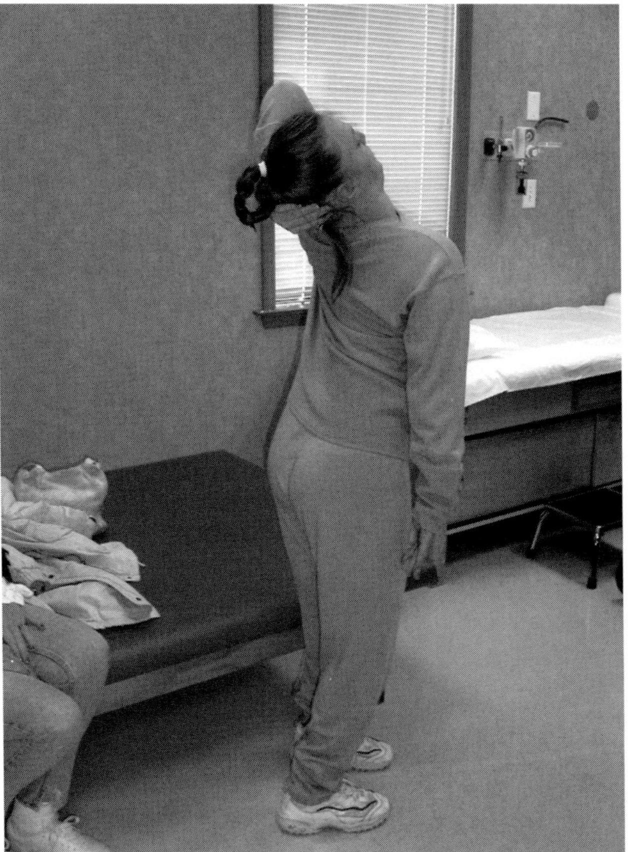

**Figure 2** Same generalized dystonia patient after implantation of bilateral GPi deep brain stimulators. *Source*: Photo courtesy Mark Stacy.

control with drugs or botulinum toxin. The results of ablative surgery targeting the globus pallidus interna (GPi) have been encouraging. One series of five patients with generalized dystonia undergoing bilateral GPi pallidotomies, reported that the four patients with idiopathic dystonia showed progressive improvement up to three months; the fifth patient with posttraumatic dystonia did not benefit beyond this time (48). Yoshor et al. reported long-term outcomes in 32 dystonia patients (49) who had either undergone thalamotomy ($n = 18$) or pallidotomy ($n = 14$). Although the two groups were not homogeneous, the authors concluded that in patients with primary dystonia, pallidotomy provided significantly better outcomes than thalamotomy. Vesper et al. report two cases of medically refractory, generalized dystonia treated by chronic high-frequency stimulation of the bilateral GPi (Fig. 2). Greater than 80% reduction in the Burke-Fahn-Marsden-Dystonia Movement Rating Scale (BFMDRS) was seen at six months and continued for 24 months (50). These findings are consistent with more recent reports on the long-term efficacy of chronic bilateral GPi stimulation. Primary dystonia patients appeared to gain greater benefit (71.2% mean improvement on BFMDRS, $n = 6$) than those with secondary dystonia (32.6%, $n = 3$). Peak benefit was reached between 6 and 12 months after surgery and appeared stable at up to three years (51). Deep brain stimulation has also shown to be of benefit in focal adult-onset primary dystonias (52,53).

## REFERENCES

1. Stacy M, Jankovic J. Differential diagnosis and treatment of childhood dystonia. Pediatr Ann 1993; 22:353–358.
2. Stacy M. Idiopathic cervical dystonia: an overview. Neurology 2000; 55(suppl 5):2–8.
3. Bressman SB, de Leon D, Brin MF, et al. Idiopathic dystonia among Ashkenazi Jews: evidence for autosomal dominant inheritance. Ann Neurol 1989; 26(5):612–620.
4. Burke RE, Brin MF, Fahn S, Bressman SB, Moskowitz C. Analysis of the clinical course of non-Jewish, autosomal dominant torsion dystonia. Mov Disord 1986; 1(3):163–178.
5. Greene P, Kang UJ, Fahn S. Spread of symptoms in idiopathic torsion dystonia. Mov Disord 1995; 10(2):143–152.
6. Pettigrew LC, Jankovic J. Hemidystonia: a report of 22 patients and a review of the literature. J Neurol Neurosurg Psychiatry 1985; 48(7):650–657.
7. Marsden CD, Obeso JA, Zarranz JJ, Lang AE. The anatomical basis of symptomatic hemidystonia. Brain 1985; 108(Pt 2):463–483.
8. Jankovic J, Fahn S. Physiologic and pathologic tremors. Diagnosis, mechanism and management. Ann Intern Med 1980; 93:460–465.
9. Rivest J, Marsden CD. Trunk and head tremor as isolated manifestations of dystonia. Mov Disord 1990; 5(1):60–65.
10. Conway D, Bain PG, Warner TT, et al. Linkage analysis with chromosome 9 markers in hereditary essential tremor. Mov Disord 1993; 8(3):374–376.
11. Obeso JA, Rothwell JC, Lang AE, Marsden CD. Myoclonic dystonia. Neurology 1983; 33(7):825–830.
12. Friedman A, Fahn S. Spontaneous remissions in spasmodic torticollis. Neurology 1986; 36(3):398–400.
13. Eldridge R, Ince SE, Chernow B. Dystonia in 61-year-old identical twins: observation over 45 years. Ann Neurol 1984; 16:356–358.
14. Nemeth AH. The genetics of primary dystonias and related disorders. Brain 2002; 125:695–721.
15. Waddy HM, Fletcher NA, Harding AE, Marsden CD. A genetic study of idiopathic focal dystonias. Ann Neurol 1991; 29:320–324.
16. Kramer PL, Heiman GA, Gasser T, et al. The DYT1 gene on 9q34 is responsible for most cases of early limb-onset idiopathic torsion dystonia in non-Jews. Am J Hum Genet 1994; 55:468–475.
17. Chuang C, Fahn S, Frucht SJ. The natural history and treatment of acquired hemidystonia: report of 33 cases and review of the literature. J Neurol Neurosurg Psychiatry 2002; 72:59–67.
18. Obeso JA, Giménez-Roldán S. Clinicopathological correlation in symptomatic dystonia. Adv Neurol 1988; 50:113–122.
19. Lorenzana L, Cabezudo JM, Porras LF, Polaina M, Rodriguez-Sanchez JA, Garcia-Yague LM. Focal dystonia secondary to cavernous angioma of the basal ganglia: case report and review of the literature. Neurosurgery 1992; 31:1108–1112.
20. Dressler D, Schonle PW. Bilateral limb dystonia due to chronic subdural hematoma. Eur Neurol 1990; 30:211–213.
21. Meyrignac C, Keravel Y, Boulu P, Nguyen JP, Degos JD. Writer's cramp and left frontal meningioma. Rev Neurol 1988; 144:378–380.
22. Messimy R, Diebler C, Metzger J. Torsion dystonia of the left upper limb probably due to a head injury. Calcification of the head of the right caudate nucleus discovered by tomodensitometric examination. Rev Neurol 1977; 133:199–206.
23. Uncini A, Di Muzio A, Thomas A, Lugaresi A, Gambi D. Hand dystonia secondary to cervical demyelinating lesion. Acta Neurol Scand 1994; 90:51–55.
24. Krauss JK, Jankovic J. Head injury and posttraumatic movement disorders. Neurosurgery 2002; 50:927–940.

25. Lee MS, Rinne JO, Ceballos-Baumann A, Thompson PD, Marsden CD. Dystonia after head trauma. Neurology 1994; 44:1374–1378.
26. Foley J. Dyskinetic and dystonic cerebral palsy and birth. Acta Pediatr 1992; 91:57–60.
27. Jankovic J. Post-traumatic movement disorders: central and peripheral mechanisms. Neurology 1994; 44:2006–2014.
28. Jones AK, Brown WD, Friston KJ, Qi LY, Frackowiak RS. Cortical and subcortical localization of response to pain in man using positron emission tomography. Proc Roy Soc Lond B Biol Sci 1991; 244:39–44.
29. Iadarola MJ, Berman KF, Byas-Smith M, et al. Positron emission tomography (PET) studies of pain and allodynia in normals and patients with chronic neuropathic pain [Abstract]. Soc Neurosci Abstr 1993; 19:1074.
30. Fahn S. High dosage anticholinergic therapy in dystonia. Neurology 1983; 33(10):1255–1261.
31. Nygaard TG, Marsden CD, Fahn S. Dopa-responsive dystonia: long-term treatment response and prognosis. Neurology 1991; 41(2 (Pt 1)):174–181.
32. Jankovic J, Orman J. Tetrabenazine therapy of dystonia, chorea, tics, and other dyskinesias. Neurology 1988; 38(3):391–394.
33. Trugman JM, Leadbetter R, Zalis ME, Burgdorf RO, Wooten GF. Treatment of severe axial tardive dystonia with clozapine: case report and hypothesis. Mov Disord 1994; 9(4):441–446.
34. Ondo W, Hanna P, Jankovic J. Tetrabenazine treatment for tardive dyskinesia: assessment by randomized videotape Protocol. Am J Psychiatry 1999; 156:1279–1281.
35. Rosenbaum F, Jankovic J. Focal task-specific tremor and dystonia: categorization of occupational movement disorders. Neurology 1988; 38:522–527.
36. Cohen LG, Hallett M, Geller BD, Hochberg F. Treatment of focal dystonias of the hand with botulinum toxin injections. J Neurol Neurosurg Psychiatry 1989; 52:355–363.
37. Rivest J, Lees AJ, Marsden CD. Writer's cramp: treatment with botulinum toxin injections. Mov Disord 1991; 6:55–59.
38. Jankovic J, Schwartz KS. Longitudinal experience with botulinum toxin injections for treatment of blepharospasm and cervical dystonia. Neurology 1993; 43(4):834–836.
39. Tsui JKC, Bhatt M, Calne S, Calne DB. Botulinum toxin in the treatment of writer's cramp: a double-blind study. Neurology 1993; 43:183–185.
40. Molloy FM, Shill HA, Kaelin-Lang A, Karp BI. Accuracy of muscle localization without EMG: implications for treatment of limb dystonia. Neurology 2002; 58(5):805–807.
41. Tintner R, Jankovic J. Focal dystonia: the role of botulinum toxin. Curr Neurol Neurosci Rep 2001; 1:337–345.
42. Hsiung GY, Das SK, Ranawaya R, Lafontaine AL, Suchowersky O. Long-term efficacy of botulinum toxin A in treatment of various movement disorders over a 10-year period. Mov Disord 2002; 17:1288–1293.
43. Skogseid IM, Roislien J, Claussen B, Kerty E. Long-term botulinum toxin treatment increases employment rate in patients with cervical dystonia. Mov Disord 2005; 20(12):1604–1609.
44. Easton JK, Ozel T, Halpern D. Intramuscular neurolysis for spasticity in children. Arch Phys Med Rehabil 1979; 60:155–158.
45. Zafonte RD, Munin MC. Phenol and alcohol blocks for the treatment of spasticity. Phys Med Rehabil Clin N Am 2001; 12:817–832.
46. Gracies JM, Elovic E, McGuire J, Simpson DM. Traditional pharmacological treatments for spasticity. Part I: local treatments. Muscle Nerve Suppl 1997; 6:S61–S91.
47. Abright AL, Barry MJ, Shafton DH, Ferson SS. Intrathecal baclofen for generalized dystonia. Dev Med Child Neurol 2001; 43:652–657.
48. Teive HA, Sa DS, Grande CV, Antoniuk A, Werneck LC. Bilateral pallidotomy for generalized dystonia. Arq Neuropsiquiatr 2001; 59:353–357.
49. Yoshor D, Hamilton WJ, Ondo W, Jankovic J, Grossman RG. Comparison of thalamotomy and pallidotomy for the treatment of dystonia. Neurosurgery 2001; 48(4):818–824; discussion 824–826.

50. Vesper J, Klostermann F, Funk T, Stockhammer F, Brock M. Deep brain stimulation of the globus pallidus internus (GPI) for torsion dystonia—a report of two cases. Acta Neurochir Suppl 2002; 79:83–88.
51. Tagliati M, Miravite J, Shils JL, Bressman SB, Saunders-Pullman R, Alterman R. Long-term efficacy of pallidal DBS for treatment of medically intractable dystonia. Mov Disord 2004; 19(suppl 9):S321–S322.
52. Bittar RG, Yianni J, Wang S, et al. Deep brain stimulation for generalised dystonia and spasmodic torticollis. J Clin Neurosci 2005; 12(1):12–16.
53. Houser M, Waltz T. Meige syndrome and pallidal deep brain stimulation. Mov Disord 2005; 20(9):1203–1205.

# 9
# Cranial Dystonia

**Pankaj Satija and William G. Ondo**
*Department of Neurology, Baylor College of Medicine, Houston, Texas, U.S.A.*

## HISTORICAL NOTE NOMENCLATURE

The earliest recognition of cranial dystonia, including blepharospasm and oromandibular dystonias (OMD), is probably found in paintings of the Flemish artist Brueghel from the 16th century, who painted subjects with apparent blepharospasm and involuntary jaw opening (JO) (1). Whether or not the subjects of these portraits actually had any medical or neurological problems is not known. The conditions were first medically described by Talkow in Germany and Wood in the United States in 1871. In 1899, Gowers described various conditions associated with tonic and clonic contractions of the neck and jaw. Henry Meige published his landmark paper on blepharospasm and OMD in 1910, and the eponym "Meige's syndrome" is often used to designate idiopathic cranial–cervical dystonia. Various authors have ascribed eponyms of Wood, Brueghel, and Blake (an artist who also painted dystonic postures) to describe this syndrome. Marsden et al. designated blepharospasm-OMD syndrome to be a variant of adult-onset torsion dystonia (2) Although often discussed together because of many similarities, they are probably distinct neurological entities. The terms blepharospasm, OMD, and cranial dystonia (combined upper and lower facial dystonia) are used throughout the chapter.

## EPIDEMIOLOGY

The prevalence of blepharospasm is estimated to be five per 100,000 (3,4) The prevalence of OMD was estimated to be 68.9 per million persons in the United States (5). These figures are viewed as a gross underestimation because of inadequate ascertainment. In the two largest series of movement disorder clinic patients in the United States, cranial dystonia (blepharospasm and OMD) was reported in approximately 25% of 8000 patients with dystonia; women outnumbered men at a ratio of about 2:1 and in two-thirds of the patients, if the movement disorder began after 50 years of age (3,5). Pooled data from eight European countries estimated prevalence rates for blepharospasm of 36 per million (6). In Italy, Defazio et al. found a prevalence of 133 per million (7). Among the patients studied, blepharospasm and apraxia of eyelid opening was found to coexist in one-third of the cases. In this review, the crude prevalence range was estimated to be from 16 to 133 per million. An early age of onset and female gender were risk factors for spread of blepharospasm to other facial musculature. Because the diagnosis is clinically based, there exists an unclear delineation between "blepharospasm" and increased blinking. If cases with increased, but not problematic, eye blinking were included in these surveys, the prevalence would greatly increase.

## CLINICAL MANIFESTATIONS

By definition, blepharospasm is a focal dystonia manifest as involuntary eyelid closure. Before the development of sustained closure of the eyelids, about a third of the patients report increased frequency of blinking. The increased blinking that precedes blepharospasm is commonly associated with a feeling of irritation in the eyes. Patients classically describe a gritty or sandy feeling under their lids. This often leads to an initial diagnosis of "dry eyes." Initially clonic and later tonic (sustained) contractions of the orbicularis oculi are the hallmark of the condition; other muscles, including the corrugator supercilii and procerus, are often involved. A small minority of patients has unilateral involvement at the onset but the opposite eye becomes involved later in essentially all patients. The intensity gradually worsens and the eventual severity varies from only a slightly annoying condition to a disabling disorder, which interferes with daily activities such as reading, watching television, and driving. Symptoms are typically aggravated by light, especially automobile headlights while driving, and stress in general. The spasms may be transiently alleviated by tactile or proprioceptive "sensory tricks" such as touching the lateral canthus, pulling on an upper eyelid or an eyebrow, pinching the neck, relaxation, reading, concentration, or looking down ("geste antagonistique") (8–10). Interestingly, talking, humming, yawning, and especially singing often reduce the eye closing.

Minor involvement of other facial muscles can be seen, but if these are primarily involved as opposed to compensating for the eye closing, then the diagnosis is changed to cranial dystonia. In addition, patients with blepharospasm may have dystonia in the limbs, trunk, and vocal cords (spasmodic dysphonia). One study identified several risk factors for spread of blepharospasm: previous head or face trauma with loss of consciousness, younger age at onset of blepharospasm, and female gender (11,12).

Psychiatric symptoms such as anxiety, depression, psychosis, may be present before or at the onset of blepharospasm, and were identified in 18% of 264 patients (3). The prevalence of obsessive compulsive symptoms often attributed to basal ganglia dysfunction in patients with blepharospasm was significantly higher than in those with hemifacial spasm (HFS), despite the clinical similarities (13). This coexistence with mild psychiatric symptoms may explain the tendency to label blepharospasm as a psychogenic problem. However, truly psychogenic forms of blepharospasm are uncommon, and there is usually little or no evidence of any meaningful psychopathology in patients with blepharospasm (14). In the author's experience, prominent functional blindness, which is reported in idiopathic blepharospasm (14), is suggestive of either a psychogenic etiology or apraxia of eyelid opening (see below).

In one survey, the diagnosis of blepharospasm was delayed by 4 to 10 years in more than half of the patients (5). Although the latency between the onset of symptoms and the diagnosis is shortening largely as a result of education of physicians and the public, there are still unacceptably long delays in correct diagnosis.

OMD is considered either a focal or a segmental dystonia resulting in sustained and patterned muscle contractions affecting the lower face, jaw, tongue, pharynx, and mouth. It usually manifests as jaw closing (JC), JO, jaw deviation (JD), jaw retraction (JR), or a combination of these. JC dystonia is the most common (15,16). Other repetitive or sustained movements may be present including facial grimacing, lip pursing, lip sucking, smacking, chewing, tongue protrusion, retraction of the corners of the mouth, contraction of platysma or the nasalis, etc. These may cause chewing difficulties, dysarthria, dysphagia, dysphonia, breathing difficulties, and involuntary vocalizations such as humming and grunting (1,17,18). Sensory tics may relieve symptoms whereas common exacerbating factors include emotional stress, talking, eating, and fatigue (19). OMD may persist during sleep or may be associated with specific tasks such as biting into hard food. Classically, it worsens with volitional activity and may in fact be task-specific to eating, chewing, or talking. It may cause severe functional disability.

In the JC-OMD subtype, spasms of the masseter and temporalis may result is trismus and bruxism (20). In a study by Wooten-Watts et al., 78.5% of OMD patients were found to have bruxism (21). Approximately, one-fourth of patients with bruxism had associated dental problems including temporomandibular joint dysfunction (21%) and tooth wear (5%) (21). OMD is more frequently associated with other dystonias compared to blepharospasm. In a study of 100 patients with OMD, however, blepharospasm was the most frequent associated feature (1,17,18). In another study by Tan and Jankovic, associated symptoms were cervical dystonia (57.4%), blepharospasm (50%), limb dystonia (21%), tremor (16%), and spasmodic dysphonia (9.9%) (16).

## ETIOLOGY

Essential blepharospasm refers to a condition with no obvious secondary cause (11). It can also occur in association with other CNS diseases such as parkinsonian conditions, Huntington's disease, and Wilson's disease. Blepharospasm has been reported in association with autoimmune diseases including myasthenia gravis, rheumatoid arthritis, and systemic lupus erythematosus (22).

The coexistence of blepharospasm with dystonia in other body segments and the occurrence of a family history of dystonia both support the hypothesis that blepharospasm and other forms of dystonia may be genetically related. A family history of dystonia was present in 9.5% of the blepharospasm patients in one series and in 14% in another (3,23). Waddy et al. found that 25% of their patients with focal dystonias including OMD had first degree relatives with dystonia (24). Jankovic and Nutt in 1988 reported that 36.5% of the 238 patients with craniocervical dystonias had at least one first- or second-degree relative with a movement disorder (23).

No specific gene for blepharospasm has been identified. Misbahuddin reported that a polymorphism for the dopamine type-5 receptor was a risk factor (25). An over expression of allele-2 with micro satellite repeat in the D5 dopamine receptor gene on chromosome-4 was found in patients with blepharospasm. They suggested that this haplotype confers susceptibility to developing blepharospasm. Genetic linkage to chromosome 18p (designated *DYT7*) has been described in a German family with adult-onset craniocervical dystonia; however, the majority of cases are sporadic without linkage to this region (26). Cranial dystonia is also seen as part of *DYT-13*. Although the most common form of genetic dystonia, *DYT1* dystonia, is almost never associated with blepharospasm, many patients with familial forms of blepharospasm have been reported (23). Studies of the *DYT1* mutation in 150 patients with dystonia found that four of 22 subjects positive for the GAG deletion had limb onset that spread to craniocervical muscles.

Most OMD patients belong to the idiopathic category. In the series studies by Tan and Jankovic, causes of OMD were classified as idiopathic (63%), drug-induced (22.8%), peripherally induced (9.3%), postanoxic (2.5%), neurodegenerative disorder (1.8%), and head injury (0.8%) (16). One-third of all patients with cranial–cervical dystonia in a series had an action tremor and one-third had a first-degree relative with tremor or dystonia (23,27) A variety of secondary cranial dystonias and other conditions that cause facial movements are listed in Table 1. The most common are drug induced, CNS lesions, and peripheral trauma.

Tardive dyskinesia (TD) is probably the most common cause of secondary cranial dystonia, including blepharospasm (28,29). TD can be more stereotypic or dystonic. Burke et al. reported that most patients with tardive dystonia also had dystonic spasms involving the orofacial muscles (30). Blepharospasm may be the initial presentation (31). Tardive dystonia may also cause dramatic opisthotonic posturing. Dopamine receptor blocking drugs such as haloperidol and thioridazine are most associated with TD, but any medication that blocks dopamine receptors such metoclopramide (Reglan®) can equally cause TD. Blepharospasm from TD cannot be distinguished from idiopathic blepharospasm, but the oral lingual movements are usually more repetitive, loose, stereotypes that improve with volitional movements, rather than worsen (32). In addition, anticholinergics, antihistamines, long-term amphetamine, and ectasy have been reported to cause OMD that is different from TD (18,33,34). Orofacial spasms and blepharospasm are also seen with treatment with levodopa, particularly in patients with multiple systems atrophy (35).

Various CNS lesions in the basal ganglia, brainstem, and thalamus, e.g., ischemia, demyelination, surgically induced lesion, hydrocephalus, have been associated with blepharospasm and other forms of cranial dystonia (36–40). These reports support the hypothesis that other subcortical and brain stem structures besides the basal ganglia play an important role in the pathophysiology of cranial dystonia.

Peripheral trauma has been implicated as a cause of dystonia and peripheral trauma may trigger dystonia in carriers of the *DYT-1* gene (41,42). Sutcher et al. described four patients with OMD that was presumably caused by ill-fitting dentures (43). The movements often improve when the dentures are not worn. Cases caused by tooth extraction and oral surgery have been reported (20). The severity and progression of symptoms were found to be more prominent in patients with peripherally induced OMD; however, they had less spread to contiguous or noncontiguous segments in comparison to patients with idiopathic OMD (20). In another series, 12% of the patients with blepharospasm reported the occurrence of ocular trauma prior to the onset of their movement disorder (3).

## PHYSIOLOGY AND PATHOLOGY

The exact neurophysiology precipitating blepharospasm and OMD is not known; however, a number of studies have illuminated some aspects. In some studies,

**Table 1** Conditions Associated with Involuntary Facial Movement

| |
|---|
| Tics |
| Physiologic/reflexive |
| Hemifacial spasm—bilateral in up to 10% of the cases |
| Facial nerve synkinesis |
| Myokymia |
| Myoclonus |
| Reticular—branchial or ocular |
| Cortical—CJD, JME |
| Seizures |
| Metabolic |
| Aceruloplasminemia, Wilson's disease, Hallervorden-Spatz syndrome, tetanus |
| Drugs |
| Tardive |
| Acute dystonic reaction |
| Dopaminergic agents in parkinsonian conditions |
| Lithium, physostigmine, alcohol |
| Extrinsic ocular irritants |
| Tear gas, pollution, environmental toxins, photophobia, foreign body, etc. |
| Intrinsic ocular irritants |
| Blepharitis, iritis, uveitis, dry eyes, corneal erosion, glaucoma |
| Eyelid Weakness, etc. |
| Peripheral nerve injury, oculomotor nerve palsy, myasthenia gravis, Eaton-Lambert syndrome, diphtheria, botulism, Guillain-Barré syndrome posttraumatic with loss of conscious |
| Dentures, dental appliances, dental extractions, etc. |
| Central nervous system lesions involving rostral brain stem |
| Vascular |
| Demyelinating disorders (multiple sclerosis) |
| Brain tumor |
| Infectious diseases |
| Malformations |
| Hydrocephalus |
| Choreiform disorders |
| Huntington's disease |
| Neuroacanthocytosis |
| Sydenham's chorea |
| Essential chorea |
| Miscellaneous neurodegenerative disorders |
| Myotonic dystrophy |
| Spinal cerebellar atrophy II |
| Postencephalitic parkinsonism |
| Progressive supranuclear palsy |
| Multiple systems atrophy |
| Schwartz–Jampel syndrome |
| Eyelid apraxia |
| Psychogenic |
| Stress, posttraumatic, conversion disorder, malingering |
| Sleep, etc. |

*Abbreviations*: CJD, Creutzfeldt-Jakob disease; JME, juvenile myoclonic epilepsy.

blepharospasms are evaluated separately while in others, they are lumped together with cranial dystonia.

The blink reflex may be elicited by electrical stimulation of the supraorbital nerve and consists of an early, first response (R1) and a late, second response (R2). Neurophysiologic studies have demonstrated increased amplitude and duration of the R1 and R2 blink response in patients with blepharospasm. In one study of 17 patients with dystonic blepharospasm and 11 age-matched controls, Gomez-Wong et al. (8,9) found that blepharospasm patients had normal prepulse inhibition occurring at 60 to 100 msec intervals but the prepulse inhibition for the R2 response was abnormally reduced in 11 (64.7%) patients, including nine who did not use sensory tricks (10). Electrophysiological studies have shown shortened silent periods of the facial muscles (3,44). Lew et al. showed that 87% of the patients with cranial–cervical dystonia display increased latency and reduced amplitude of the acoustic reflex (45). These studies indicate that some cases of blepharospasm result from hyperexcitability of cortical neurons and brainstem interneurons, or a lack of inhibition of neurons that supply the facial muscles, possibly as a result of dysfunction of descending basal ganglia pathways.

Positron emission tomographic (PET) measurements of regional cerebral flow or metabolism, either at rest or during activation, have provided key insights into the pathophysiology of dystonia. Measuring metabolism by using F-18 fluorodeoxyglucose PET in patients with idiopathic blepharospasm, Esmaeli-Gutstein et al. showed significantly increased activity in the striatum and thalamus and Hutchinson et al. found increased metabolic activity in the pons and cerebellum (46,47). In another study using PET before and after vibration applied to the lower face, Feiwell et al. showed that the normal activation of the primary sensorimotor area significantly decreased following vibration in patients with blepharospasm (48). Interestingly, abnormal cortical sensory responses to vibration in dopa-responsive dystonia may normalize after levodopa administration, suggesting that sensory motor processing at the cortical level is influenced by dopaminergic pathways, most likely through basal ganglia cortical circuits (49). Lack of cortical inhibition rather than abnormal excitation is thought to best explain the excessive movement in patients with dystonia (50,51). PET measurement of the in vivo binding of the dopaminergic radioligand [$^{18}$F]spiperone in the putamen of 21 patients with cranial and hand dystonia revealed a significant 29% mean decrease in a binding index in dystonic subjects compared to normal controls. These findings are consistent with decreased dopamine D2-like binding in the putamen (49).

Few patients with cranial dystonia, including blepharospasm, have been studied at autopsy (37,52,53). Normal findings or nonspecific abnormalities are present in nearly all brains from patients with idiopathic blepharospasm. Jankovic et al. reported a 68-year old patient with metastatic adenocarcinoma and a seven year history of progressive blepharospasm, spasmodic dysphonia, and cervical dystonia, whose brain was collected within 30 minutes of her death and examined histologically as well as biochemically. There were no abnormalities noted on histological examination, but the norepinephrine levels were markedly increased in the brainstem (199.6% in red nucleus and 415.2% in substantia nigra). Two patients with atypical cranial dystonia were found to have a mosaic neuronal cell loss and gliosis in the striatum (54). Neuronal cell loss in the substantia nigra and other brainstem nuclei was reported in three patients, two of whom had associated Lewy bodies (55).

Animal studies have found that serotonin [5-hydroxytryptamine (5-HT)] facilitates the excitability of facial motor neurons through 5-HT2 receptors, which are densely concentrated in the facial nucleus. Serotonin agonists produce blepharospasm and serotonin antagonists reduce blink frequency (56). Furthermore, the normal prepulse inhibition of the trigeminal reflex is abnormal in some patients with blepharospasm. It is postulated that in these patients, the normal sensory gating on trigeminal afferents are disturbed, the normal contact-induced reduction in the gain of trigeminal–facial reflexes is lost (9,10). Schicatano et al. proposed a two-factor model based on the observation that dopamine depletion reduces the tonic inhibition of trigeminal blink circuit, thus creating "a permissive environment within the trigeminal blink circuits," which along with an external ophthalmic insult (second factor), precipitates blepharospasm (57). They suggest that this model may also be applicable to the genesis of other dystonias.

## DIFFERENTIAL DIAGNOSIS

"Eyelid opening apraxia" or "eyelid freezing" is related to the lack of contractions or inhibition of the levator palpebrae muscles. This condition may occur in isolation or may be associated with patients with other parkinsonian syndromes, Huntington's disease, hemispheric cerebral vascular disease, and neuroacanthocytosis. Compensatory contractions of the frontalis muscles are a frequent phenomenon (58,59). Based on clinical and electrophysiological observations in six patients, Elston argued that this sign was caused by isolated contraction of the pretarsal orbicularis oculi (60). Krack et al. generally corroborated this finding and posited that "apraxia of eyelid opening" is not a true apraxia but rather a dystonia (59). They advocated treatment with botulinum toxin (BoTN) injections around the pretarsal area of the orbicularis oculi, further supporting a dystonic physiology. Electromyographic (EMG) recording from the levator palpebrae and orbicularis oculi muscles, however, may help differentiate this persistent pretarsal orbicularis oculi contraction from the levator inhibition seen in some cases (61,62). Apraxia associated with parkinsonian syndromes may respond to levodopa (63).

Blinking is probably the most common motor tic, present in 70% of patients with Tourette's syndrome. They may strongly mimic blepharospasm and even possess similar sensory symptoms. Often eye-closing tics are associated with other eye movements, especially oculomotor deviation or at least other facial tics. Tics are usually partially suppressible and typically begin in childhood.

Involuntary eye closure may also be caused by ophthalmologic disorders affecting contractions of the orbicularis oculi, possibly mediated by the trigeminal–palpebral reflex (e.g., blepharitis, conjunctivitis, keratitis, iritis, uveitis) or the opticopalpebral reflex (e.g., albinism, achromatopsia, maculopathies) (1). It can be difficult, however, to differentiate dry eyes from the sensory component of blepharospasm.

Reflex blepharospasm is also seen in premature infants, patients with parkinsonian syndromes, lesions in the nondominant temporoparietal lobe (Fisher's sign), and in response to loud noise (cochleopalpebral reflex), sudden free fall (vestibulopalpebral reflex), and gag (palatopalpebral reflex).

HFS, a form of segmental myoclonus, is characterized by involuntary, paroxysmal, tonic or clonic contractions of the muscles on one side of the face (64). In contrast to blepharospasm, the symptoms are unilateral; however, bilateral facial spasms have been reported (65). In one study, magnetic resonance tomographic angiography showed that 64.9% of patients with HFS had ipsilateral vascular compression (66). The presumed pathophysiologic mechanism of HFS involves the generation of ortho- and antidromic impulses by a damaged area of the facial nerve. Typically HFS begins with twitches in the eyelids that eventually progress to involve the lower face. The contractions are often triggered by action (smiling, talking, eating, and blinking). Patients with HFS often exhibit paradoxical raising of the eyebrow as the eye closes (the "other" Babinski sign) (67). In rare cases, HFS may be associated with trigeminal neuralgia (tic convulsive) or glossopharyngeal neuralgia (68,69).

The phenomenology of aberrant facial regeneration or facial synkinesis is similar to HFS, but the onset usually follows facial palsy. Studies in macaque monkeys show that following facial nerve injury, the orbicularis oculi motoneurons innervate the perioral muscles causing cocontraction (synkinesia) of eyelid and perioral muscles (70). Blepharospasm has been also reported after Bell's palsy (71,72). Hemimasticatory spasm is a rare disorder whose underlying mechanism is similar to HFS but the trigeminal rather than the facial nerve is involved (73). Facial myokymia, a rapid undulation, and flickering of the facial muscles from the frontalis to the platysma is thought to be due to an intramedullary lesion close to the facial motor nucleus. Multiple sclerosis is probably the most common cause, but intra-axial tumors, Guillain-Barré syndrome, spinal–cerebellar ataxia type-2, and facial nerve injuries have also been described as associated with this movement disorder. Blepharoclonus refers to rhythmic contractions of the orbicularis oculi closely resembling tremor, which is present during gentle closure of the eyelids. Although no apparent cause can be identified in many cases, blepharoclonus is occasionally associated with multiple sclerosis, obstructive hydrocephalus, and Arnold–Chiari malformation (74,75). In addition to gastrointestinal symptoms, patients with Whipple's disease typically exhibit supranuclear ophthalmoparesis and rhythmic contractions of the eyelids, face, and mouth in synchrony with convergent eye oscillations. This oculomasticatory myorhythmia is usually associated with contractions of neck, pharyngeal, and proximal and distal musculature.

OMD is frequently misdiagnosed as TMJ dysfunction and bruxism. Delay in appropriate treatment may lead to TMJ dislocation as well as other TMJ-related problems (76,77). The issue of whether bruxism is a separate entity from OMD is controversial. The American Academy of Orofacial Pain defines bruxism as a diurnal or nocturnal parafunctional activity including clenching, grinding, bracing, and gnashing of teeth (78). This definition may be too general and encompassing. Prevalence estimates of bruxism in adult population vary from 5% to 96% (79,80). However, while some patients with OMD clench and grind their teeth, these patients appear differently from people with nocturnal bruxism, frequently seen in the general population (21,81). Wooten-Watts et al. demonstrated that the majority of OMD patients had diurnal bruxism, with symptoms disappearing during sleep (21). Only 13% of these patients had nocturnal bruxism. Severe diurnal bruxism is frequently associated with organic brain disease such as Huntington's disease and Rett Syndrome (69,82).

Tetanus is caused by tetanus toxin, a product of Clostridium tetani, and it is characterized by hyperactivity of motor neurons, which causes forceful closure of the eyelids or trismus (jaw spasm). Although rare in the United States, it still remains a major public health problem in underdeveloped areas. Involvement of other body parts gives clues to the diagnosis. Similarly, tonic spasms of facial muscles in multiple sclerosis are associated with limb dystonia and other neurological signs (83,84). Focal motor seizures involving the facial muscles sometimes presenting as increased blinking are abrupt in onset and may become secondarily generalized (85). Malignant hyperthermia can also present with jaw spasm, but is quickly followed by temperature elevation.

## PROGNOSIS AND COMPLICATIONS

Once present, blepharospasm is generally persistent. In most studies, fewer than 3% of the patients experienced prolonged spontaneous remission, but the remission rates have been reported to be as high as 10%, usually within the first five years (3,5,86,87). Typically, symptoms progressively worsen during the first months to years after onset followed by stabilization. In a minority with blepharospasm, the dystonia will later spread to involve other facial, oromandibular, pharyngeal, laryngeal, and cervical muscles (cranial–cervical dystonia). It would be very rare for this to spread past that segment of the body. Complications of chronic, untreated blepharospasm includes dermatochalasis (abnormal looseness of the eyelid skin due to constant pulling on the eyelids) and xerophthalmia "dry eyes." The dermatochalasis often requires blepharoplasty as the excess skin can drape over the eye and impair vision.

## MANAGEMENT

Therapy for blepharospasm and cranial dystonia, in general, can be divided into oral agents, BoTN injections, surgical procedures, and complimentary therapy such as sunglasses. One problem regarding blepharospasm treatment research is the absence of any validated scale. Many studies have used the Fahn Blepharospasm Rating Scale and the Blepharospasm Disability scale, but these have never been well validated (30,88,89). Many studies have employed their own rating scales and global impressions.

As with the other forms of dystonia, many oral medications have been used to treat blepharospasm and OMD. Poor pathophysiological understanding of cranial dystonia hampers rational drug development, but a variety of muscle relaxants and other medications have been reported to help blepharospasm in open label trials. Fewer reports discuss oral mandibular dystonia. Generally of modest efficacy, these agents have dose limitations due to side effects. Interestingly, many drugs that work reciprocally have been reported to benefit individual patients. Some examples are anticholinergics [e.g., trihexyphenidyl (Artane®), benztropine (Cogentin®), orphenadrine (Norflex®), ethopropazine (Parsidol®)], and cholinergic drugs (e.g., choline, deanol); dopaminergic agents (e.g., levodopa and dopamine agonists) and antidopaminergic drugs (e.g., haloperidol, tetrabenazine). Other categories that have been used include gamma aminobutyric acid (GABA)-ergic drugs (e.g., baclofen, tizanadine), benzodiazepines (e.g., lorazepam, clonazepam, diazepam), anticonvulsants (e.g., carbamazepine, lamotrigine), cyproheptadine, cannabidiol, mexiletine, and lithium (90–95). Large open label series tend to favor anticholinergics, benzodiazepines, and tetrabenazine.

There are only a few small controlled trials for blepharospasm and none for oral–mandibular dystonia. Orphenadrine, apomorphine, tetrabenazine have shown benefit whereas trihexyphenidyl, deanol, bromocriptine were not superior to placebo (96).

The effectiveness of BoTN A in blepharospasm was first demonstrated in a double-blind, placebo-controlled trial in 1987 (92). In a subsequent trial of 477 patients with various dystonias and HFS, Jankovic et al. (97) reviewed the results in 90 patients injected with Botox® for blepharospasm. Moderate or marked improvement was noted in 94% of the patients. Pretarsal injections, particularly into the Riolan's part of the pretarsal orbicularis oculi seemed to provide the most benefit (98–100). The average latency from the time of the injection to the onset of improvement was two to five days and the average duration of maximum benefit was three to four months. In addition to the observed functional improvement, there was usually a meaningful amelioration of discomfort and social stress. The most common adverse events were ptosis, blurring of vision or diplopia, tearing, and local hematoma, all of which lessen with subsequent injections (101). This may, in part, be explained by greater experience and improvements in injection techniques.

All of the BoTN (type A: Botox and Dysport®, type B: Myobloc® and Neurobloc®, and type F) improve blepharospasm in controlled trials. BoTN F has a shorter duration of benefit (102,103). In a double-blind comparative study of 212 patients with essential blepharospasm who received one injection of Botox and one injection of Dysport in two separate treatment sessions, using an empirical ratio Botox: Dysport of 1:4 (IU), the average dose of Botox per treatment was 45.4 IU ± 13.3 and of Dysport 182.1 IU ± 55.1. There was no difference in the duration of the effect, but side effects, particularly ptosis, were more frequent with Dysport as compared to Botox (24.1% vs. 17.0%), ($p < 0.05$).

BoTN treatment is now considered as the treatment of choice for blepharospasm (American Academy of Ophthalmology 1989; American Academy of Neurology 1990) (104). Apraxia of eyelid opening is more difficult to treat than blepharospasm, but some patients with apraxia of eyelid opening improve with BoTN injections into the pretarsal orbicularis oculi, particularly if it is triggered by blepharospasm (105).

Patients who fail to obtain satisfactory control of their blepharospasm with BoTN may be candidates for surgical treatment. Facial nerve ablation and orbicularis oculi myectomy are used much less than in the past because of postoperative complications such as ectropion, exposure keratitis, facial droop, and postoperative swelling and scarring (106,107). Myectomy usually results in some ptosis but is often effective. Patients with severe apraxia of eyelid opening may benefit from frontalis suspension combined with blepharoplasty (108). Chemomyectomy with muscle necrotizing drugs such as doxorubicin, has been tried in some patients with blepharospasm. Severe local irritation currently limits the usefulness of this therapy. However, a modification of the procedure using a combination of bupivacaine/hyaluronidase and Doxil (Sequus, Menlo Park, CA), a liposome-encapsulated form of doxorubicin, may be more effective and safer (109). Blockade of the superior sympathetic ganglion with local anesthetic has been reported to improve light-induced eyelid spasm and, as such, may be possibly useful as a therapeutic modality in patients with blepharospasm (110). One report suggested that the administration of a combination of linoleic acid and alphalinoleic acid, which presumably modifies the composition and function of neuronal membranes, has improved blepharospasm in a catecholamine-depleted rat model (111). This combination has yet not been tested in patients with blepharospasm.

Several nonpharmacological or surgical treatments should be noted. Eyelid crutches on glasses have been reported to be helpful in some patients with blepharospasm, usually after BoTN injections (112). Sunglasses, have been demonstrated to help some cases. Biofeedback and other muscle relaxation techniques and stress management may be helpful, particularly for those patients in whom stress exacerbates the symptoms (113).

BoTN is also considered the treatment of choice for OMD. Many investigators have reported the effectiveness of BoTN A in relieving symptoms of OMD (17,87,92,97,114–122). In 1987, a double-blind, placebo-controlled trial found that 37.5% of a small series of OMD cervical dystonia patients improved after BoTN A treatment (92). In an open label design study, Blitzer et al. demonstrated that

BoTN A yielded a 50% improvement in 20 patients with OMD (116). Most of these patients had previously failed a variety of pharmacological treatments.

## SELECTION OF MUSCLES FOR OROMANDIBULAR DYSTONIAS

Ideally, one should be able to determine which muscles are primarily involved in the abnormal movements, inject these muscles with the appropriate dose of BoTN, and thus affect only those actions involved in the production of the abnormal movement or posture. The masseters and temporalis represent targets for JC-OMD, and the submentalis complex, comprising of the digastrics, geniohyoid and mylohyoid muscles, or the lateral pterygoid muscles for JO-OMD. Palpation may be helpful in this approach, but EMG may be required to inject nonpalpable muscles. In some forms of focal dystonia, the pattern of muscle involvement may change over time (123). Studies directly comparing various modes and dosage of BoTN administration remain to be done. The doses of BoTN used depend on the clinical severity. In most patients, the dose has to be titrated according to the clinical response and any toxin-related complications after an initial modest dose.

Botox was used in the two largest studies of OMD (15,16). In the Baylor prospective study, 162 patients satisfied the study inclusion criteria. The masseters and submentalis complex were the only two muscle groups injected with BoTN in this group of patients. More than half the patients had JC dystonia. The mean doses of BoTN (per side) were 54.2 ± 15.2 U for the masseters and 28.6 ± 16.7 U for the submentalis complex. The mean total duration of response was 16.4 ± 7.1 weeks. The mean global effect of BoTN was 3.1 ± 1.0 (range, 0–4, where 4 equals the complete abolition of dystonia), with the JC dystonia patients responding best. Fifty-one patients (31.5%) reported adverse effects with BoTN in at least one visit. Complications such as dysphagia and dysarthria were reported in 135 (11.1%) of all treatment visits. There was a poorer response and higher complication rate with JOD than with the other types of OMD.

The New York group studied 96 patients, 72.9% women, with a mean age of symptoms onset of 43.9 years ± 2.0 years (15). The median doses of BoTN given for the jaw muscles were masseter, 24.5; temporalis, 18.5; medial pterygoid, 16.3; lateral pterygoid, 15.9 and anterior digastric, 9.8 units. The percentage improvement after BoTN was: JC (45%), JO (44%), and JD (37%). Dysphagia was the most common compliant seen in 40% of the patients with JO–OMD; however, in patients with JC-OMD, some complaints included weakened chewing, soreness and pain at injection suite, facial swelling, and headache.

Certain sensory tricks may transiently improve the symptoms of OMD. For instance, touching the lips may relieve jaw spasm, touching the chin may aid in JC. Dental assessment may help patients with associated TMJ dysfunction. Speech therapy may facilitate speech and help to relieve swallowing difficulties. Various forms of relaxation and biofeedback therapies are useful in patients whose symptoms are aggravated by stress or anxiety. Acupuncture is another alternative form of treatment; however, relief of symptoms such as pain, if any, is usually transient.

Overall, OMD is more difficult to treat and unlike blepharospasm, BoTN usually does not result in a complete remission of symptoms. JO and JR are particularly difficult to treat. Nevertheless, BoTN remains the most effective therapy for OMD. Peripheral ablative surgeries do not exist and even CNS neurosurgeries such as pallidotomy and pallidal stimulation used in generalized dystonia, seldom improve this anatomic area (124,125).

## REFERENCES

1. Jankovic J. Etiology and differential diagnosis of blepharospasm and oromandibular dystonia. Adv Neurol 1988; 49:103–116.
2. Marsden CD. Blepharospasm-oromandibular dystonia syndrome (Brueghel's syndrome): a variant of adult-onset torsion dystonia? J Neurol Neurosurg Psychiatry 1976; 59:1204–1209.
3. Grandas F, Elston J, Quinn N, Marsden CD. Blepharospasm: a review of 264 patients. J Neurol Neurosurg Psychiatry 1988; 51:767–772.
4. Nutt JG, Muenter MD, Aronson A, et al. Epidemiology of focal and generalized dystonia in Rochester, Minnesota. Mov Disord 1988; 3:188–194.
5. Jankovic J, Orman J. Blepharospasm: demographic and clinical survey of 250 patients. Ann Ophthalmol 1984; 16:371–376.
6. The Epidemiological Study of Dystonia in Europe (ESDE) Collaborative Group. A prevalence study of primary dystonia in eight European countries. The Epidemiological Study of Dystonia in Europe (ESDE) Collaborative Group. J Neurol 2000; 247:787–792.
7. Defazio G, Livrea P, De Salvia R, et al. Prevalence of primary blepharospasm in a community of Puglia region, Southern Italy. Neurology 2001; 156:1579–1581.
8. Gomez-Wong E, Marti MJ, Tolosa E, Valls-Sole J. Sensory modulation of the blink reflex in patients with blepharospasm. Arch Neurol 1998; 55:1233–1237.
9. Gomez-Wong E, Marti MJ, Cossu G, et al. The geste antagonistique induces transient modulation of the blink reflex in human patients with blepharospasm. Neurosci Lett 1998; 24:125–128b.
10. Jankovic J, Fahn S. Dystonic disorders. In: Jankovic J, Tolosa E, eds. Parkinson's Disease Movement Disorders. 4th ed. Philadelphia, PA: Lippincott Williams and Wilkins, 2002.
11. Defazio G, Livrea P. Epidemiology of primary blepharospasm. Mov Disord 2002; 17:7–12.
12. Defazio G, Berardelli A, Abbruzzese G, et al. Risk factors for spread of primary adult-onset blepharospasm: A multicenter investigation of the Italian movement disorders study group. J Neurol Neurosurg Psychiatry 1999; 67:613–619.
13. Broocks A, Thiel A, Angerstein D, Dressler D. Higher prevalence of obsessive compulsive symptoms in patients with blepharospasm than in patients with hemifacial spasm. Am J Psychiatry 1998; 155:555–557.
14. Scheidt CE, Schuller B, Rayki O, et al. Relative absence of psychopathology in benign essential blepharospasm and hemifacial spasm. Neurology 1996; 47:43–45.
15. Brin MF, Blintzer A, Herman S, et al. Oromandibular dystonia: treatment of 96 patients with botulinum toxin A. In: Jankovic J, Hallett M, eds: Therapy with Botulinum Toxin. New York: Marcel Dekker, 1994:429–435.
16. Tan EK, Jankovic J. Botulinum toxin A in patients with oromandibular dystonia: long term follow up. Neurology 1999; 53:2102–2108.
17. Charles PD, Davis TL, Shannon KM, et al. Tongue protrusion dystonia: treatment with botulinum toxin. South Med J 1997; 90:522–525.
18. Tolosa E, Marti MJ. Blepharospasm-oromandibular dystonia (Meige's syndrome): clinical aspects. Adv Neurol 1988; 49:73–84.
19. Jankovic J, Ford J. Blepharospasm and orofacial-cervical dystonia: clinical and pharmacological findings in 100 patients. Ann Neurol 1983; 13:402–411.
20. Sankhla C, Lai EC, Jankovic J. Peripherally induced oromandibular dystonia. J Neurol Neurosurg Psychiatry 1998; 65:722–728.
21. Wooten-Watts M, Tan EK, Jankovic J. Bruxism and cranio-cervical dystonia: is there a relationship? Cranio 1999; 17:196–201.
22. Nilaver G, Whiting S, Nutt JG. Autoimmune etiology for cranial dystonia. Mov Disord 1990; 5:179–180.
23. Jankovic J, Nutt JG. Blepharospasm and cranial-cervical dystonia (Meige's syndrome): familial occurrence. Adv Neurol 1988; 49:117–123.
24. Waddy HM. Fletcher NS, Harding AE, et al. A genetic study of idiopathic dystonias. Ann Neurol 1991; 29:320–324.

25. Misbahuddin A, Placzek MR, Chaudhuri KR, et al. A polymorphism in the dopamine receptor DRD5 is associated with blepharospasm. Neurology 2002; 58:124–126.
26. Leube B, Hendgen T, Kessler KR, et al. Sporadic focal dystonia in Northwest Germany: Molecular basis on chromosome 18p. Ann Neurol 1997; 42:111–114.
27. Jankovic J. Essential tremor: a heterogenous disorder. Mov Disord 2002; 17:638–644.
28. Jankovic J. Tardive syndromes and other drug-induced movement disorders. Clin Neuropharmacol 1995; 18:197–214.
29. Mauriello JA, Carbonaro P, Dhillon S, et al. Drug-associated facial dyskinesias - a study of 238 patients. J Neurophthalmol 1998; 18:153–157.
30. Burke RE, Fahn S, Marsden CD, et al. Validity and reliability of a rating scale for the primary torsion dystonias. Neurology 1985; 35:73–77.
31. Sachdev P. Tardive blepharospasm. Mov Disord 1998; 13:947–951.
32. Tan EK, Jankovic J. Tardive and idiopathic oromandibular dystonia: a clinical comparison. J Neurol Neurosurg Psychiatry 2000; 68(2):186–190.
33. Jankovic J. Drug induced and other orofacial-cervical dyskinesias. Ann Intern Med 1981; 94:788–793.
34. Powers JM. Decongestant-induced blepharospasm and orofacial dystonia. JAMA 1982; 247:3244–3255.
35. Weiner WJ, Nausieda P. Meige's syndrome during long-term dopaminergic therapy in Parkinson's disease. Arch Neurol 1982; 39:451–452.
36. Aramideh M, de Visser O, Holsege G, et al. Blepharospasm in association with a lower pontine lesion. Neurology 1996; 46:476–478.
37. Hallett M, Daroff RB. Blepharospasm: Report of a workshop. Neurology 1996; 46:1213–1218.
38. Jankovic J. Blepharospasm with basal ganglia lesions. Arch Neurol 1986; 43:866–868.
39. Miranda M, Millar A. Blepharospasm associated with bilateral infarcts confined to the thalamus: case report. Mov Disord 1998; 13:616–617.
40. Verghese J, Milling C, Rosenbaums DM. Ptosis, blepharospasm, and apraxia of eyelid opening secondary to putaminal hemorrhage. Neurology 1999; 53:652.
41. Jankovic J. Posttraumatic movement disorders: Central and peripheral mechanisms. Neurology 1994; 44:2008–2014.
42. Jankovic J. Can peripheral trauma induce dystonia and other movement disorders? Yes! Mov Disord 2001; 16:7–12.
43. Sutcher HD, Underwood RB, Beatty RA, et al. Orofacial dyskinesia: a dental dimension. JAMA 1971; 216:1459–1463.
44. Grandas F, Traba A, Alonso F, Esteban A. Blink reflex recovery cycle in patients with blepharospasm unilaterally treated with botulinum toxin. Clin Neuropharmacol 1998; 21:307–311.
45. Lew H, Jordan C, Jerger J, Jankovic J. Acoustic reflex abnormalities in cranial-cervical dystonia. Neurology 1992; 42:594–597.
46. Esmaeli-Gutstein B, Nahmias C, Thompson M, et al. Positron emission tomography in patients with benign essential blepharospasm. Ophthal Plast Reconstr Surg 1999; 15: 23–27.
47. Hutchinson M, Nakamura T, Moeller JR, et al. The metabolic topography of essential blepharospasm. A focal dystonia with general implications. Neurology 2000; 55:673–677.
48. Feiwell RJ, Black KJ, McGee-Minnich LA, et al. Diminished regional cerebral blood flow response to vibration in patients with blepharospasm. Neurology 1999; 52:291–297.
49. Perlmutter JS, Stambuk MK, Markham J, et al. Decreased [18F] spiperone binding in putamen in idiopathic focal dystonia. J Neurosci 1997; 17:843–850.
50. Hallett M. Is dystonia a sensory disorder? Ann Neurol 1995; 38:139–140.
51. Hallett M. Physiology of dystonia. Adv Neurol 1998; 78:11–18.
52. Gibb WR, Lees AJ, Marsden CD. Pathological report of four patients presenting with cranial dystonias. Mov Disord 1988; 3:211–221.
53. Hallett M. Blepharospasm: Recent advances. Neurology 2002; 59:1306–1312.

54. Hayes MW, Ouvrier RA, Evans W, Somerville E, Morris JG. X-linked Dystonia-Deafness syndrome. Mov Disord 1998; 13(2):303–308.
55. Mark MH, Sage JI, Dickson DW, et al. Meige syndrome in the spectrum of Lewy body disease. Neurology 1994; 44:1432–1436.
56. LeDoux MS, Lorden JF, Smith JM, Mays LE. Serotonergic modulation of eye blinks in cat and monkey. Neurosci Lett 1998; 253:61–64.
57. Schicatano EJ, Basso, Evinger C. Animal model explains the origins of the cranial dystonia benign essential blepharospasm. J Neurophysiol 1997; 77:2842–2846.
58. Golbe LI, Davis PH, Lepore FE. Eyelid movement abnormalities in progressive supranuclear palsy. Mov Disord 1989; 4:297–302.
59. Krack P, Marion MH. "Apraxia of lid opening." A focal eyelid dystonia: Clinical study of 32 patients.
60. Elston JS. A new variant of blepharospasm. J Neurol Neurosurg Psychiatry 1992; 55:369–371.
61. Aramideh M, Ongerboer de Visser BW, Koelman JHTM, et al. Motor persistence of orbicularis oculi muscle in eyelid-opening disorders. Neurology 1995; 45:897–902.
62. Tozlovanu V, Forget R, Iancu A, Boghen D. Prolonged orbicularis oculi activity. A major factor in apraxia of lid opening. Neurology 2001; 57:1013–1018.
63. Dewey RB, Maraganore DM. Isolated eyelid-opening apraxia: Report of a new levodopa-responsive syndrome. Neurology 1994; 44:1752–1754.
64. Wang A, Jankovic J. Hemifacial spasm: Clinical findings and treatment. Muscle Nerve 1998; 21:1740–1747.
65. Burke RE, Fahn S, Jankovic J, et al. Tardive dystonia: late-onset and persistent dystonia caused by antipsychotic drugs. Neurology 1982; 32:1335–1346.
66. Adler CH, Zimmerman RA, Savino PJ, et al. Hemifacial spasm: evaluation by magnetic resonance imaging and magnetic resonance tomographic angiography. Ann Neurol 1992; 32:502–506.
67. Devoize JL. "The other" Babinski's sign: paradoxical raising of the eyebrow in hemifacial spasm. J Neurol Neurosurg Psychiatry 2001; 70:516.
68. Kobata H, Kondo Am Iwasaki K, et al. Combined hyperactive dysfunction syndrome of the cranial nerves: trigeminal neuralgia, hemifacial spasm and glossopharyngeal neuralgia: 11 year experience and review. Neurosurgery 1998; 43:1351–1361.
69. Tan EK, Jankovic J, Ondo W. Bruxing behavior in Huntington' disease. Mov Disord 2000; 15:171–173.
70. Baker RS, Stava MW, Nelson KR, et al. Aberrant reinnervation of facial musculature in a subhuman primate: A correlative analysis of eyelid kinematics, muscle synkinesis, and motoneuron localization. Neurology 1994; 44:2165–2173.
71. Baker RS, Sun WS, Hasan SA, et al. Maladaptive neural compensatory mechanisms in Bell's palsy-induced blepharospasm. Neurology 1997; 49:223–229.
72. Chuke JC, Baker RS, Porter JD. Bell's palsy-associated blepharospasm relieved by aiding eyelid closure. Ann Neurol 1996; 39:263–268.
73. Auger RG, Litchy WJ, Cascino TL, Ahlskog JE. Hemimasticatory spasm: clinical and electrophysiologic observations. Neurology 1992; 42:2263–2266.
74. Jacome DE. Blepharoclonus and Arnold-Chiari malformation. Acta Neurol Scand 2001; 104:113–117.
75. Jacome DE. Blepharoclonus in multiple sclerosis. Acta Neurol Scand 2001; 104:380–384.
76. Gray AR, Barker GR. Idiopathic blepharospasm-oromandibular dystonia syndrome (Meige's syndrome) presenting as chronic temporo-mandibular joint dysfunction. Br J Oral Maxillofac Surg 1991; 29:97–99.
77. Verma RK, Gupta BK, Kochar SK, et al. Meige's syndrome. J Assoc Physicians India 1993; 41:173–174.
78. McNeil C. Temporomandibular disorders: Guidelines for Classification, Assessment and Management. Chicago: The American Academy of Orofacial Pain, Quintessence, 1993.

79. Tan EK, Jankovic J. Treatment of severe bruxism with botulinum toxin. J Am Dent Assoc 2000; 131:211–216.
80. Thompson BA, Blount BW, Krumholz TS. Treatment approaches to bruxism. Am Fam Physician 1994; 49:1617–1622.
81. Rugh JD, Harlan JA. Nocturnal bruxism and temporomandibular disorders. Adv Neurol 1988; 49:329–341.
82. FitzGerald PM, Jankovic J, Percy AK. Rett Syndrome and associated movement disorders. Mov Disord 1990; 5:195–202.
83. Berger JR, Sheremata WA, Melamed MD. Paroxysmal dystonia as the initial manifestation of multiple sclerosis. Arch Neurol 1984; 41:747–750.
84. Thompson PD, Obeso JA, Delgado G, et al. Focal dystonia of the jaw and the differential diagnosis of unilateral jaw and masticatory spasm. J Neurol Neurosurg Psychiatry 1986; 49:651–656.
85. Benbadis SR, Kotagal P, Klem GH. Unilateral blinking: A lateralizing sign in partial seizures. Neurology 1996; 46:45–48.
86. Castelbuono A, Miller NR. Spontaneous remission in patients with essential blepharospasm and Meige syndrome. Am J Ophthalmol 1998; 126:432–435.
87. Mauriello JA Jr, Dhillon S, Leone T, et al. Treatment selections of 239 patients with blepharospasm and Meige syndrome over 11 years. Br J Ophthalmol 1996; 80:1073–1076.
88. Lindeboom R, De Haan R, Aramideh M, Speelman JD. The blepharospasm disability scale: An instrument for the assessment of functional health in blepharospasm. Mov Disord 1995; 10:444–449.
89. Fahn S. Rating scales for blepharospasm. Adv Ophthalmic Plast Reconstr Surg 1985; 4:97–101.
90. Gimenez Roldan S, Mateo D, Orbe M, et al. Acute pharmacological tests in cranial dystonia. Adv Neurol 1988; 49:451–465.
91. Greene P, Shale H, Fahn S. Analysis of open-label trials in torsion dystonia using high doses of anticholinergics and other drugs. Mov Disord 1988; 33:46–60.
92. Jankovic J, Orman J. Botulinum A toxin for cranial-cervical dystonia: a double blind, placebo-controlled study. Neurology 1987; 37:616–623.
93. Jankovic J, Orman J. Tetrabenazine therapy of dystonia, chorea, tics, and other dyskinesias. Neurology 1988; 38:391–394.
94. Klawans HL, Tanner CM. Cholinergic pharmacology of blepharospasm with oromandibular dystonia (Meige's syndrome). Adv Neurol 1988; 49:443–449.
95. Verma A, Miller P, Carwile ST, et al. Lamotrigine-induced blepharospasm. Pharmacotherapy 1999; 19:877–880.
96. Balash Y, Giladi N. Efficacy of pharmacological treatment of dystonia: evidence-based review including meta-analysis of the effect of botulinum toxin and other cure options. Eur J Neurol 2004; 11(6):361–370.
97. Jankovic J, Schwartz K, Donovan DT. Botulinum toxin treatment of cranial-cervical dystonia, spasmodic dysphonia, other focal dystonias and hemifacial spasm. J Neurol Neurosurg Psychiatry 1990; 53:633–639.
98. Jankovic J. Pretarsal injection of botulinum toxin for blepharospasm and apraxia of eyelid opening. J Neurol Neurosurg Psychiatry 1996; 60:704.
99. Kowal L. Pretarsal injections of botulinum toxin improve blepharospasm in previously unresponsive patients. J Neurol Neurosurg Psychiatry 1997; 63:556.
100. Mackie IA. Riolan's muscle: action and indications for botulinum toxin injection. Eye 2000; 14:347–352.
101. Jankovic J, Schwartz K. Longitudinal experience with botulinum toxin injections for treatment of blepharospasm and cervical dystonia. Neurology 1993; 43:834–836.
102. Mezaki T, Kaji R, Kohara N, et al. Comparison of therapeutic efficacies of type A and F botulinum toxins for blepharospasm: a double-blind, controlled study. Neurology 1995; 45:506–508.

103. Racette BA, Stambuk M, Perlmutter JS. Secondary Nonresponsiveness to new bulk botulinum toxin A (BCB2024). Mov Disord 2002; 17(5):1098–1100.
104. Tucha O, Naumann M, Berg D, et al. Quality of life in patients with blepharospasm. Acta Neurol Scand 2001; 103:49–52.
105. Forget R, Tozlovanu V, Iancu A, Boghen D. Botulinum toxin improves lid opening in blepharospasm-associated apraxia of lid opening. Neurology 2002; 58:1843–1846.
106. Anderson RL, Patel BC, Holds JB, Jordan DR. Blepharospasm: past, present, and future. Ophthal Plast Reconstr Surg 1998; 14:305–317.
107. Chapman KL, Bartley GB, Waller RR, Hodge DO. Follow-up of patients with essential blepharospasm who underwent eyelid protractor myectomy at the Mayo Clinic from 1980 through 1995. Ophthal Plast Reconstr Surg 1999; 15:106–110.
108. De Groot V, De Wilde F, Smet L, Tassignon MJ. Frontalis suspension combined with blepharoplasty as an effective treatment for blepharospasm associated with apraxia of eyelid opening. Ophthal Plast Reconstr Surg 2000; 16:34–38.
109. McLoon LK, Wirtschafter JD. Doxil-induced chemomyectomy: effectiveness for permanent removal of orbicularis oculi muscle in monkey eyelid. Invest Ophthalmol Vis Sci 2001; 42:1254–1257.
110. McCann JD, Gauthier M, Morschbacher R, et al. A novel mechanism for benign essential blepharospasm. Ophthal Plast Reconstr Surg 1999; 15:384–389.
111. Mostofsky DI, Yehuda S, Rabinovitz S, Carasso R. The control of blepharospasm by essential fatty acids. Neuropsychobiology 2000; 41:154–157.
112. Hirayama M, Kumano T, Aita T, Nakagawa H, Kuriyama M. Improvement of apraxia of eyelid opening by wearing goggles. Lancet 2000; 356:1413.
113. Tarbox AR, Jankovic J, Wilkins RB. Effects of electromyographic biofeedback in the treatment of blepharospasm. In: Bosniak SL, ed. Blepharospasm. New York: Pergamon Press, 1985:243–260.
114. Behari M, Singh KK, Seshadri S, et al. Botulinum toxin A in blepharospasm and hemifacial spasm. J Assoc Physicians India 1994; 42:205–208.
115. Berardelli A , Formica A, Mercuri B, et al. Botulinum toxin treatment in patients with focal dystonia and hemifacial spasm. A multicenter study of the Italian movement disorder group. Ital J Neurol Sci 1993; 14:361–367.
116. Blitzer A, Greene PE, Brin MF, et al. Botulinum toxin for treatment of oromandibular dystonia. Ann Otol Rhinol Laryngol 1989; 98:93–97.
117. Brin MF, Fahn S, Moskowitz C, et al. Localized injections of botulinum toxin for treatment of focal dystonia and hemifacial spasm. Mov Disord 1987; 2:237–254.
118. Heise GJ, Mullen MP. Oromandibular dystonia treated with botulinum toxin: report of case. J Oral Maxillofac Surg 1995; 53:332–335; 335–337.
119. Hermanowicz N, Truong DD. Treatment of oromandibular dystonia with botulinum toxin. Laryngoscope 1991; 101:1216–1281.
120. Maurri S, Brogelli S, Alfieri G, et al. Use of botulinum toxin in Meige's disease. Riv Neurol 1988; 58:245–248.
121. Poungvarin N, Devahastin V, Chaisevikul R, et al. Botulinum A toxin treatment for blepharospasm and Meige syndrome: report of 100 patients. J Med Assoc Thai 1997; 80:1–8.
122. Van den Bergh P, Francart J, Mourin S, et al. Five-year experience in the treatment of focal movement disorders with low-dose Dysport botulinum toxin. Muscle Nerve 1995; 18:720–729.
123. Gelb DJ, Yoshimura DM, Olney RK, Lowerstein DH, Aminoff MJ. Change in pattern of muscle activity following botulinum toxin injections for torticollis. Ann Neurol 1991; 29:370–376.
124. Ondo WG, Desaloms JM,Jankovic J, et al. Pallidotomy for generalized dystonia. Mov Disord 1998; 13:693–698.
125. Tronnier VM, Fogel W. Pallidal stimulation for generalized dystonia: report of three cases. J Neurosurg 2000; 92:453–456.

# 10
# Cervical Dystonia

**Khashayar Dashtipour**
*Department of Neurology, Loma Linda University, Loma Linda, California, U.S.A.*

**Mark Lew**
*Department of Neurology, University of Southern California, Los Angeles, California, U.S.A.*

## DEFINITION

Cervical dystonia (CD) is a simultaneous and sustained contraction of both agonist and antagonist muscles of the neck. Based on head posture and positioning, CD can be described as torticollis (neck rotation), anterocollis (head-forward flexion or pulled forward), retrocollis (head-posterior extension or pulled backward) or laterocollis (head tilt or lateral flexion). Combinations of the above postures are also common (Figs. 1 and 2 )

## BACKGROUND

In the 16th century, Rabelais applied the term "torty colly" to elucidate the term wry-neck (1). More than 200 years later, in 1911, Oppenheim, impressed with the abnormalities in tone seen with these patients, coined the definition of dystonia. In this way, he contributed the nomenclature of dystonia musculorum deformans, the precursor appellation of generalized dystonia.

## EPIDEMIOLOGY

CD is the most common form of focal dystonia. Few epidemiological studies exist that estimate the incidence and prevalence of CD. Separate studies of different geographical locations and times show the prevalence between 9 and 30 per 100,000 in the United States (2–4). Currently, the prevalence of CD in the United States is estimated to be greater than 90,000. Other studies show that its prevalence differs among ethnic groups (5–7). Claypool et al., in 1995, reported an incidence of 1.2 per 100,000 (3) while an incidence of 5.4 per 100,000 was published in a practice-based survey of dystonia in Munich (7).

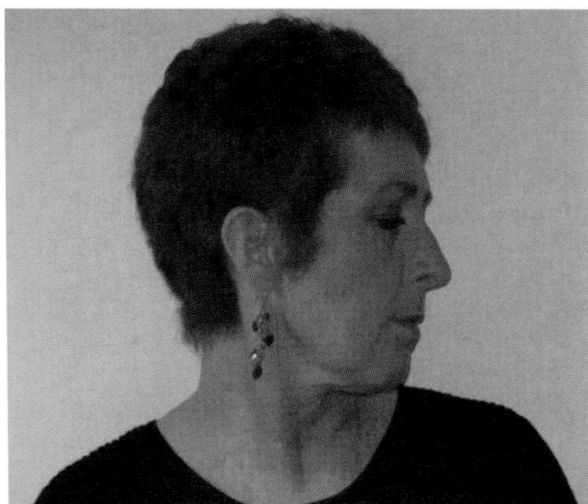

**Figure 1** A patient with Torticollis, full range rotation to the left 90°.

Women are affected 1.3- to 2-fold more often than men. CD can occur at any time of life but most individuals experience their first symptoms in middle age. Chan et al. reviewed the clinical details of CD in 266 patients (8). In their study, the median age of onset was 41 years old with a female to male ratio of 1.9 to 1. They found a familial history of dystonia in 12% of the cases. Remission was achieved in 9.8% of the patients (8).

## PATHOPHYSIOLOGY

The pathophysiology of idiopathic CD is not well understood. Recent studies have explained the pathogenesis of CD at the peripheral and central nervous system level. Although any muscle in the neck may be involved, Table 1 lists the common muscles associated with abnormal head posture (9,10). Currently, the main focus is on decreased inhibition, sensory deficit, and sensorimotor mismatch, aberrant neuroplasticity, and basal ganglia discharge. CD, like other focal dystonias, is a syndrome of abnormality in central motor processing.

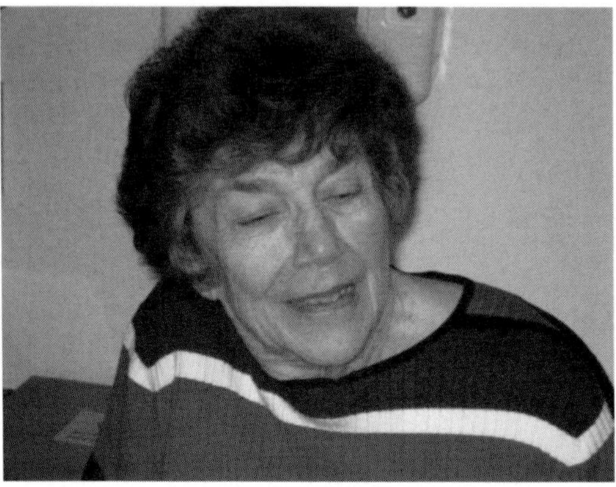

**Figure 2** A patient with a combination of left rotation, right tilt, and right shoulder elevation.

**Table 1** Commonly Injected Muscles in Treating Cervical Dystonia

| Muscle | Origin | Insertion | Action | Innervation |
|---|---|---|---|---|
| Sternocleidomastoid | Anterior surface of manubrium, medial-third of clavicle | Mastoid processes of temporal bone | Unilateral–Ipsilateral flexion and contralateral rotation. Bilaterally—Head and neck flexion | Spinal portion of accessory nerve and two cervical root |
| Splenius capitis | Spinous processes of seventh cervical and upper-third or fourth thoracic vertebrae | Mastoid process of temporal bone and lateral part of superior nuchal line | Bilateral—extends neck and head. Unilateral—flexes and rotates the head slightly to the same side | Lateral branches of posterior primary rami of middle and lower cervical roots |
| Semispinalis capitis | Transverse processes, upper-sixth or -seventh thoracic, seventh cervical, articular processes fourth to sixth cervical vertebrae | Occipital bone between superior and inferior nuchal lines | Extension, lateral flexion, and rotation of neck | Posterior primary rami of the spinal nerves |
| Scalenes | | | | |
| Anterior | Anterior–transverse processes C3–C6 | Anterior-first rib | Bilateral—elevate ribs during inhalation | Anterior—5–8 cervical roots |
| Medius | Middle–transverse processes of C2–C7 | Middle-first rib | Unilateral–ipsilateral neck flexion, contralateral rotation | Middle—3–4 cervical roots |
| Posterior | Posterior–transverse processes of C4–C6 | Posterior-second rib | Anterior—neck flexion | Posterior—lower-fourth cervical roots, branches of 3–4 cervical |
| Levator scapulae | Transverse processes of upper-fourth cervical vertebrae | Posterior border of scapula above the root of the spine | Elevates the superior angle of the scapula | 3–4 cervical nerves |
| Trapezius upper | External occipital protuberance, spinous process of the seventh cervical vertebrae | The outer-third of the posterior border of the clavicle | Elevates, retracts, and rotates scapula | Spinal accessory nerve and 3–4 cervical nerves |

## HYPOTHESES UNDERLYING POTENTIAL CAUSES OF CERVICAL DYSTONIA

### Loss of Inhibition in Dystonia

There is some evidence showing that dystonia is generated by decreased central inhibition (11). Currently, the concept of surround inhibition has been accepted in sensory physiology, similar to what has been elaborated in the visual system (12). This hypothesis suggests that with a directed movement, a certain area of the motor cortex activates for the desired movement and unwanted movements are inhibited by a similar concept of surround inhibition (11). Several electrophysiologic studies have shown that reciprocal inhibition is reduced in different types of dystonia including torticollis (13–16). Ikoma et al., by applying Transcranial Magnetic Stimulation (TMS) to the motor cortex contralateral to the side of electromyographic (EMG) recording, showed that cortical motor excitability was increased in dystonia and that this was most likely secondary to a decrease of inhibition (17). By using a $\gamma$-aminobutyric acid (GABA) antagonist in primates, Matsumura developed an animal model with cocontraction of antagonist muscles as is seen in dystonia (18). Further evidence supporting this hypothesis comes from the observation of Levy and Hallet in 2002, who found impaired brain GABA level in focal dystonia via applying magnetic resonance spectroscopy (19). Several electrophysiologic and imaging studies have provided evidence that the basal ganglia exert influence on cortical inhibition (20). Low striatal D2 receptor binding, as assessed by [$^{123}$I] Iodobenzamide (IBZM) single photon emission computed tomography (SPECT), was shown in patients with focal dystonia (21). Using SPECT, Naumann et al. concluded that disturbance of the indirect pathway causes disinhibition of thalamocortical circuitry in torticollis (22).

### Sensory Deficit and Sensorimotor Mismatch

Tactile sensation, or a "geste antagonistique/sensory trick," is a well-known sensory phenomenon used to improve abnormal postures in torticollis and other forms of focal dystonia. The pathophysiology of this sensory trick is unknown. An abnormal sensory input such as trauma, however, can be a precedent to focal dystonia such as torticollis (23). These two examples and other information suggest that dystonia is at least in part a sensory related disorder (24). Molloy et al. in 2003 evaluated sensory spatial discrimination in the hands of patients with focal dystonia. They showed involvement of the dominant and nondominant somatosensory cortices, and hypothesized that abnormal sensory processing is a fundamental disturbance in focal dystonia (25). Earlier, Bara Jimenez et al. showed abnormal spatial discrimination in patients with writer's cramp, supporting the theory of sensory dysfunction in focal dystonia (26). The above studies suggest that improper sensory assistance in a motor activity may be the cause of the cocontraction of agonist and antagonist muscles seen in focal dystonia.

### Aberrant Neuroplasticity

The capacity of the nervous system for neural adaptation and network reorganization has already been shown in several studies. In different pathological dynamics, the maladaptive reorganization can occur in response to brain injury or external stimuli. Electrophysiologic mapping techniques in primates and computational models suggest the presence of neuroplasticity in focal dystonias (27–30). Recently, Bara Jimenez et al. showed an abnormal somatosensory homunculus in dystonia of the hand (31). Using magnetic source imaging, other laboratories such as Elberta et al. revealed similar results (32). They showed a fusion of digital representations in somatosensory cortex for the affected hand in focal hand dystonia. This maladaptive neural network or aberrant neuroplasticity in focal hand dystonia can be reversed by using botulinum toxin injections (33). Using TMS, the reversible reorganization of the motor cortex was shown for non–task-specific focal dystonias such as torticollis (34). This study provided evidence showing that aberrant neuroplasticity is widespread beyond the motor cortex and correlated to affected cervical muscles.

### Basal Ganglia Discharge

There is much evidence supporting the role of basal ganglia in dystonic posture but the mechanisms are poorly understood (35–38). Sanghera et al. reported data analyzing basal ganglia neuronal discharge in patients who underwent posteroventral pallidotomy for the treatment of primary genetic, secondary, or idiopathic dystonia (39). On comparison of the discharge rates and neuronal pattern in parkinsonian patients versus patients with dystonia, they found that: (i) in both dystonia and Parkinson's disease (PD), the discharge rates in the putamen are very low but discharge rates are much lower in the globus pallidus neurons in dystonia than in PD. (ii) In dystonia, there are no differences in discharge rates and patterns of neurons in globus pallidus, but in PD patients Globus Pallidus externa (GPe) recording shows lower rates than Globus Pallidus interna (GPi). Recently Zhuang et al. analyzed neuronal discharge in the GPi, ventral thalamic nuclear group, ventral oral posterior/ ventral intermediate, and subthalamic nucleus in patients with dystonia (37). Their result was consistent with previous studies to support an association of dystonia and alteration in neuronal discharge in the basal ganglia and thalamus. Based on their findings, focal dystonia involves only small regions of the basal ganglia. However, patients with generalized dystonia show changes throughout the nuclei (37).

## CLINICAL MANIFESTATION

CD, like other forms of focal dystonia, begins in a single body part with simultaneous cocontraction of agonist and antagonist muscles. In a minority of the cases, CD can spread to adjacent body parts representing a segmental dystonia. Interestingly, for a given dystonic head position, the pattern of muscle activity may be changed following botulinum toxin injection (40). Using EMG for a series of four consecutive injections, these authors demonstrated an evolving pattern of muscle involvement. While decreased EMG activity was shown in the injected muscles as expected, in muscles that had not been injected, there was a tendency for increased electrical activity in adjacent muscles. This changing pattern of muscle involvement also occurred in subjects not benefiting from injection sessions (40). Head tremor and neck spasms are cardinal clinical features in patients with CD (8,41). The majority of affected patients complain of pain, which is not common in other types of focal dystonia other than writer's cramp. Hand and arm tremor may be seen in patients with torticollis (41–43). In certain cases, head, arm, or trunk tremor can be the initial presenting symptom and, sometimes, the isolated manifestation of torticollis (44).

Most patients with torticollis find a sensory trick a useful tool to control or eliminate their symptoms. As previously mentioned, a sensory trick has been called a *geste antagoniste* and is a unique feature of dystonia. Typically, placing the hand on the chin, side of the face, or the back of the neck reduces muscle contraction in

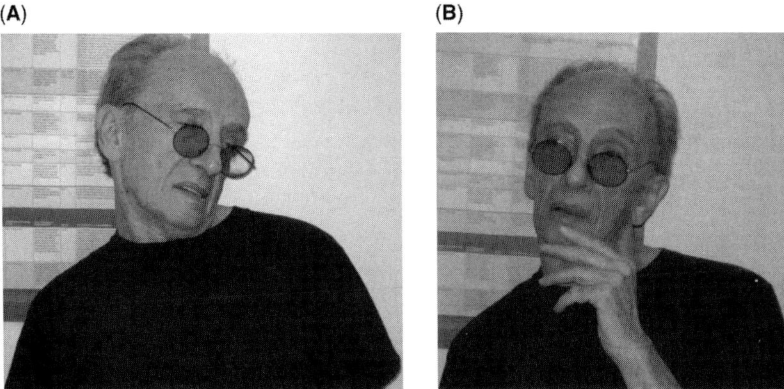


**Figure 3** (**A**) A patient with prominent left rotation, left tilt, and shoulder elevation. (**B**) Same patient using a sensory trick by touching his left hand to his chin showing greatly diminished dystonia.

CD without applying mechanical pressure (Fig. 3 A and B). In some patients, just thinking about a "*geste antagoniste*" eliminates or diminishes their symptoms the same as actually performing the sensory trick (45). Although the use of a "geste antagoniste" is reported in more than 50 percent of patients with CD (41), its mechanism of action is still unknown.

In addition to sensory–motor signs and symptoms, patients with torticollis also show a high incidence of psychiatric comorbidities. A recent study showed that depression and anxiety disorders occur in patients with CD with a 3.7-fold increase compared to a matched group with similar body image dissatisfaction (46). Therefore, the authors concluded that psychiatric comorbidity is not just secondary to chronic disease and disfigurement and may have its own pathogenesis primarily related to dystonia. Furthermore, some patients with CD complain of worsening of their symptoms with stress, emotion, self-consciousness, walking, carrying objects, writing, running, social situations, fatigue, and lack of sleep (47). On the other hand, some patients reported sleep, lying on their back or side, relaxation, and a "*geste antagoniste*" as ameliorating factors (47).

There are several reports presented separately showing CD as the initial manifestation or presenting sign of diseases such as multiple sclerosis (48), spinocerebellar ataxia 17 (49) and systemic onset juvenile rheumatoid arthritis (50). While it is clear that this is a very uncommon event, CD can be secondary and due to a variety of identifiable pathologies (Table 2) (51–63).

## MANAGEMENT

### Medical Therapy

The efficacy of oral drug therapy is limited and many different medication trials show a low rate of success to control the symptoms of CD (64).

#### *Anticholinergic Agents*

Trihexyphenidyl was approved by the Food and Drug Administration (FDA) in 1949. It is a tertiary antimuscarinic agent that penetrates the central nervous system

**Table 2** Differential Diagnosis of Torticollis

| |
|---|
| Wilson's disease |
| Progressive supranuclear palsy |
| Corticobasal ganglionic degeneration |
| Tardive dystonia |
| Spinal cord ependymoma |
| Posterior fossa tumor |
| Pseudotumor cerebri |
| Systemic lupus erythematosus |
| Huntington's disease |
| Langerhans cell histiocytosis |
| Hemorrhagic and ischemic stroke |
| Cerebellopontine angle tumors |
| Intramedullary glioma |
| Cerebellar cavernous angioma |
| Syrinx |
| Retropharyngeal abscess |
| Ocular pathology |
| Electrical injury |
| Arteriovenous malformation |
| Multiple sclerosis |
| Pantothenate kinase-associated neurodegeneration |
| Ataxia–telangiectasia |
| Psychogenic dystonia |

(CNS). It antagonizes cholinergic receptors in the CNS and smooth muscle. Trihexyphenidyl has antispasmodic action on smooth muscles. In a double-blinded, randomized, placebo-controlled trial, it was shown to be effective in treating segmental and generalized dystonia (65). CNS disturbances are common side effects of anticholinergic agents, especially in the elderly. Trihexyphenidyl needs to be discontinued slowly in order to prevent neuroleptic malignant syndrome, which has been reported rarely (66,67).

*Benzodiazepines*

Benzodiazepines such as lorazepam are commonly used to treat dystonia. Chlordiazepoxide was the first benzodiazepine released in 1960, later diazepam in 1965, clonazepam in 1975, and lorazepam in 1977. Benzodiazepines work through enhancement of GABA receptors causing CNS depression, sedation, and muscle relaxation. There are no controlled trials to show their effectiveness but there is an open label study reported by Greene et al. (68). Clonazepam is the most commonly prescribed medication for the treatment of CD.

*Mexiletine*

Mexiletine is an antiarrhythmic agent whose effectiveness in treatment of CD was shown in an open label case study (69). The dose range is 450 to 1200 mg/day but it is not approved by the FDA to treat CD and efficacy in controlled trials is lacking.

*Riluzole*

Riluzole is a glutamate antagonist that is believed to modulate glutamate release. Several open label studies showed success in the treatment of torticollis with riluzole by improving symptoms (70). Again, placebo-controlled trials have not been performed.

*Baclofen*

Baclofen is an oral muscle relaxant. It is a GABA-B agonist and works mainly at spinal cord level by inhibiting firing of motor neurons. It is used commonly in the treatment of dystonia. There are no controlled trials available on the successful use of baclofen in CD but some reports showed beneficial effects with the treatment of CD by infusion of intrathecal baclofen (71).

*Tetrabenazine*

Tetrabenazine, a benzoquinolizine derivative, is a presynaptic catecholamine depleting agent that is effective and a relatively safe medication for the treatment of hyperkinetic movement disorders. Jankovic and Beach treated more than 500 patients with hyperkinetic movement disorders over 15 years and analyzed the long-term effects of tetrabenazine in those patients (72). They showed marked improvement in 62.9% of patients with idiopathic dystonia. Its efficacy has also been shown in a retrospective chart review study in patients with truncal dystonia including torticollis (129). Tetrabenazine was used for treating abnormal movements in patients with tardive dystonia (130). Serious side effects can occur with the use of tetrabenazine such as parkinsonism, sedation, depression, anxiety, insomnia, and akathisia. Tetrabenazine is not currently available in the United States.

*Other Agents*

Other medications that have been reported to be used in treatment of CD include, benzotropine, valproate, olanzapine, clozapine and ethanol injection (131–133,73,74). In a pilot trial, clozapine was shown to have no effect on dystonic posture of patients with CD but decreased the associated jerky head movements by 50% (131). Olanzapine was shown to be effective in tardive dystonia in the cervical region that was induced by antipsychotic drugs (73). The beneficial effect of valproate in torticollis was shown in a case report in 1984 when it was used in combination with baclofen (72). A significant improvement of the symptoms was reported by injecting ethanol every other week repeatedly with a mean of 10 times in 14 patients with torticollis (74).

## Botulinum Toxin

Seven different serotypes of botulinum toxin have been identified. Their specific action is at cholinergic synapses to block presynaptic release of acetylcholine. By inhibiting the release of acetylcholine at the neuromuscular junction, it decreases inappropriate cocontraction of agonist and antagonist muscles in dystonia. Over the last 15 years, intramuscular injection of botulinum toxin has become the treatment of choice for patients with CD. Injection of toxin into appropriate neck muscles relieves torticollis symptoms. A 30-gauge needle may be used for superficial injection and a larger 25- to 27-gauge needle for deeper musculature. Various controlled trials show 60% to 90% improvement following intramuscular toxin injection (75–81). Patients usually notice improvement of their symptoms in 5 to 10 days after injection with lasting benefit for three to four months. Two distinct serotypes of botulinum toxin types A and B, are available for the treatment of dystonia.

*Botulinum Toxin Type A*

Botulinum toxin type A is effective and safe and has been shown to be more effective than medical therapy such as trihexyphenidyl in controlling symptoms of CD with a better side effect profile (82). Currently, three formulations of type A toxin are available in clinical practice, Botox$^{TM}$, Merz NT 201, and Dysport.

**Botox$^{TM}$.** The efficacy and safety of Botox$^{TM}$ has been established in several clinical trials, with 70% to 90% of the patients with CD benefiting from this formulation (76,77,83,84). The mean dose in clinical studies was between 198 and 300 units divided among affected muscles. There is concern about the possibility of developing neutralizing antibodies with repeated therapy. In general, avoidance of using high doses (Botox$^{TM}$ above 400 units) and extending the interdose interval to a minimum of three months' duration is the accepted norm. In some reports, neutralizing antibodies have been shown in up to the 17% of the patients but Jankovic et al., using the current formulation of botulinum toxin type A, did not detect the presence of blocking antibodies in a three-year open label observation (85).

Specialized local injection techniques such as EMG-guided injection may be used to increase the magnitude of benefit (86). Just prior to injection, Botox$^{TM}$ should be reconstituted using sterile nonpreserved normal saline. Reconstituted medication should not be stored more than four hours in a refrigerator because the potency is reported to wane substantially thereafter (87). Botox$^{TM}$ is a pregnancy category-C medication and is supplied in the United States in 100-unit vials as a lyophillized preparation.

The effect of Botox$^{TM}$ may be potentiated by other drugs that interfere with neuromuscular transmission such as aminoglycoside antibiotics and other neuromuscular blockers. One study showed antagonistic action of chloroquine with botulinium toxin (88) by preventing internalization of the toxin. Multiple studies have shown Botox$^{TM}$ to be a safe medication in the hands of trained physicians (76,77,83). Adverse effects such as dysphagia, neck weakness, local pain, lethargy, dysphonia, and xerostomia are temporary but can last for weeks or months prior to waning (89).

**Dysport.** Dysport is another A type toxin (not available in the United States) shown to be safe and effective for more than a decade of use in Europe (90,91). There are several studies comparing Botox$^{TM}$ and Dysport directly. Odergren et al. showed similar improvements and safety profile in patients treated with Botox$^{TM}$ or Dysport (90). In 2002, Ranoux et al. demonstrated that although Dysport had a higher incidence of adverse effects, it was more effective than Botox$^{TM}$ for both impairment and pain in CD (91). A multicenter double-blind randomized controlled trial in the United States recently confirmed previous reports that Dysport is safe, effective, and well tolerated in patients with CD (92).

To compare the safety, effectiveness, and duration of the clinical effect of Botox$^{TM}$ and Dysport, a single arm, crossover-design study was performed in 48 patients with CD, blepharospasm, and hemifacial spasm (93). This study showed that therapeutic effectiveness, safety, and duration of action are enhanced with Botox$^{TM}$. A pivotal, randomized, double-blind, placebo-controlled study of Dysport for the treatment of CD is ongoing in the United States.

**Merz NT 201.** NT 201 is a new compound from MERZ pharmaceuticals. It is a lyophillized preparation of botulinum toxin type A, free of other potentially immunogenic proteins of clostridial origin. Recently, a double-blind noninferiority trial compared the efficacy and safety of NT 201 with Botox$^{TM}$ in 420 patients with CD in 11 European centers (94). This study showed noninferiority of the NT 201 versus Botox$^{TM}$ with a similar safety and tolerability profile.

In a separate randomized controlled trial, the efficacy and tolerability of NT 201 was compared with Botox$^{TM}$ in 14 healthy volunteers (95). After injecting four units of Botox$^{TM}$ and NT 201 into the extensor digitorum brevis muscle, reduction of compound muscle action potential was observed in both groups. The maximal effect was found between 7 and 14 days with no significant differences between groups for efficacy, time to onset of action, duration of action, and tolerability. This compound is only available in Germany but trials are currently ongoing in the United States.

*Botulinum Toxin Type B*

**Myobloc.** Myobloc was the first toxin approved by the FDA for the treatment of CD in December 2000. Myobloc has been shown effective by reducing the pain, severity, and disability associated with CD in both botulinum toxin type A-responsive and type A-resistant patients (79–81,96). Botulinum toxins inhibit acetylcholine release at the neuromuscular junction by binding to receptors on presynaptic cholinergic nerve terminals via a multiple stage process (97). Myobloc specifically cleaves synaptic vesicle associated membrane protein, also known as synaptobrevin (98). This cleavage blocks docking and fusion of the synaptic vesicles, a necessary step for neurotransmitter release. Botox$^{TM}$ cleaves another target protein, synaptosome-associated protein of 25 kDa (98). Controlled trials have shown that patients notice the benefit of Myobloc injection within four weeks, with a median duration of action between 12 and 16 weeks (99). The recommended initial dose is between 2500 and 5000 units divided among injected neck muscles. Maximal reported doses have been as high as 25,000 to 28,000 units (100,101). Dry mouth, dysphagia, and injection site pain are the most common reported side effects with Myobloc.

Myobloc and Botox$^{TM}$ have been compared in at least two studies in patients both naive and previously treated with Botox$^{TM}$. These trials revealed that both toxins provide equivalent benefit in patients with CD and have comparable side effect profiles except that Myobloc caused more dry mouth (102,103).

## Surgery

Surgical procedures for the treatment of CD are considered in the uncommon case of toxin inefficacy or the development of resistance to both serotypes of toxin and failure of medical therapy. Both central and peripheral nervous system procedures have been used to treat CD recalcitrant to medical intervention. To date, surgical therapy strictly remains an option when other treatments fail or become ineffective.

*Brain Lesioning*

Since the early 1940s, brain lesioning as a treatment for CD has been undertaken with variable results. Several targets have been explored in the basal ganglia and thalamus to treat movement disorders. Meyers reported a surgical procedure for postencephalitic tremor in 1941 (104). Afterward, he reported his 10 years' experience of operation to treat movement disorders including dystonia by creating lesions in selected regions of the basal ganglia and thalamus (105). These results have been replicated by placing lesions in various regions of basal ganglia (106). Thalamotomy as a traditional stereotactic therapy for CD shows controversial results (107). Bilateral thalamatomy can be modestly effective to treat symptoms in CD but can cause serious side effects including weakness and dysphagia, in contrast to the unilateral thalamotomy, which shows less beneficial response but a more favorable safety profile (64). Lesioning of globus palidus was later reported as a treatment for CD (106).

The posteroventral medial pallidotomy targets the pallidothalamic pathway and is hypothesized to interrupt abnormal neurocircuitry involved in CD (106). Interestingly, most reports show gradual improvements in dystonic patients following pallidotomy over several months (64). Yoshor et al. compared pallidotomy and thalamotomy to treat patients with different forms of intractable dystonia. The long-term outcome with pallidotomy was significantly better than thalamotomy for all patients with dystonia including CD (108). Several reports show thalamotomy as a more effective procedure for secondary dystonia than primary dystonia (108–110).

#### *Brain Stimulation*

Deep brain stimulation (DBS) is being used to treat several types of movement disorders. It has advantages over brain lesioning because it is reversible and adjustable. DBS was used initially in the 1960s to control chronic pain and decades later it was used for various movement disorders such as PD, tremor, and dystonia (111). Several studies showed DBS as a relatively safe procedure and a very useful therapeutic option for disabling CD in patients who do not respond to medical therapy and botulinum toxin injection (112–114). The mechanism of action of DBS in dystonia is poorly understood. The target used for DBS in dystonia is located in the posteroventral lateral GPi, a target also used in PD. Several investigators are in favor of bilateral DBS over unilateral DBS because of the evidence showing bilateral basal ganglia dysfunction in patients with CD (112,115,116). Postoperative improvement has been reported to be gradual, sometimes several weeks or months after surgery, but progressive and sustained in nature (117). Compared to DBS for other movement disorders such as PD, initial settings require higher voltages and pulse widths, followed by gradual increment of intensity (117). Prospective studies have shown up to two years of follow-up with ongoing benefit in a gradual and exponential manner (113,117,118).

#### *Peripheral Surgical Intervention*

A peripheral surgical approach is one of the alternative options for treatment of patients with botulinum-toxin–resistant CD. There are various types of peripheral surgical techniques, but selective peripheral denervation is the most commonly performed procedure. In 1987 and 1988, Bertrand et al. reported their observations and analysis with significant success rate in patients with CD who underwent selective denervation (119,120). There are several well-established procedures for selective peripheral denervation such as denervation of the accessory nerve and the posterior rami of the cervical spinal nerves and, more recently, levator scapulae muscle with wide range of response rates (121–126). In an open label study, Ford et al. concluded that the best candidates for selective ramisectomy were those patients with secondary botulinum toxin failure (127). In contrast, Cohen et al., in a retrospective analysis, concluded that outcome was not predicted by preoperative head position, severity, and duration of symptoms or response to botulinum toxin (128).

## PROGNOSIS

CD can be sustained, may spread to other muscles, or go into remission. Developing segmental or rarely generalized dystonia has been reported in some cases (63). Chan et al. reported remission in 9.8% of their cases but spontaneous remissions in up to

20% of the patients also were observed in some reviews (8). In general, this is not a progressive disorder and most patients experience stabilization of symptoms within the first five years of toxin therapy.

## SUMMARY

CD is the most common form of focal dystonia that affects more than 90,000 people in the United States. Its pathophysiology is not well understood but several hypotheses detail involvement at the central and peripheral level. In addition to sustained neck spasms, which result in abnormal head posture, the majority of affected patients complain of head tremor and pain. One of the interesting and unique features of CD is the *geste antagoniste*.

Several medications are used in the treatment of CD but the efficacy of oral drug therapy is limited with a low rate of success. Over the last decade, chemodenervation with botulinum toxin opened a new chapter in treatment of CD. Two types of botulinum toxin, types A and B, are being used for treatment of CD with equivalent benefit. In cases when medical therapy fails, surgery is an option. Several trials are currently ongoing in the United States and Europe to evaluate the efficacy of DBS in CD. Additionally, trials evaluating efficacy and safety of new type A toxins are underway.

## REFERENCES

1. Tibbetts RW. Spasmodic torticollis. J Psychosom Res 1971; 15(4):461–469.
2. Nutt JG, Muenter MD, Aronson A, et al. Epidemiology of focal and generalized dystonia in Rochester, Minnesota. Mov Disord 1988; 3(3):188–194.
3. Claypool DW, Duane DD, Ilstrup DM, et al. Epidemiology and outcome of cervical dystonia (spasmodic torticollis) in Rochester, Minnesota. Mov Disord 1995; 10(5):608–614.
4. Cardoso F, Jankovic J. Dystonia and dyskinesia. Psychiatr Clin North Am 1997; 20(4):821–838.
5. Asgeirsson H, Jakobsson F, Hjaltason H, et al. Prevalence study of primary dystonia in Iceland. Mov disord 2006; 21(3):293–298.
6. Nakashima K, Kusumi M, Inoue Y, et al. Prevalence of focal dystonias in the western area of Tottori prefecture in Japan. Mov Disord 1995; 10(4):440–443.
7. Konkiewitz CE, Trender-Gerhard I, Kamm C, et al. Service-based survey of dystonia in munich. Neuroepidemiology 2002; 21(4):202–206.
8. Chan J, Brin MF, Fahn S. Idiopathic cervical dystonia: clinical characteristics. Mov disord 1991; 6(2):119–126.
9. Warfel JH. The head, neck and trunk. 5th ed. Philadelphia, PA: Lea & Febiger, 1985: 34–56.
10. Gray H. Anatomy, descriptive and surgical. The unabridged running press ed. Philadelphia, PA: Running Press, 1974:336–346.
11. Hallett M. Dystonia: abnormal movements result from loss of inhibition. Adv Neurol 2004; 94:1–9.
12. Srinivasan MV, Laughlin SB, Dubs A. Predictive coding: a fresh view of inhibition in the retina. Proc R Soc Lond B Biol Sci 1982; 216(1205):427–459.
13. Rothwell JC, Day BL, Obeso JA, et al. Reciprocal inhibition between muscles of the human forearm in normal subjects and in patients with idiopathic torsion dystonia. Adv Neurol 1988; 50:133–140.
14. Panizza ME, Hallett M, Nilsson J. Reciprocal inhibition in patients with hand cramps. Neurology 1989; 39(1):85–89.

15. Nakashima K, Rothwell JC, Day BL, et al. Reciprocal inhibition between forearm muscles in patients with writer's cramp and other occupational cramps, symptomatic hemidystonia and hemiparesis due to stroke. Brain 1989; 112 (Pt 3):681–697.
16. Deuschl G, Seifert C, Heinen F, et al. Reciprocal inhibition of forearm flexor muscles in spasmodic torticollis. J Neurol Sci 1992; 113(1):85–90.
17. Ikoma K, Samii A, Mercuri B, et al. Abnormal cortical motor excitability in dystonia. Neurology 1996; 46(5):1371–1376.
18. Matsumura M, Sawaguchi T, Oishi T, et al. Behavioral deficits induced by local injection of bicuculline and muscimol into the primate motor and premotor cortex. J Neurophysiol 1991; 65(6):1542–1553.
19. Levy LM, Hallett M. Impaired brain GABA in focal dystonia. Ann Neurol 2002; 51(1):93–101.
20. Priori A, Berardelli A, Inghilleri M, et al. Motor cortical inhibition and the dopaminergic system. Pharmacological changes in the silent period after transcranial brain stimulation in normal subjects, patients with Parkinson's disease and drug-induced parkinsonism. Brain 1994; 117(Pt 2):317–323.
21. Horstink CA, Praamstra P, Horstink MW, et al. Low striatal D2 receptor binding as assessed by [123I]IBZM SPECT in patients with writer's cramp. J Neurol Neurosurg Psychiatry 1997; 62(6):672–73.
22. Naumann M, Pirker W, Reiners K, Lange KW, Becker G, Brucke T. Imaging the pre- and postsynaptic side of striatal dopaminergic synapses in idiopathic cervical dystonia: a SPECT study using [123I] epidepride and [123I] beta-CIT. Mov Disord 1998; 13(2):19–23.
23. Jankovic J. Can peripheral trauma induce dystonia and other movement disorders? Yes! Mov Disord 2001; 16(1):7–12.
24. Hallett M. Is dystonia a sensory disorder? Ann Neurol 1995; 38(2):139–140.
25. Molloy FM, Carr TD, Zeuner KE, et al. Abnormalities of spatial discrimination in focal and generalized dystonia. Brain 2003; 126 (Pt 10):2175–2182.
26. Bara Jimenez W, Shelton P, Hallett, M. Spatial discrimination is abnormal in focal hand dystonia. Neurology 2000; 55(12):1869–1873.
27. Byl NN, Merzenich MM, Jenkins WM. A primate genesis model of focal dystonia and repetitive strain injury: I. Learning-induced dedifferentiation of the representation of the hand in the primary somatosensory cortex in adult monkeys. Neurology 1996; 47(2):508–520.
28. Byl NN, Merzenich MM, Cheung S, et al. A primate model for studying focal dystonia and repetitive strain injury: effects on the primary somatosensory cortex. Phys Ther 1997; 77(3):269–284.
29. Sanger TD, Merzenich MM. Computational model of the role of sensory disorganization in focal task-specific dystonia. J Neurophysio 2000; 84(5):2458–2464.
30. Blake DT, Byl NN, Cheung S, et al. Sensory representation abnormalities that parallel focal hand dystonia in a primate model. Somatosen Mot Res 2002; 19(4):347–357.
31. Bara-Jimenez W, Catalan MJ, Hallett M, Gerloff C. Abnormal somatosensory homunculus in dystonia of the hand. Ann Neurol 1998; 44:828–831.
32. Elbert T, Candia V, Altenmuller E, et al. Alteration of digital representations in somatosensory cortex in focal hand dystonia. Neuroreport 1998; 9(16):3571–3575.
33. Byrnes ML, Thickbroom GW, Wilson SA, et al. The corticomotor representation of upper limb muscles in writer's cramp and changes following botulinum toxin injection. Brain 1998; 121 (Pt 5):977–988.
34. Thickbroom GW, Byrnes ML, Stell R, et al. Reversible reorganisation of the motor cortical representation of the hand in cervical dystonia. Mov Disord 2003; 18(4):395–402.
35. Vitek JL, Chockkan V, Zhang JY, et al. Neuronal activity in the basal ganglia in patients with generalized dystonia and hemiballismus. Ann Neurol 1999; 46:22–35.
36. Vitek JL. Pathophysiology of dystonia: a neuronal model. Mov Disord 2002; 17(suppl. 3): S49–S62.

37. Zhuang P, Li Y, Hallett M. Neuronal activity in the basal ganglia and thalamus in patients with dystonia. Clin Neurophysiol 2004; 115(11):2542–2557.
38. DeLong MR. Primate models of movement disorders of basal ganglia origin. Trends Neurosci 1990; 13:281–285.
39. Sanghera MK, Grossman RG, Kalhorn CG, et al. Basal ganglia neuronal discharge in primary and secondary dystonia in patients undergoing pallidotomy. Neurosurgery 2003; 52(6):1358–1370; discussion 1370.
40. Gelb DJ, Yoshimura DM, Olney RK, et al. Change in pattern of muscle activity following botulinum toxin injections for torticollis. Ann Neurol 1991; 29(4):370–376.
41. Jankovic J, Leder S, Warner D, et al. Cervical dystonia: clinical findings and associated movement disorders. Neurology 1991; 41(7):1088–1091.
42. Couch JR. Dystonia and tremor in spasmodic torticollis. Adv Neurol 1976; 14:245–258.
43. Deuschl G, Heinen F, Guschlbauer B, et al. Hand tremor in patients with spasmodic torticollis. Mov Disord 1997; 12(4):547–552.
44. Rivest J, Marsden CD. Trunk and head tremor as isolated manifestations of dystonia. Mov Disord 1990; 5(1):60–65.
45. Muller J, Wissel J, Masuhr F, et al. Clinical characteristics of the geste antagoniste in cervical dystonia. J Neurol 2001; 248(6):478–482.
46. Gundel H, Wolf A, Xidara V, et al. High psychiatric comorbidity in spasmodic torticollis: a controlled study. J Nerv Ment Dis 2003; 191(7):465–473.
47. Jahanshahi M. Factors that ameliorate or aggravate spasmodic torticollis. J Neurol Neurosurg Psychiatry 2000; 68(2):227–229.
48. Ruegg SJ, Buhlmann M, Renaud S, et al. Cervical dystonia as first manifestation of multiple sclerosis. J Neurol 2004; 251(11):1408–1410.
49. Hagenah JM, Zuhlke C, Hellenbroich Y, et al. Focal dystonia as a presenting sign of spinocerebellar ataxia 17. Mov Disord 2004; 19(2):217–220.
50. Uziel Y, Rathaus V, Pomeranz A, et al. Torticollis as the sole initial presenting sign of systemic onset juvenile rheumatoid arthritis. J Rheumatol 1998; 25(1):166–168.
51. Silberbauer C, Rittmannsberger H. Torticollis spasmodicus as a manifestation of tardive dystonia. Fortschritte der Neurologie Psychiatrie 1995; 63(10):388–392.
52. Cammarota A, Gershanik OS, Garcia S, et al. Cervical dystonia due to spinal cord ependymoma: involvement of cervical cord segments in the pathogenesis of dystonia. Mov Disord 1995; 10(4):500–503.
53. Marmor MA, Beauchamp GR, Maddox SF. Photophobia, epiphora, and torticollis: a masquerade syndrome. J Pediatr Ophthalmol Strabismus 1990; 27(4):202–204.
54. Baquis GD, Rosman NP. Pressure-related torticollis: an unusual manifestation of pseudotumor cerebri. Pediatr Neurol 1989; 5(2):111–113.
55. Rajagopalan N, Humphrey PR, Bucknall RC. Torticollis and blepharospasm in systemic lupus erythematosus. Mov Disord 1989; 4(4):345–348.
56. Kajiwara A, Kobayashi H. Torticollis as a manifestation of Huntington's disease. Folia Psychiatr Neurol Jpn 1961; 63:44–49.
57. Kostaridou S, Anastasopoulos J, Veliotis C, et al. Recurrent torticollis secondary to langerhans cell histiocytosis: a case report. Acta Orthop Belg 2005; 71(1):102–106.
58. Tranchant C, Maquet J, Eber AM, et al. Cerebellar cavernous angioma, cervical dystonia and crossed cortical diaschisis. Rev Neurol 1991; 147:599–602.
59. Kiwak KJ, Deray MJ, Shields WD. Torticollis in three children with syringomyelia and spinal cord tumor. Neurology 1983; 33:946–948.
60. LeDoux MS, Brady KA. Secondary cervical dystonia associated with structural lesions of the central nervous system. Mov Disord 2003; 18(1):60–69.
61. Vazquez Lopez ME, Gonzalez Gomez FJ, Fernandez Iglesias JL, et al. Torticollis secondary to retropharyngeal abscess. An Esp Pediatr 2001; 55(3):288–289.
62. Williams CR, Clarke NM, Morris RJ. Torticollis secondary to ocular pathology. J Bone Joint Surg 1996; 78(4):620–62.
63. Langlois M, Richer F, Chouinard S. New perspectives on dystonia. Can J Neurol Sci 2003; 30(Suppl 1):S34–S44.

64. Adler CH, Kumar R. Pharmacological and surgical options for the treatment of cervical dystonia. Neurology 2000; 55(12):S9–S14.
65. Burke RE, Fahn S, Marsden CD. Torsion dystonia: a double-blind, prospective trial of high-dosage trihexyphenidyl. Neurology 1986; 36:160–164.
66. Spivak B, Gonen N, Mester R, et al. Neuroleptic malignant syndrome associated with abrupt withdrawal of anticholinergic agents. Int Clin Psychopharmacol 1996; 11(3):207–209.
67. Spivak B, Weizman A, Wolovick L, et al. Neuroleptic malignant syndrome during abrupt reduction of neuroleptic treatment. Acta Psychiatr Scand 1990; 81(2):168–169.
68. Greene P, Shale H, Fahn S. Analysis of open-label trials in torsion dystonia using high dosages of anticholinergics and other drugs. Mov Disord 1988; 3(1):46–60.
69. Lucetti C, Nuti A, Gambaccini G, et al. Mexiletine in the treatment of torticollis and generalized dystonia. Clinical Neuropharmacol 2000; 23(4):186–189.
70. Muller J, Wenning GK, Wissel J, et al. Riluzole therapy in cervical dystonia. Mov Disord 2002; 17(1):198–200.
71. Dykstra DD, Mendez A, Chappuis D, et al. Treatment of cervical dystonia and focal hand dystonia by high cervical continuously infused intrathecal baclofen: a report of 2 cases. Arch Phys Med Rehabil 2004; 86(4):830–833.
72. Jankovic J, Beach J. Long-term effects of tetrabenazine in hyperkinetic movement disorders. Neurology 1997; 48(2):358–362.
73. Kuniyoshi M, Ohyama S, Otsuka M, et al. Treatment of cervical dystonia by olanzapine. Hum Psychopharmacol 2003; 18(4):311–312.
74. Hasegawa O, Nagatomo H, Suzuki Y. Local alcoholisation treatment of spasmodic torticollis. Rinsho Shinkeigaku 1990; 30(7):718–722.
75. Jankovic J, Schwartz K. Botulinum toxin injections for cervical dystonia. Neurology 1990; 40(2):277–280.
76. Balash Y, Giladi N. Efficacy of pharmacological treatment of dystonia: evidence-based review including meta-analysis of the effect of botulinum toxin and other cure options. Eur J Neurol 2004; 11(6):361–370.
77. Tsui JK, Eisen A, Stoessl AJ, et al. Double-blind study of botulinum toxin in spasmodic torticollis. Lancet 1986; 2(8501):245–247.
78. Zesiewicz TA, Stamey W, Sullivan KL, et al. Botulinum toxin A for the treatment of cervical dystonia. Expert Opin Pharmacother 2004; 5(9):2017–2024.
79. Brashear A, Lew MF, Dykstra DD, et al. Safety and efficacy of NeuroBloc (botulinum toxin type B) in type A-responsive cervical dystonia. Neurology 1999; 53(7):1439–1446.
80. Brin MF, Lew MF, Adler CH, et al. Safety and efficacy of NeuroBloc(botulinum toxin type B) in type A-resistant cervical dystonia. Neurology 1999; 53(7):1431–1438.
81. Lew MF, Brashear A, Factor S. The safety and efficacy of botulinum toxin type B in the treatment of patients with cervical dystonia: summary of three controlled clinical trials. Neurology 2000; 55(12):S29–S35.
82. Costa J, Espírito-Santo C, Borges A, et al. Botulinum toxin type A versus anticholinergics for cervical dystonia. Cochrane Database Syst Rev 2005; (1):CD004312.
83. Data on file, Allergan, Inc. A randomized, multicenter, double-blind, placebo-controlled study of intramuscular BOTOX$^{TM}$ (botulinum toxin type A) purified neurotoxin complex (original 79–11 BOTOX$^{TM}$) for the treatment of cervical dystonia, 1998.
84. Costa J, Espírito-Santo C, Borges A, et al. Botulinum toxin type A therapy for cervical dystonia. Cochrane Database of Syst Rev 2005; (1):CD003633.
85. Jankovic J, Vuong KD, Ahsan J. Comparison of efficacy and immunogenicity of original versus current botulinum toxin in cervical dystonia. Neurology 2003; 60(7):1186–1188.
86. Comella CL, Buchman AS, Tanner CM, et al. Botulinum toxin injection for spasmodic torticollis: increased magnitude of benefit with electromyographic assistance. Neurology 1992; 42(4):878–882.
87. Botox$^{TM}$ package insert. Allergan Pharmaceuticals.
88. Deshpande SS, Sheridan RE, Adler M. Efficacy of certain quinolines as pharmacological antagonists in botulinum neurotoxin poisoning. Toxicon 1997; 35(3):433–445.

89. Comella CL, Jankovic J, Brin MF. Use of botulinum toxin type A in the treatment of cervical dystonia. Neurology 2000; 55(12):S15–S21.
90. Odergren T, Hjaltason H, Kaakkola S, et al. A double blind, randomised, parallel group study to investigate the dose equivalence of Dysport and Botox$^{TM}$ in the treatment of cervical dystonia. Neurol Neurosurg Psychiatry 1998; 64(1):6–12.
91. Ranoux D, Gury C, Fondarai J, et al. Respective potencies of Botox$^{TM}$ and Dysport: a double blind, randomised, crossover study in cervical dystonia. J Neurol Neurosurg Psychiatry 2002; 72(4):459–462.
92. Truong D, Duane DD, Jankovic J, et al. Efficacy and safety of botulinum type A toxin (dysport) in cervical dystonia: results of the first US randomized, double-blind, placebo-controlled study. Mov Disord 2005; 20(7):783–791.
93. Bihari K. Safety, effectiveness, and duration of effect of BOTOX$^{TM}$ after switching from Dysport for blepharospasm, cervical dystonia, and hemifacial spasm. Curr Med Res Opin 2005; 21(3):433–438.
94. Benecke R, Jost WH, Kanovsky P et al. A new botulinum toxin type A free of complexing proteins for treatment of cervical dystonia. Neurology 2005; 64(11):1949–1951.
95. Jost WH, Kohl A, Brinkmann S, et al. Efficacy and tolerability of a botulinum toxin type A free of complexing proteins (NT201) compared with commercially available botulinum toxin type A (BOTOX$^{TM}$) in healthy volunteers. J Neural Transm 2005; 112(7):905–913.
96. Costa J, Espírito-Santo C, Borges A, et al. Botulinum toxin type B for cervical dystonia. Cochrane Database of Syst Rev 2005; (1):CD004315.
97. Setler P. The biochemistry of botulinum toxin type B. Neurology 2000; 55(12) (Suppl 5): S22–S28.
98. Dressler D et al. Botulinum toxin: mechanisms of action. Eur Neurol 2005; 53:3–9.
99. Lew MF. Duration of effectiveness of botulinum toxin type B in the treatment of cervical dystonia. Adv Neurol 2004; 94:211–215.
100. Factor SA, Molho ES, Evans S, et al. Efficacy and safety of repeated doses of botulinum toxin type B in type A resistant and responsive cervical dystonia. Mov Disord 2005; 20(9):1152–1160.
101. Berman B, Seeberger L, Kumar R. Long-term safety, efficacy, dosing, and development of resistance with botulinum toxin type B in cervical dystonia. Mov Disord 2005; 20(2):233–237.
102. Comella C, Jankovic J, Shannon KM, et al. Comparison of botulinum toxin serotypes A and to B for the treatment of cervical dystonia. Neurology 2005; 65(9):1423–1429.
103. Cleveland P, Leong M, Royal M. A review of adult adverse events associated with botulinum toxin type B (Myobloc®). Poster, Basic and Therapeutic Aspects of Botulinum and Tetanus Toxins, Denver, CO, 2005.
104. Meyers R. Surgical procedure for postencephalitic tremor, with notes on the physiology of premotor fibers. Arch Neurol Psychiatry 1940; 44:455–458.
105. Meyers R. Surgical experiments in the therapy of certain 'extrapyramidal' diseases: a current evaluation. Acta neurol Scand Suppl 1951; 67:1–42.
106. Ford B. Pallidotomy for generalized dystonia. Adv Neurol 2004; 94:287–299.
107. Vitek JL. Surgery for dystonia. Neurosurg Clin N Am 1998; 9(2):345–366.
108. Yoshor D, Hamilton WJ, Ondo W, et al. Comparison of thalamotomy and pallidotomy for the treatment of dystonia. Neurosurgery 2001; 48(4):818–824, discussion 824.
109. Tasker RR, Doorly T, Yamashiro K. Thalamotomy in generalized dystonia. Adv Neurol 1988; 50:615–631.
110. Yamashiro K, Tasker RR. Stereotactic thalamotomy for dystonic patients. Stereotact Funct Neurosurg 1993; 60(1–3):81–85.
111. Laitinen LV. Personal memories of the history of stereotactic neurosurgery. Neurosurgery 2004; 55(6):1420–1428; discussion 1428.
112. Krauss JK, Yianni J, Loher TJ, et al. Deep brain stimulation for dystonia. J Clin Neurophysiol 2004; 21(1):18–30.

113. Bittar RG, Yianni J, Wang S, et al. Deep brain stimulation for generalised dystonia and spasmodic torticollis. J Clin Neurosci 2005; 12(1):12–16.
114. Kiss ZH, Doig K, Eliasziw M, et al. The Canadian multicenter trial of pallidal deep brain stimulation for cervical dystonia: preliminary results in three patients. Neurosurg focus 2004; 17(1):E5.
115. Magyar-Lehmann S, Antonini A, Roelcke U, et al. Cerebral glucose metabolism in patients with spasmodic torticollis. Mov Disord 1994; 12:704–708.
116. Krauss JK. Deep brain stimulation for cervical dystonia. J Neurol Neurosurg Psychiatry 2003; 74(11):1598.
117. Yianni J, Bain PG, Gregory RP, et al. Post-operative progress of dystonia patients following globus pallidus internus deep brain stimulation. Eur J Neurol 2003; 10(3): 239–247.
118. Yianni J, Bain PG, Giladi N, et al. Globus pallidus internus deep brain stimulation for dystonic conditions: a prospective audit. Mov Disord 2003; 18(4):436–442.
119. Bertrand C, Molina Negro P, Bouvier G, et al. Observations and analysis of results in 131 cases of spasmodic torticollis after selective denervation. Appl Neurophysiol 1987; 50(1):319–323.
120. Bertrand CM, Molina Negro P. Selective peripheral denervation in 111 cases of spasmodic torticollis: rationale and results. Adv Neurol 1988; 50:637–643.
121. Taira T, Kobayashi T, Hori T. Selective peripheral denervation of the levator scapulae muscle for laterocollic cervical dystonia. J Clin Neurosci 2003; 10(4):449–452.
122. Taira T, Kobayashi T, Takahashi K, et al. A new denervation procedure for idiopathic cervical dystonia. J Neurosurg 2002; 97(2 Suppl):201–216.
123. Bertrand CM. Selective peripheral denervation for spasmodic torticollis: surgical technique, results, and observation in 260 cases. Surg Neurol 1993; 40(2):96–103.
124. Munchau A, Palmer JD, Dressler D, et al. Prospective study of selective peripheral denervation for botulinum-toxin resistant patients with cervical dystonia. Brain 2001; 124 (Pt):769–783.
125. Chen X, Ma A, Liang J, et al. Selective denervation and resection of cervical muscles in the treatment of spasmodic torticollis: long-term follow-up results in 207 cases. Stereotact Funct Neurosurg 2000; 75(2):96–102.
126. Braun V, Richter HP. Selective peripheral denervation for spasmodic torticollis: 13-year experience with 155 patients. J Neurosurg 2002; 97(2):207–212.
127. Ford B, Louis ED, Greene P, et al. Outcome of selective ramisectomy for botulinum toxin resistant torticollis. J Neurol Neurosurg Psychiatry 1998; 65(4):472–478.
128. Cohen-Gadol AA, Ahlskog JE, Matsumoto JY, et al. Selective peripheral denervation for the treatment of intractable spasmodic torticollis: experience with 168 patients at the Mayo Clinic. J Neurosurg 2003; 98(6):1247–1254.
129. Paleacu D, Giladi N, Moore O, et al. Tetrabenazine treatment in movement disorders. Clin Neuropharmacol 2004; 27(5):230–233.
130. Jankovic J, Orman J. Tetrabenazine therapy of dystonia, chorea, tics, and other dyskinesias. Neurology 1988; 38(3):391–394.
131. Burbaud P, Guehl D, Lagueny A, et al. A pilot trial of clozapine in the treatment of cervical dystonia. J Neurol 1998; 245(6):329–331.
132. Pakkenberg H, Pedersen, B. Medical treatment of dystonia. Psychopharmacology 1985; 2:111–117.
133. Sandyk R. Beneficial effect of sodium valproate and baclofen in spasmodic torticollis. A case report. S Afr Med J 1984; 65(2):62–63.

# 11
# Limb Dystonia

**Barbara I. Karp**
*National Institute of Neurological Disorders and Stroke, National Institutes of Health, Bethesda, Maryland, U.S.A.*

## INTRODUCTION

Limb dystonia can be a primary, isolated focal disorder or can arise in association with more widespread involvement of multiple body areas. When dystonia involves the limbs, it can be particularly disabling. Hand use and walking require finely coordinated patterned movements, so that even a mild degree of dystonia can severely disrupt function.

Hemidystonia, dystonic involvement of the upper extremity, lower extremity, and face on the same side, is often secondary to an underlying structural cerebral lesion. When dystonia involves at least two adjacent body areas, such as the limbs and more proximal limb girdle muscles, it is referred to as segmental dystonia. Upper extremity, lower extremity, and limb segmental dystonia will be discussed in this chapter.

## FOCAL HAND DYSTONIA

Upper extremity dystonia tends to affect the distal muscles of the forearm and hand rather than the proximal muscles of the upper arm. Focal hand dystonia was first recognized and named by its characteristic impairment of specific tasks and tendency to cluster in those practicing particular occupations. One of the earliest descriptions, Ramazzini's 1713 treatise on maladies associated with various occupations, "De Morbis Artificum" (Diseases of Workers) (1), depicted the "morbid affections" of scribes and notaries:

> "Furthermore, incessant driving of the pen over paper causes intense fatigue of the hand and the whole arm because of the continuous and almost tonic strain on the muscles and tendons, which in course of time results in failure of power in the right hand."

The task specificity of "scrivener's palsy" was further noted by Solly in the *Lancet*, in 1864 (2):

> "[The disease] shows itself outwardly in a palsy of the writing powers. The muscles cease to obey the mandate of the will. It comes on very insidiously, . . . these unnatural sensations subside during the hours of rest and sleep, to return with the writer's work on the next day . . . The paralysed scrivener, though he cannot write . . . can do almost anything he likes, except earn his daily bread as a scribbler."

W. C. Gowers provided a more complete description of such "occupational neuroses" in "*A Manual of Diseases of the Nervous System*" (3), published 1886–1888, noting the insidious onset typically in middle age, task specificity, possible association with limb trauma, and the tendency for involvement of the nondominant hand in those who switched hands for writing. As well as arising in those who wrote for a living, Gowers reported similar symptoms in

> ". . . pianoforte players, violin players, seamstresses, telegraphers, smiths, harpists, artificial flower makers, turners, watchmakers, knitters, engravers, masons, compositors, enamellers, cigarette makers, shoemakers, milkers, money counters, and zither players"

or in those with, as Ramazzini commented, "particular posture of the limbs or unnatural movements of the body called for while they work."

The task specificity of focal hand dystonia is reflected even in today's nomenclature. Although all forms can be called "focal task-specific hand dystonia," names applied to task-specific variants have included writer's cramp, musician's cramp, typist cramp, occupational cramp or golfer's cramp (the "yips"). Writer's cramp is the most common focal hand dystonia in the general population.

## Signs and Symptoms

The first symptom of focal hand dystonia is usually a feeling of tightness or loss of facility with a previously easily performed action, often accompanied by fatigue and aching in the affected hand and forearm that worsen with continued hand use. The discomfort and difficulty using the hand resolve with rest but return quickly when the eliciting activity resumes. Symptoms may evolve over months to years, with the progressive development of uncontrolled, involuntary muscle contraction, abnormal position of the fingers and wrist, loss of control and impaired motor performance (Fig. 1). With writer's cramp, many patients report an excessively tight grip on the pen. The writing process becomes slow and tedious and the quality of handwriting deteriorates, worsening as writing continues (Fig. 2). In some patients, including approximately 50% of those with writer's cramp, the dystonia is exquisitely task-specific ("simple cramp"), leaving other tasks, even those performed with same muscles, unaffected (4,5). For example, some musicians severely impaired in playing one instrument, can play a second, even related instrument, with ease (6). In other patients, the dystonia progresses to involve other skilled tasks ("dystonic cramp"). When most severe, there is dystonic posturing at rest (Fig. 3). Focal hand dystonia may remain simple, but sometimes generalizes as "progressive cramp" that can spread to involve more proximal arm muscles, the neck, or lower face (5,7,8). Dystonia can also spread to involve the opposite limb (5,8).

The particular pattern of focal hand dystonia varies widely from individual to individual and may involve various combinations of distal and proximal muscles, flexors and extensors, and supinators or pronators. Certain patterns are more common than others and tend to be characteristic of patient occupation or other activities. In writer's cramp, the dominant hand is affected more frequently than the nondominant

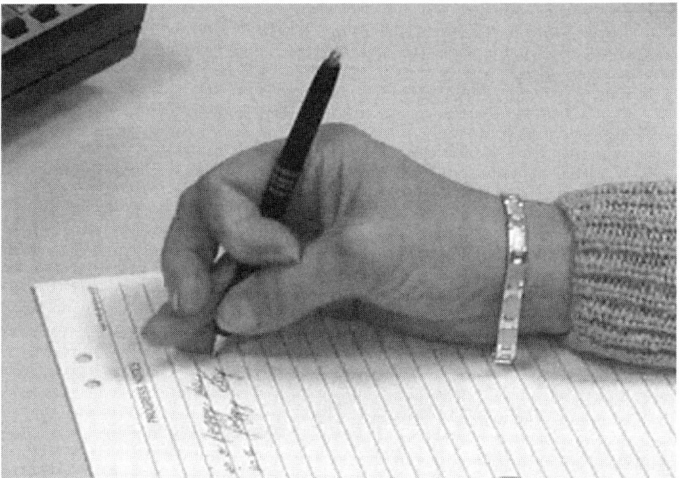

**Figure 1** Writer's cramp.

hand, flexors more commonly than extensors, and distal more commonly than proximal muscles. In typists, either one hand or both hands may become dystonic. In musicians, the pattern of dystonia reflects the muscles relied on most for instrumental play (9–11). In pianists, about 75% have right-hand involvement; fourth and fifth finger hyperflexion is particularly common. In violinists, the nonbowing left hand is affected in 60%, often with hyperflexion of the fourth and fifth fingers as in pianists. When the bowing hand is affected, the dystonia involves the wrist rather than the fingers. The third finger often flexes uncontrollably in guitar players, but extends in clarinetists.

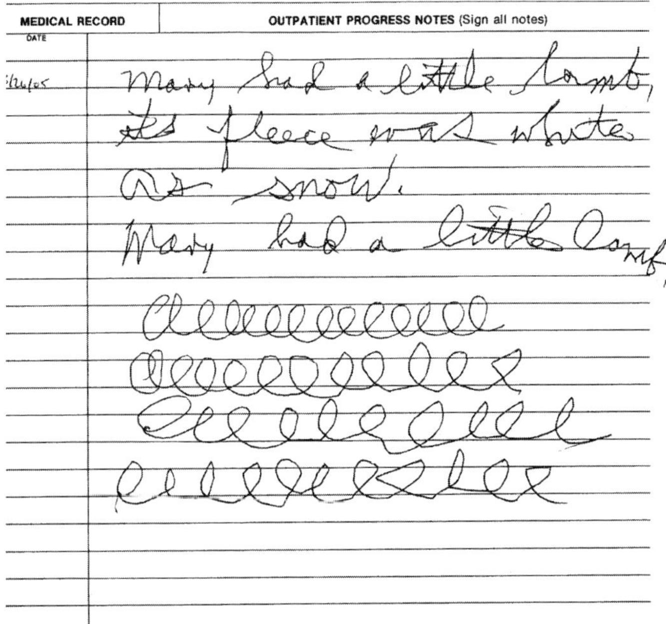


**Figure 2** Writing sample from a patient with writer's cramp. Quality deteriorates the longer writing continues.

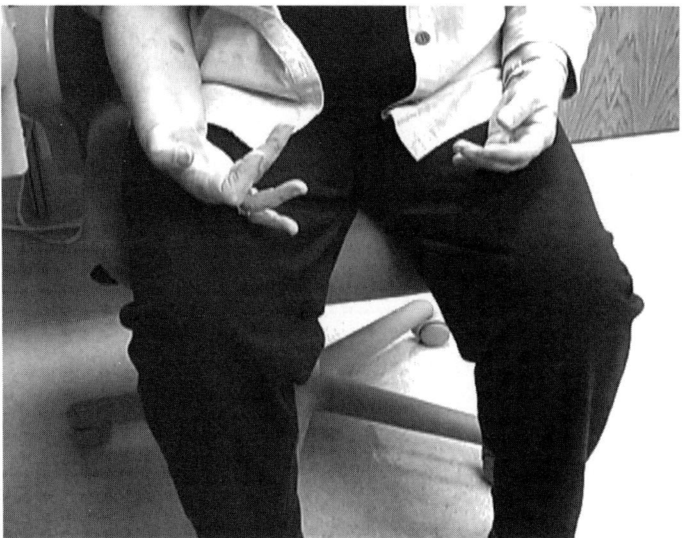

**Figure 3** Writer's cramp: abnormal dystonic hand posture at rest.

In woodwind players, the right hand, which has to both support and play the instrument, is more frequently affected than the left.

Primary sensory modalities are intact, although impaired spatial or temporal discrimination may be identified if specifically sought (12,13). Strength is normal, as are deep tendon reflexes. Actions eliciting the dystonia may be performed slowly and irregularly, but there is no ataxia. Additional signs may include myoclonic jerks, increased muscle tone, or loss of arm swing on the affected side. Dystonic muscles may hypertrophy over time. Tremor is present in up to 48% of patients with focal hand dystonia, usually unilateral in the affected arm, and may be task-specific (5,14). Primary writing tremor, task-specific tremor present only during writing, shares physiologic features with dystonia and can respond to similar medications, including botulinum toxin. It thus may be a variant of dystonia in some patients (15,16).

## Epidemiology

Focal hand dystonia has an incidence of 1.7 to 14 and a prevalence of 7 to 69 per million population (17–19). The prevalence of musician's dystonia is estimated to be between 0.2% and 0.5% (20), affecting as many as 5% to 24% of musicians presenting for evaluation of hand complaints (9,21,22). The typical age of focal hand dystonia onset is the fourth decade (4,5). In contrast to most other adult-onset focal dystonias that are more frequent in women, writer's cramp and musician's cramp affect men three times more frequently than women (6,9,17). Musicians with dystonia tend to be male (74%–83%), professional, classical musicians, and may have a slightly younger age of onset than the general focal hand dystonia population (6,9). Pianists, string players, and woodwind players are especially prone to develop hand dystonia.

## Genetics

Five percent to 20% of those with writer's cramp and 9% of those with musician's cramp have a family member with dystonia, suggesting a genetic component (7,11,23). Identical twins discordant for focal hand dystonia have been reported (9).

Genes associated with focal hand dystonia are increasingly being identified. Focal hand dystonia can be found in a few patients with the *DYT1* mutation of idiopathic torsion dystonia, and thus may be a "forme fruste" in some circumstances (24,25). Upper extremity and lower extremity dystonia are not uncommonly presenting symptoms of *DYT1* dystonia, with generalization ensuing over the following years (8). However, the *DYT1* gene is not frequent in either writer's cramp (26) or musician's cramp (27). Focal hand dystonia has also been reported in *DYT6* (28), *DYT7* (29), and *DYT13* (30) families. Bhidayasiri reported three brothers with writer's cramp onset in the sixth decade, linked to chromosome 18p, as are *DYT7* and *DYT15* (31).

## Pathophysiology

The initial characterization of abnormal patterns of muscle contraction in dystonia focused on writer's cramp. Surface EMG during writing revealed cocontraction of agonists and antagonists, prolonged muscle bursts, and lack of muscle selectivity with overflow contraction of muscles not ordinarily activated by writing (32–34).

Physiologic studies focused on hand dystonia have demonstrated a variety of central nervous system deficits including impaired intracortical inhibition, abnormal cortical excitability, and aberrant sensorimotor plasticity that likely contribute to the overcontraction of muscles and loss of motor control characteristic of this disorder (35–38). The way these identified abnormalities combine to result in a particular manifestation of the dystonic symptoms is not well understood. Some physiologic abnormalities are present bilaterally despite apparently unilateral symptomatology, and others are present independent of whether dystonia is activated. Many do not correlate with the severity of dystonic symptoms. However, Chen was able to demonstrate loss of cortical inhibition with transcranial magnetic stimulation that was specific to the symptomatic hand (39). Odergren found abnormally increased activation of primary sensorimotor cortex, premotor cortex, thalamus, and cerebellum, which paralleled worsening disability during sustained writing (40). Pujol elicited dystonia by having musicians play a modified guitar during fMRI scanning and found decreased activation in premotor areas with increased activation of primary sensorimotor cortex contralateral to the dystonic hand. The decrease in premotor activation was less prominent when the musicians played with the nondystonic hand (41).

Somatosensory system abnormalities are well demonstrated in focal hand dystonia. Sensory maps for the hand are distorted with overlapping finger representation (42–45). Defects are also present in temporal and spatial sensory discrimination, although it is not clear if the sensory abnormalities cause or result from dystonia (12,13,42,46–48). Simultaneous stimuli applied to different digits lead to blending of cortical receptive fields for those fingers, while temporally separate stimulation does not. Thus, defects in temporal discrimination of sensory stimuli could lead to cortical dedifferentiation of sensory maps (49).

Rosenkranz et al. proposed that different mechanisms may play a role in the genesis of focal hand dystonia in writers, who use their hands no more than the average worker, and in others, such as musicians, where there is clearly prolonged, repetitive, stressful use of the hands. They demonstrated physiologic differences in intracortical inhibition between writer's cramp and musician's cramp, with less influence of sensory input on motor output in writer's cramp and more loss of short-latency intracortical inhibition from vibratory stimulation in musician's cramp. Interestingly, nondystonic musicians had a decrease in intracortical inhibition compared to normals, but it was less severe than in those with dystonia, supporting the possibility of aberrant plasticity in those with dystonia (50). Similarly, Lim found an increase in the amplitude of the late component of the contingent negative variation in musicians' cramp, consistent with an increase in corticomotor excitability or loss of inhibition that differed from the decrease in amplitude reported in CNV studies of writer's cramp (51).

Although brain structure appears normal on anatomic examination or structural MRI, Garraux, using voxel-based morphometry, found increased gray matter in hand territories of primary somatosensory and motor cortex in patients with focal hand dystonia (52). A similar finding in the hemisphere contralateral to the unaffected hand suggested that the change was not a secondary effect of the dystonia.

## Etiology

As noted in the earliest medical description of focal hand dystonia, symptoms appear to first arise with prolonged repetitive use of the small muscles of the hand. Musicians often report the onset of symptoms during a period of particularly intense practice or when approaching especially difficult works. A role for excessive hand use in the development of focal hand dystonia is further supported by the pattern of dystonic muscle involvement. Focal hand dystonia tends to develop on the side and in the muscles used most frequently. Thus, writers develop dystonia in the dominant writing hand. About 74% of pianists develop dystonia in the right hand that handles more technically demanding parts than the left, while it affects the fingering left hand in 60% of violinists (9,20,53,54). Dystonia in both pianists and violinists has a predilection for the fourth and fifth fingers. These fingers may be particularly vulnerable because their relative weakness requires more effort during playing than other fingers and because they have relatively little independence of movement compared to the other fingers (53). Individual anatomic factors, such as joint immobility or intertendinous connections, may also play a role in susceptibility to focal hand dystonia (55).

The "overuse" hypothesis is further supported by a monkey model in which attended, highly repetitive hand movements produced a movement disorder similar to focal hand dystonia. There was, in addition, remodeling of primary somatosensory cortex with enlarged and overlapping cortical receptive fields for the digits that correlated with severity of the motor abnormality, similar to aberrations of sensory cortical field representation found in focal hand dystonia (56,57).

Limb overuse, however, cannot be the sole factor eliciting dystonia, since many people, including most professional musicians, use their hands extensively and do not develop dystonia. Jedynak found that fewer than half of the patients with writer's cramp had a history of writing intensively before the dystonia onset (4). The expression of focal hand dystonia may therefore require both an underlying predisposition and a trigger. Personality, genetics, prior cerebral injury, and aspects of performance may combine with a trigger, such as prolonged hours of use, to lead to the development of focal hand dystonia (35,58,59).

Although controversial (60,61), one possible trigger for focal hand dystonia is trauma. Focal hand dystonia can follow acute or remote, even minor, trauma to the dystonic limb (59,62–66). Complex regional pain syndrome [(CRPS) (also known as reflex sympathetic dystrophy)] may, but need not, be present. Five to ten percent of those with writer's cramp and a few musicians report prior trauma to the affected limb (4,5,7,9,14). Spinal injuries and conditions such as thoracic outlet syndrome have also been reported as precipitants (67–69). Although rare, isolated focal hand dystonia can follow brain injury, sometimes as a late sequela (70,71).

Peripheral nerve dysfunction may also contribute to the development of dystonic symptoms (72). Charness reported uncontrolled finger flexion, especially of the fourth and fifth digits, in musicians with ulnar neuropathy, characterized by defective agonist/antagonist activation and prolonged muscle bursts on EMG (73,74). Similar EMG abnormalities were present in nondystonic patients with ulnar neuropathy, even in muscles not innervated by the ulnar nerve, suggesting that the ulnar neuropathy had altered central motor processing. Most patients with focal hand dystonia, however, have neither symptoms nor physiologic evidence of ulnar nerve dysfunction.

## Differential Diagnosis

The diagnosis of idiopathic focal hand dystonia relies on clinical evaluation identifying features consistent with dystonia and excluding secondary causes. Patients with other disorders may present similar complaints, but the combination of painless, task-specific uncontrolled spasm and the pattern of abnormal posture should suggest dystonia.

Repetitive stress injury (RSI) or "overuse syndrome" is a commonly diagnosed occupational cause of hand pain and disability that can be mistaken for dystonia (75,76). The hallmark of RSI is pain in the affected hand and arm. RSI symptoms may progress from pain present only during limb use to pain persisting despite rest and may be accompanied by swelling or other signs of inflammation. Similar to dystonia, RSI can be precipitated by stressful, repetitive hand use, and among its risk factors are the use of high force, awkward joint positions, and prolonged unnatural postures (77). Unlike dystonia, however, function is preserved except as impeded by pain. RSI is due to tenosynovitis, often with microtears in the soft tissue and stress fractures. About 2% of RSI patients have nerve impairment, such as carpal tunnel or other pressure neuropathy.

Therapy for RSI includes rest, splinting, ice, elevation, nonsteroidal anti-inflammatory medications, and local steroid injections, all aimed at decreasing pain and inflammation. Similar to focal hand dystonia, preventing exacerbation entails changing limb posture, altering hand use techniques, and improved ergonomic design of work tools.

CRPS (previously "reflex sympathetic dystrophy") causes pain, autonomic dysfunction, and trophic changes, usually following injury to the affected extremity. In type I CRPS, there is no identifiable nerve injury, while type 2 CRPS (previously called "causalgia") is associated with identifiable peripheral nerve damage. The pathogenesis of CRPS is believed to entail both central nervous system processes and peripheral neurogenic inflammation. Motor abnormalities occur in up to 97% of patients with CRPS (78) and include weakness, hyper-reflexia, difficulty initiating movement, tremor, and irregular myoclonic jerks (79,80). Dystonia is present in 10% to 30% of patients with CRPS, especially those with type 2 (78,81). Jankovic found CRPS in 9 of 18 patients with dystonia following peripheral trauma (59). The dystonia may precede other CRPS symptoms, but is especially likely in those with long-standing CRPS. Unlike idiopathic dystonia that associated with CRPS may be fixed, painful, and persist during sleep (79). Prolonged muscle contraction and cocontraction of agonists and antagonists on EMG and H-reflex abnormalities indicating loss of inhibition, similar to that in idiopathic dystonia, are also present in CRPS-associated dystonia (79,82). The treatment of CRPS focuses on control of pain, the most disabling symptom. Early on, the dystonic symptoms may respond to sympathetic blockade or sympathectomy. Medications such as benzodiazepines or lioresal may also be helpful.

Nerve entrapment may be mistaken for focal hand dystonia or can arise subsequent to it. Carpal tunnel syndrome does not commonly cause hand dystonia, but hand dystonia may predispose to the development of carpal tunnel syndrome (72). Although the forearm and hand discomfort associated with focal hand dystonia could be mistaken for carpal tunnel syndrome, hand weakness, sensory loss, Tinel's sign, and Phalen's sign should be absent.

The relationship between ulnar neuropathy and focal hand dystonia is less clear. As noted above, patients with ulnar neuropathy may develop finger hyperflexion similar to dystonia. Charness found symptoms and EMG evidence of ulnar neuropathy in 40% of 73 musicians with occupational cramp, needing near-nerve recording since surface EMG detected the ulnar nerve abnormality in only one-third of cases (73). Even though musician's dystonia is more common in men, ulnar neuropathy was more likely in women with musician's cramp. Ulnar neuropathy is not present in most patients with focal hand dystonia, but it should be carefully excluded by physical examination and EMG, with near-nerve recording if warranted.

In the early literature, dystonia was attributed to cerebral dysfunction. In "A note on scrivener's palsy," Pearce includes the analysis of Sir Charles Bell (1830) (83):

> "The nerves and muscles are capable of their proper functions and proper adjustments; the defect is in the imperfect exercise of the will, or in the secondary influence the brain has over the relations established in the body."

In the 19th century, however, focal hand dystonia was often considered a neurotic or hysterical disorder (5). While most patients with focal hand dystonia have no demonstrable psychopathology, limb dystonia is not uncommonly a presentation of psychogenic dystonia. Psychogenic dystonia should be considered when there is abrupt onset, rapid progression to fixed posture, prominent pain, other psychogenic neurologic signs, and multiple somatizations (84,85).

In symptomatic or secondary dystonias, hand and arm involvement are frequently associated with dystonia of the leg or trunk muscles (hemidystonia) or more proximal muscles (segmental dystonia) on the same side. Secondary dystonia is rarely expressed as isolated focal hand or arm dystonia. However, it has been reported with cerebral lesions, usually involving the contralateral basal ganglia, as well as with spinal cord, nerve root, or brachial plexus lesions (71,86). Symptomatic dystonias are usually recognized by the additional signs and symptoms, reflective of the underlying disorder, that are not otherwise present in idiopathic dystonia.

## Natural History

Spontaneous remission of focal hand dystonia is rare and often only temporary (7). In most patients, the symptoms evolve over a few months to years and then stabilize, although later progression has been reported (8,87). Hand dystonia can interfere with activities of daily living or occupation, but is rarely disabling (5). Only 10% to 15% of those with writer's cramp were unable to continue their usual occupation or writing with the dominant hand. The situation is different, however, in professional musicians for whom even a minor degree of dystonia can be disabling. Only 36% to 53% of affected professional musicians are able to continue playing professionally, even with treatment and changes in technique or repertoire (9,87).

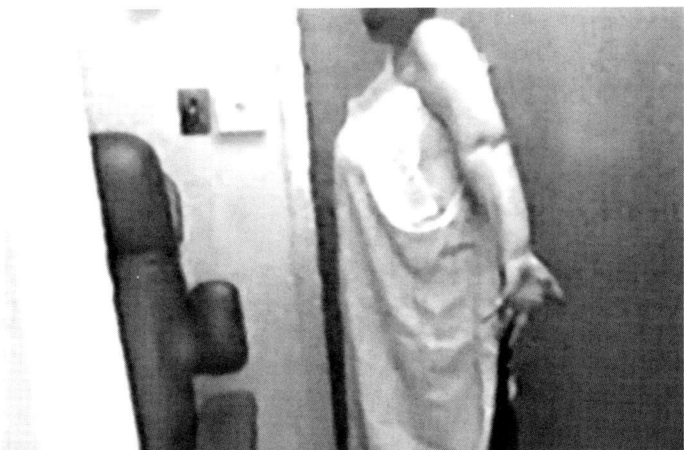

**Figure 4** Segmental dystonia with typical pattern of shoulder elevation, arm adduction, and internal rotation.

## SEGMENTAL DYSTONIA

Segmental dystonia involves not only the limb but also the contiguous proximal limb girdle musculature. Primary segmental dystonia may be a little more frequent than focal hand dystonia (17,19). In the upper limbs, segmental dystonia often causes a characteristic posture of shoulder elevation with adduction and internal rotation of the arm (Fig. 4). Segmental dystonia can also be an expression of the *DYT1* mutation (88). Similar to hemidystonia, segmental dystonia is often symptomatic of an underlying brain, spinal cord, root, or nerve lesion and can follow peripheral trauma (89–92). Delayed dystonia after childhood or adult brain damage is often segmental (93). Similar to other dystonias, when segmental dystonia occurs in the presence of a central lesion, the most common location is the contralateral basal ganglia. Stathis reported a patient with a putaminal stroke, but no residual hand weakness, who developed segmental dystonia following arm fracture and casting three years later, supporting the idea that peripheral trauma may be a trigger in someone with an underlying susceptibility, such as a basal ganglia lesion (94).

## LEG AND FOOT DYSTONIA

The leg and foot are often affected along with other parts of the body in generalized dystonia, dystonia-plus syndromes, and psychogenic dystonia (85). Symptomatic leg dystonia can also be seen with brain, spinal, or radicular lesions (70,71,95–97) or following peripheral trauma with or without CRPS (79,92). Leg involvement, as a presenting sign of early-onset dystonia, signals a likelihood of generalization, with spread to the trunk and arms following within months to years. Leg dystonia in patients with dopa-responsive dystonia (DRD) improves with rest and responds to low doses of l-dopa. In adults, leg dystonia can be an initial sign of Parkinson's disease, occurring before the onset of bradykinesia, tremor, or rigidity. In this case, the dystonia may respond to l-dopa. Later in the course of Parkinson's disease, limb dystonia can arise as a complication of l-dopa therapy (98).

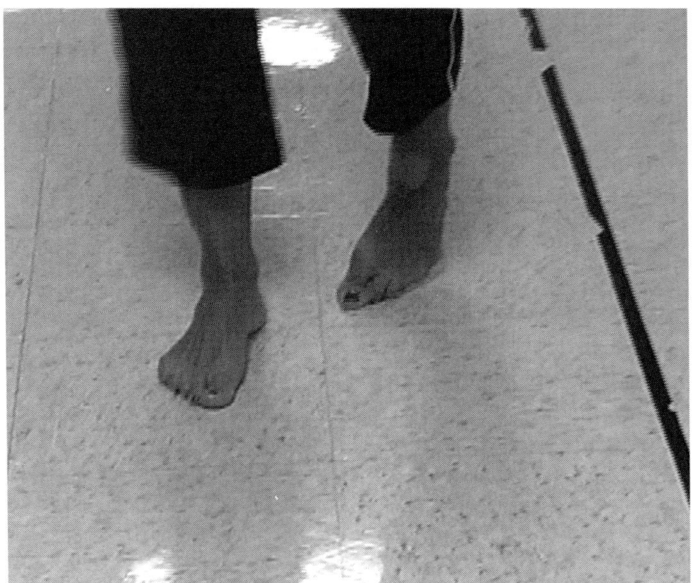

**Figure 5** Lower extremity dystonia with typical internal rotation of foot.

Idiopathic focal leg dystonia is uncommon. The incidence is not known; only single cases and a small series have been reported (99–102). Singer reviewed four of his own cases and three in the literature (103). In those seven patients, the mean age of leg dystonia onset was 57 +/− 12 years. The main dystonic pattern was foot or leg inversion and plantar flexion, as seen in one of our patients (Fig. 5). Foot dorsiflexion was less frequent. The toes flexed in some patients but extended in others. Symptoms were less obvious on walking backwards. Idiopathic leg and foot dystonia was action-induced, occasionally seen at rest, and caused mild-to-moderate gait impairment.

A number of reasons may explain why lower limb dystonia occurs less frequently than upper limb dystonia. One is that the underlying pathologic cause of dystonia may have a predilection for anatomically specific areas of the brain. Other explanations may be that less area is devoted to representation of the lower limb than the hand and arm in brain regions important in dystonia, or because specific triggers, such as overuse, rarely affect the leg.

## EVALUATION OF LIMB DYSTONIA

### Physical Examination

The first step in evaluating limb dystonia is a complete neurologic examination. Signs of radiculopathy, peripheral neuropathy, parkinsonism, and other disorders that can secondarily cause dystonia should be sought. The examination may then focus on the dystonia itself.

To determine the full extent of dystonic involvement, patients need to be examined in a variety of conditions, including rest, sustained posture, during activities that provoke the dystonia, and while performing other activities. Most patients with limb dystonia have normal resting posture. However, the dystonia, sometimes

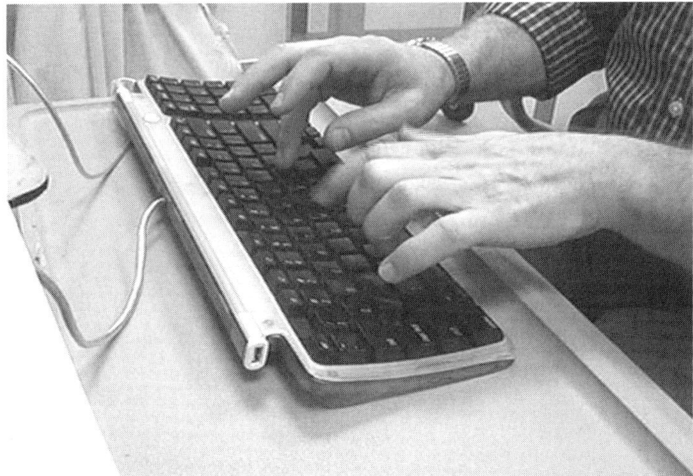

**Figure 6** Typist cramp affecting both hands.

with choreiform movements of the fingers, is obvious at rest in the most severely affected patients.

One of the most important aspects of the examination is observation during performance of the tasks eliciting the dystonia. For example, typists should be observed at a keyboard (Fig. 6), and those with writer's cramp should be examined during writing, using both whatever adaptive grip they have developed to cope with the dystonia and their premorbid grip. Musicians need to be examined while playing their instruments, both with and without any adaptations that they may have made (Fig. 7).

There are few validated rating scales for dystonia and none specifically for writer's cramp or musician's cramp. Methods of assessment for writer's cramp have

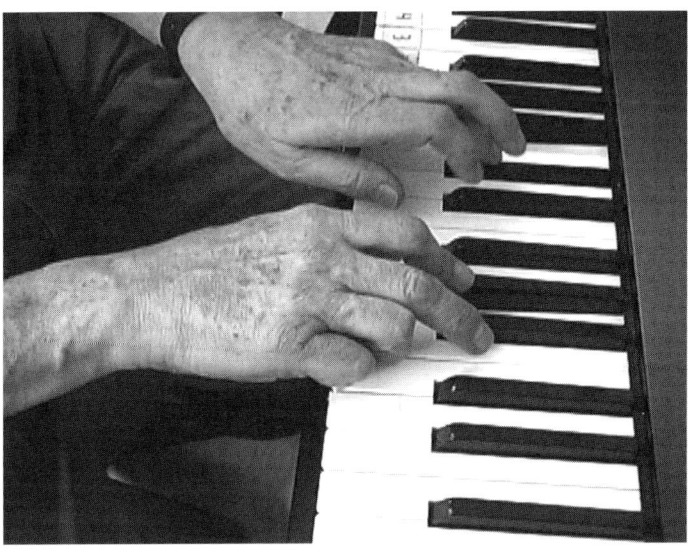

**Figure 7** Musician's cramp: fourth and fifth finger hyperflexion in a pianist.

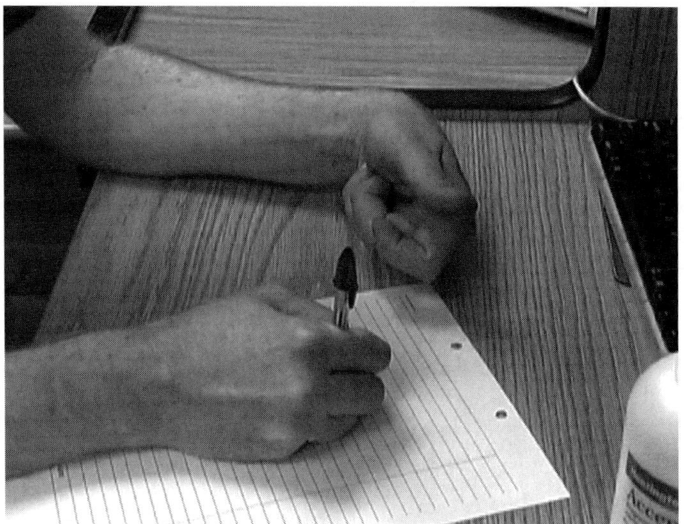

**Figure 8** Mirror dystonia in the dominant left hand during writing with the nondominant right hand.

included judging the quality of writing samples of either words or repeated loops, timed tasks such as the number of words or letters written in a set period of time, speed of writing a particular passage, qualitative descriptions, analysis of digitized movement parameters, and visual analog scales. Music performance can similarly be analyzed objectively, but no uniformly accepted, validated method is available. Assessment more commonly relies on expert judgment of performance or self-report.

If botulinum toxin treatment is being considered, it is important to delineate the specific muscles involved in the dystonia in order to select muscles for injection. The determination of affected muscles may not be straightforward. Dystonia may not be present at rest and the performance of actions that elicit the dystonia is often complicated by the presence of compensatory movements that may not be consciously adopted. Patients should be asked to perform without compensating for the dystonia, when possible. Observing tasks other than the primary eliciting task may allow observation of dystonic patterns without compensation. For example, 5% to 40% of patients have mirror dystonic posturing in the dominant hand when writing with the nondominant hand (Fig. 8) (4,7). Observing mirror dystonia allows one to detect the pattern of muscle involvement without the confound of compensatory movements and may be helpful in selecting muscles for botulinum toxin injection (104). Additional tasks that may be helpful in focal hand dystonia are to have the patient draw a spiral with outstretched fingers rather than while gripping the pen or to tap on a table with each finger sequentially (Fig. 9).

Segmental dystonia of the upper limb is often best seen during walking, as is dystonia of the leg and foot. Patients with leg dystonia should be examined walking, both with and without whatever shoes or orthotics they commonly wear.

## Ancillary Studies

Routine EMG is not helpful in the diagnosis of focal limb dystonias other than to eliminate an underlying neuropathy or radiculopathy. Its use can, therefore, be

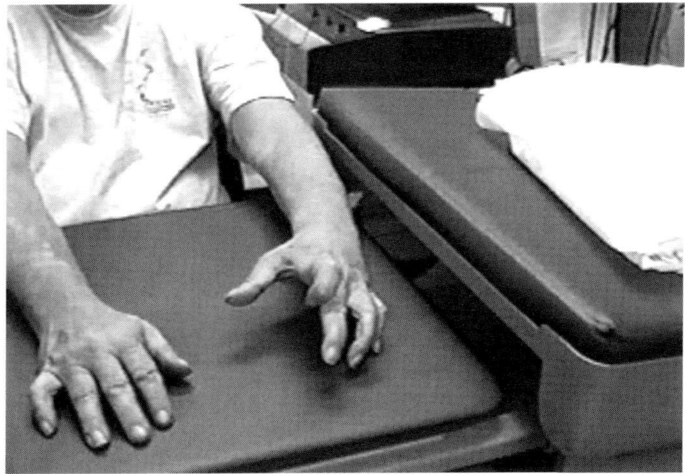

**Figure 9** Focal hand dystonia: symptoms elicited by sequential finger tapping.

reserved for patients with sensory or motor signs on examination. Near-nerve recording may be needed to detect occult neuropathies. Multiple wire EMG recorded during dystonic activation may be helpful in determining the affected muscles, especially those deep or not obvious on clinical inspection. Brain or spinal cord imaging is not routinely obtained but should be done whenever there are atypical features or signs other than dystonia on examination. In addition, imaging can be helpful in segmental dystonia, a condition more frequently associated with a structural lesion. Similarly, genetic testing is not routinely performed for those with focal hand dystonia, but *DYT1* or DRD testing should be considered in those with suggestive clinical features, early onset limb dystonia, or a family history of dystonia.

## TREATMENT

The main goal of treatment in limb dystonia is usually functional improvement in the use of the limb. However, correction of abnormal posture and relief of discomfort are also important to some patients. With the development of hand dystonia, most patients try to alter hand use or their environment to minimize functional disability. For example, those with writer's cramp try thicker pens, change their handgrip, or switch to writing with the nondominant hand. Unfortunately, 25% to 50% of patients who switch hands will eventually develop dystonia in the nondominant hand (4,7). Musicians, attributing the early symptoms of dystonia to problems with technique or inadequate practice, therefore often first practice more intensely, refinger music, adjust hand and wrist positions, or modify their instrument. Those with leg dystonia try new shoes or orthotics.

Some patients pursue massage therapy, psychotherapy, relaxation therapy, splinting, biofeedback, chiropractory, hypnosis, or acupuncture (105,106). However, these approaches rarely produce sustained relief. Herbal therapies, such as geranium oil, almond oil, and amylase enzyme treatment, and implements, such as specially designed pens, are of no proven benefit. Physical and occupational therapy, including the use of splints or other devices, benefit some patients but are rarely adequate treatment by themselves.

The development of new therapies for hand dystonia has recently focused on the evolving understanding of cerebral plasticity and the role that aberrant cerebral remodeling may play in the expression of dystonic symptoms. Both movement and sensory-based retraining focus on trying to reverse maladapted plasticity. Sensory-based approaches specifically try to restore normal sensory representation of the hand and digits in the dedifferentiated cortex of dystonic subjects.

Byl had 12 patients with hand dystonia practice sensory discrimination tasks, combining nonsimultaneous attended sensory stimulation of the fingertips with mental imagery, muscle biofeedback to eliminate cocontraction, and movements practiced under mirror observation (107). In this uncontrolled study, 80% of patients had 30% to 70% improvement in both sensory and motor function after three to six months of training.

Zeuner chose Braille reading, which requires attended, nonrepetitive movement and tactile discrimination, as a sensorimotor task for dystonia rehabilitation. While blindfolded, 10 patients with writer's cramp trained the finger most affected by dystonia and the two adjacent fingers to read Braille. At the end of eight weeks, five patients had improved writing and sensory discrimination. Continued practice was needed to sustain benefit up to 20 weeks (108).

For "sensory retuning therapy" of musician's dystonia, a primarily affected "focal dystonic finger" is identified and rehabilitated by the performance of repetitive movements with other digits, one at a time, while the remaining fingers are splinted and immobilized. Musical play without the splints resumes after a week and is increased as tolerated. Of 11 musicians treated with sensorimotor retuning, none of the 3 woodwind players improved. The remaining 8 (6 pianists and 2 guitarists) had improved music performance after three months of therapy. Some patients had sustained benefit for over a year even though their training lapsed after a few months. In others, continued practice with isolation and immobilization of the fingers was needed to maintain benefit (109,110). Improvement in cortical somatosensory derangements accompanied improved performance (111).

Priori, taking advantage of "inactivity-dependent neuroplasticity," explored the benefit of four to five weeks of limb immobilization as therapy for dystonia, based on the observation that prolonged immobilization shrinks limb motor cortical representation in nondystonic subjects (112). Weakness and clumsiness of the immobilized limb, present immediately after the splint was removed, was followed one week later by improved motor performance and diminished dystonia. Seven of eight splinted patients had at least moderate improvement for as long as 24 weeks.

Therapeutic modification of motor function has also been preliminarily explored. Siebner applied 1 Hz repetitive transcranial magnetic stimulation (rTMS), which can decrease cortical excitability, over the motor cortex of 12 patients with writer's cramp. Intracortical inhibition improved, as well as clarity of handwriting and drawing, but improvement lasted less than a day (113). Murase compared 0.2 Hz rTMS of motor cortex, premotor cortex, and supplementary motor area (SMA). Stimulation of premotor cortex, but not of motor cortex or SMA, improved writing performance (114). Tinazzi used transcutaneous electrical nerve stimulation (TENS), applied to forearm flexor muscles in 10 patients with writer's cramp over 10 sessions of 20 minutes each (115). Writing time and handwriting clarity improved for as long as three weeks. It was suggested that TENS activated muscle large fiber afferents, which modulated the balance between central excitation and inhibition of agonist and antagonist muscles.

Peripheral nerve surgery may relieve nerve compression symptoms, if present, but does not reverse the dystonia, except in a few patients with coexistent ulnar nerve palsy. Charness reported that in some of the patients with dystonic symptoms and ulnar neuropathy, symptoms of both improved when the neuropathy was treated. Others, however, have found no improvement in dystonia with ulnar nerve release in patients with coexistent dystonia and ulnar neuropathy (66). Carpal tunnel surgery does not relieve dystonia even in patients with carpal tunnel syndrome. In leg dystonia, tendonotomy or tendon transfer may improve posture or gait (116). Limb amputation has been performed in severe circumstances (117).

The current experience with stereotactic brain surgery for focal limb dystonia is limited. Stereotactic ventro-oralis (Vo) complex thalamotomy has been used, largely in Japan, to disrupt abnormal activity in pallido-thalamo-cortical motor loops. Goto reported remarkable improvement in hand function sustained at least six months in a single patient with dystonic hand cramp (118), and Shibata (119) reported improvement in dystonic writing tremor following such surgery. Taira performed Vo complex thalamotomy in 12 patients with task-specific focal hand dystonia refractory to oral medication; botulinum toxin injections had not been available (120). All patients had immediate resolution of dystonic symptoms on lesion placement, which was sustained 13 months later. Two patients had partial recurrence, which responded to a second thalamotomy. Iacono et al. reported improvement in leg dystonia in patients with atypical parkinsonism who underwent unilateral pallidotomy (121). The use of deep brain stimulation for idiopathic hand dystonia has not yet been reported.

In limb dystonia, oral medications are largely reserved for those with severe dystonia or widespread involvement. Medications for focal limb dystonia, including anticholinergic drugs, dopamine agonists and antagonists, baclofen, clonazepam or other benzodiazepines, and muscle relaxants, are rarely effective (54,122). Anticholinergic medication, such as trihexyphenidyl, may be the most effective oral medications for idiopathic limb dystonia, especially for young patients with segmental dystonia (122). Unfortunately, even anticholinergic medication is seldom more than minimally helpful, and its toxicity often outweighs the limited benefit (123). Oral or intrathecal baclofen may be helpful in relieving limb dystonia in patients with CRPS, and l-dopa can successfully treat dystonia in both DRD and Parkinson's disease.

Options for neuromuscular blockade or neurolysis include phenol or botulinum toxin injection. Phenol, which can only be used on pure motor nerves, is not an option for focal hand dystonia, but may be helpful in lower limb dystonia. A case report described a patient with leg dystonia who responded to phenol but not botulinum toxin injection (101).

The treatment of choice for focal limb dystonia is currently botulinum toxin injection. It has been 15 years since the initial reports demonstrating efficacy of botulinum toxin for limb dystonia (124–126). Botulinum toxin has been shown to be safe and effective without the systemic effects of oral medications. Botulinum toxin injections may also be safely combined with oral medications and nonpharmacological therapies.

When used for limb dystonia, proper selection of muscles for injection is crucial. A single muscle or combinations of muscles is chosen for injection on the basis of clinical examination, patient report of tightness, and, if needed, EMG evidence of excessive muscle activation. When using botulinum toxin for limb dystonia, it is not always necessary to inject every muscle involved in the dystonia. Some patients respond well to injection of one or a few of the muscles that are the main source of disability or discomfort. For focal hand dystonia, forearm muscles, especially wrist and finger flexors, most often require injection; treatment of proximal muscles is needed less frequently. Segmental dystonia of the upper extremity, however, requires injection of proximal arm, shoulder, and chest wall muscles. Since the pattern of internal rotation and adduction of the arm with shoulder elevation is common, the muscles most frequently injected are teres major, latissimus dorsi, trapezius, and pectoralis major. When injecting muscles of the chest wall, particular care must be taken not to pierce the pleura, causing a pneumothorax. Since the most common pattern of leg dystonia is foot inversion and plantar flexion, the most frequently injected muscles for leg dystonia are tibialis posterior and flexor digitorum longus. A high dose of toxin is often needed for these large leg muscles. Higher doses than might be predicted on the basis of muscle size may be required for injection of foot intrinsic muscles such as the flexor digitorum. The use of electromyographic guidance enhances the accuracy of injection localization in limb muscles (127).

While the efficacy of botulinum toxin in limb dystonia may largely be due to its peripheral action, neuromuscular junction blockade, there is also evidence of central effects. Botulinum toxin injection can at least temporarily reverse some central physiologic abnormalities characteristic of dystonia including the loss of long latency inhibition (128), cortical motor map distortion (45), and intracortical inhibition (129).

Sixty percent to 80% of patients treated for focal hand dystonia have more than minimal improvement lasting approximately three months (130–134). After three to four injection sessions, most patients have a stable response to treatment and, in the absence of antibody development, benefit can be maintained for years with repeated injections, usually with little change in the muscles injected or in dose. Thirty percent to 50% of patients continue botulinum toxin injection for limb dystonia for longer than two to five years (130,131,134,135). Other than atrophy in the injected or adjacent muscles, there have been no reports of long-term, adverse effects with repeated botulinum toxin injections.

Although botulinum toxin helps with excessive tightness and abnormal posture, it is less effective in correcting the loss of fine motor control present in dystonia. Hence, musicians may not be able to continue professional performance, even if the dystonia is greatly improved (123).

There are no controlled studies of botulinum toxin for lower limb dystonia, but such patients have been described in case reports and included in larger studies of botulinum toxin use. Singer, in a description of adult-onset leg dystonia, noted benefit from botulinum toxin in both of two patients treated (103). Botulinum toxin appears to be equally effective for idiopathic and symptomatic leg dystonia, including that associated with Parkinson's disease and levodopa treatment (100,102,126,136,137). Similar to the treatment of arm dystonia, symptoms usually begin improving within one to two weeks, and the benefit lasts about four months (137).

The botulinum toxin treatment of hand and arm dystonia, but not leg dystonia, is usually accompanied by muscle weakness that may be as disabling as the dystonia. There is no correlation between the degree of weakness and magnitude of the benefit produced—the balance between benefit and weakness in a given individual is unpredictable. Some patients have almost complete relief of symptoms with little weakness; others have pronounced weakness with only minimal improvement in their dystonia. Therefore, the acceptability of botulinum toxin treatment lies with the patient who needs to decide if the benefit achieved outweighs any transient weakness incurred.

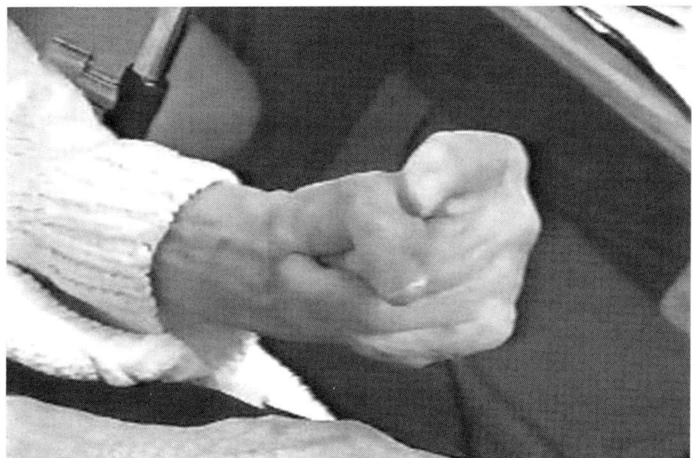

**Figure 10** Dystonic, clenched fist in patient with corticobasal ganglionic degeneration.

Patients with symptomatic secondary dystonia, such as corticobasal ganglionic degeneration, Parkinson's disease, CRPS, or poststroke dystonia, may develop tightly clenched fists (Fig. 10). Even though hand function cannot be restored, botulinum toxin injection may allow the hand to be opened, enhancing patient comfort and allowing improved palmar hygiene (138,139). Higher doses of toxins may be required in patients with symptomatic secondary dystonia than in those with idiopathic hand dystonia.

## SUMMARY

Limb dystonia may arise as an idiopathic focal disorder, usually of adult onset, as part of generalized idiopathic dystonia or as secondary dystonia. Significant progress has been made in recent years in understanding the pathophysiology of focal hand dystonia, particularly the importance of somatosensory involvement and the aberrant sensorimotor remodeling that occurs with repeated use of the hand and fingers. This knowledge is now being applied to the development of novel therapies that address the underlying cerebral basis of the dystonia. Until the potential of such therapies is realized, botulinum toxin injection remains the most effective treatment for limb dystonia.

## REFERENCES

1. Ramazzini B. Diseases of Scribes and Notaries. In: Diseases of Workers. New York: Hafner Publishing Company, 1713:421–425.
2. Solly S. Scrivener's palsy, or the paralysis of writers. Lancet 1864; 2:709–711.
3. Gowers WR. A Manual of Diseases of the Nervous System. In: American ed. Philadelphia: P. Blakiston, Son & Co, 1888.
4. Jedynak PC, Tranchant C, de Beyl DZ. Prospective clinical study of writer's cramp. Mov Disord 2001; 16(3):494–499.
5. Sheehy MP, Marsden CD. Writer's cramp- a focal dystonia. Brain 1982; 105:461–480.

6. Altenmuller E, Focal dystonia: advances in brain imaging and understanding of fine motor control in musicians. Hand Clin 2003; 19:(3) 523–538, xi.
7. Marsden CD, Sheehy MP. Writer's cramp. Trends Neurosci 1990; 13:148–153.
8. Greene P, Kang UJ, Fahn S. Spread of symptoms in idiopathic torsion dystonia. Mov Disord 1995; 10(2):143–152.
9. Brandfonbrener AG, Robson C. Review of 113 musicians with focal dystonia seen between 1985 and 2002 at a clinic for performing artists. Adv Neurol 2004; 94: 255–256.
10. Newmark J, Hochberg F. Isolated painless manual incoordination in 57 musicians. J Neurol Neurosurg Psychiatry 1987; 50:291–295.
11. Altenmuller E. Causes and cures of focal limb dystonia in musicians. Int Soc Study Tension Perform J 1998; 9:13–17.
12. Bara-Jimenez W, Shelton P, Sanger TD, Hallett M. Sensory discrimination capabilities in patients with focal hand dystonia. Ann Neurol 2000; 47(3):377–380.
13. Sanger TD, Tarsy D, Pascual-Leone A. Abnormalities of spatial and temporal sensory discrimination in writer's cramp. Mov Disord 2001; 16(1):94–99.
14. Rosenbaum F, Jankovic J. Focal task-specific tremor and dystonia: categorization of occupational movement disorders. Neurology 1988; 38:522–527.
15. Byrnes ML, Mastaglia FL, Walters SE, et al. Primary writing tremor: motor cortex reorganisation and disinhibition. J Clin Neurosci 2005; 12(1):102–104.
16. Singer C, Papapetropoulos S, Spielholz NI. Primary writing tremor: report of a case successfully treated with botulinum toxin A injections and discussion of underlying mechanism. Mov Disord 2005; 20(10):1387–1388.
17. The Epidemiological study of dystonia in Europe (ESDE) collaborative group. A prevalence study of primary dystonia in eight European countries. J Neurol 2000; 247(10):787–792.
18. Nutt JG, Muenter MD, Aronson A, et al. Epidemiology of focal and generalized dystonia in Rochester, Minn. Mov Disord 1988; 3(3):188–194.
19. Duffey PO, Butler AG, Hawthorne MR, et al. The epidemiology of the primary dystonias in the north of England. Adv Neurol 1998; 78:121–125.
20. Frucht SJ. Focal task-specific dystonia in musicians. Adv Neurol 2004; 94:225–230.
21. Hochberg FH, Leffert RD, Heller MD, et al. Hand difficulties among musicians. JAMA 1983; 249(14):1869–1872.
22. Lederman RJ. Neuromuscular problems in musicians. Neurology 2002; 8(3):163–174.
23. Waddy HM, Fletcher NA, Harding AE, et al. A genetic study of idiopathic focal dystonias. Ann Neurol 1991; 29:320–324.
24. Leube B, Kessler KR, Ferbert A, et al. Phenotypic variability of the DYT1 mutation in German dystonia patients. Acta Neurol Scand 1999; 99(4):248–251.
25. Gasser T, Windgassen K, Bereznai B, et al. Phenotypic expression of the DYT1 mutation: a family with writer's cramp of juvenile onset. Ann Neurol 1998; 44(1):126–128.
26. Kamm C, Naumann M, Mueller J, et al. The DYT1 GAG deletion is infrequent in sporadic and familial writer's cramp. Mov Disord 2000; 15(6):1238–1241.
27. Friedman JR, Klein C, Leung J, et al. The GAG deletion of the DYT1 gene is infrequent in musicians with focal dystonia. Neurology 2000; 55(9):1417–1418.
28. Almasy L, Bressman SB, Raymond D, et al. Idiopathic torsion dystonia linked to chromosome 8 in two Mennonite families. Ann Neurol 1997; 42:670–673.
29. Leube B, Hendgen T, Kessler KR, et al. Sporadic focal dystonia in northwest Germany: molecular basis on chromosome 18p. Ann Neurol 1997; 42(1):111–114.
30. Valente EM, Bentivoglio AR, Cassetta E, et al. DYT13, a novel primary torsion dystonia locus, maps to chromosome 1p36.13–36.32 in an Italian family with cranial-cervical or upper limb onset. Ann Neurol 2001; 49(3):362–366.
31. Bhidayasiri R, Jen JC, Baloh RW. Three brothers with a very-late-onset writer's cramp. Mov Disord 2005; 20(10):1375–1377.
32. Cohen LG, Hallett M. Hand cramps: clinical features and electromyographic patterns in a focal dystonia. Neurology 1988; 38:1005–1012.

33. Farmer SF, Sheehan GL, Mayston MJ, et al. Abnormal motor unit synchronization of antagonist muscles underlies pathological co-contraction in upper limb dystonia. Brain 1998; 121:801–814.
34. Von Reis G. Electromyographical studies in writer's cramp. Acta Med Scand 1954; 149:253–260.
35. Hallett M. Physiology of dystonia. Adv Neurol 1998; 78:11–18.
36. Hallett M. The neurophysiology of dystonia. Arch Neurol 1998; 55(5):601–603.
37. Berardelli A, Rothwell JC, Hallett M, et al. The pathophysiology of primary dystonia. Brain 1998; 121:1195–1212.
38. Kaji R, Urushihara R, Murase N, et al. Abnormal sensory gating in basal ganglia disorders. J Neurol 2005; 252 (Suppl) 4:iv13–iv16.
39. Chen R, Wassermann EM, Canos M, et al. Impaired inhibition in writer's cramp during voluntary muscle activation. Neurology 1997; 49(4):1054–1059.
40. Odergren T, Stone-Elander S, Ingvar M. Cerebral and cerebellar activation in correlation to the action-induced dystonia in writer's cramp. Mov Disord 1998; 13(3):497–508.
41. Pujol J, Roset-Llobet J, Rosines-Cubells D, et al. Brain cortical activation during guitar-induced hand dystonia studied by functional MRI. Neuroimage 2000; 12(3):257–267.
42. Byl N, Wilson F, Merzenich M, et al. Sensory dysfunction associated with repetitive strain injuries of tendonitis and focal hand dystonia: a comparative study. J Orthop Sports Phys Ther 1996; 23(4):234–244.
43. Bara-Jimenez W, Catalan MJ, Hallett M, et al. Abnormal somatosensory homunculus in dystonia of the hand. Neurology 1998; 44:828–831.
44. McKenzie AL, Nagarajan SS, Roberts TP, et al. Somatosensory representation of the digits and clinical performance in patients with focal hand dystonia. Am J Phys Med Rehabil 2003; 82(10):737–749.
45. Byrnes ML, Thickbroom GW, Wilson SA, et al. The corticomotor representation of upper limb muscles in writer's cramp and changes following botulinum toxin injection. Brain 1998; 121:977–988.
46. Molloy FM, Carr TD, Zeuner KE, et al. Abnormalities of spatial discrimination in focal and generalized dystonia. Brain 2003; 23:23.
47. Lim VK, Bradshaw JL, Nicholls ME, et al. Perceptual differences in sequential stimuli across patients with musician's and writer's cramp. Mov Disord 2003; 18(11): 1286–1293.
48. Tinazzi M, Frasson E, Bertolasi L, et al. Temporal discrimination of somesthetic stimuli is impaired in dystonic patients. Neuroreport 1999; 10(7):1547–1550.
49. Wang X, Merzenich MM, Sameshima K, J et al. Remodelling of hand representation in adult cortex determined by timing of tactile stimulation. Nature 1995; 378(6552):71–75.
50. Rosenkranz K, Williamon A, Butler K, et al. Pathophysiological differences between musician's dystonia and writer's cramp. Brain 2005; 128(Pt 4):918–931.
51. Lim VK, Bradshaw JL, Nicholls ME, et al. Abnormal sensorimotor processing in pianists with focal dystonia. Adv Neurol 2004; 94:267–273.
52. Garraux G, Bauer A, Hanakawa T, et al. Changes in brain anatomy in focal hand dystonia. Ann Neurol 2004; 55(5):736–739.
53. Amadio PC, Russotti GM. Evaluation and treatment of hand and wrist disorders in musicians. Hand Clin 1990; 6(3):405–416.
54. Lederman RJ. Neuromuscular and musculoskeletal problems in instrumental musicians. Muscle Nerve 2003; 27(5):549–561.
55. Leijnse JN. Anatomical factors predisposing to focal dystonia in the musician's hand-principles, theoretical examples, clinical significance. J Biomech 1997; 30(7):659–669.
56. Byl NN, Merzenich MM, Cheung S, et al. A primate model for studying focal dystonia and repetitive strain injury: effects on the primary somatosensory cortex. Phys Ther 1997; 77(3):269–284.
57. Byl NN, Merzenich MM, Jenkins WM. A primate genesis model of focal dystonia and repetitive strain injury. Neurology 1996; 47:508–520.

58. Lim VK, Altenmuller E, Bradshaw JL. Focal dystonia: current theories. Hum Mov Sci 2001; 20(6):875–914.
59. Jankovic J, Van Der Linden C. Dystonia and tremor induced by peripheral trauma: predisposing factors. J Neurol Neurosurg Psychiatry 1988; 51:1512–1519.
60. Jankovic J. Can peripheral trauma induce dystonia and other movement disorders? Yes! Mov Disord 2001; 16(1):7–12.
61. Weiner WJ. Can peripheral trauma induce dystonia? No! Mov Disord 2001; 16(1):13–22.
62. Fletcher NA, Harding AE, Marsden CD. The relationship between trauma and idiopathic torsion dystonia. J Neurol Neurosurg Psychiatry 1991; 54:713–717.
63. Bhatia KP, Bhatt MG, Marsden CD. The causalgia-dystonia syndrome. Brain 1993; 116:843–851.
64. Adler CH, Caviness JN. Dystonia secondary to electrical injury: surface electromyographic evaluation and implications for the organicity of the condition. J Neurol Sci 1997; 148(2):187–192.
65. Tarsy D, Sudarsky L, Charness ME. Limb dystonia following electrical injury. Mov Disord 1994; 9(2):230–232.
66. Frucht S, Fahn S, Ford B. Focal task-specific dystonia induced by peripheral trauma. Mov Disord 2000; 15(2):348–349.
67. Quartarone A, Girlanda P, Risitano G, et al. Focal hand dystonia in a patient with thoracic outlet syndrome. J Neurol Neurosurg Psychiatry 1998; 65(2):272–274.
68. Hill MD, Kumar R, Lozano A, et al. Syringomyelic dystonia and athetosis. Mov Disord 1999; 14(4):684–688.
69. Tamburin S, Zanette G. Focal hand dystonia after cervical whiplash injury. J Neurol Neurosurg Psychiatry 2003; 74(1):134.
70. Obeso JA, Gimenez-Roldan S. Clinicopathological correlation in symptomatic dystonia. Adv Neurol 1988; 50(2):113–122.
71. Choi YC, Lee MS, Choi IS. Delayed-onset focal dystonia after stroke. Yonsei Med J 1993; 34(4):391–396.
72. Scherokman B, Husain F, Cuetter A, et al. Peripheral dystonia. Arch Neurol 1986; 43:830–832.
73. Charness ME, Ross MH, Shefner JM. Ulnar neuropathy and dystonic flexion of the fourth and fifth digits: clinical correlation in musicians. Muscle Nerve 1996; 19(4):431–437.
74. Ross MH, Charness ME, Lee D, et al. Does ulnar neuropathy predispose to focal dystonia? Muscle Nerve 1995; 18:606–611.
75. Pitner MA. Pathophysiology of overuse injuries in the hand and wrist. Hand Clin 1990; 6(3):355–364.
76. Rettig AC. Wrist and hand overuse syndromes. Clin Sports Med 2001; 20(3):591–611.
77. Verdon ME. Overuse syndromes of the hand and wrist. Prim Care 1996; 23(2):305–319.
78. Birklein F, Riedl B, Sieweke N, et al. Neurological findings in complex regional pain syndromes-analysis of 145 cases. Acta Neurol Scand 2000; 101(4):262–269.
79. Schwartzman R, Kerrigan J. The movement disorder of reflex sympathetic dystrophy. Neurology 1990; 40(1):57–61.
80. Deuschl G, Blumberg H, Lucking CH. Tremor in reflex sympathetic dystrophy. Arch Neurol 1991; 48(12):1247–1252.
81. Wasner G, Schattschneider J, Binder A, et al. Complex regional pain syndrome-diagnostic, mechanisms, CNS involvement and therapy. Spinal Cord 2003; 41(2):61–75.
82. Koelman JH, Hilgevoord AA, Bour LJ, et al. Soleus H-reflex tests in causalgia-dystonia compared with dystonia and mimicked dystonic posture. Neurology 1999; 53(9):2196–2198.
83. Pearce JM. A note on scrivener's palsy. J Neurol Neurosurg Psychiatry 2005; 76(4):513.
84. Fahn S, Williams DT. Psychogenic dystonia. Adv Neurol 1988; 50:431–455.
85. Lang AE. Psychogenic dystonia: a review of 18 cases. Can J Neurol Sci 1995; 22(2):136–143.
86. Uncini A, Di Muzio A, Thomas A, et al. Hand dystonia secondary to cervical demyelinating lesion. Acta Neurol Scand 1994; 90(1):51–55.

87. Scheuele SU, Lederman RJ. Long-term outcome of focal dystonia in instrumental musicians. Adv Neurol 2004; 94:261–266.
88. Im JH, Ahn TB, Kim KB, et al. DYT1 mutation in Korean primary dystonia patients. Parkinsonism Relat Disord 2004; 10(7):421–423.
89. Munchau A, Filipovic SR, Oester-Barkey A, et al. Spontaneously changing muscular activation pattern in patients with cervical dystonia. Mov Disord 2001; 16(6):1091–1097.
90. Bhatia KP, Marsden CD. The behavioural and motor consequences of focal lesions of the basal ganglia in man. Brain 1994; 117(4):859–876.
91. Pettigrew LC, Jankovic J. Hemidystonia: a report of 22 patients and a review of the literature. J Neurol Neurosurg Psychiatry 1985; 48(7):650–657.
92. Schott GD. The relationship of peripheral trauma and pain to dystonia. J Neurol Neurosurg Psychiatry 1985; 48:698–701.
93. Scott BL, Jankovic J. Delayed-onset progressive movement disorders after static brain lesions [see comments]. Neurology 1996; 46(1):68–74.
94. Stathis P, Hampipi C. Dystonia after a bone fracture of the arm in a patient with a history of striato-pallidal ischemic stroke: a case report. Parkinsonism Relat Disord 2005; 11(3):195–198.
95. Berardelli A, Thompson PD, Day B, et al. Dystonia of the legs induced by walking or passive movement of the big toe in a patient with cerebellar ectopia and syringomyelia. Neurology 1986; 36:40–44.
96. Blunt SB, Richards PG, Khalil N. Foot dystonia and lumbar canal stenosis. Mov Disord 1996; 11(6):723–725.
97. Munchau A, Mathen D, Cox T, et al. Unilateral lesions of the globus pallidus: report of four patients presenting with focal or segmental dystonia. J Neurol Neurosurg Psychiatry 2000; 69(4):494–498.
98. Jankovic J, Tintner R. Dystonia and parkinsonism. Parkinsonism Relat Disord 2001; 8(2):109–121.
99. Koller WC. Adult-onset foot dystonia. Neurology 1984; 34:703.
100. Duarte J, Sempere AP, Coria F, et al. Isolated idiopathic adult-onset foot dystonia and treatment with botulinum toxin. J Neurol 1995; 242(2):114–115.
101. Kim JS, Lee KS, Ko YJ, et al. Idiopathic foot dystonia treated with intramuscular phenol injection. Parkinsonism Relat Disord 2003; 9(6):355–359.
102. Sherman AL, Willick SP, Cardenas DD. Management of focal dystonia of the extensor hallucis longus muscle with botulinum toxin injection: a case report. Arch Phys Med Rehabil 1998; 79:1303–1305.
103. Singer C, Papapetropoulos S. Adult-onset primary focal foot dystonia. Parkinsonism Relat Disord 2006; 12(1):57–60.
104. Singer C, Papapetropoulos S, Vela L. Use of mirror dystonia as guidance for injection of botulinum toxin in writing dysfunction. J Neurol Neurosurg Psychiatry 2005; 76(11):1608–1609.
105. O'Neill MA, Gwinn KA, Adler CH. Biofeedback for writer's cramp. Am J Occup Ther 1997; 51(7):605–607.
106. Deepak KK, Behari M. Specific muscle EMG biofeedback for hand dystonia. Appl Psychophysiol Biofeedback 1999; 24(4):267–280.
107. Byl NN, McKenzie A. Treatment effectiveness for patients with a history of repetitive hand use and focal hand dystonia: a planned, prospective follow-up study. J Hand Ther 2000; 13(4):289–301.
108. Zeuner KE, Bara-Jimenez W, Noguchi PS, et al. Sensory training for patients with focal hand dystonia. Ann Neurol 2002; 51(5):593–598.
109. Candia V, Elbert T, Altenmuller E, et al. Constraint-induced movement therapy for focal hand dystonia in musicians [letter]. Lancet 1999; 353(9146):42.
110. Candia V, Schafer T, Taub E, et al. Sensory motor retuning: a behavioral treatment for focal hand dystonia of pianists and guitarists. Arch Phys Med Rehabil 2002; 83(10):1342–1348.

111. Candia V, Wienbruch C, Elbert T, et al. Effective behavioral treatment of focal hand dystonia in musicians alters somatosensory cortical organization. Proc Natl Acad Sci U S A 2003; 100(13):7942–7946.
112. Priori A, et al. Limb immobilization for the treatment of local occupational dystonia. Neurology 2001; 57(3):405–409.
113. Siebner HR, Auer C, Ceballos-Baumann A, et al. Has repetitive transcranial magnetic stimulation of the primary motor hand area a therapeutic application in writer's cramp? Electroencephalogr Clin Neurophysiol Suppl 1999; 51:265–275.
114. Murase N, Rothwell JC, Kaji R, et al. Subthreshold low-frequency repetitive transcranial magnetic stimulation over the premotor cortex modulates writer's cramp. Brain 2005; 128(Pt 1):104–115.
115. Tinazzi M, Farina S, Bhatia K, et al. TENS for the treatment of writer's cramp dystonia: a randomized, placebo-controlled study. Neurology 2005; 64(11):1946–1948.
116. Moore TJ, Evans W, Murray D. Operative management of foot and ankle equinovarus associated with focal dystonia. Foot Ankle Int 1998; 19(4):229–231.
117. Moberg-Wolff EA. An aggressive approach to limb dystonia: a case report. Arch Phys Med Rehabil 1998; 79:589–590.
118. Goto S, Tsuiki H, Soyama N, et al. Stereotactic selective Vo-complex thalamotomy in a patient with dystonic writer's cramp. Neurology 1997; 49(4):1173–1174.
119. Shibata T, Hirashima Y, Ikeda H, et al. Stereotactic Voa-Vop complex thalamotomy for writer's cramp. Eur Neurol 2005; 53(1):38–39.
120. Taira T, Harashima S, Hori T. Neurosurgical treatment for writer's cramp. Acta Neurochir Suppl 2003; 87:129–131.
121. Iacono RP, Kuniyoshi SM, Schoonenberg T. Experience with stereotactics for dystonia: case examples. Adv Neurol 1998; 78:221–226.
122. Balash Y, Giladi N. Efficacy of pharmacological treatment of dystonia: evidence-based review including meta-analysis of the effect of botulinum toxin and other cure options. Eur J Neurol 2004; 11(6):361–370.
123. Jabusch HC, Zschucke D, Schmidt A, et al. Focal dystonia in musicians: Treatment strategies and long-term outcome in 144 patients. Mov Disord 2005; 20(12):1623–1626.
124. Cohen LG, Hallett M, Geller BD, et al. Treatment of focal dystonias of the hand with botulinum toxin injections. J Neurol Neurosurg Psychiatry 1989; 52:355–363.
125. Tsui JKC, Bhatt M, Calne S, et al. Botulinum toxin in the treatment of writer's cramp: A double blind study. Neurology 1993; 43:183–185.
126. Yoshimura DM, Aminoff MJ, Olney RK. Botulinum toxin therapy for limb dystonias. Neurology 1992; 42:627–630.
127. Molloy FM, Shill HA, Kaelin-Lang A, et al. Accuracy of muscle localization without EMG: implications for treatment of limb dystonia. Neurology 2002; 58(5):805–807.
128. Naumann M, Reiners K. Long-latency reflexes of hand muscles in idiopathic focal dystonia and their modification by botulinum toxin. Brain 1997; 120:409–416.
129. Gilio F, Curra A, Lorenzano C, et al. Effects of botulinum toxin type A on intracortical inhibition in patients with dystonia. Ann Neurol 2000; 48:20–26.
130. Mari Z, Karp B, Hallett M. Long-term botulinum toxin treatment for focal hand dystonia. Ann Neurol 2005; 58:S20.
131. Schuele S, Jabusch HC, Lederman RJ, et al. Botulinum toxin injections in the treatment of musician's dystonia. Neurology 2005; 64(2):341–343.
132. Jankovic J, Schwartz K, Donovan DT. Botulinum toxin treatment of cranial-cervical dystonia, spasmodic dysphonia, other focal dystonias and hemifacial spasm. J Neurol Neurosurg Psychiatry 1990; 53:633–639.
133. Lees AJ, Turjanski N, Rivest J, et al. Treatment of cervical dystonia, hand spasms and laryngeal dystonia with botulinum toxin. J Neurol 1992; 239:1–4.
134. Karp BI, Cohen LG, Cole R, et al. Long-term botulinum toxin treatment of focal hand dystonia. Neurology 1994; 44:70–76.

135. Hsiung GY, Das SK, Ranawaya R, et al. Long-term efficacy of botulinum toxin A in treatment of various movement disorders over a 10-year period. Mov Disord 2002; 17(6):1288–1293.
136. Heinen F, Korinthenberg R, Stucker R, et al. Dystonic posture of the lower extremities associated with myelomeningocele: successful treatment with botulinum A toxin in a six-month-old child. Neuropediatrics 1995; 26:214–216.
137. Pacchetti C, Albani G, Martignoni E, et al. "Off" painful dystonia in Parkinson's disease treated with botulinum toxin. Mov Disord 1995; 10(3):333–336.
138. Cordivari C, Misra VP, Catania S, et al. Treatment of dystonic clenched fist with botulinum toxin. Mov Disord 2001; 16(5):907–913.
139. Muller J, Wenning GK, Wissel J, et al. Botulinum toxin treatment in atypical parkinsonian disorders associated with disabling focal dystonia. J Neurol 2002; 249(3):300–304.

# 12
# Spasmodic Dysphonia

**Tanya K. Meyer**
*Department of Otorhinolaryngology, Head and Neck Surgery, University of Maryland Medical Center, Baltimore, Maryland, U.S.A.*

**Andrew Blitzer**
*New York Center for Voice and Swallowing Disorders, Head and Neck Surgical Group, St. Luke's Roosevelt Medical Center, New York, New York, U.S.A.*

## INTRODUCTION

Spasmodic dysphonia (SD) is considered a focal laryngeal dystonia in which a patient experiences inappropriate laryngeal muscular contractions during speech. The most common form, adductor SD, produces inappropriate muscle contraction causing excessive glottal closure and a strained and strangled speaking pattern. Abductor SD is less common, and results in a persistently open glottal configuration with breathy breaks or a whispering speaking pattern. Although the task specificity for focal laryngeal dystonia has been observed mostly for speech, there is a low incidence of adductor breathing dystonia that may produce inspiratory stridor. The etiology of laryngeal dystonia falls into the same categories as forms affecting other areas of the body. Drug-induced glottic dystonic reactions have been described causing acute upper airway obstruction necessitating intubation (1,2,2a).

The gold standard of treatment for laryngeal dystonia is electromyography (EMG)-guided botulinum toxin (BTX) injections into the affected musculature. Medications may also ameliorate symptoms, but rarely have a significant impact. Multiple surgical interventions have been performed, many of which have fallen out of favor as recidivism is seen over time. Selective denervation–reinnervation procedures have shown promising preliminary data, but long-term results are still to be evaluated.

## HISTORY AND BACKGROUND

Traube first described SD in 1871 within a treatise detailing the effects of typhus on the larynx:

> The spastic type of nervous (neurologic) hoarseness was observed by Professor Traube in a hysterical young girl. The very hoarse, almost aphonic patient could, with great strain, only produce very high, whistle-like sounds (3). (Translation from German courtesy of A.F. Jahn, MD).

Critchley provided a similar description in 1939: "there results a peculiarly forced character in the speech, which appears difficult of accomplishment, almost as though the patient were trying to talk whilst being choked" (4). These and similar descriptions promoted the assumption that this was a psychological disturbance, an unfortunate categorization that may have been further supported by the unique characteristics of the disease such as task and even word specificity, fluctuation of symptoms, co-occurrence of anxiety and depression, female preponderance, worsening in stressful situations, and relief with anxiolytics.

Aronson (5) reviewed SD and other hyperfunctional voice disorders in detail and proposed that this symptom complex could arise from a neurologic etiology. This conclusion was based on the high incidence of associated neurologic signs—including tremor and other cranial dystonias. Additionally, psychological testing did not discriminate between patients with SD and normal controls, indicating an organic as opposed to a psychiatric etiology. Dedo (6) reported a dramatic and immediate normalization of voice among individuals after transection of the recurrent laryngeal nerve (RLN), further suggesting an organic cause. Abnormalities in autonomic function (7) and abnormal V-wave latencies from brainstem auditory-evoked potential testing (8–10) implied a central defect, further supported by the lack of consistent abnormalities in histologic studies of the RLN (11,12), and intrinsic laryngeal muscles (13). Functional studies with EMG show that electrical patterns during whispering and non-speech tasks were not different between affected individuals and normal controls (14), and during speech, if aphonic intervals were excluded, electrical patterns were otherwise normal (15). In general, neuroimaging studies have failed to identify consistent anatomic abnormalities among individuals with SD (16,17).

In 1980, Jacome and Yanez (18) postulated that SD was a disorder of the extrapyramidal system based on the frequent coexistence with other cranial dystonias and tremor, and the lack of morphometric abnormalities of the RLN in these patients. Marsden and Sheehy (19) in 1982 again noted the frequent coexistence of SD with Meige disease and further concluded, "since SD may occur in the same syndrome, it is quite likely that isolated SD itself may be a sole focal manifestation of dystonia" and classified cases of SD as examples of isolated focal laryngeal dystonia. Blitzer et al. in 1985 reviewed EMGs of the laryngeal musculature in focal and generalized dystonia, further supporting SD as a focal dystonia (20).

The exact etiology of dystonia remains unknown. Dedo felt that proprioceptive abnormalities might exist in these individuals who might be altered after unilateral section of the RLN (6) and might account for bilateral amelioration of spasmodic activity. Bielamowicz and Ludlow noted an improved EMG signal in contralateral thyroarytenoid and cricothyroid muscle groups after unilateral BTX injections and hypothesized that a central reduction in motor neuron activity due to altered sensorimotor feedback could explain these findings (21). Additionally, successful BTX injections given to one dystonic muscle group often is associated with improvement of spasms in other muscle groups without treatment. Currently, most theories implicate SD as a disorder of motor circuitry rather than a structural defect in a particular cortical or subcortical structure (22).

## EPIDEMIOLOGY

Blitzer and Brin (23) published one of the largest studies of SD in 1998, reviewing a 12-year experience of 901 cases of laryngeal dystonia treated with injections of BTX.

Of these cases, 70% were isolated to laryngeal involvement and the remainder with either segmental cranial or generalized dystonia. The majority (82.5%) were classified as a primary dystonia. There was a 63% female preponderance and 12% had a family history of dystonia. In this group, 82% were of the adductor type, 17% of the abductor type, and 1% had adductor breathing dystonia. The average age of onset was 39 years. Of patients with primary laryngeal involvement, 14% to 16% (23,24) had eventual spread to other areas of the body; therefore, patients with laryngeal dystonia should be examined on a regular basis.

## DIAGNOSIS

The diagnosis of SD relies on clinical history, voice analysis, and physical exam including flexible fiberoptic laryngoscopy. SD is a chronic adult onset disorder, although some children with generalized dystonia may have laryngeal involvement. Patients often first notice their symptoms after an illness, during a period of increased stress, or during a public speaking venue. Some individuals describe a gradual onset with symptoms noted only during periods of stress or increased speaking demands, others describe a sudden occurrence that may be related to an illness or life event. Almost all individuals remark that symptoms are markedly exacerbated or more acutely perceived when speaking on the telephone. Speech may be better on awakening in the morning or after an alcoholic drink. Although the symptoms can wax and wane, there is almost always some sense of presence of the disorder. Certain words or combinations of words will be more difficult to say, depending on the type of SD. Individuals usually report that singing, laughing, yelling, and falsetto are relatively spared. Cough and swallow, along with other vegetative laryngeal tasks, are preserved. Vocal tremor is frequently coexistent.

Vocal characteristics vary depending on the type of SD. Patients with adductor SD have a characteristic strained, strangled, effortful speech with vocal breaks and frequency shifts. There is often a reduction in loudness and prosody. These individuals have spasmodic hyperadduction during tasks in which the vocal folds are already adducted to create voiced sounds such as vowels. So, instead of creating the appropriate degree of glottic closure to allow controlled airflow past the vocal folds, creating vocal fold vibration and consequently sound, the larynx squeezes shut, completely interrupting the airflow through the glottis, thereby precluding sound formation. These patients will have difficulty with sentences containing a predominance of voiced consonants and vowels such as "We mow our lawn all year" or counting from 80 to 90.

Patients with abductor SD have a breathy, although still effortful, voice quality with aphonic whispered segments. These are particularly marked when attempting to phonate a vowel after a voiceless consonant such as /p/, /f/, /t/, /s/, /d/, /k/, or /h/. During the voiceless consonant, the cords are held apart so that no vocal cord vibration is created and the sound is thereby formed, not at the glottic level, but rather at the lips (/p/,/f/), tongue/teeth (/t/, /s/, /d/, /k/), or oropharynx (/h/). To experience the difference between voiceless and voiced sounds try saying a prolonged /f/ and then transitioning to a /v/. The oral cavity, tongue, and pharyngeal articulators are held in the same position with the two sounds, but when transitioning from /f/ to /v/, the glottis is engaged to add phonation. The same can be experienced when transitioning from /s/ to /z/. Abductor SD patients have hyperabduction of the vocal folds during the voiceless consonant and then have trouble overcoming this opening spasm to bring the folds together to create a voiced vowel sound. Examples of sentences that these individuals have particular difficulty with are "Harry had a hard head," "The puppy bit the tape," or "Taxi."

Patients experiencing spasms in both adductor and abductor groups are occasionally seen. These individuals can be quite challenging, as appropriate treatment may only be determined after treatment of the individual muscle groups singly has failed. Cannito and Johnson proposed that abductor and adductor abnormalities exist in all patients and the final symptoms depend on the net abnormal activity of the laryngeal musculature (25).

Some individuals with SD exhibit compensatory behavior in an effort to overcome their spasms. This is most common in adductor SD in which individuals will exhibit compensatory abduction producing a breathy voice by whispering or incomplete contraction of the vocal folds. Compensatory adduction in abductor dysphonia is rare. These behaviors can create diagnostic confusion with functional voice disorders such as muscle tension dysphonia in which there is no neurologic defect and often responds to speech therapy and psychological counseling. In an effort to find better diagnostic markers, Sapienza et al. performed acoustic analysis of 10 patients with SD compared to 10 patients with muscle tension dysphonia and found voice breaks only in the SD group (26). Other experienced clinicians firmly believe that. While voice breaks may be a pathognomonic sign of SD, these are not a requirement for the condition (Bastian RW. Personal communication).

Adductor breathing dystonia is a rare laryngeal movement disorder that, unfortunately, is task specific for breathing. Patients have a normal voice, cough, and swallow but have adduction of the vocal folds during inspiration and with sniffing. Although individuals can exhibit alarming inspiratory stridor, they rarely become hypoxic and their breathing is normal during sleep.

On flexible fiberoptic laryngeal exam, the patient should have normal anatomy with no evidence of extreme inflammatory mucosal disease. In general, the patient should exhibit a normal glottic aperture and movement with vegetative laryngeal tasks such as sniffing, coughing, and swallowing. The patient is then asked to perform eliciting speech tasks as described above. For adductor SD, the patients will have excessive glottal closure with false vocal fold approximation (Fig. 1). For abductor SD, the patient will have hyperabduction of the vocal folds with the appearance of a delay in closure of the vocal fold or "hanging" of the arytenoid with speech tasks. Patients with adductor breathing dystonia will have vocal fold adduction with inspiration and with sniffing maneuvers, but this will not affect speech or swallowing.

It is strongly suggested that all patients exhibiting signs and symptoms of SD be evaluated by both a neurologist and an otolaryngologist with an interest or specialization in movement disorders to confirm the diagnosis, exclude other body part involvement, examine for additional neurological signs or symptoms, and discover causative disorders (e.g., Wilson's disease, multiple sclerosis, and storage diseases).

## TREATMENTS

### Botulinum Toxin

Transcutaneous EMG-guided injection of BTX is the gold standard for the treatment of SD. Most individuals will report an excellent effect, and it can temporarily restore the voice to near normal with both a reduction in voice breaks and an effort required for speaking. The specific adductor or abductor muscle groups responsible

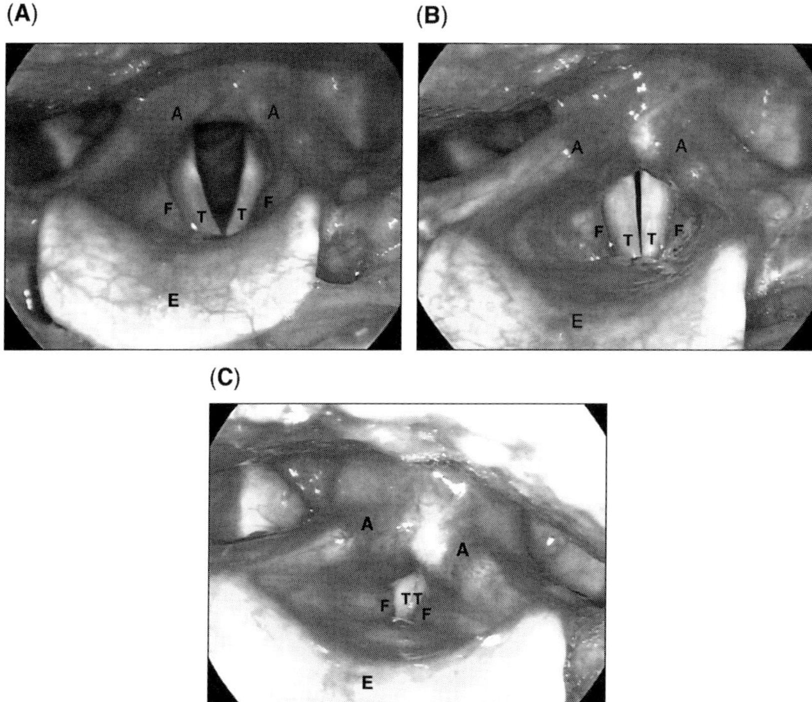


**Figure 1** (**A**) Normal vocal fold abduction, as for inspiration. (**B**) Normal vocal fold adduction, as during phonation. Note that the true vocal folds approximate but do not squeeze together overly tightly, thus permitting controlled airflow past the true vocal folds to create sound. (**C**) Laryngeal spasm or hyperadduction, as with adductor SD. Note the tight, almost overlapping closure of the true vocal folds, and also the closure of the false folds over the true folds. The larynx also appears shortened in the anterior–posterior diameter due to the sphincteric contraction of the supraglottic structures. *Note*: E, epiglottis; A, arytenoid; F, false vocal fold; T, true vocal fold. *Abbreviation*: SD, spasmodic dysphonia.

can be targeted and the dose can be titrated to produce just enough weakness to relieve spasm in target muscles without causing unnecessary weakness in neighboring muscles resulting in dysphagia, prolonged breathiness (adductor), or airway compromise (abductor). Rarely is the dose high enough to cause frank paralysis of the targeted muscle group.

The thyroarytenoid or lateral cricoarytenoid are usually targeted for adductor SD (Fig. 2). If too high of a dose is given, the patient may experience excessive breathiness from an inability to fully adduct the vocal folds, or dysphagia from diffusion of toxin to the pharyngeal constrictors. The initial dose is one unit bilaterally, which can be titrated up or down depending on each individual's response weighed against their side effect profile. Some patients are remarkably sensitive and we have successfully used doses of less than 0.1 units to achieve spasm amelioration. Some patients do well with a higher dose given unilaterally, alternating the side and decreasing the injection interval. In especially refractory patients, injection of supraglottic musculature, the cricothyroid (27), or the interarytenoideus has shown success (28).

The posterior cricoarytenoid muscle is targeted for abductor SD (Fig. 3). Although there are differences in technique, most authors favor doses only unilaterally during a session because bilateral abductor weakness can lead to stridor and

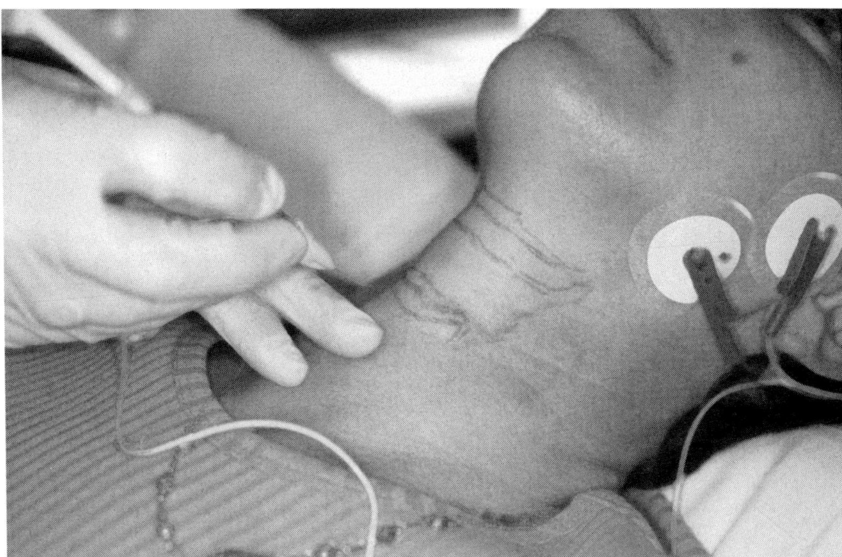

**Figure 2** This image shows the laryngeal landmarks drawn on the skin and the technique for injection of the thyroarytenoid muscle for adductor spasmodic dysphonia (SD). The needle electrode is inserted at the midline through the cricothyroid membrane, the tip is directed submucosally, in a rostral and lateral direction toward the superior thyroid cornu. Correct placement is verified with phonation.

airway obstruction requiring tracheotomy. All patients are evaluated with flexible fiberoptic exam prior to any injection to determine which cord has the strongest abductor spasms and verify an adequate glottic aperture. The usual starting dose is 3.75 units unilaterally. If abductor spasms are satisfactorily ameliorated, the patient can return in two weeks for reevaluation at which time a booster can be given to the original side, or a carefully planned dose can be given to the contralateral side. Individuals requiring injection of bilateral posterior cricoarytenoid muscles for speech benefit may be treated in a staggered fashion at a two-week interval, always evaluating the airway endoscopically prior to injection to assure an adequate glottal aperture.

Excellent results from adductor SD toxin injections are well accepted. In a series (23) of 901 patients treated over 12 years evaluating 6280 injection sessions, the average dose was one unit bilaterally producing an effect in 2.4 days and achieving a rate of nearly 90% of normal function (37% average improvement) lasting 15 weeks. Mild breathiness occurred in 35% of patients lasting for less than one week and 15% described mild coughing when drinking fluids.

In the same series, abductor SD was successfully treated with staggered injections to the posterior cricoarytenoid (PCA) muscle in 80% and unilateral injections in 20%. The average dose was 3.2 units to one side and 0.6 to 2.5 units to the contralateral side two weeks later. The effect lasted 10.5 weeks and achieved a rate of 70% of normal function (43% average improvement). Because these patients did not achieve the same degree of voice normalization, 30% received additional systemic agents including clonazepam, trihexiphenidyl, or baclofen.

Although no cases of resistance due to antibody formation in patients injected solely for laryngeal dystonia have been reported, some patients may respond to one isoform of toxin better than another. For this reason, if subjects do not demonstrate

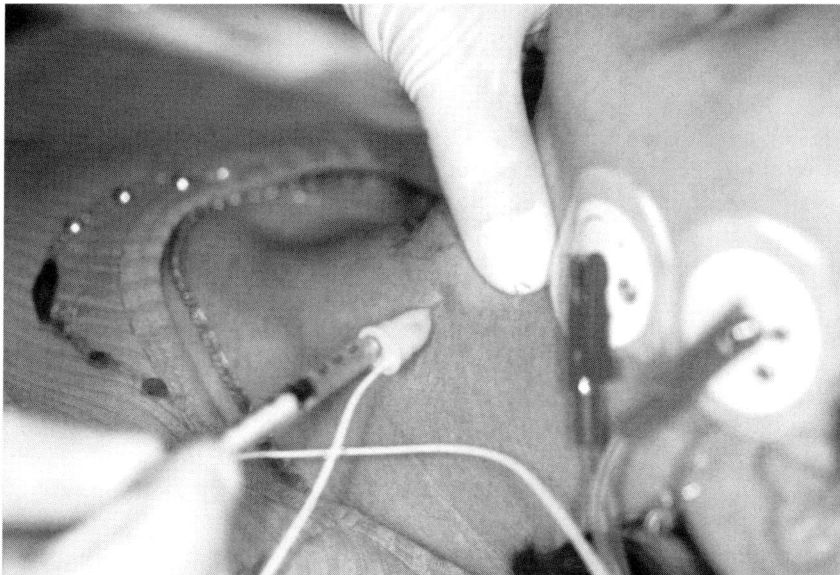

**Figure 3** This image demonstrates rotation of the larynx to allow injection of the posterior cricoarytenoid muscle for abductor spasmodic dysphonia (SD). The thumb of the noninjecting hand is hooked behind the posterior edge of the thyroid lamina to rotate the larynx away and expose the posterior aspect. The needle is inserted at the level of the cricoid ring, transversing the inferior constrictor until it stops against the rostrum of the cricoid cartlage. Correct placement is verified with the sniffing maneuver.

good response with BTX, type A, a trial of BTX, type B should be considered (29). The relative toxin potencies are a bit different with dose ratio being approximately 55:1 (Myobloc units:Botox units) with an onset of two days, benefit of 10 weeks, and a more abrupt offset (30).

## Oral Medications and Voice Therapy

Oral medications such as muscle relaxants, anxiolytics, anticholinergic drugs, or beta-blockers are usually not effective as primary therapy, but may be useful as an adjunct, or agent to prolong the duration of improvement from BTX injection. Voice therapy is generally unsuccessful as a sole treatment, although may be essential to diagnosis and prevention of unwanted compensatory patterns. Use of breath support strategies and easy onset phonation may prolong the duration of benefit from toxin in patients with adductor SD (31).

## Surgery

The first surgical therapy for adductor SD was the RLN section by Dedo, first reported in 1976 (6). Initially, patients demonstrated a dramatic normalization of voicing, although over time a failure rate of up to 64% was noted (32). Overcompensation of the normal cord with central exaggeration of the dystonic symptoms was implicated, as the cause of recurrent spasms and thinning of the vocal fold with lasers was used as salvage (33), although with only temporary success. Neural regeneration was discovered during re-exploration (34), but even with subsequent avulsion of a segment of the recurrent nerve, significant recidivism was seen over long-term follow-up (35).

Several procedures designed to mechanically relax the vocal folds through alterations in the laryngeal framework have been attempted (36,37). Although successful in isolated centers, the results are not widely reproducible and have not gained general acceptance.

In 1999, Berke developed a selective adductor denervation/reinnervation surgery, which has shown promising preliminary results (38). This procedure involves section of the adductor branch of the RLN, which supplies the thyroarytenoid and lateral cricoarytenoid muscles of the glottis (the adductor muscles that are targeted by routine BTX injections) and immediate reinnervation using microsurgical technique to a branch of the ansa cervicalis (originating from the cervical spinal nerves C2 to C4 and the hypoglossal nerve). The procedure is performed bilaterally at the same sitting. Gross vocal fold mobility is preserved because the RLN branches are divided distal to the interarytenoideus (adductor) and posterior cricoarytenoid (abductor) branches. Postoperatively all patients can expect three to six months of moderate breathiness, and 10% experience temporary aspiration. Because this procedure creates a permanent alteration in laryngeal function and significant short-term vocal dysfunction, it should only be performed in patients with relatively severe symptoms.

The premise of this operation is intriguing. Re-anastamosis of the recurrent nerve with a different nerve accomplishes three things: (i) prevents reinnervation by neighboring branches of the vagal plexus, which is a potential cause of failure of the RLN section procedure, (ii) permits reinnervation by a nerve that is controlled by a different part of the brain than that causing the laryngeal dystonia, (iii) preserves tone to the vocal fold, thereby preventing muscular atrophy. The original report described 19 of 21 patients with "absent to mild" dysphonia and a median follow-up of 36 months. Other groups have duplicated the surgery, although with a slight decrement in success rate (39). Long-term follow-up is still pending on this procedure.

Another procedure with promising initial results is surgical thinning and resection of the dystonic muscles. This has been predominantly performed for adductor SD. The original studies were performed in rabbits in which a portion of the thyroarytenoid muscle was resected via a window in the thyroid cartilage causing permanent decrease in the muscle mass without disturbing the vibratory edge (40). This has been performed with promising preliminary results under local anesthesia in humans (41). One concern that has been raised is that eye, limb, and cervical dystonias have never been successfully treated with muscular resection, which often causes an initial amelioration of symptoms with an eventual expression of dystonic contractions in another muscle group. Long-term follow-up needs to be evaluated before the true efficacy of these procedures can be determined.

Very preliminary reports have theorized potential applications of the vagal nerve stimulator (42) and deep brain stimulation for SD, although no formal studies are available to date.

## CONCLUSIONS

SD is classified as a focal laryngeal dystonia. To date, the majority of interventions is targeted at the end organ and provides only symptomatic control. As in the classical *geste antagoniste*, the central nervous system eventually adapts to the change created in the neural inputs by these interventions and returns to sending out an inappropriate signal to the involved muscles. Future developments will hopefully target the central nervous system through medical or surgical means in hope of durable cure.

## REFERENCES

1. Warren J, Thompson P. Drug-induced supraglottic dystonia and spasmodic dysphonia. Mov Disord 1998; 13(6):978–979.
2. Newton-John H. Acute upper airway obstruction due to supraglottic dystonia induced by a neuroleptic. BMJ 1988; 297(6654):964–965.
2a. Grillone G, Blitzer A, Brin MF. Treatment of Adductor Breathing Dystonia with botilinum toxib. Larynseope 1994; (104):30–33.
3. Traube L. Zur Lehre von den larynxaffectionen beim ileotyphus. Berlin: Verlag Van August Hisschwald, 1871:674–678.
4. Critchley M. Spastic dysphonia "inspiratory speech". Brain 1939; 62:96–103.
5. Aronson AE et al. Spastic dysphonia I. Voice, neurologic, and psychiatric aspects. J Speech Hear Disord 1968; 33(3):203–218.
6. Dedo HH. Recurrent laryngeal nerve section for spastic dysphonia. Ann Otol Rhinol Laryngol 1976; 85(4 Pt 1):451–459.
7. Schaefer SD. Neuropathology of spasmodic dysphonia. Laryngoscope 1983; 93(9):1183–1204.
8. Feldman M et al. Abnormal parasympathetic vagal function in patients with spasmodic dysphonia. Ann Intern Med 1984; 100(4):491–495.
9. Finitzo-Hieber T et al. Auditory brainstem response abnormalities in adductor spasmodic dysphonia. Am J Otolaryngol 1982; 3(1):26–30.
10. Schaefer SD et al. Brainstem conduction abnormalities in spasmodic dysphonia. Ann Otol Rhinol Laryngol 1983; 92(1 Pt 1):59–64.
11. Carlsoo B et al. The recurrent laryngeal nerve in spastic dysphonia. A light and electron microscopic study. Acta Otolaryngol 1987; 103(1–2):96–104.
12. Ravits JM et al. No morphometric abnormality recurrent laryngeal nerve in spastic dysphonia. Neurology 1979; 29(10):1376–1382.
13. Chhetri DK et al. Histology of nerves and muscles in adductor spasmodic dysphonia. Ann Otol Rhinol Laryngol 2003; 112(4):334–341.
14. Roark RM et al. Time-frequency analyses of thyroarytenoid myoelectric activity in normal and spasmodic dysphonia subjects. J Speech Hear Res 1995; 38(2):289–303.
15. Van Pelt F, Ludlow CL, Smith PJ. Comparison of muscle activation patterns in adductor and abductor spasmodic dysphonia. Ann Otol Rhinol Laryngol 1994; 103(3):192–200.
16. Aronson AE, Lagerlund TD. Neuroimaging studies do not prove the existence of brain abnormalities in spastic (spasmodic) dysphonia. J Speech Hear Res 1991; 34(4):801–811.
17. Schaefer S et al. Magnetic resonance imaging findings and correlations in spasmodic dysphonia patients. Ann Otol Rhinol Laryngol 1985; 94(6 Pt 1):595–601.
18. Jacome DE, Yanez GF. Spastic dysphonia and Meigs disease. Neurology 1980; 30(4):349.
19. Marsden CD, Sheehy MP. Spastic dysphonia, meige disease, and torsion dystonia. Neurology 1982; 32(10):1202–1203.
20. Blitzer A et al. Electromyographic findings in focal laryngeal dystonia (spastic dysphonia). Ann Otol Rhinol Laryngol 1985; 94(6 Pt 1):591–594.
21. Bielamowicz S, Ludlow CL. Effects of botulinum toxin on pathophysiology in spasmodic dysphonia. Ann Otol Rhinol Laryngol 2000; 109(2):194–203.
22. Pearson EJ, Sapienza CM. Historical approaches to the treatment of Adductor-type spasmodic dysphonia (ADSD): review and tutorial. NeuroRehabilitation 2003; 18(4):325–338.
23. Blitzer A, Brin MF, Stewart CF. Botulinum toxin management of spasmodic dysphonia (laryngeal dystonia): a 12-year experience in more than 900 patients. Laryngoscope 1998; 108(10):1435–1441.

24. Greene P, Kang UJ, Fahn S. Spread of symptoms in idiopathic torsion dystonia. Mov Disord 1995; 10(2):143–152.
25. Cannito MP, Johnson JP. Spastic dysphonia: a continuum disorder. J Commun Disord 1981; 14(3):215–233.
26. Sapienza CM, Walton S, Murry T. Adductor spasmodic dysphonia and muscular tension dysphonia: acoustic analysis of sustained phonation and reading. J Voice 2000; 14(4): 502–520.
27. Bielamowicz S et al. Unilateral versus bilateral injections of botulinum toxin in patients with adductor spasmodic dysphonia. J Voice 2002; 16(1):117–123.
28. Hillel AD et al. Treatment of the interarytenoid muscle with botulinum toxin for laryngeal dystonia. Ann Otol Rhinol Laryngol 2004; 113(5):341–348.
29. Adler CH et al. Safety and efficacy of botulinum toxin type B (Myobloc) in adductor spasmodic dysphonia. Mov Disord 2004; 19(9):1075–1079.
30. Blitzer A. American Academy of Otolaryngology 2004, Presentation.
31. Murry T, Woodson GE. Combined-modality treatment of adductor spasmodic dysphonia with botulinum toxin and voice therapy. J Voice 1995; 9(4):460–465.
32. Aronson AE, De Santo LW. Adductor spastic dysphonia: three years after recurrent laryngeal nerve resection. Laryngoscope 1983; 93(1):1–8.
33. Dedo HH, Izdebski K. Evaluation and treatment of recurrent spasticity after recurrent laryngeal nerve section. A preliminary report. Ann Otol Rhinol Laryngol 1984; 93(4 Pt 1): 343–345.
34. Netterville JL et al. Recurrent laryngeal nerve avulsion for treatment of spastic dysphonia. Ann Otol Rhinol Laryngol 1991; 100(1):10–14.
35. Weed DT et al. Long-term follow-up of recurrent laryngeal nerve avulsion for the treatment of spastic dysphonia. Ann Otol Rhinol Laryngol 1996; 105(8):592–601.
36. Isshiki N, Yamamoto I, Fukagai S. Type 2 thyroplasty for spasmodic dysphonia: fixation using a titanium bridge. Acta Otolaryngol 2004; 124(3):309–312.
37. Tucker HM. Laryngeal framework surgery in the management of spasmodic dysphonia. Preliminary report. Ann Otol Rhinol Laryngol 1989; 98(1 Pt 1):52–54.
38. Berke GS et al. Selective laryngeal adductor denervation-reinnervation: a new surgical treatment for adductor spasmodic dysphonia. Ann Otol Rhinol Laryngol 1999; 108(3):227–231.
39. Allegretto M et al. Selective denervation: reinnervation for the control of adductor spasmodic dysphonia. J Otolaryngol 2003; 32(3):185–189.
40. Genack SH et al. Partial thyroarytenoid myectomy: an animal study investigating a proposed new treatment for adductor spasmodic dysphonia. Otolaryngol Head Neck Surg 1993; 108(3):256–264.
41. Koufman JA. Combined Otolaryngology Spring Meeting 2005, Presentation.
42. Lundy DS et al. Effects of vagal nerve stimulation on laryngeal function. J Voice 1993; 7(4):359–364.

# 13
# Embouchure and Other Task-Specific Musician's Dystonias

**Steven E. Lo and Steven J. Frucht**
*The Neurological Institute, Columbia University Medical Center, New York, New York, U.S.A.*

## INTRODUCTION

Embouchure and hand dystonias are the two major forms of focal dystonia affecting musicians. Both fall under the category of focal task-specific dystonias (FTSDs), which by definition affect only one part of the body and are triggered solely during performance of specific activities (1). Depending on the task involved, FTSD can be a functionally devastating disorder for patients who derive their livelihood from the task. In the case of musicians, especially those who are professional performers or instructors, this can be a particularly disabling condition that may lead to loss of confidence and career. Unlike most other FTSDs, the manifestations of musicians' dystonia are both audible and visible (1).

The embouchure refers to the complex pattern of lower cranial muscles used by woodwind and brass musicians to play their instruments by exquisitely controlling the amplitude and force of airflow into the mouthpiece (2,3). It consists of 11 perioral muscles as well as the tongue and various jaw muscles (Fig. 1) (1). Hand dystonias affecting musicians typically involve fingers, the wrist, or any combination of distal extremity structures. The end result in both embouchure and hand dystonia is the loss of automatic, coordinated motor performance. Musicians of virtually every instrument have been affected, including bowed string instruments (violin, viola, and cello), plectrum or plucked strings (guitar, banjo, lute, mandolin, harp, and Japanese koto), keyboard (piano, accordion, organ, and harpsichord), woodwinds (flute, clarinet, saxophone, oboe, and bassoon), brass (French horn, trumpet, trombone, and tuba), and percussion instruments (drums and tablas) (1,4).

In this chapter, we review the historical background and discuss the epidemiology, clinical features, and predisposing factors for these two forms of musician's dystonia. We also review the long-term course, proposed pathophysiologic mechanisms and potential therapies for this intriguing disorder.

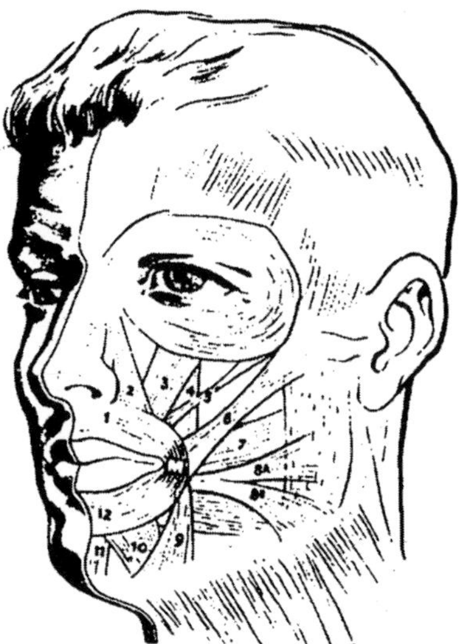

**Figure 1** A lateral view of the muscles of the embouchure. *Key*: M, modiolus; *1* and *12*, orbicularis oris; *2*, levator labii sup. alaeque nasi; *3*, levator labii superioris; *4*, levator anguli oris; *5*, zygomaticus minor; *6*, zygomaticus major; *7*, buccinator; *8a*, risorius (masseteric strand); *8b*, risorius (platysma strand), *9*, depressor anguli oris; *10*, depressor labii inferioris; *11*, mentalis. *Source*: From Ref. 3.

## HISTORICAL BACKGROUND

FTSDs were first described nearly 300 years ago, when the Italian physician Bernardino Ramazzini revised the treatise, *Diseases of Workers*, in 1713 (5–7). Sir Charles Bell also reported a case of focal dystonia in 1830, (1) and several decades later in 1864 Samuel Solly described scrivener's palsy, or what is now referred to as writer's cramp. Throughout the rest of the 19th century, reports of other occupational hand cramps surfaced, such as those affecting shoemakers, tailors, and telegraphists. These occupational cramps were also referred to as "craft palsies," "occupational neuroses," "occupational spasms," and "professional impotence" (8,9).

For musicians, it appears that the first case was reported in 1853 by Romberg, who described a pianist with task-specific thumb flexion (10). This patient had been treated by Stromeyer in 1840, apparently successfully, with a tenotomy (6,11). In addition, Bianchi reported in 1878 a flutist with left fourth digit cramping while playing, who was allegedly cured with a combination of galvanic current to the spine and injections of nitrate of strychnia (11,12).

In 1888, an amazingly detailed account of writer's cramp is given in Sir William R. Gowers' book, *A Manual of Diseases of the Nervous System* (13). Gowers defined occupational cramps as "a group of maladies in which certain symptoms are excited by the attempt to perform some often-repeated muscular action, commonly one that is involved in the occupation of the sufferer." Gowers also mentions the many occupations that have exhibited focal hand cramps, including musicians:

> Among other occupations which have been known to lead to the development of cramp and have given names to special varieties, are those of ... pianoforte players, violin players, seamstresses, telegraphists, smiths, harpists, artificial flower

> makers, turners, watchmakers, knitters, engravers, masons, compositors, enamellers, cigarette makers, shoemakers, milkers, money counters and zither players.

Although Gowers was the first to use the term "occupational neurosis" in writings, it is doubtful that Gowers was implying a psychological mechanism for these hand disabilities (6,8). Nonetheless, at points in time in the first-half of the 20th century, FTSDs were indeed viewed as psychogenic (6,14).

One year prior to the publication of Gowers' book, George Vivian Poore published the first large series of musicians with professional disability, focusing in particular on pianists (15). Although all of the musicians were clearly impaired, Poore was astute enough to recognize that the vast majority of the cases did not actually fit the pattern for a FTSD (1). Citing the task-specific nature of writer's cramp, Poore noted that the pianists had a general disability of their affected limb for nearly all tasks, as well as prominent pain, and hence Poore cast doubt on the similarity between musicians' disability and true FTSDs. Despite this, Poore did recognize the devastating impact any form of hand impairment could have on musicians:

> When I use the word "minor," please remember that they are minor only to our eye, and in a pathological sense; they are often of maximum importance to the sufferer, who possibly sees his livelihood in jeopardy, because his hand has forgotten its cunning.

Twentieth century detective work by J. Garcia de Yebenes suggests that the great 19th century pianist and composer Robert Schumann had a task-specific pianist hand cramp (16). Schumann, born in 1810, was a gifted pianist but by his early 20s was forced to give up piano performance due to an intermittent task-specific impairment of right second and third fingers. The cause for this focal difficulty remains unknown, and Schumann considered reasons such as excessive practice time and practicing on a very hard wooden clavier. Others have attributed Schumann's hand and finger dysfunction to use of a finger-stretching device, known as a "cigar," which was used by many piano students at the time. However, de Yebenes provided historical evidence that suggests a dystonic process, citing Schumann's complaints of pain and rigidity in fingers with twisting overflow to adjacent muscles, its apparent manifestation only with piano playing and its fluctuation in relation to stress, and the possible progression later in life to affect handwriting, as all being features of idiopathic dystonia. de Yebenes also argues against other possible etiologies, such as entrapment neuropathies, fractures, and syphilis. Although we may never ultimately know what ailed Robert Schumann, the possibility of a focal hand dystonia being the culprit remains an intriguing hypothesis.

In more recent times, the public announcement of pianist Gary Graffman in 1981 that he was afflicted with FTSD spurred an interest in performing arts medicine (17). The first American performing arts medicine clinic was started at the Massachusetts General Hospital where Graffman was diagnosed, and within a few years the Performing Arts Medicine Association was created (18). And after nearly 30 years of suffering without a clear diagnosis, world-renown pianist Leon Fleisher was finally given a diagnosis of focal dystonia in 1991, also of right hand. For decades, Maestro Fleisher had all but confined repertoire to musical pieces for the left hand alone. After receiving botulinum toxin (BoTN) injections at the National Institutes of Health, Fleisher has regained enough control and flexibility of right hand and fingers to allow Fleisher to once again play with two hands. Maestro Fleisher now serves as a major spokesperson and Musical Advisory board member for Musicians with Dystonia, a program entity of the Dystonia Medical Research Foundation (19).

## EPIDEMIOLOGY

The epidemiology of FTSD has not been well studied. Nutt and colleagues estimated the incidence of focal dystonia to be 24 per million per year, with a prevalence of 295 per million (20). However, only 13% of their focal dystonia cases had writer's cramp, and there was no mention of musician's dystonia (11). For musician's dystonia, epidemiologic data are derived from the experience of specialized performing arts medical centers.

### Embouchure Dystonia

Compared to focal hand dystonias in musicians, embouchure dystonia (ED) is much rarer. Although there is no formal study comparing the two forms of musician's dystonia, by pooling the data of several major series reporting dystonia among musicians, approximately 600 cases of limb involvement may be compared to nearly 100 cases of embouchure involvement. The first detailed series of musicians with ED was reported by Lederman, (6) whose four musicians (all male) had an average age of dystonia onset of 36.5 years. Brandfonbrener later described 11 patients (eight males and three females) whose mean onset was 39.8 years (21). Charness and colleagues also briefly mentioned three cases of oromandibular dystonia in their large musicians series, but details were not given (22). More recently, Frucht and colleagues reported the largest detailed series of ED patients, with 20 male and 6 female musicians and a mean onset age of 37.9 years (3). Since publication of this paper, these authors have collected an additional 50 patients with ED.

The average of onset for ED was comparable in the above three series. There was also a clear male predominance, which is replicated in the data for hand dystonias. The majority of instruments in these ED series were brass, with 33 brass compared to 8 woodwinds. Although there may be a degree of referral bias from one center to another, there appears to be a clear predominance of brass instrument involvement. It is possible that brass musicians have a particular vulnerability to developing ED, given the significantly high pressure placed on brass mouthpieces compared to those in woodwind reeds.

### Hand Dystonia

The prevalence of hand dystonia in musicians is unknown but estimated to be between 0.5% and 1% of performing musicians (11,23,24). There have been multiple large series of musicians with hand dystonias, again primarily arising from performing arts medical centers. Approximately, 5% to 15% of musicians who seek care at performing arts medical centers present with a focal dystonia, with the majority of these related to the hand (6,8,25–27).

The majority of patients in these series were professional musicians, usually performers or teachers. The mean age of dystonia onset in these series ranged from 31 to 34 years (range 16–70 years) (6,8,9,11,22,25,26). This is comparable to data from writer's cramp patients, where the mean onset age was 38.4 years (Table 1) (28).

There is a significant male predominance seen, with male to female (M:F) ratios generally ranging from 2:1 to 3:1, but as high as 7:1 in one recent large series (27). This gender predisposition is particularly striking when compared to all other playing-related disorders, where the M:F ratio is approximately 1:1.6 (11). Charness and colleagues reported 28 musicians with FTSD and evidence of ipsilateral ulnar neuropathy, evident clinically and/or by electrophysiologic testing (22). In this

**Table 1** Summary of Case Series of Musicians with Dystonia

| Study (year published) | Sample years | Sample size | Male:female ratio (number of males and females) | Mean age at onset (range) (in years) | Mean age at evaluation (range) (in years) | Mean duration of symptoms (range) (in years) | Number of keyboard | Number of bowed strings | Number of plectrum (plucked) instruments | Number of woodwind | Number of brass | Number of percussion |
|---|---|---|---|---|---|---|---|---|---|---|---|---|
| Newmark-Hochberg (1987) | 1980–1985 | 57–59 | 2.5:1 (42,17) | — | 41.7(17–70) | 7.7(0.25–24) | 35 | 6 | 7 | 9 | 1 | 1 |
| Lederman (1988) | 1979–1986 | 21 | 2:1 (14,7) | 34(18–68) | 38(19–70) | 4(0.2–21) | 4 | 6 | 3 | 4 | 3 | 1 |
| Lederman (1991) | 1979–1990 | 42 | 2.2:1 (29,13) | 33.9(19–68) | ~39 | ~5(0.1–27) | 9 | 9 | 5 | 11 | 5 | 3 |
| Schuele-Lederman (2004) | 1985–2001 | 45 | 2.8:1 (33,12) | 34(18–68) | Long-term data provided | 4.1(0.6–22) | 0 | 21 | 0 | 24 | 0 | 0 |
| Jankovic-Shale (1989) | Unclear | 11 | 11:0 (all males) | 31.1(17–50) | 40.4(19–60) | 9.3 (1–40) | 3 | 2 | 2 | 2 | 2 | 0 |
| Brandfonbrener (1995) | 1985–1995 | 58 | 2.9:1 (43,15) | 38(21–58) | — | — | 16 | 7 | 8 | 17 | 7 | 3 |
| Brandfonbrener (2004) | 1985–2002 | 113 | 2.9:1 (84,29) | "Fourth decade" | — | — | 34 | 15 | 20 | 26 | 13 | 5 |
| Charness et al. (1996) | 1984–1995 | 28 | 1:0.9 (13:15) | [a] | [a] | [a] | 14 | 6 | 4 | 4 | 0 | 0 |
| Frucht et al. (2001) | 1997–2000 | 26 | 3.3:1 (20,6) | 37.9(16–66) | 46.3(17–73) | 8.4(1–28) | 0 | 0 | 0 | 3 | 23 | 0 |
| Lim-Altenmuller (2003) | 1994–2000 | 183 | 5.3:1 (154,29) | 33.8 | — | — | 54 | 31 | 34 | 42 | 22 | 0 |
| Jabusch et al. (2005) | 1994–2001 | 144 | 4.1:1 (116,28) | 33 | Long-term data provided | 5.1 | 40 | 22 | 29 | 37 | 16 | 0 |
| Rosset-Llobet et al. (2005)[b] | Over 4 yr, prior to 2005 | 86 | 7:1 | ? | ? | ? | 4 | 5 | 36 | ? | ? | ? |

[a]Data provided for 69 patients in total study population, not the sample of 28 patients as reported in the paper.
[b]Data from abstract; article currently unavailable.

group there was loss of the male predominance; in fact, the M:F ratio significantly reversed to 0.87:1 when compared with the dystonic patients without ulnar neuropathy. The significance of this change in gender prevalence in this group with a corresponding peripheral lesion is uncertain, but may suggest that these patients are inherently different than other musicians who develop hand dystonia without a suspected cause or trigger.

## CLINICAL FEATURES

### Embouchure Dystonia

In order to discuss dystonia of the embouchure, we must first review the basic features of this unique anatomical–functional region. Most nonmusicians, and indeed even many nonbrass/woodwind musicians, do not appreciate the extraordinary demands that brass/woodwind instruments; place on the muscles of the lower face and tongue (29,30). The embouchure not only is responsible for the considerable force needed for sound production, but also exquisitely modulates airflow, changing the timbre, pitch, and articulation of that sound (31). Brass instrumentalists position both upper and lower lips inside the ring of the mouthpiece, and as air passes through the narrow opening the lips vibrate. Brass players control the pitch of each note by minutely changing the tension and size of the lip opening. The perioral muscles involved in exquisitely controlling lip opening/tension include the paired levator and depressor anguli oris, the levator labii superioris, depressor labii inferioris, zygomaticus major and minor, and the buccinator (Figs. 1 and 2). The tongue assists in articulating separation of notes. Any deviation of lip closure or jaw positioning that lead to air leakage in the embouchure will lead to impaired sound production (2,3).

In the first reported small series of ED patients, Lederman described four musicians (trombone, French horn, trumpet, and bassoon) with symptoms of lip and cheek spasm as they attempted to play, leading to diminished embouchure control (6). The bassoonist actually had segmental involvement, with tongue, lips, jaw, and larynx involved. Loss of embouchure seal around the mouthpiece was particularly problematic for the French horn musician. Later, Lederman reported seven more ED patients, (11) and with Schuele described six additional ED cases (two bassoon, two clarinet, and two flute), with symptoms of tremulous jaw movements, lateral pulling of the chin, involuntary jaw closure, and tongue protrusion (32). Brandfonbrener had 11 initial patients

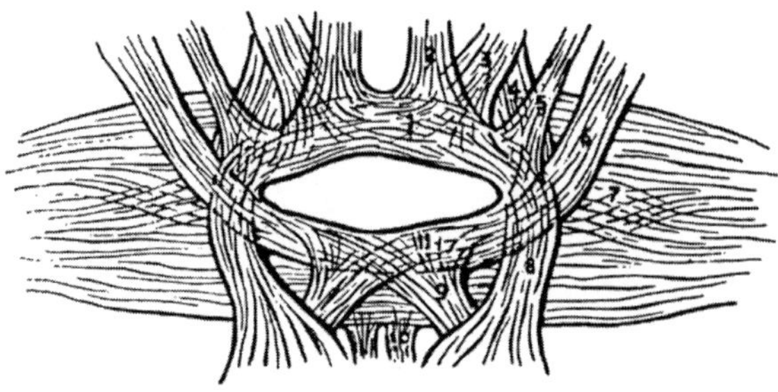

**Figure 2** A frontal view of the muscles of the embouchure. *Key*: M, modiolus; *1* and *12*, orbicularis oris; *2*, levator labii sup. alaeque nasi; *3*, levator labii superioris; *4*, levator anguli oris; *5*, zygomaticus minor; *6*, zygomaticus major; *7*, buccinator; *8a*, risorius (masseteric strand); *8b*, risorius (platysma strand), *9*, depressor anguli oris; *10*, depressor labii inferioris; *11*, mentalis. *Source*: From Ref. 3.

with ED (seven brass, one clarinet, and one flute) and later provided updated data on 16 patients (13 brass and 3 flutists) (21,25).

In recent years, Frucht and colleagues have reported with significant detail several cases of ED (31,33). In two cases of French horn ED, the major complaint was an insidious decline in ability to play with loss of precision due to task-specific lip separation, which resulted in loss of air seal. The patients illustrated many common features of ED, including lack of pain, lack of an identifiable sensory trick, and presence of a change in technique shortly prior to ED onset. Both horn players also developed a similar disability with drinking from a soda bottle, with separation of lips leading to dribbling of liquid. This suggests that the soda bottle opening resembled French horn mouthpieces sufficiently enough that it also served as a task-specific trigger for the dystonia.

Frucht and colleagues later presented the largest and most comprehensively studied series of ED patients, a total of 26 musicians (11 French horns, 5 trumpets, 5 tubas, 2 trombones, 2 flutes, and 1 clarinet) (3). The most common complaint was "difficulty performing," with loss of embouchure control, lip fatigue or tremor, and/or involuntary lower facial movements. Although 11 musicians (42%) complained of discomfort, only three (12%) had frank oral pain. A significant number of musicians had dystonia specific to certain registers (65%) or certain styles of playing (35%).

Although each patient had slightly different movements, five general patterns of ED were noted: lip tremor (eight musicians), lateral pulling (5), lip-lock (4), jaw movements (4), and Meige syndrome (2). Lip tremor was found to be rapid and involved both upper and lower lips. Lateral pulling referred to movements of one or both lips in a particular direction leading to loss of air seal. Lip-lock referred to involuntary lip closure leading to airflow obstruction. The jaw movements included jaw closure, deviation, and tremor. In two trumpet players Meige syndrome developed separately after task-specific embouchure involvement.

There were some other intriguing findings in this series of patients. Although the numbers were small, there appeared to be a register-specific tendency for two of the noted patterns; that is, all five lateral pulling ED patients played high-register brass instruments (four French horns and one trumpet), and all four lip-lock ED patients played low-register brass instruments (three tubas and one trombone). Because lateral pulling may be a compensatory way to deal with the high mouthpiece pressures of high-register brass instruments, and lip closure is a normal preparatory maneuver for low-register brass instruments, Frucht and colleagues postulated that perhaps these particular patterns were inappropriate alterations of normal motor program. In the two patients with jaw-closure ED, it was discovered that placing a straw between clenched teeth served as a sensory trick to improve dystonic closure. However, a concerning feature in the jaw ED patients was that three of the four experienced spread of dystonic movements to other more basic oral activities, such as talking and chewing. This spread of dystonia to other oral tasks was also seen in two of four patients reported by Lederman (6). Finally, three of the patients had dystonic hand involvement prior to onset of their ED, with preceding symptoms as far back as 19 years.

Finally, there was a long delay between onset of symptoms and appropriate diagnosis in that series, not dissimilar to other case series of musician's dystonia. Possible reasons for this include a reluctance in musicians to seek medical attention, musicians' belief that lack of practice is the cause, and the relative unfamiliarity of dystonias, embouchure anatomy, and musicians' techniques among most health care professionals.

## Hand Dystonia

The most common complaint that musicians with FTSD of the hand have is an inadequate ability to control parts of their hand, thereby interfering with the playing of their instruments (6,8). The first reported large series of musicians with FTSD came from the Massachusetts General Hospital, where 57 cases of isolated single limb manual incoordination were reported by Newmark and Hochberg (8). In this series, speed and volume of sound were most commonly affected, pianists had difficulty with ascending arpeggios while other instrumentalists had problems with fast-scale passages. Guitarists reported difficulty with sustaining tremolo evenly, woodwind instrumentalists noted hands rising off their instruments, and other keyboard players noted trouble crossing over fingers. None of the musicians had pain, numbness or paresthesias as part of their complaints. Otherwise manual activities of daily living were normal in the majority of the patients, with a few noting difficulty with writing and typing. There was no spread of incoordination to other body parts.

Newmark and Hochberg also noted three stereotyped patterns of dysfunction that they felt were related to instrument type: flexion of the fourth and fifth digits in pianists (22 cases), flexion of the third digit in plectrum instruments (five cases), and extension of the third digit with flexion of digits 4 and 5 in clarinetists (five cases). The remaining musicians in their series had a wide variety of other involuntary hand movements.

In 1988, Lederman first reported 21 cases of focal dystonia out of 134 musicians evaluated, 17 with upper extremity involvement (six violinists, four pianists, three guitarists, two clarinetists, and one flutist) (6). At that time, Lederman noted the tendency for lateralization of symptoms based on instruments, with predominant left upper extremity involvement in violinists (five of six) and right upper extremity involvement in pianists (three of four). This finding would be later replicated in larger, updated series (11,23). The most frequent complaint was impaired control and dexterity, and other complaints included stiffness, cramping, tightness, and fatigue. Many patients also had involuntary movements or dystonic postures, including hand tremor. Pain was not common, occurring in less than 20% of the patients, although several reported aching or uncomfortable sensations. Lederman's patients did not appear to show the stereotyped patterns associated with specific instrument groups as described by Newmark and Hochberg.

In two earlier studies, (6,11) Lederman showed that the majority (57–67%) of musicians with hand FTSD were purely task specific. Some cases were so highly specific that mimicking the action without the instrument did not lead to the same dystonic spasms. In three patients with hand dystonia writing was also affected, and two patients had dystonic spasms with any manual task. Between 17% and 24% of Lederman's patients noted sensory tricks that helped temporarily ameliorate their dystonia. These included lightly touching the affected hand with the unaffected hand, modifying the position of the affected hand/arm, and even taping a popsicle stick to a finger to prevent finger flexion.

In later publications, Lederman reported long-term follow-up data on 21 bowed string instruments and 24 woodwinds (23,26,32). Among the bowed string musicians, 16 (76%) had left-hand involvement (i.e., their fingering hand) and five (24%) had right-hand involvement (i.e., their bowing arm). In the group with right/bowing-sided symptoms, there was a wide range of abnormalities, including forced pressure, tremor, and involuntary proximal arm movements (wrist flexion and forearm pronation). In the woodwind musicians, 18 (75%) had hand involvement and six (25%) had embouchure involvement. Although numbers were small, seven of the eight (88%) clarinetists and all three oboe players had right-hand involvement, while six of nine flutists and bagpipers had left-hand involvement. Schuele and Lederman therefore felt that instrument-specific stresses on the hand and fingers appear to determine the laterality—the more complicated and/or demanding the motor task for that side, the more likely it will be the side affected by dystonia. Predominance (>70%) of left or fingering hand dystonia in bowed string instruments and right-hand dystonia in keyboard players (>75%) have been seen in other large series (8,25). Following this hypothesis, woodwinds would not be expected to have a significant lateralization, and this is borne out in the more balanced percentages in 25 clarinetists and flutists (44% left hand and 54% right hand) (1).

Charness and colleagues reported a series of 73 cases of focal dystonia occurring in a total of 69 musicians. Their series focused on the high incidence of nerve entrapments found ipsilateral to the dystonic limb in their patients (40 of 73 cases, 55%), and in particular reported on 28 of these patients with ulnar neuropathy (22). However, the relatively surprising high prevalence of peripheral lesions found is likely related to highly sensitive neurophysiologic tests, including near-nerve recordings and quantitative electromyography. There were three common patterns of dystonic finger posturing noted: flexion of digits 4 and 5 (31 cases), extension of one or more digits (23 cases), and flexion of one or more of digits 1, 2, and 3 (12 cases). They noted that a finding of ulnar neuropathy strongly predicted the pattern of dystonic posturing, with flexion of digits 4 and 5 (the digits most affected by ulnar weakness) occurring in 24 of 28 cases (86%) of dystonia with ulnar neuropathy. In comparison, this same pattern occurred only in 8 of 45 cases (18%) of dystonia without ulnar neuropathy. The other two major dystonic finger patterns seen, with mainly median or radial innervation patterns, were infrequently associated with concurrent ulnar neuropathy.

Finally, it is interesting to note that bilateral hand involvement in musicians with FTSD is quite rare. After reviewing the multiple available case series in the literature, only nine musicians with bilateral focal limb dystonia appear to have been reported (6,9,23,25,34). Task specificity on both sides could not be verified in all of the cases. In the four patients in whom some history is described, it appears that in all cases only one limb was affected at first, with the second limb becoming affected years later (range 2–14 years) (23,25). For example, Schuele and Lederman described a violinist with initial left-sided fingering symptoms who later developed right-sided symptoms 11 years after switching to right hand for fingering.

## DIAGNOSIS

The diagnosis of FTSD in musicians is usually not difficult, once clinicians are aware of the general features, and a thorough history and full neurological examination are performed. Indeed, the biggest hurdle for many clinicians, who are not movement disorder specialists or who do not have a rudimentary music background, is to simply know that such an unusual disorder exists. Careful attention should be spent on the affected body part, testing strength, sensation, tone, and range of motion. In the majority of cases all these should be normal; exceptions include those dystonias induced by a trauma or a peripheral lesion, which we will discuss later.

Because of the task specificity, it is critical that patients demonstrate the abnormal posturing or movements with their actual instruments. Although most of the time the abnormality is easily visible and/or audible, an adequate amount of time and patience is necessary to discern more subtle difficulties. If appropriate, patients may be asked to play scales, play at slow and fast tempos, play with different qualities of notes (such as short staccato or legato notes), or play in high and low registers (especially for brass instruments). A search for sensory tricks may also be helpful during the evaluation, as they may prove useful as part of the treatment.

Overall, general laboratory and imaging studies, including rheumatologic, will be normal. Electrophysiologic testing with electromyography and nerve conduction studies may prove useful if there is clinical or historical suspicion for a peripheral lesion.

## PREDISPOSING FACTORS AND TRIGGERS

### Embouchure Dystonia

There are little data for predisposing factors or known triggers related to ED onset. None of the 26 patients described by Frucht and colleagues had exposure to neuroleptic medications or a family history of dystonia. However, three musicians had writer's cramp prior to ED, suggesting that in some patients there may be a predisposition to develop focal dystonia. In no patients was there a history of major dental work in the year prior to onset of symptoms. Only three patients (12%) changed their embouchure and only two (8%) altered their instrument within the year preceding dystonia onset. Only one patient had prior facial trauma that occurred several days prior to dystonia onset (3,35). Although numbers are likely too small for direct correlation, it is known that peripheral trauma can trigger oromandibular dystonia (36). Hence, an injury to the mouth, jaw, or other parts of the lower face could conceivably trigger ED, as we suspect occurred in the above patient.

Although it appears that male gender is a significant risk factor for ED, given the high M:F ratio, one must consider the baseline gender bias for brass instruments. Brass instruments are more commonly played by men than women, and ED tends to develop more frequently in brass players than woodwind players. This hypothesis appears to be confirmed by an analysis of instruments and gender differences, which showed that brass instruments are the only instrumental group without a gender bias for symptoms (37).

### Hand Dystonia

More attention has been paid to possible predisposing factors or triggers in focal hand dystonias. In the series by Newmark and Hochberg, 37 out of a total 59 musicians had histories of trauma (four cases of acute hand injury), surgery, inflammation (such as tendonitis/tenosynovitis), or increased demands upon the hand (17 noted significant increases in practice time) preceding onset of their hand incoordination (8). Although the precise temporal relation of these various events to the hand dystonia is not listed, the range was in the matter of "acute" onset to years. Likewise, Lederman had 60% to 67% of the musicians describe a predisposing factor or triggering mechanism near the onset of symptoms, including excessive practice, change in technique or new instrument, trauma, and unusual emotional stress (6,11). This differs from Brandfonbrener's series, which found no clear-cut risk or immediate precipitant in 67% of patients (25).

It is clear that male gender is a risk factor for musician's dystonia in the hand, given the greater than 2:1 M:F ratios seen. This was statistically verified by Lim and

Altenmuller, who showed that male musicians are more likely than females to develop musician's cramp within nearly all instrument types (except brass) (37).

The majority of musicians with dystonia do not have a family history or dystonia or other movement disorders (1). In a small series of 18 musicians, Friedman and colleagues found no cases of *DYT1* gene mutations. However, they postulated that an as yet unknown susceptibility gene might still contribute to dystonia development in certain patients, citing a positive family history of tremor or dystonia in 5 of 17 (29%) unrelated patients (34). Brandfonbrener had only two patients with any family history of a movement disorder (one with a father with cervical dystonia and another whose father had Parkinson's disease) (25), and in many series there was no family history of dystonia at all. However, Brandfonbrener did report a particularly fascinating subset of patients that appears to defy both genetics and environmental factors or triggers. Two sets of identical twins played the same instrument (one pair played piano and one pair viola), had the same music teachers, and in each set only one twin had focal dystonia. The set of pianist twins has been followed for over a decade with no "dystonia conversion" in the unaffected twin.

Charness and colleagues reported a large series of focal hand dystonias thought to be related to ulnar neuropathy. They do admit that in their cases the ulnar neuropathy was usually mild, making it difficult to determine the temporal relationship between neuropathy and dystonia. However, there did appear to be some indirect evidence of a causative relationship, in that the clinical course of digits 4 and 5 flexion tended to mirror that of ulnar neuropathy; 13 of 14 (93%) patients with improved neuropathy also had sustained improvement of the dystonia (22). They suggest that ulnar neuropathy can predispose to a particular pattern of hand dystonia. This was indeed seen by Frucht and colleagues in a professional bagpipe player with ulnar neuropathy from peripheral trauma that lead to left-hand dystonia, with flexion of digits 4 and 5 (35).

Others have been unable to demonstrate nerve entrapments as common causes for hand dystonias in musicians. Lederman had five patients with nerve entrapments that could not account for their disability; one musician who later underwent surgical release of the nerve had no dystonia benefit (11). In 18 woodwind instrumentalists with hand dystonia, 14 underwent electrophysiologic studies, with only four abnormal studies found. None of the three patients who underwent nerve decompression surgery had dystonia improvement (32). One consideration, however, is that Charness and colleagues used highly sensitive electrophysiologic techniques in addition to normal surface recordings, and may have picked up more subtle signs of ulnar involvement.

## LONG-TERM COURSE AND PROGNOSIS

### Embouchure Dystonia

In the Frucht ED series long-term data were not available, but it appears that ED carries a persistent, unfavorable prognosis. ED symptoms did not improve or remit, with seven musicians disabled within four months of dystonia onset, and 17 unable to continue playing at a high enough level to maintain a career. Only two musicians had mild enough symptoms to allow them to maintain their professional performance schedule. Spread of dystonia to other oral tasks occurred in seven patients (27%), including drinking, speaking, and eating. It may, therefore, be advisable to recommend some ED patients to reduce or abstain from instrument playing, particularly those with jaw movements (3).

Lederman reported persistence of ED despite cessation of playing for years. One of Lederman's patients with ED with a French horn had not played for several years prior to the evaluation by Lederman. Within the first few attempts to play, the patient's lower facial muscles began to pull to the left, resulting in loss of seal (6).

The obvious impact of ED in the majority of cases was significant psychological stress, with loss of self-esteem and confidence, as well as depression in some. The particularly devastating aspect of musician's dystonia is that it tends to occur after the period of fine motor skill acquisition, with onset usually at the peak time of a musician's performing career. Many of the ED patients had already committed their lives to a career in performance, with social and family contacts revolving around music. And in this series, few had adequate disability insurance (3).

### Hand Dystonia

In the series from Newmark and Hochberg, the mean duration of symptoms was 7.7 years, with a range of 4 months to 24 years (8). In Lederman's first series the duration of symptoms at time of initial evaluation ranged from 2 months to 21 years (mean duration four years) (6). Lederman later reported that only 4 of 42 patients were playing with minimal or no impairment, with 24 playing with mild-to-moderate impairment, and 14 unable to play at all (11).

Most recently, Schuele and Lederman published long-term outcome data. They used a questionnaire as part of follow-up, sent out on average 10.4 and 7.7 years after their first evaluation for a group of string and woodwind instrumentalists, respectively (23). They were thereby able to provide long-term information on a group of musicians who have dealt with their symptoms on average between 12 and 15 years. Most cases had insidious onset with gradual progression within the first year, with a tendency to plateau thereafter. In general, remissions, fluctuations, and spread to other body regions were rare, and the prognosis overall appeared unfavorable. About 20% to 33% of musicians complained of problems with other activities. Only a few felt that there was any mild improvement over the 5 to 10 years following their first evaluation. Only 5 of 11 (45%) bowed string musicians with hand dystonia were able to continue to perform, three of them by changing techniques or refingering certain music passages. None of the musicians with dystonia involving the bowing arm were able to continue as professional musicians (26). Of 15 woodwind musicians, only 8 were able to remain professional performers (5 of 9 hand dystonia and 3 of 6 ED) (23,32).

Brandfonbrener also provided extended follow-up of 54 patients, 14 of whom had their initial evaluation 12 or more years earlier. Thirty-six of 54 were professional musicians, of whom 19 were still actively playing. Many had to make significant changes to technique or switch their repertoire. Seventeen professionals were unable to continue to work as musicians, and in no patient did symptoms resolve or improve to a significant degree (25).

## PATHOPHYSIOLOGY AND MECHANISMS

Recent evidence supports the idea that focal dystonia is a central disorder of motor control, with the end result at the muscle level of cocontraction of agonist and antagonist muscles. However, there are physiologic abnormalities in focal dystonia that are evident at various levels of the nervous system, from the muscle spindle extending all the way up the neuraxis to the cortex. Abnormalities at the muscle spindle afferent level have been demonstrated, based on studies that showed that sensory input to a resting limb of a patient with FTSD can provoke dystonic contractions. This similar peripherally triggered dystonic spasm could be reduced with local injections of lidocaine that reduces muscle spindle afferent activity (38). Although no study has shown direct basal ganglia physiologic abnormalities in musicians with hand dystonia, Delmaire recently showed basal ganglia abnormalities in patients with writer's cramp, another FTSD of the hand. They showed that the somatotopic representation of the body in the putamen contralateral to the affected limb in patients with writer's cramp was disrupted, suggesting dedifferentiation of normally segregated striatal sensorimotor maps (39).

There is a significant amount of physiologic and functional imaging evidence to suggest that patients with FTSD harbor significant cortical abnormalities. These abnormalities include a disturbed central processing of sensory information, impaired integration between sensory and motor processes, inappropriate areas of activation, decreased cortical inhibition, reorganization of the sensorimotor cortex, and distorted cortical representations of motor function (23,40).

At the cortex there is evidence that corticomotor excitation is significantly increased in patients with FTSD compared to controls, (41–43) and this increased cortical excitability may be due to reduced intracortical inhibition (44). Recent work with magnetic resonance spectroscopy by Hallett suggests that reduced intracortical inhibition may be due to decreased levels of $\gamma$-aminobutyric acid in FTSD patients (45). Physiologic studies and functional imaging for brain mapping have shown abnormal sensory maps in musicians with dystonia. Elbert and colleagues used magnetoencephalography (MEG) to show that the distance between cortical sensory representation of digit pairs was smaller in musicians with dystonia compared with normal controls or musicians without dystonia (46). Bara-Jiminez and colleagues used somatosensory-evoked potentials to show fusion of the cortical representation of the digits in the primary somatosensory cortex of patients with FTSD. They also showed inversion of digits 1 and 5 positions in the sensory homunculus in these patients compared to controls (47). Meunier and colleagues used MEG to show that there was bilateral disorganization of finger representations in the primary sensory cortex of patients with writer's cramp, with greater disorganization on the side contralateral to the unaffected limb. Despite unilateral symptoms, the nondystonic hemisphere is originally affected by the disease as well (48). Thus, representation of the hand in primary sensory cortex is markedly disordered bilaterally in dystonic patients.

There have been a limited number of studies done specifically for musician's dystonia. Hirata and colleagues examined the somatosensory homuncular representation of eight brass players with ED, comparing them to control subjects, and reported digit representation shifts in a lateral direction toward the lip zone in those ED patients. As this cortical asymmetry was absent in the control subjects, they hypothesized that this homuncular reorganization may contribute to the development of ED (49). Pujol and colleagues similarly demonstrated abnormal cortical activity in musicians with FTSD of the hand. They used functional magnetic resonance imaging (MRI) and a specially adapted MRI-compatible guitar to demonstrate abnormal brain activation in five guitarists with task-specific dystonia. Compared to nondystonic guitar controls, there was significantly increased primary sensorimotor cortex activation contralateral to the dystonic hand, as well as decreased premotor area activation (50,51).

Charness and Schlaug evaluated brain activation patterns in pianists with hand dystonia, normal pianists, and nonmusicians. Using the same finger-tapping task, they were able to show that normal pianists had increased activation of the dorsolateral precentral gyrus and reduced supplementary motor area activation compared to the afflicted pianists and the nonmusicians. This suggested that pianists with dystonia had regression of activation patterns (52).

How does one now combine the above abnormal findings and hypotheses with the features of musician's dystonia that have been described in clinical series? For example, the mean age of onset for FTSD in musicians appears to be in the first-half of the third decade. Yet, the majority of these musicians have already been learning and practicing their craft for years before onset of symptoms. Thus, FTSD arises mainly in musicians who have already attained a high level of skill, rarely developing during the acquisition of this skill. Charness believes that focal dystonias emerge through an alteration of the plastic neural processes that accompany the rehearsal of highly skilled movements. However, because FTSDs occur only in a small percentage of musicians, "experience-related neural plasticity" is by itself insufficient for FTSD to develop (40). One thought then is that perhaps an as yet undefined genetic predisposition in select musicians allows for cortical disorganization to occur as musicians rehearse repeatedly.

Another clinical feature that raises question is how can an increase in practice time lead to a greater risk for focal dystonia? One hypothesis that may explain the apparent risk is that repetitive hand movements can lead to cortical reorganization (40). Byl and colleagues used New World owl monkeys to show that repetitive hand movements can lead to dystonic-appearing hand movements with associated somatosensory cortex reorganization (enlargement and overlap of receptive fields) (53). This cortical reorganization may lead to the generation of inappropriate motor programs or inappropriate digit movements.

Finally, Charness and colleagues noted that their study revealed that weakness in ulnar-innervated muscles appeared to initiate a dystonia mediated by median-innervated superficial flexors. They suggest that several of their cases of dystonia with ulnar neuropathy may be an involuntary and maladaptive compensatory maneuver (22). They also proposed another theory—as peripheral nerve injury has been shown to induce cortical reorganization beyond the territory of the injured nerve, ulnar nerve injury may therefore increase cortical representations of median superficial flexors, leading to inappropriate flexion of digits 4 and 5.

## TREATMENT

After a diagnosis of dystonia is made and initial questions answered, the next critical issue on patients' minds is treatment. Unfortunately, the benefit from current available treatments is generally moderate at best, with a significant percentage of musicians forced to leave professional performance careers. As has been demonstrated in various reported case series, resolution of dystonia is rare, except for those cases clearly related to nerve entrapments. Tables 2 and 3 list therapies that have been used by musicians, mostly without a great deal of success.

### Embouchure Dystonia

Compared to treatment of patients with hand dystonia, therapeutic options are more limited for ED, simply based on anatomy. For example, rehabilitation therapies such

**Table 2** Treatments Used for Embouchure Dystonia

| Little or no success | Modest-to-moderate success |
|---|---|
| Botulinum toxin injections | Embouchure retraining/rebuilding |
| Prolonged rest/cessation of playing | Alteration in technique (change to different embouchure/mouthpiece) |
| Dental prosthetic | Sensory trick device (single case) |
| Medications (anticholinergic and dopaminergic) | Technical exercises |
| Biofeedback | Changing instruments |
| Psychotherapy | |
| Acupuncture or herbal therapy | |

as immobilization and constraint-induced therapy would not be applicable to the embouchure. And unfortunately, ED appears to be inherently more resistant to treatments than task-specific hand dystonias. In their series, Jabusch and colleagues showed that the response rate to nearly every form of treatment modality was inferior for ED patients compared to patients with limb dystonia. The overall percentage of patients with ED who had improvement was 15% (3 of 20 patients) compared to 50% (62 of 123 patients) with limb dystonia. None of the ED patients who tried trihexyphenidyl (five patients), BoTN (three patients), ergonomic aid (two patients), or pedagogical retraining (two patients) as therapies had any improvement. Only 6 of 11 ED patients (54%) reported some improvement with nonspecific technical exercises, which was comparable to the rate in musicians with hand dystonia who used this strategy (24).

Frucht and colleagues reported the most success with embouchure retraining to minimize abnormal movements, as well as alteration of technique by changing to a different embouchure and/or using a different type of mouthpiece (such as switching to a trombone-type embouchure/mouthpiece) (3). The success rate unfortunately was modest at best, helping mainly those musicians with lateral pulling ED but not those with lip tremor (31). Schuele and Lederman also had two patients improve with rebuilding the embouchure, which included changes in size, configuration, placement of the mouthpiece, and retraining through "buzzing" exercises. One flutist

**Table 3** Treatments Used for Task-Specific Hand Dystonias in Musicians

| Little or no success | Modest success | Moderate success |
|---|---|---|
| Prolonged rest, cessation of playing | Anticholinergic medications (e.g., trihexyphenidyl) | Botulinum toxin injections |
| Biofeedback | Refingering music passages | Surgery for nerve entrapment-induced cases |
| Psychotherapy | Ergonomic changes (instrument modification) | Immobilization/splinting (in one small series) |
| Dopaminergic medications | Alteration in techniques or retraining | Sensory motor retuning (constraint-induced therapy) |
| Transcutaneous nerve stimulation | Change in teacher or instrument | |
| | Use of sensory tricks | |

*Source*: Modified from Ref. 23.

with mild dystonia was able to continue to play after retraining and switching to a different flute (23,32).

Many other therapies, both traditional and nontraditional, were tried by patients. Alternative/complementary therapies such as acupuncture, herbal therapy, chiropractic treatment, and massage were generally ineffective. Dental prosthetics were used in five musicians without benefit in Frucht's large series. However, in a single case report one French horn player who responded to a sensory trick (clenching a straw between left rear molars) and who experienced spread of dystonia to speech and drinking had near resolution of these symptoms with a dental prosthesis that mimicked the sensory trick (33).

Finally, seven patients in Frucht and colleague's series received BoTN injections to perioral muscles, resulting in unacceptable weakness or minimal functional improvement in most, and functionally significant improvement in only a single patient with jaw-closure ED (3). Similarly, Schuele and colleagues had three ED patients undergo BoTN injections, and all three actually felt worse after the first injection (54). Given the extreme force requirements needed for brass embouchures and therefore the vulnerability to even the slightest bit of excess weakness, it is not surprising that even musicians who had some dystonia improvement would choose not to continue BoTN injections. It appears, therefore, that BoTN is simply not a practical treatment for ED.

## Hand Dystonias

In their series of musicians, Newmark and Hochberg reported several ineffective therapies tried by their patients, including surgical procedures (tendon release, carpal tunnel release, and nerve release), pharmacologic trials (dopaminergic medications, diazepam, steroids, and propanolol), psychotherapy, transcutaneous nerve stimulation, acupuncture, and physical/occupational therapy. There was also no benefit with rest or cessation of instrument playing up to three years. Their own treatment strategies were only slightly more successful; specific physical therapy to strengthen distal extensors/interossei/lumbrical groups had significant improvement in only three patients, and trihexyphenidyl helped only two patients (8).

These results were similarly reported by Lederman. Exercises, biofeedback, modification of instruments (such as changing shoulder rests in violinists and thumb rest in a clarinet), psychotherapy, anticholinergics (up to 40 mg of trihexyphenidyl), and dopamine agonists were of no significant benefit. Prolonged rest was ineffective and largely impractical (6). Four of 18 woodwind players with hand dystonia had benefit from immobilization with splints or casting (32).

BoTN injection for musicians with FTSD generally offers moderate benefit for many, but the improvement in dystonia always needs to be balanced with resultant muscle weakness. Because musicians depend on exquisite motor control for perfect performance, any dystonia improvement that is achieved at the expense of focal weakness usually proves unacceptable for performers (9). Cohen and colleagues were among the first to enroll musicians with dystonia and writer's cramp in open-label trials of BoTN; they showed subjective moderate-to-major improvement in cramping and motor performance in 72% to 81% of their subjects (55,56). Later, a double-blind trial of BoTN with a placebo phase for each subject (10 patients with FTSD of the hand, including a pianist and a bagpiper) objectively verified the true efficacy of BoTN in the treatment of focal hand dystonias (57).

In the past two years, several series of musician's dystonia describing long-term treatment outcomes have been published. Among Schuele and Lederman's 21 patients, four tried BoTN: two had no improvement, one had variable response, and one has derived benefit and continues to be injected with 50 to 70 units of BoTN Type A (26). Schuele and colleagues described the long-term outcome of BoTN therapy in 84 musicians (81 hand and 3 ED). They reported that 58 of 84 musicians (69%) experienced benefit (defined as $\geq$ mild degree of improvement), and 38 of 84 (45%) had enough improvement to notice better performance ability. However, 98% of the musicians noticed some degree of weakness. Twenty-four musicians continued to receive BoTN over a mean of 36 months (range 9–76 months), with a mean number of 11.7 injections (range 3–29). Six of 11 hand dystonia patients who discontinued BoTN did so because they had sustained benefit and no longer felt the need for more treatment. Unfortunately, there were 23 hand dystonia patients (28%) who had no response to BoTN or who felt worse with treatment (54).

The most recent and largest series describing long-term treatment outcomes comes from Jabusch and colleagues. A total of 144 musicians (116 males and 28 females) were retrospectively studied for their response to treatment, with 124 of them (86%) having limb dystonia. The major categories of therapy tried were trihexyphenidyl (33% of patients with improvement), BoTN injections (57% of patients who had more than one injection reported improvement), ergonomic changes such as with splints or instrument modification (63% with improvement), pedagogical retraining (50% with improvement), and use of nonspecific technical exercises (56% with improvement). As expected, trihexyphenidyl was the least tolerated because of frequent side effects. BoTN injections were most beneficial for those musicians with limited demand for lateral finger motion (woodwinds and right hand in guitarists). The behavioral therapies appeared to be comparable to chemodenervation with BoTN, and hence the authors recommended it be tried in all applicable cases (24).

Charness and colleagues found that among the dystonic patients with ulnar neuropathy, three benefited from supportive therapies such as rest or splinting, and 11 out of 12 patients who underwent ulnar decompression surgery had significant and sustained improvement of dystonia. They suggest therefore that all musicians with flexion dystonia of digits 4 and 5 be carefully evaluated for ulnar neuropathy (22). Lederman had a similar case of surgical reversal of FTSD apparently due to nerve entrapment, in which one patient found to have carpal tunnel syndrome had resolution of dystonia after carpal tunnel release surgery was performed (6).

In addition to BoTN injections and behavioral modifications (retraining, refingering passages, and instrument changes), several rehabilitation approaches have been developed as potential therapies. The main idea of these therapies is to try to modify the cortical representation of the affected limb through immobilization (1). Priori and colleagues showed in a small series of patients with FTSD of the hand (7 musician's dystonia and 1 writer's cramp) that prolonged immobilization of the affected limb for four to five weeks led to significant improvements in dystonia severity and performance in motor tasks. At the six-month follow-up, seven of the eight patients had at least moderate improvement (three had 20–33% improvement from baseline objective scores and four had >70% improvement from baseline scores) (58). There was no worsening of the dystonia from splint immobilization, and there appeared to be persistent benefit months after removal of the splint. Priori and colleagues concluded that limb immobilization may be a safe, inexpensive, and effective treatment for focal occupational limb dystonias. Several trials designed to replicate this finding are in progress.

Candia and colleagues presented long-term data in 11 musicians who used sensory motor retuning, also known as constraint-induced therapy. In this treatment modality, the finger(s) that exhibit dystonia are left unrestrained while one or several compensatory fingers are immobilized, and extensive regular practice of specific finger tasks are employed over a year. The hypothesis is that a behavioral intervention focusing on movement may improve the use-dependent alteration in the cortical representations of digits seen in patients with focal hand dystonias. Their prospective series showed benefit in six pianists, two guitarists, but none in three woodwind players (59). Although further data are needed, the results revealed a promising alternative therapy to be tried.

Finally, as part of the supportive therapies offered to musicians with embouchure or hand dystonia, a clinician may bring to their attention the existence of the Musicians with Dystonia program. Founded in 2000 as part of the Dystonia Medical Research Foundation, it offers practical support to musicians, raises awareness of dystonia to the musical community, and facilitates research collaborations. Interested musicians and clinicians may find out more information about the program in Ref. (60).

## CONCLUSIONS

FTSDs can have a far-reaching impact on musicians. Beyond the often-dramatic physical effects, there are often social and emotional ramifications that impact the livelihood and passions of patients suffering with this disorder. In addition, there may be significant financial implications for those unable to continue in their careers as professional musicians (1). For the clinician, the first step in helping this unique patient population is recognition and understanding this debilitating disorder. From there, appropriate diagnostic steps and treatments can be offered. A referral to a performing arts medical center, especially one that has a large experience with focal dystonias, may be warranted. Despite our best efforts, however, embouchure and hand dystonias in musicians remain a mysterious and difficult entity to treat.

## REFERENCES

1. Frucht SJ. Focal task-specific dystonia in musicians. Adv Neurol 2004; 94:225–230.
2. Farkas P. The art of brass playing. Rochester, NY: Wind Music Inc, 1962.
3. Frucht SJ, Fahn S, Greene PE, et al. The natural history of embouchure dystonia. Mov Disord 2001; 16:899–906.
4. Ragothaman M, Sarangmath N, Jayaram S, et al. Task-specific dystonia in tabla players. Mov Disord 2004; 19:1254–1256.
5. Ramazzini B. Diseases of Workers (1713) Revised and translated by Wright WC. Chicago: University of Chicago, 1940:420–425.
6. Lederman RJ. Occupational cramp in instrumental musicians. Med Probl Perform Art 1988; 3:45–51.
7. Altschuler EL. Ramazzini and writer's cramp. Lancet 2005; 365:938.
8. Newmark J, Hochberg FH. Isolated painless manual incoordination in 57 musicians. J Neurol Neurosurg Psychiatry 1987; 50:291–295.
9. Jankovic J, Shale H. Dystonia in Musicians. Semin Neurol 1989; 9:131–135.
10. Romberg MH. A manual of the nervous diseases of man. In: Translated by Sieveking EH. 1. London: Syndenham Society, 1853:320–324.

11. Lederman RJ. Focal dystonia in instrumentalists: clinical features. Med Probl Perform Art 1991; 6:132–136.
12. Bianchi L. A contribution on the treatment of the professional dyscinesiae. Br Med J 1878; 1:87–89.
13. Gowers WR. A manual of diseases of the nervous system. Philadelphia: P. Blakiston, 1888.
14. Crisp AH, Moldofsky H. A psychosomatic study of writers' cramp. Br J Psychiatry 1965; 111:841–858.
15. Poore GV. Clinical lecture on certain conditions of the hand and arm which interfere with the performance of professional acts, especially piano-playing. Br J Med J 1887; 1:441–447.
16. de Yebenes JG. Did Robert Schumann have dystonia? Mov Disord 1995; 10:413–417.
17. Graffman G. Doctor, can you lend an ear? Med Probl Perform Art 1986; 1:3–6.
18. Newmark J. Musicians' dystonia: the case of Gary Graffman. Semin Neurol 1999; 19(suppl 1):41–45.
19. Pullman SL, Hristova AH. Musician's dystonia. Neurology 2005; 64:186–187.
20. Nutt JG, Muenter MD, Melton LJ III, Aronson A, Kurland LT. Epidemiology of dystonia in Rochester, Minnesota. Adv Neurol 1988; 50:361–365.
21. Brandfonbrener AG. Musicians with focal dystonia: a report of 58 cases seen during a ten-year period at a performing arts medicine clinic. Med Probl Perform Art 1995; 10: 121–127.
22. Charness ME, Ross MH, Shefner JM. Ulnar neuropathy and dystonic flexion of the fourth and fifth digits: clinical correlation in musicians. Muscle Nerve 1996; 19:431–437.
23. Schuele SU, Lederman RJ. Long-term outcome of focal dystonia in instrumental musicians. Adv Neurol 2004; 94:261–266.
24. Jabusch HC, Zschucke D, Schmidt A, et al. Focal dystonia in musicians: treatment strategies and long-term outcome in 144 patients. Mov Disord 2005; 20:1623–1626.
25. Brandfonbrener AG, Robson C. Review of 113 musicians with focal dystonia seen between 1985 and 2002 at a clinic for performing artists. Adv Neurol 2004; 94:255–256.
26. Schuele S, Lederman RJ. Long-term outcome of focal dystonia in string instrumentalists. Mov Disord 2004; 19:43–48.
27. Rosset-Llobet J, Fabregas i Molas S, Rosines i Cubells D, et al. [Clinical analysis of musicians' focal hand dystonia. Review of 86 cases] Neurologia 2005; 20:108–115. [Article in Spanish].
28. Sheehy MP, Rothwell JC, Marsden CD. Writer's cramp. Adv Neurol 1988; 50:457–472.
29. Bouhuys A. Lung volumes and breathing patterns in wind-instrument players. J Appl Physiol 1964; 19:967–975.
30. Lederman RJ. Questions and answers: trumpet player's neuropathy. JAMA 1987; 257:1526.
31. Frucht S, Fahn S, Ford B. French horn embouchure dystonia. Mov Disord 1999; 14: 171–173.
32. Schuele S, Lederman RJ. Focal dystonia in woodwind instrumentalists: long-term outcome. Med Probl Perform Art 2003; 18:15–20.
33. Frucht S, Fahn S, Ford B, Gelb M. A geste antagoniste device to treat jaw-closing dystonia. Mov Disord 2000; 14:883–886.
34. Friedman JR, Klein C, Leung J, et al. The GAG deletion of the DYT1 gene is infrequent in musicians with focal dystonia. Neurology 2000; 55:1417–1418.
35. Frucht S, Fahn S, Ford B. Focal task-specific dystonia induced by peripheral trauma. Mov Disord 2000; 15:348–350.
36. Sankhla C, Lai EC, Jankovic J. Peripherally induced oromandibular dystonia. J Neurol Neurosurg Psychiatry 1998; 65:722–728.
37. Lim VK, Altenmuller E. Musician's cramp: instrumental and gender differences. Med Probl Perform Art 2003; 18:21–26.
38. Kaji R, Rothwell JC, Katayama M, et al. Tonic vibration reflex and muscle afferent block in writer's cramp. Ann Neurol 1995; 38:155–162.

39. Delmaire C, Krainik A, Tezenas du Montcel S, et al. Disorganized somatotopy in the putamen of patients with focal hand dystonia. Neurology 2005; 64:1391–1396.
40. Charness ME, Schlaug G. Brain mapping in musicians with focal task-specific dystonia. Adv Neurol 2004; 94:231–238.
41. Siebner HR, Auer C, Conrad B. Abnormal increase in the corticomotor output to the affected hand during repetitive transcranial magnetic stimulation of the primary cortex in patients with writer's cramp. Neurosci Lett 1999; 262:133–136.
42. Ikoma K, Samii A, Mercuri B, et al. Abnormal cortical motor excitability in dystonia. Neurology 1996; 46:1371–1376.
43. Lim VK, Bradshaw JL, Nicholls ME, et al. Abnormal sensorimotor processing in pianists with focal dystonia. Adv Neurol 2004; 94:267–273.
44. Ridding MC, Sheean G, Rothwell JC, et al. Changes in the balance between motor cortical excitation and inhibition in focal, task specific dystonia. J Neurol Neurosurg Psychiatry 1995; 59:493–498.
45. Levy LM, Hallett M. Impaired brain GABA in focal dystonia. Ann Neurol 2002; 51: 93–101.
46. Elbert T, Candia V, Altenmuller E, et al. Alteration of digital representations in somatosensory cortex in focal hand dystonia. Neuroreport 1998; 9:3571–3575.
47. Bara-Jimenez W, Catalan MJ, Hallett M, et al. Abnormal somatosensory homunculus in dystonia of the hand. Ann Neurol 1998; 44:828–831.
48. Meunier S, Garnero L, Ducorps A, et al. Human brain mapping in dystonia reveals both endophenotypic traits and adaptive reorganization. Ann Neurol 2001; 50:521–527.
49. Hirata Y, Schulz M, Altenmuller E, et al. Sensory mapping of lip representation in brass musicians with embouchure dystonia. Neuroreport 2004; 15:815–818.
50. Pujol J, Roset-Llobet J, Rosines-Cubells D, et al. Brain cortical activation during guitar-induced hand dystonia studied by functional MRI. Neuroimage 2000; 12:257–267.
51. Pascual-Leone A. The brain that plays music and is changed by it. Ann N Y Acad Sci 2001; 930:315–329.
52. Charness ME, Schlaug G. Cortical activation during finger movements in concert pianists, dystonic pianists, and non-musicians. Neurology 2000; 54(suppl 3):A221.
53. Byl NN, Merzenich MM, Jenkins WM. A primate genesis model of focal dystonia and repetitive strain injury: learning-induced dedifferentiation of the representation of the hand in the primary somatosensory cortex in adult monkeys. Neurology 1996; 47:508–520.
54. Schuele S, Jabusch HC, Lederman RJ, et al. Botulinum toxin injections in the treatment of musician's dystonia. Neurology 2005; 64:341–343.
55. Cohen LG, Hallett M, Geller BD, Hochberg F. Treatment of focal dystonias of the hand with botulinum toxin injections. J Neurol Neurosurg Psychiatry 1989; 52:355–363.
56. Cole RA, Cohen LG, Hallett M. Treatment of musician's cramp with botulinum toxin. Med Probl Perform Art 1991; 6:137–143.
57. Cole R, Hallett M, Cohen LG. Double-blind trial of botulinum toxin for treatment of focal hand dystonia. Mov Disord 1995; 10:466–471.
58. Priori A, Pesenti A, Cappellari A, et al. Limb immobilization for the treatment of focal occupational dystonia. Neurology 2001; 57:405–409.
59. Candia V, Schafer T, Taub E, et al. Sensory motor retuning: a behavioral treatment for focal hand dystonia of pianists and guitarists. Arch Phys Med Rehabil 2002; 83: 1342–1348.
60. www.dystonia-foundation.org, or via e-mail: musicians@dystonia-foundation.org.

# 14

# Sports-Related Task-Specific Dystonia: The Yips

**Charles H. Adler**
*Department of Neurology, Mayo Clinic, Scottsdale, Arizona, U.S.A.*

## INTRODUCTION

While dystonia affecting athletes has not been researched or written about to the same degree as other focal dystonias, this may well be due to a previous lack of awareness or interest among both physicians and athletes. Because dystonia and occupational cramps affect people who write, type, and play a musical instrument, it is logical to believe that dystonia also affects people who play sports. This review represents an attempt to specifically focus on sports-related dystonia, and provide the clinician a rational approach to define the patient with the potential for benefit from emerging treatments for this interesting focal dystonia.

## GOLFER'S CRAMP: YIPS

Golfers all know about the "yips," a term that is often not spoken or only said with a whisper. The lay press has made common use of this term when describing professional golfers who miss key putts in tournaments. It is also used to describe golfers who are in a "slump" (1). There are numerous definitions for the term "yips" including that found in Merriam-Webster Online Dictionary "a state of nervous tension affecting an athlete (as a golfer) in the performance of a crucial action <had a bad case of the *yips* on short putts>" (26). It is unclear how this term first came to be used. Some have said that Sam Snead, a famous golfer who developed difficulty putting, first used the term yips. Although this term seems consistent with the penchant for colloquialism, and certainly captures the sense of an abrupt and fleeting movement to ruin a putt, there is no published evidence attributing the term to Sneed. Tommy Armour, another golf champion, also developed the yips and popularized the term. Other golfers who have discussed their difficulties with the yips include Johnny Miller, Mark O'Meara, and Bernhard Langer (27,28).

The possibility that the yips may be an occupational cramp was initially proposed by Foster (2) in the description of the involuntary movements suffered by both Ben Hogan and Sam Snead. The report drew from Gower's descriptions of spasms during certain occupational actions, especially writer's cramp (2). Ben Hogan is also the subject of one chapter in Klawans' entertaining book on sports and neurology (3). Here it describes how Hogan first developed a dystonic extension of a finger during the 71st hole of the U.S. Open and lost the tournament (3). In a broad discussion of the focal dystonias, Marsden described occupational cramps that affect golfers as well as billiard and dart players (4).

### What Causes the Yips?

Much has been written in the lay literature about the yips. Most, if not all, of these descriptions suggest that the yips are a psychological disorder (29). Many have referred to the yips as a form of "choking," an extreme manifestation of performance anxiety, associated with reduction of performance under pressure circumstances (5). Despite the potential for the yips being an occupational cramp, the majority of golfers, and those who work with golf professionally, believe that the yips are a psychological disorder. Most golf psychologists and golf instructors have only written about the psychological nature of the yips without consideration of possible neurological issues. This is quite similar to how other focal dystonias have been perceived, including torticollis and spasmodic dysphonia. Typical therapeutic recommendations include a variety of techniques to overcome the yips, most having to do with the psychology of putting (6). Others postulate that choking results from an athlete spending too much time focusing on the movement and the worsening of that in the setting of anxiety (5). A more extreme interpretation described the yips as a sports performance phobia (7). However, the first attempt to objectify this phenomenon was initiated by Crews who used electroencephalogram brain mapping to suggest that choking was due to overactivity of the left hemisphere in the presence of anxiety while putting (30). In addition, systematic retrospective analysis of putting data from professional golf tournaments (men's and women's) also suggests that choking is not an issue (8,9).

Dave Pelz, a recognized putting teacher for many competitive golfers in the Professional Golf Association (PGA), proposes that the yips are due to the golfer momentarily losing consciousness while putting (10). Dave Pelz postulates that the golfer has a period of unconsciousness lasting less than 1/1000 of a second. This period occurs just before impact of the putter with the golf ball, and that the jerk (yip) occurs as the golfer recovers awareness. While there are many issues and limitations to this hypothesis, Dave Pelz is the first recognized golf teacher to move the yips from a psychological disorder to, perhaps, a neurological disorder. It remains the responsibility of the neurology community to educate the public regarding the phenomenological classification of the movement disorder.

## NEUROLOGIC STUDY OF THE YIPS

Kachi et al. initiated the first neurologic evaluation of a golfer with a movement disorder (11). As part of a larger study of primary writing tremor, one subject with tremor while swinging a golf club was included (11). This 29-year-old man reported tremor while golfing for the past four years, but did not exhibit tremor with any other activity. The tremor was described as jerky, and could be elicited with wrist tendon percussion. During electrophysiological testing, as the man began the backswing, surface electromyographic (EMG) recordings revealed a 5 to 6 Hz alternating tremor between the finger flexors and extensors with no tremor in the biceps or triceps (11). The patient had no benefit from alcohol, and administration of 2 mg of propranolol intravenously did not change the tremor (11).

One of the first careful assessments to address the yips in a golfer was undertaken by McDaniel et al. in 1988 (12). The patient was a professional golfer who developed the yips at the age of 23. Symptoms occurred only during putting and only during tournament play. There was no evidence of involuntary movements with any other activity and no abnormality on examination. Changes in grip and a trial of propranolol were not effective, but the patient compensated for the problem by changing to a left-handed putting approach.

The same report summarized results from a 69-item questionnaire study of 750 professional (300 male PGA Tour, 200 male PGA Senior Tour, 250 female LPGA Tour) and 300 male amateur golfers (12). While only 335 (42%) men and 25 (10%) women responded, 28% of the male golfers reported the yips. The mean age of onset of golfers indicating this symptom was 35.9 years and duration of golfing prior to yips onset was 20.9 years. The majority of subjects reported the yips only when putting (54%), while others reported symptoms when putting plus chipping or driving (40%), chipping alone (5%), and driving alone (2%). These golfers described movements such as jerks, spasms, and tremor occurring in the distal arm mainly when putting, as well as freezing episodes especially during the forward stroking of the ball. The yips affected play during tournaments in 99% of respondents, intensified with anxiety in 77%, and occurred during practice in 46%. Compensatory strategies helped 52% of the golfers, and included changes in grip, conversion to a long putter, and changes in posture or approach (changing from right handed to left handed). Interestingly, 24% reported that other tasks were affected and 25% stated that other body regions were affected, suggesting that the yips may be one of many dystonic movements in these individuals. When compared to unaffected golfers, the golfers with the yips were older and had been golfing longer. Additionally, golfers with the yips had a higher score on one item related to obsessional thinking compared to the unaffected golfers. Interestingly, no differences between affected and nonaffected golfers were seen in responses to questions assessing the frequency or severity of anxiety-related symptoms (12).

Sachdev has carefully evaluated 20 patients who reported symptoms of the yips while golfing, and compared them to age, sex, and golfing-matched controls (13). He has proposed the following criteria to diagnosis the yips (13):

1. > five years of golfing with > one year at a high level of proficiency
2. Development of an involuntary movement or freezing while putting or chipping
3. The sparing of long strokes (i.e., driving) at least at initial onset
4. No history of dystonia, Parkinson's disease, or other neurologic disorder
5. Normal neurologic and musculoskeletal examination
6. Either benefit from a trick, fluctuating symptoms, or similar symptoms with another task-specific activity

The mean age for all golfers was 54.5 years, but the group differed in that two yips subjects were professional golfers, while the control group did not contain any golfer at this level of proficiency. The mean age of onset of the yips was 35.1 years and the mean duration of golf prior to development of the yips was 16.1 years. Most described the problem as occurring with putts shorter than 3 m. The majority (75%) had the symptoms only during competitive play. Compensatory strategies included changes in putter type, grip, and position. By history, writing was affected in two subjects, tennis and table tennis in two, cricket bowling in one, and shooting pool in one. Neurological examinations were unremarkable except for one subject diagnosed with mild essential tremor.

No differences in neuropsychological or cognitive testing were found between the two groups (13). Assessments included self-rating of anxiety, Spielberger Anxiety Scale, Zung Depression Scale, and Leyton's Obsessional Inventory. While these data differ from the observations of McDaniel et al. (12), Sachdev did suggest that anxiety and arousal factors may play a role in the yips, but are not the primary cause of the disorder (13).

Smith et al. (14) have also surveyed a population of 2630 advanced golfers (handicap <12) registered for tournaments with the Minnesota Golf Association. A total of 1031 (39%) golfers (986 men and 45 women) responded, and a surprisingly high, and perhaps falsely elevated, number of respondents (541 or 52%) reported experiencing the yips. From the survey data 359 yips-affected and 278 unaffected golfers controlled for mean age (46.2 years), playing experience (30 years), best handicap (4.5), and male gender were identified. The mean duration of the yips was six years. As in previous studies it was the short putts (<2 m) that were most affected. In addition, this group indicated that fast, downhill, and left-to-right breaking putts were most affected, perhaps suggesting forearm supination or pronation plays a role.

In the same investigation, four yips-affected golfers and three unaffected golfers were studied using EMG, grip force, and heart rate evaluations during putting (14). The yips-affected golfers had higher heart rates, more grip force on the putter, and increased EMG activity in some forearm muscles. Additionally, the yips-affected golfers made fewer putts and missed putts by greater distances than the unaffected golfers, although no statistical calculations were used to determine whether these differences reached significance (14).

Given that the yips has evolved from the golfing community, and may be a term frequently ascribed to a golfer with any number of difficulties with putting, it is not surprising that both organic and psychological factors may be considered the same. Smith et al. have proposed that the yips represent a continuum between focal dystonia (organic) and choking (psychological) (15). Following a questionnaire completed by 72 yips-affected golfers (69 males), these investigators separated the group based on survey responses. The mean age of the golfers was 52 years and mean handicap was 6.7. Based on the subjects' responses to descriptors of yips as jerking, freezing, and shaking versus nervousness or lack of confidence, each golfer was categorized: likely dystonia ($n = 40$), likely choking ($n = 16$), and not determined ($n = 16$). Although the study was greatly limited by the lack of clinical evaluations, it does suggest that the term is used broadly in the golf community (15).

Similar to the work by Kachi (11), Adler et al. studied three golfers using surface EMG recordings (16). The first golfer had a normal examination yet had EMG trains of 6 to 7 Hz rhythmic, co-contractions of the left deltoid and bicep while standing over a putt. These movements only occurred while addressing the ball and stopped once the putter was moved. The second golfer had very mild writer's cramp involving the right thumb and index finger. Surface EMG was normal when writing but revealed abnormal trains of 6 to 8 Hz rhythmic co-contracting with 75 msec bursts of EMG activity lasting 500 to 1000 msec in the right deltoid and wrist flexors when putting. The third golfer had very mild rest and terminal tremor of the hands. Surface EMG revealed trains of 4 to 7 Hz rhythmic co-contracting 150 msec bursts in the right deltoid and biceps lasting 500 to 1000 msec when holding the putter (16). This data suggested that the yips may be a dystonia, but, because it was occurring in two cases that had evidence of a movement disorder when they were not putting, further research was needed.

Adler et al. have collected pilot data utilizing surface EMG recordings in 10 yips-affected golfers and 10 unaffected golfers matched for age (mean = 50 years) and current handicap (mean = 7.2) (17). In this study, the yips-affected golfers had been golfing for a longer time (37.6 vs. 25.9 years, $p = 0.03$) and had a better best handicap (3.5 vs. 6.3, $p = 0.01$). All golfers studied were male and all used a right-hand, traditional, low putting grip. All subjects had a normal neurological examination, and no other evidence of a movement disorder. Subjects were monitored at rest, while writing, and with arms outstretched using surface EMG recordings of bilateral proximal and distal upper extremity muscles. No tremor or dystonia was detected in any subject. They were then asked to complete 75 putts (30 at 2 m, 10 at 1 m, then 35 at 2.5 m) on an indoor, artificial, flat putting green surface. EMG recordings were made while they held the putter at rest and then during each putt, with an electronic photocell recording the initiation of each stroke and the time of putter/golf ball impact (Fig. 1).

During the putting study, only 2/10 yips-affected golfers felt like they were experiencing the yips (17). By observation it appeared to the investigators that all 10 yips-affected golfers, and none of the unaffected golfers, were having a visible jerk of the wrist or twist of the forearm at the time of the forward swing of the putting stroke. When the EMG data were analyzed, there were no differences between groups in right or left forearm EMG activity, wrist flexor or extensor activity, or phasic flexor or extensor bursts of motor activity. However, at 200 msec prior to putter/ball impact, 5/10 yips-affected golfers demonstrated co-contractions of the wrist flexor and extensor muscles, a phenomenon not seen in any of the 10 unaffected golfers ($p = 0.06$, exact McNemar test) (17). This finding was consistent in all the putting conditions studied. When comparing the yips-affected golfers who had co-contraction

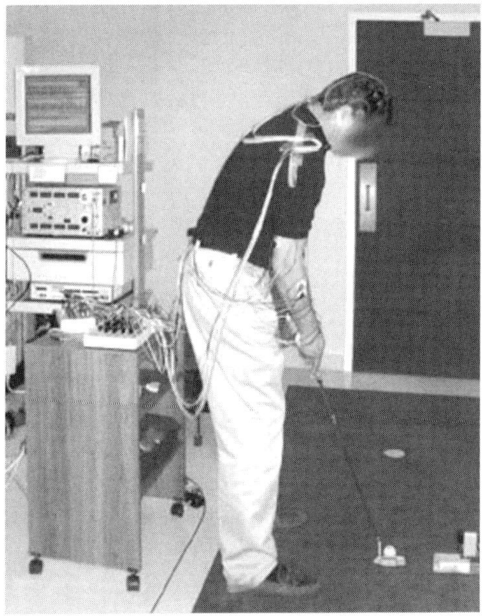

**Figure 1** Set-up for yips study.

($n = 5$) with those who did not have co-contraction ($n = 5$) there was a trend for the co-contracting golfers to be older (58 vs. 42 years), have higher handicaps (9.2 vs. 4.0), have yips for fewer years (5.5 vs. 9.2 years), have more error in terms of distance in missed putts (4.8 vs. 3.2 cm), and make fewer total putts (61% vs. 67%).

Somatosensory evoked potential (SEP) testing also demonstrated differences between the yips-affected and yips-unaffected subjects. There was evidence for higher-amplitude N30 waves in the yips-affected group that was statistically significant at one electrode with a trend at two other electrodes. Similar SEP data have been reported for cervical dystonia (18) and writer's cramp (19).

Adler et al. have concluded that the presence of co-contraction of the wrist flexor and extensor muscles in half of the yips-affected golfers but none of the unaffected golfers suggests that the yips are a focal dystonia in some cases (17). Of those with co-contractions, only two of the cases felt that they were having the yips during the study, the other three stated that they were not having any problem putting. The finding of co-contraction is known to be a hallmark for dystonia, although it is not diagnostic (20–22). Further work is therefore needed to determine whether the 50% occurrence of co-contraction is present in a larger population of yips-affected golfers. Additionally, further study of unaffected golfers to determine patterns of EMG activation is needed for comparison purposes. Studies comparing yips-affected golfers who have co-contractions with those who do not are needed, and assessment of anxiety and psychological factors should be included. Finally, attempts at treating the yips should be undertaken with monitoring of surface EMG patterns to determine subjective as well as objective response to intervention.

In terms of pathophysiology, the cause of the yips in golf remains unclear. Unfortunately, the same holds for most cases of dystonia and tremor. There are no data on the genetics or hereditary patterns of yips-affected individuals. While some authors postulate that occupational cramps (writer's and musician's cramp and other focal dystonias) are due to an overuse syndrome, this hypothesis may not be as valid for putting a golf ball. The teaching and goal of all golfers is to hold the putter with the arms swinging as a pendulum, with no movement of the hands or wrists. Yet, most golfers with the yips describe abnormal movement affecting the forearms and wrist, regions that should not be moving. Thus, this should not be overused, because the regions affected by the yips should not be moving when performing the task. Additionally, those affected by the yips do not describe any pain. There is no description of discomfort or strain as is often found.

## OTHER SPORT-RELATED DYSTONIAS

Like the yips, the recognition of sports-related cramps evolves, because physicians and athletes become more aware of the potential disorder. In addition, cultural differences may also limit the awareness and generalization of these phenomena to particular sports. However, in some settings, these symptoms are gaining diagnostic acceptance.

### Cricket

A first-person account of the yips in cricket bowling is written by Gavin Hamilton (31). Hamilton does not describe any twitch or jerk, just an inability to control the bowling. Bawden and Maynard evaluated eight athletes who were cricket bowlers (23). Mean age was 23.4 years (range 18–32) and four were amateurs, four were semiprofessionals. Average bowling experience was 11 years. The subjects all had contacted the investigators for psychological advice to overcome their loss of performance (23). All participants were interviewed in detail and none of the cricket bowlers had complaints prior to the onset of the yips. The investigators concluded that at the onset there was a physical rather than psychological problem, similar to that of the focal dystonia described in golfers (23). However, over time the investigators state that the yips of bowling became more consistent with choking and sports performance phobias, with increased anxiety and self-consciousness (5,7,23). These authors concluded that the symptoms suffered by these athletes were most consistent with a psychological rather than an organic disorder. However, there is no published neurologic evaluation of these athletes to determine if there could be an involuntary movement disorder present.

## Tennis

There is a single case report of a tennis player with bilateral segmental dystonia (24). This 34-year-old male professional tennis player began to have involuntary movements in the dominant left arm and shoulder at the age of 16. As with other dystonias, this patient was sent for months of physical therapy, psychotherapy, and had shoulder surgery. Examination revealed bilateral hand tremor, decreased fine-motor control of the left hand, and writer's cramp. Analysis of the tennis playing showed no difficulty with simulated movement or with swinging the racket freely, but when swinging at a ball there was dystonic posturing of the arm. A diagnosis of segmental dystonia was made and this patient experienced a good response to trihexiphenidyl, 10 mg/d (24). These authors also postulate that one reason for the lack of information regarding dystonia in sports may relate to the fact that other than in golf, professional athletes usually finish their careers at a fairly early age. Additionally, many sports do not require fine-motor activity of the arms, which may be the more likely region for dystonia to develop (24).

## Darts

Other athletes who have had dystonias include billiard players and dart throwers (4,25). Eric Bristow, a 5-time World Champion dart thrower, developed "dartitis" or the yips of dart throwing in his 30s (32).

## Baseball

Baseball players, mainly pitchers, have also been associated with the yips. Although there have been no scientific publications regarding the yips in baseball players several cases might be candidates for more careful study. Steve Blass of the Pittsburgh Pirates and Rick Ankiel of the St. Louis Cardinals both rather suddenly lost pitching control and had their careers ended or threatened (33). As a result of these original observations, baseball lexicon now refers to a sudden, unexplainable loss of pitching control as "Steve Blass Disease" (34). Other position players, including catchers, have had this problem. Dale Murphy began his career as a catcher with the Atlanta Braves but developed the inability to throw back to the pitcher with occasional overthrows reaching the center fielder (35). Once moved to the outfield, Dale Murphy became an all-star. Other baseball players who developed throwing difficulties included Mackey Sasser of the New York Mets, Steve Sax of the Los Angeles Dodgers, and Chuck Knoblauch of the New York Yankees (36). Knoblauch was a Gold

Glove winning second baseman who developed an inability to throw to first base (37). While some players moved from positions requiring short throws (catcher, infield) to positions requiring longer throws (outfield), this did not always keep their careers alive. Additionally, most were treated from a psychological perspective and unfortunately did not undergo movement disorders evaluation at the time to potentially improve symptoms of a highly task-specific dystonia.

## SUMMARY

In summary, there is evidence to suggest that some athletes, especially golfers, may develop a task-specific dystonia. As with some other forms of dystonia, the extent of organic and psychological factors remains unanswered. It is likely that some athletes suffer from performance anxiety alone while others have an involuntary movement disorder that is worsened by anxiety. Multidisciplinary approaches to athletes with dystonia are needed. Further research is necessary to determine the extent of this disorder as well as potential treatment options.

## REFERENCES


1. Palmer A, Dobereiner P. Arnold Palmer's Complete Book of Putting. New York: Atheneum, 1986.
2. Foster JB. Putting on the agony. World Med 1977:26–27.
3. Klawans HL. The Bantam: Ben Hogan in why Michael couldn't hit and other tales of the neurology of sports. New York: W. H. Freeman, 1996:83–108.
4. Marsden CD. The focal dystonias. Clin Neuropharmacol 1986; 9(Suppl 2):S49–S60.
5. Baumeister RF. Choking under pressure: self-consciousness and paradoxical effects of incentives on skillful performance. J Pers Soc Psychol 1984; 46(3):610–620.
6. Kingston K, Madill M, Mullen R. Yielding to internal performance stress? The yips in Golf: A review with a commentary from a player's perspective, in Science and Golf IV. Thain E, ed. London: Routledge, 2002:268–283.
7. Silva JM. Sport performance phobias. Int J Sport Psychol 1994; 25:100–118.
8. Clark RD 3rd. Evaluating the phenomenon of choking in professional golfers. Percept Mot Skills 2002; 95(3 Pt 2):1287–1294.
9. Clark RD 3rd. Do professional golfers "choke"? Percept Mot Skills 2002; 94(3 Pt 2): 1124–1130.
10. Pelz D. In: Putt like the pros. New York: Harper Perennial, 1989.
11. Kachi T et al. Writing tremor: its relationship to benign essential tremor. J Neurol Neurosurg Psychiatry 1985; 48(6):545–550.
12. McDaniel KD, Cummings JL, Shain S. The "yips": a focal dystonia of golfers. Neurology 1989; 39(2 Pt 1):192–195.
13. Sachdev P. Golfers' cramp: clinical characteristics and evidence against it being an anxiety disorder. Mov Disord 1992; 7(4):326–332.
14. Smith AM et al. A multidisciplinary study of the 'yips' phenomenon in golf: An exploratory analysis. Sports Med 2000; 30(6):423–437.
15. Smith AM et al. The 'yips' in golf: a continuum between a focal dystonia and choking. Sports Med 2003; 33(1):13–31.
16. Adler CH, Caviness JN, Crews D. The yips: an electophysiologic evaluation. Mov Disord 2002; 17(Suppl 5):S307–S308.
17. Adler CH et al. Abnormal co-contraction in yips-affected but not unaffected golfers: evidence for focal dystonia. Neurology 2005; 64(10):1813–1814.

18. Kanovsky P et al. Lateralization of the P22/N30 component of somatosensory evoked potentials of the median nerve in patients with cervical dystonia. Mov Disord 1997; 12(4):553–560.
19. Reilly JA, Hallett M, Cohen LG. The N30 component of somatosensory evoked potentials in patients with dystonia. Electroencephalogr Clin Neurophysiol 1992; 84:243–247.
20. Ghez C, Gordon J, Hening W. Trajectory control in dystonia. Adv Neurol 1988; 50: 141–155.
21. Day BL et al. Reciprocal inhibition between the muscles of the human forearm. J Physiol 1984; 349:519–534.
22. Marsden CD, Rothwell JC. The physiology of idiopathic dystonia. Can J Neurol Sci 1987; 14(Suppl 3):521–527.
23. Bawden M, Maynard I. Towards an understanding of the personal experience of the 'yips' in cricketers. J Sports Sci 2001; 19(12):937–953.
24. Mayer F et al. Bilateral segmental dystonia in a professional tennis player. Med Sci Sports Exerc 1999; 31(8):1085–1087.
25. Sheehy MP, Rothwell JC, Marsden CD. Writer's cramp, in Dystonia 2. In: Fahn S, Marsden CD, Calne DB, eds. Advances in Neurology. New York: Raven Press, 1988: 457–472.
26. http://www.merriam-webster.com, accessed October 2005.
27. http://www.golfdigest.com/search/index.ssf?/instruction/gd200410puttingyips.html, accessed November 2005.
28. http://sport.guardian.co.uk/golf/story/0,1071594,00.html, accessed November 2005.
29. http://www.finleyongolf.com/articles/YipesIveGottheYips.htm, accessed November 2005.
30. http://www.golfonline.com/golfonline/print/0,18068,468914,00.html, accessed November 2005.
31. http://observer.guardian.co.uk/osm/story/0,1182705,00.html, accessed November 2005.
32. http://observer.guardian.co.uk/osm/story/0,626797,00.html, accessed November 2005.
33. www.doubletongued.org/index.php/dictionary/yips, accessed October, 2005.
34. http://sportsillustrated.cnn.com/baseball/mlb/2001, accessed November, 2005.
35. http://www.oaklandfans.com/coopconf17.html, accessed June 2005.
36. http://www.oaklandfans.com/coopconf17.html, accessed June 2005.
37. http://www.usatoday.com/sports/bbw/2001–03–21/2001–03–21-specialchuck.htm, accessed October 2005.

# 15
# Dopa-Responsive Dystonia

**Masaya Segawa and Yoshiko Nomura**
*Segawa Neurological Clinic for Children, Tokyo, Japan*

**Nobuyoshi Nishiyama**
*Department of Laboratory of Chemical Pharmacology, Graduate School of Pharmaceutical Sciences, The University of Tokyo, Tokyo, Japan*

## INTRODUCTION

Dopa-responsive dystonia (DRD) is a clinical term first proposed by Nygaard et al. (1) and later modified by Calne (2). Initially, this term was used to describe an autosomal-dominant DRD, now termed autosomal-dominant guanosine triphosphate cyclohydrolase I (AD GCH-I) deficiency. However, it is now used more comprehensively, and refers to all dystonias responding to levodopa. This chapter will review the clinical characteristics of the DRD, but will emphasize AD GCH-I deficiency and autosomal-recessive tyrosine hydroxylase (TH) deficiency.

## AUTOSOMAL-DOMINANT GUANOSINE 5′-TRIPHOSPHATE (GTP) CYCLOHYDROLASE I (AD GCH-I) DEFICIENCY (SEGAWA DISEASE): DOMINANT-TYPE *DYT5*

### Introduction

The proper term for autosomal-dominant *DYT5* or Segawa disease is AD GCH-I deficiency. The dystonic symptoms associated with an AD GCH-I deficiency are caused by mutation of *GCH-I* gene, located on chromosome 14.q22.1 to q22.2. This disease was initially reported as hereditary progressive dystonia with marked diurnal fluctuation (HPD), an autosomal dominantly inherited generalized, postural dystonia. The hallmarks of this syndrome included onset in childhood, diurnal fluctuation of symptoms, and marked and sustained response to levodopa (3–5). Prior to molecular identification of the causes of HPD, Deonna et al. (6) termed this disorder Segawa syndrome. The descriptions included AD GCH-1 deficiency and also recessive TH deficiency or recessive *DYT5*. In 1988, Nygaard et al. (1) proposed the term DRD; the criteria later defined by Calne (2) was the same as that of HPD. Because of these reports, the literature of the 1990s uses the terms DRD or HPD/DRD in most English language journals.

Prior to the identification of the *GCH-I* gene, the symptoms of HPD had already been known to be highly age related (7), and presence of adult-onset patients without dystonia were known (7). Since the discovery of the causative gene, the phenotypical variations have been markedly expanded (8,9). Some childhood-onset patients were shown to have focal (8), segmental (10), or action dystonia (11). Other neurological conditions associated with this allele include psychiatric disorders, autism, depression, and migraine; furthermore, a group of subjects found to be compound heterozygotes showed hypotonia, failure in locomotion, and delay in mental and motor development in infancy (12). Additionally, a family with a dopa-responsive myoclonus-dystonia syndrome has been reported (13).

## Clinical Signs and Symptoms

The clinical characteristics of AD GCH-I deficiency are based on the long-term care of 14 personal cases of the authors (5,14), and the review of an additional 46 familial and 19 sporadic Japanese cases reported from 1971 to 1990 (Table 1) (7).

The initial descriptions have been expanded with continued follow-up of childhood-onset cases (15), and the phenotypic variation has been modified by studies of late-onset cases and by cases identified after the discovery of the causative gene (Table 2) (8,10–12,16).

The age of onset assessed in 43 childhood-identified cases ranged from 1 to 11 years. All but one had symptom onset of within the first decade, and the average age at onset was 6.1 +/− 2.4 years (familial cases 6.3 +/− 2.2 years and sporadic cases 5.9 +/− 2.7 years). An additional eight cases belonged to the parental generation, with an age of onset ranging from 2.6 to 34 years, including three cases with onset at 11, 18, and 34 years. Recently, a 58-year-old father of a female patient with action dystonia with onset at eight years was discovered (10). The age of onset in the remaining six patients, grandparents of affected children, ranged from 50 to 65 years, except for one subject who reported symptoms at age eight years.

Of 51 cases with onset in the first decade, the initial symptom was postural dystonia of one leg with gait disturbance in 46 cases (90.2%). The remaining

**Table 1** Clinical Characteristics of Autosomal-Dominant Guanosine Triphosphate Cyclohydrolase I Deficiency

| |
|---|
| Onset in the first decade with foot dystonia. A few cases have onset in adulthood with postural tremor |
| Marked diurnal fluctuation, which, however, attenuates with age |
| Apparent progression in the first two decades, attenuates with age; progression becomes unapparent after the fourth decade |
| The main symptom is postural dystonia with lower extremity predominance. Postural retrocollis may occur. In a few cases, action dystonia with action retrocollis with or without oculogyric crisis, focal or segmental dystonia are observed. No patients show axial torsion |
| Tremor: postural tremor with frequency of 8–10 Hz, occurring in one upper extremely and expand to all limbs and neck muscles by the fourth decade. No parkinsonian resting tremor of 4–5 Hz |
| Bradykinesia appears later. Locomotion is preserved |
| Deep tendon reflexes exaggerated in all, some with ankle clonus or striatal toe, no Babinski sign |
| Levodopa shows marked and sustained response without any unfavorable side effects. The dose of levodopa can be reduced later |
| Asymmetry is observed, in most patients with left-side predominance |
| Female predominance |
| Stagnation of the growth of body length in childhood-onset patients |
| Autosomal-dominant inheritance with low penetrance |

**Table 2** Phenotypical Variation Clarified after Detection of the Causative Gene

| |
|---|
| Focal dystonia: writer's cramp and guitarist's finger |
| Action dystonia |
| Paroxysmal dystonia |
| Spontaneous reduction and exacerbation of dystonia |
| Dystonic spasm with or without pain |
| Oculogyric crisis |
| Muscle hypotonia with delay in development in crawling |
| Delay in development of language |
| Complete recovery only after the administration of 5-hydrosytryptophan or tetrahydrobiopterin |
| Psychological symptoms: autism and depression |
| Migraine |

five cases (9.8%) presented with postural dystonia of the hand (three), hand tremor (one), or leaning of the trunk (one). In eight late-onset cases, postural tremor, gait disturbance, or both were the initial symptoms. Tremor was observed in 13 cases (20%). Although tremor did occur before 10 years in 3 of 13 cases, in most instances tremor developed beyond the age of 10 years; four developed tremor prior to the age of 20 years and six after 30 years of age. Tremor is not observed in patients receiving levodopa prior to 10 years of age. Slowness in movement or bradykinesia was observed in all cases, and with progression, showed retropulsion, hypomimia, and dysarthria.

Diurnal fluctuation of symptoms is observed in all with onset in childhood. The neurological symptoms aggravate toward the evening and recover markedly in the morning after sleep. In the early stages of childhood, there was almost a complete recovery, but the grade of fluctuation of dystonia attenuated with age. In cases with onset in early childhood body length fails to grow normally with the onset of dystonia and becomes short stature in the ages of late teen.

## Neurological Examinations

With the exception of the motor examination, the neurological examination in people with DRD is essentially unremarkable. The tendon reflexes are brisk and ankle clonus may be observed, but the plantar reflexes are flexor. Although, some patients exhibit sustained dorsiflexion of the toe, this "striatal toe sign" is not elicited by plantar stimulation, and is associated with basal ganglia involvement. Although muscle stretch reflexes demonstrate a rigid hypertonus, there is no plastic rigidity, and repeated testing will produce fluctuations in tone. There may be a high-frequency postural tremor (8–10 Hz), but a Parkinson-type, resting tremor has not been reported. These clinical signs show asymmetry, but the pattern of involvement of the sternocleidomustoideus (SCM) differs between rigidity and tremor. That is, the side of predominant affected in the SCM is contralateral to that of extremities in rigidity, while it is ipsilateral in tremor. Bradykinesia or postural instability may emerge with advancing symptoms of dystonia. Freezing phenomena or the "marche a petit pas" of Parkinson's disease (PD) is not seen, and locomotion is preserved throughout the course of illness. There are neither cerebellar signs nor sensory disturbances.

## Clinical Course

The clinical symptoms of AD GCH-I deficiency vary with age of onset. Typically, symptoms begin in childhood with a postural dystonia involving a lower extremity, mostly as *pes equinovarus*. This symptom often expands to all limbs by 10 to 15 years of age with aggravation of dystonic hypertonus. Around the age of 10 years, the postural tremor appears in one upper extremity. Dystonia progression tends to slow with age and becomes almost stationary by the fourth decade. Postural tremor continues to spread to other limbs; around the fourth decade, it appears on all extremities, including the neck muscles. Importantly, the diurnal fluctuation, particularly that associated with dystonia, declines with age. It may not be readily apparent by the age of 20 years, and almost disappears in the fourth decade. However, the asymmetry of symptoms persists throughout the course of illness.

It is noteworthy that the progression of this disease also varies with the age of onset. Patients developing symptoms in the second decade tend to start with dystonia of the upper limbs with or without postural tremor. Those with onset in adulthood start with hand tremor without dystonia and diurnal fluctuation. Although there is mild rigid hypertonus, it shows no apparent progression. Exaggeration of tendon reflexes is a characteristic feature of child patients, and short stature is not observed in patients with onset after late childhood or adolescence. The asymmetry of symptoms is commonly observed without any relation to the age of onset (17).

## Clinical Variation

Besides the phenotypical variation related to age at onset, the discovery of the gene has greatly expanded the spectrum of this presentation (Table 2) (7). While postural dystonia is the hallmark of AD GCH-I deficiency, there were families with some patients who show action dystonia involving the upper extremity or the neck, usually as retrocollis. In a review of 28 gene-proved patients from 15 families, five patients from three families had action dystonia besides postural dystonia. Furthermore, paroxysmal dystonia, dystonic cramp, and oculogyric crisis were observed in patients with action dystonia (10,17). This suggests a possibility of effects of the loci of mutation in the *GCH-I* gene on this phenotypical variation (10,17). Other symptoms, such as depression, migraine, autism, hypotonia, failure in locomotion, and delay in mental and motor development may be related to depletion of serotonin (5HT) in early developmental course, which could occur with marked deficiency of GCH-I. The heterogeneity of symptoms in this disorder appears to be related to age at onset, pathophysiological differences probably due to the loci of mutation, and the grade of the involvement of serotonergic neurons (10).

## Treatment and Prognosis

In most cases, a dose of 20 mg/kg per day of levodopa without decarboxylase inhibitor alleviates the symptoms completely (14,15). With decarboxylase inhibitors, the corresponding doses are 4 to 5 mg/kg per day. Some patients starting treatment with plain levodopa without decarboxylase inhibitor before 10 years tend to decrease the responsiveness to plain levodopa after around 13 years (15). Older-onset subjects do not always respond to levodopa alone. To these patients levodopa with decarboxylase inhibitor is recommended. In a few cases choreic movements develop by a rapid increase of dosage or by administration of a higher dose of levodopa in initial stage of treatment, but these symptoms respond to dosage reduction (14). In cases with action dystonia, action retrocollis and oculogyric crisis may be aggregated by initial doses. In cases with compound heterozygote, aggravation of dystonia by initial dosage is prominent (12). In these patients after titration to an optimal dosage, the effect of levodopa is sustained, rarely requiring adjustment, and usually without unfavorable side effects (12,14,15). Levodopa is effective in almost all cases, and often, may be reduced after the age of 30 years (15).

Anticholinergic drugs may have a marked and prolonged effect, but do not afford a complete relief, either clinically or polysomnographically. However, anticholinergic drugs are helpful in cases with oculogyric crisis (15). Amantadine has proven beneficial for levodopa-related chorea (18). Bromocriptine is also effective but does not provide complete relief (19). Tetrahydrobiopterin ($BH_4$) treatment was attempted on HPD/DRD patients, (20–24) but with the exception of one case report, no favorable effects have been obtained with $BH_4$ monotherapy (21). In a case with compound heterozygote, administration of $BH_4$ is necessary for complete recovery (12).

Prior to the introduction of levodopa as a treatment regimen, unilateral stereotactic pallidotomy and nucleus ventralis lateralis (VL) thalamotomy were performed in one female patient. Lifetime follow-up information was available in this patient with the onset of dystonia at the age of six years, later proved to have a mutation of *GCH-I gene* (25). The pallidotomy performed at 30 years improved postural dystonia and dystonic spasm. Ipsilateral VL thalamotomy seven years later was effective on postural tremor. However, the effect of the pallidotomy on postural dystonia was incomplete, and the VL thalamotomy showed no further beneficial effects on the postural dystonia that remained after the pallidotomy. Levodopa started at the age of 41 years showed marked effects. The effect was complete on the non operated side, while it was not complete on the operated side. These effects continued without any side effects until 71 years when she was deceased.

## Investigation

### *Biochemical studies*

Serial spinal fluid examination of catecholamine metabolites reveals low levels of homovanillic acid (HVA) throughout the day, but afternoon concentrations were less than that in samples collected in the early morning (26–29). Both biopterin and neopterin levels in the cerebrospinal fluid (CSF) are markedly below (20%) the normal range (24,30–32). Moderate reduction of these substances is also observed (about 30–50% of normal levels) in CSF of asymptomatic carriers of AD GCH-I deficiency (33).

Ichinose et al. (34) estimates the activity of GCH I in the mononuclear blood cells of patients with AD GCH-I deficiency to be less than 20% of those in normal individuals, while asymptomatic carriers reached 30% to 40% of normal levels. Phenylalanine-loading tests in both child and adult patients reveal a six-hour increase in phenylalanine levels (35). In addition, the phenylalanine to tyrosine ratio levels remain elevated during the postloading period, while biopterin levels decline, suggesting that the decrease in liver phenylalanine hydroxylase activity may be due to defective $BH_4$.

### *Neuroimaging*

MRI and CT scans of the brain show no abnormalities, while PET scanning demonstrates normal or low normal ($^{18}$F) dopa uptake levels (36–38). Patients with onset at older ages (39) and an asymptomatic carrier (40) also showed normal levels. These results suggest a functional deficit of dopamine (DA) metabolism, specifically concerning decrease in the hydroxylation of tyrosine and preservation of the activities of aromatic acid decarboxylase (36). While $^{[11}$C$^{]}$ raclopride PET shows normal activity in symptomatic subjects (41), $^{[11}$C$^{]}$ N-spiperone PET reveals mild increase in receptor binding (42,43). Interestingly, no increase in receptor binding was demonstrated in follow-up PET analysis after seven months of levodopa therapy (42). Thus, the increase of DA $D_2$-receptor binding is not considered a factor determining the clinical state of AD GCH-I deficiency (42). Furthermore, ($^{123}$I) ß-CIT SPECT scanning is normal in this condition, suggesting that impairment of the DA transporter molecule does not seem to play a role in this disease (44).

*Neurophysiological Studies*

Polysomnography (PSG) in subjects who were later shown to have heterozygous for the *GCH-I* gene mutation revealed abnormalities of the DA regulated, phasic components of sleep. These changes include a decrease in the number of gross movements and twitch movements (TMs), and an increase in rapid eye movement (REM) activity. Sleep structure, percent sleep stages, and other parameters modulated by the brainstem aminergic neurons remain normal (4,45,46). The phasic components of sleep are modulated by the basal ganglia and the nigrostriatal (NS)-DA neuron, while the number of TM during REM sleep reflect NS-DA neuronal activity (45,46). Normally, REM-associated TM decline with age and decremental nocturnal variation with sleep cycle.

In AD GCH-I deficiency age and the nocturnal variations of the TM are preserved, but the amount of TM decline to approximately 20% of normal values (16,47). In addition, horizontal REM demonstrate side preference toward the side with predominantly affected limbs (16,47,48). Although similar findings have been noted in case of hemi-parkinsonism, (16,47) studied on four subjects with hemidystonia demonstrated horizontal REM directed away from the affected side (16,47,48).

Other neurophysiologic assessments include measurement of saccadic eye movements and magnetic stimulation. Neuro-ophthalmologic evaluation reveals abnormalities in both visually guided and memory-guided voluntary saccades, and implicates involvement of both the direct and the indirect pathways (49,50). Besides hyperactive nigro-collicular inhibition associated with slowing in both memory-guided and visually guided saccades, disinhibition of the superior colliculi has been postulated by failure in suppression of unnecessary saccade in memory-guided task. Supracranial magnetic stimulation was normal, showing preservation of the corticospinal tract (51).

*Brain pathology and histochemistry*

Neuropathological and neurohistochemical study was available of an 18-year-old woman with DRD who died in a traffic accident, (52,53) and later proven to be AD GCH-I deficiency by DNA analysis (54). Neuropathological examination revealed no abnormalities except decrease in melanin pigmentation of the neuron of the pars compacta of the substania nigra, particularly in the ventral tier of it. Histochemically, DA content was reduced in the pars compacta in the substantia nigra and striatum. Similar to PD, the reduction was greater in the putamen than in the caudate nucleus, and subregionally, more in the rostral caudate and the caudal putamen. In contrast to PD this case showed a greater DA loss in the ventral subdivision of the rostral caudate than its dorsal counterpart, and the activity and protein content of TH was decreased only in the striatum, while it was within the normal range in the substantia nigra (53).

Furukawa et al. (55) report similar findings in two autopsied brains. Although the DA content in the striatum was not reported, these investigators did show marked reduction of total biopterin (84%) and neopterin (62%) in the putamen, despite normal concentration of aromatic acid-decarboxylase, DA transporter and vesicular monoamine transporter. Additional postmortem study of an asymptomatic carrier by these investigators found modest reduction of TH protein (52%) and DA (44%), despite marked reduction of striatal biopterin (by 82%) (56).

*Molecular Biological Studies*

Nygaard et al. (57) mapped the DRD locus to a 22cM region, between *D14S47* (14q11.2-q22) and *D 14S63* (14q11-q24.3) on chromosome 14q. Ichinose et al. (34) examined patients with AD GCH-I deficiency and confirmed this mutation involved the *GCH-I gene* located on 14q22.1-q22.2 (57). Although more than 100 independent mutations have now been identified in the coding region of *GCH-I*, no changes are seen within affected pedigrees, which differs among families but is identical in one family (8,34,58). The rate of mutant GCH-I mRNA production against normal RNA was 28% in a patient but it was 8.3% in the asymptomatic carrier (59,60). The extensive genetic evaluation, combined with spinal fluid study of the biopterin and neopterin levels and mononucleocyte GCH-I levels in asymptomatic carriers, have confirmed that HPD/DRD is an autosomal dominantly inherited GCH-I deficiency with low penetrance (34,40,61).

Molecular analysis remains unable to determine mutations of the coding region of the gene in approximately 40% of subjects with GCH-I deficiency (62). In some of these subjects abnormalities in intron genomic deletion, (58,63) a large gene deletion, (64) an intragenic duplication or inversion of *GCH-I*, or mutation in as yet undefined regulatory gene modifying enzyme function may be important (62).

## Pathophysiology

Although the pathogenetic mechanisms for dominant inheritance are unknown, a classic dominant-negative effect (65,66) and destabilizing effect have been considered (67). The wide variations in clinical expression depend on a number of factors, including the locus of the genetic mutation and ratio of mutant versus normal gene in the area of active neurological substrate. The ratio of mutant/wild-type GCH-I mRNA in lymphocytes was higher in an affected individual than an unaffected heterozygote, and varies depending on the locus of the mutation (60,67,68). Furthermore, the ratio differed among affected individuals in some families, depending on the locus of the mutation (60,68). This suggests that the degree and the pattern of inactivation of normal enzyme by mutant gene differ among the locus of mutation (60,68) and may cause inter- and intrafamilial variation of the phenotype as well as the rate of penetrance as the locus of mutation differs among families.

GCH-I is the rate-limiting enzyme for the synthesis of $BH_4$, the coenzyme for synthesis of TH and also tryptophan hydroxylase. In AD GCH-I deficiency the TH appears to be preferentially affected when compared to tryptophan hydroxylase. This could be explained by the difference in distribution of GCH-I mRNA in DA and 5HT neurons (69) or the destabilization of the molecule of TH or impairment of axonal transport (56). There is the difference of $K_m$ value for TH and tryptophan hydroxylase (70). With heterozygotic mutant gene, the $BH_4$ decreases partially in AD GCH-I deficiency. Thus, TH with higher affinity to $BH_4$ is affected rather selectively. In molecular conditions with marked decrease of $BH_4$, both tryptophan hydroxylase and TH are affected, producing symptoms induced by deficiencies of the 5HT neurons.

Complete and sustained response to levodopa, especially given the absence of morphological changes, further suggests that the lesion in AD GCH-I deficiency is restricted to the NS-DA neurons (5,14). The onset in the first decade of life and the age-related clinical course correlates to the decremental age variation of the activities of TH at the terminals of the NS-DA neuron in the caudate nucleus (71). Neurohistochemistry studies confirm the decrease of the TH protein and its activities at the terminal, and the PSGs suggested that the TH activities at the terminal follow the decremental age and nocturnal variation of normal individuals with low levels but without progressive decrement of the activities (16,47). TH activity of the NS-DA neurons also shows circadian oscillation in the terminals (71). However, these age- (71) and state-dependent variations (71,72) are not observed in the substantia nigra or the perikaryon of the nigrostriatal DA neuron (71,72). These features suggest that AD GCH-I deficiency is not a progressive or degenerative disorder and the NS-DA neurons preserve their fundamental functions.

Study of GCH-I activity in stimulated mononuclear blood cells show age dependent, decreasing activity in the first three decades of life (73). Furukawa and Kish (74) measured brain biopterin levels in 57 normal subjects ranging in age from one day to 92 years and have demonstrated increasing putamenal biopterin levels in the postnatal period, reaching a plateau at 1 to 13 years of age, before declining in adulthood. In addition, pteridine metabolism has a critical period beginning early in infancy and extending to early childhood (75). These results imply important roles for GCH-I and $BH_4$ for neuronal development in the first and the second decades of life.

Studies on the compartmental substructure of the human striatum revealed that within the rostral caudate, in particular, the medial/ventral portions, the striosomes/patches, or $D_1$-direct pathways are more numerous, whereas in the dorsal/lateral portions the matrix compartment is more homogenous (76,77). Hornykiewicz (53) suggests that the DA loss in AD GCH-I deficiency is more prominent in the striosomes/patches compartment, the terminal for the $D_1$ receptor. Clinically, it is suggested that the $D_1$-direct pathways mature earlier than the $D_2$-indirect pathways (78). However, dopa-responsive growth arrest seen in children with AD GCH-I deficiency is a reflection of the tuberoinfundibular $D_4$-receptor involvement. The $D_4$ receptor belongs to the $D_2$-receptor family, which, however, matures early among $D_2$ families (79). Thus, the DA neuron in which the DA synthesis is modulated by pteridine metabolism might regulate DA receptors that mature early in the developmental course.

Tremor is levodopa responsive but develops independently, from symptoms of dystonia. The side predominance of tremor is identical to dystonic hypertonus in the extremities while it is contralateral in the SCM. These suggest a different pathophysiology of tremor from that of dystonia and postulate locus of responsible lesion in the downstream of the striatum. Kreis et al. showed that the DA neuron mediates the subthalamic nucleus (STN) via the $D_1$ receptor located on the nucleus (80,81). Thus, for tremor the DA neuron innervating to the STN with $D_1$ receptor is postulated to be involved (10,48). For generation of the rhythmic discharge of tremor the circuits consisted with the STN and two globus pallidusis are considered. In addition, response of the tremor to stereotactic VL thalamotomy suggests involvement of the ascending pathway to the VL nucleus of the thalamus (10,25). Given that ascending pathways to the thalamus develop later than the descending pathways (76), increasing age may be a factor for development of tremor. Further support for the $D_1$-receptor-mediated hypothesis stems from PET findings of preserved function of $D_2$ receptors, (41–43) and suggests that the striatal indirect pathway does not play a role in the generation of symptoms.

However, PSGs of AD GCH-I deficiency patients with action dystonia suggested DA-receptor supersensitivity besides the involvements of the indirect pathways (46). The same situation as the hypersensitivity of the $D_2$ receptor could be explained by the hypofunction of the STN. Thus for development of the action dystonia, and related phenotypes, hypofunction of the DA neurons projecting to the STN with $D_1$ receptor is postulated.

Although neurochemically distinct from AD GCH-I deficiency, neurophysiologic procedures in *DYT1* patients may provide evidence for understanding pathway involvement in postural and action dystonia (82). Altering the descending pathway of basal ganglia to the brainstem reticular formation through posteroventral pallidotomy (83) or deep brain stimulation to the pallidum is effective in treating symptoms of postural dystonia. For action dystonia the ventralis oralis posterior thalamotomy is effective (10,11,84).

Thus, for postural dystonia the descending pathway of the basal ganglia to the brainstem reticular formation and for action dystonia the ascending pathways of the basal ganglia to the specific nucleus, e.g., the Voa nucleus of the thalamus are considered to be involved (10,11).

The 5HT neuron involves modulation of locomotion and postural tone as well as of behavioral function. The hypotonia and failure in locomotion, that is, crawling observed in patients with compound heterozygotes (12) are associated with deficiency of the 5HT-regulated activities. Preservation of interlimb coordination or locomotion in AD GCH-I deficiency may depend on the preservation of the descending output of the basal ganglia to the pedunculo pontine nucleus (PPN) (10,48,85). Moreover, early disturbance of the postural tone and locomotion may affect the PPN that induces dysfunction of the DA neurons of the substantia nigra and the ventrotegmental area (86). This may induce DA dysfunction other than that caused by GCH-I deficiency and may relate severity of symptoms and the early occurrence of dyskinesia in these patients.

Although there is loss of striatal TH protein, in the substantia nigra TH protein was normal in two autosomal-dominant GHC-I deficiency patients. Furukawa et al. (55) suggest that $BH_4$ may control protein stability rather than expression. Leff et al. (87) presented gene transfer data and suggested a role for stabilization of TH protein by coexpression of *GCH-I* in vivo. Sumi-Ichinose et al. (88) showed loss of TH protein but not of TH mRNA in the brains of $BH_4$-deficient mice.

These extensive and diverse data suggest that AD GCH-I deficiency leads to the decrease of the TH protein or DA in the ventral area of the striatum. This in turn causes disfacilitation of the $D_1$ striatal direct pathway, and disinhibits the output projection of the internal segment of the globus pallidus and pars reticulata of the substantia nigra, which suppress the reticulospinal tract and the superior colliculus. Reticulospinal tract suppression may cause postural dystonia with exaggeration of the tendon reflexes without extensor plantar reflexes. However, the output projection to the PPN may not be affected, so the locomotion is preserved. Whereas, with involvement of the DA neuron innervating to the STN with $D_1$ receptor, the ascending outputs to the thalamus are disfacilitated and develop tremor and action dystonia. Focal and segmental dystonia observed in patients with action dystonia may be caused by dysfunction of the motor cortex due to disinhibition of the thalamocortical pathway. This process may also involve the failure in suppression of unnecessary saccade in memory-guided task.

The pathophysiologies of AD GCH-I deficiency are shown in Figure 1, type of postural dystonia in (a) and that of action dystonia in (b).

Ichinose et al. (34) showed that the base levels of GCH-I in the mononuclear blood cells were higher in males, but this has yet to be confirmed. Furukawa et al. (89) showed a much higher penetrance in females (87%) than in males (38%), and similar results have

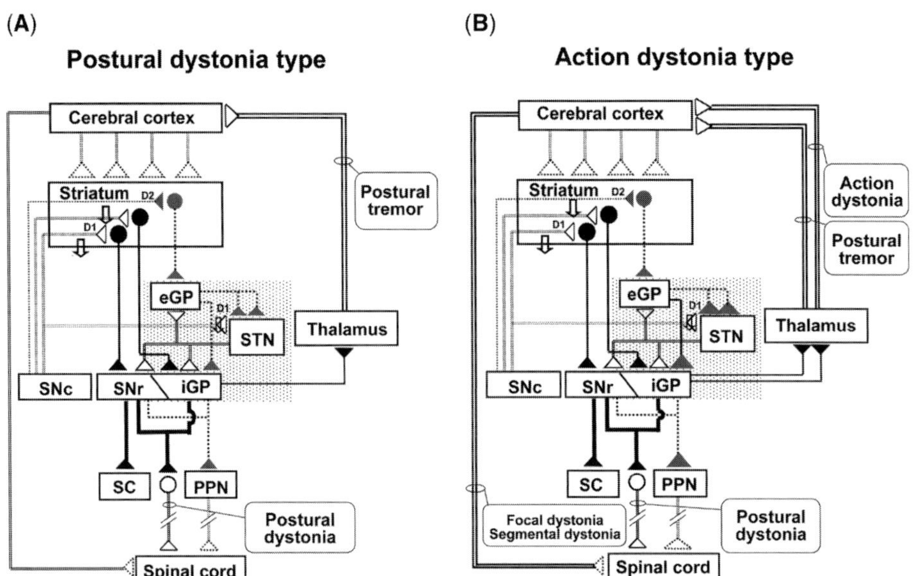


**Figure 1** (**A**) Postural dystonia type. (**B**) Action dystonia type. *Abbreviations*: eGP, external segment of globus pallidus; iGP, internal segment of globus pallidus; STN, subthalamic nucleus; SNc, substantia nigra pars compacta; SNr, substantia nigra pars reticulata; SC, superior colliculus; PPN, pedunculopontine nucleus. *Symbols*: solid, single and open lines denote pathways involved in pathophysiology; the width shows degree of activities, dotted lines denote pathways not involved in pathophysiology; single line denotes inhibitory neuron; open line denotes excitatory neuron; closed triangle denotes inhibitory neuron; open triangle denotes excitatory neuron; shaded region with dots denotes the area of the circuit for postural tremor.

been seen in the authors' 47 subjects: the ratios of symptomatic carriers were 26/30 (87%) in females and 6/17 (35%) in males. Thus, marked female predominance might depend on a genetically determined gender difference of the DA neuron (90).

Further studies are necessary to confirm these speculations. In addition, it is necessary to clarify the pathophysiology with which a heterozygous maturation of the *GCH-I* gene decreases TH protein in the striatum and affects particular NS-DA neurons and the neuronal pathways of the basal ganglia depending on the locus of the mutation.

## Diagnosis

Confirming the diagnosis of DRD is usually not difficult in the setting of characteristic clinical symptoms. The phenylalanine-loading test is helpful, but may yield a false-negative result, while the estimation of GCH-I activity in peripheral nucleated cells is more accurate, but technically complicated. Thus, estimation of neopterin and biopterin levels in CSF is the most reliable for diagnosis.

## Differential Diagnosis

All children with gait disturbance and limb dystonia should be evaluated for AD GCH-I deficiency. Other conditions with this clinical presentation may include Wilson's disease, Hallervorden–Spatz disease, hereditary spastic paraplegia, and cerebral palsy. AD GCH-I deficiency is often misdiagnosed as hereditary spastic paraplegia. In addition, Duchenne muscular dystrophy, psychological reaction, or hysteria has been considered as an initial diagnosis. However, the differentiation of AD GCH-I deficiency from these disorders is usually not difficult with careful clinical examination, but for atypical patients estimation of CSF pteridine metabolites is recommended (61).

Cases with axial torsion dystonia, including early-onset autosomal-dominant torsion dystonia (*DYT1*), differ clinically from AD GCH-I deficiency in the pattern of involvement of the SCM and muscles of the extremities; the side of the SCM predominantly affected is contralateral to that of the limb muscles in AD GCH-I deficiency, while it is ipsilateral in dystonias with axial torsion (11,45,46). This difference in the side preference reflects changes in the NS-DA neurons in AD GCH-I deficiency instead of the striatum or the pallidum in torsion dystonia. With a functional or morphological lesion in the striatum or the pallidum cases with torsion dystonia show axial torsion and consequently do not respond to levodopa. However, it should be taken into consideration that AD GCH-I deficiency and also *DYT1* may appear with focal or segmental dystonia without general dystonia in adolescence or adulthood.

### Dopa-Responsive Dystonia Other Than Autosomal-Dominant Guanosine Triphosphate Cyclohydrolase I Deficiency

This group includes recessive disorders of pteridin metabolism and recessive TH deficiencies (recessive *DYT5*). All of the inherited disorders of pteridine metabolism develop levodopa-responsive dystonia caused by decrease of $BH_4$ in infancy and early childhood as in AD GCH-I deficiency (91). However, they show postural hypotonia and psychological disturbances caused by the deficiency of 5HT activities.

### Dopa-Responsive Dystonia Parkinsonism

All of juvenile parkinsonism (JP) is included in this group. They show parkinsonian plastic rigidity and/or resting tremor predominantly, but appear as dystonia when they occur in childhood to early teens. Although dystonia of JP responds briskly to levodopa, dyskinesia develops soon after levodopa is started. Among JPs that are caused by the parkin gene (*PARK II*) it is particularly important to differentiate from AD GCH-I deficiency.

In addition, some patients with AD GCH-I deficiency develop symptoms later in life (e.g., the 50s and 60s). In this population, tremor and gait disturbance are the primary signs, and dystonia is absent or not prominent (7,92). In these patients diurnal fluctuation is not observed (7,92), and often misdiagnosed as PD (7,10,14). However, the tremor in these cases is mainly postural and their clinical features are milder with minimal progression. ($^{18}$F) Dopa Positron Emission tomography (PET) scan and ($^{11}$C) spiperone PET scan in these late-onset adult cases reveal normal uptake rate, as observed in childhood-onset AD GCH-I deficiency (10). In these patients, all symptoms including tremor, exhibit marked and sustained responses to small doses of levodopa.

## RECESSIVE DISTURBANCE OF PTERIDINE METABOLISM

Metabolic maps of pteridine metabolism and its relation to synthesis of dopamine are shown in Figure 2.

The enzymes deficiency of which cause DRD are shown with wide letters. Details of each deficiency are shown below.

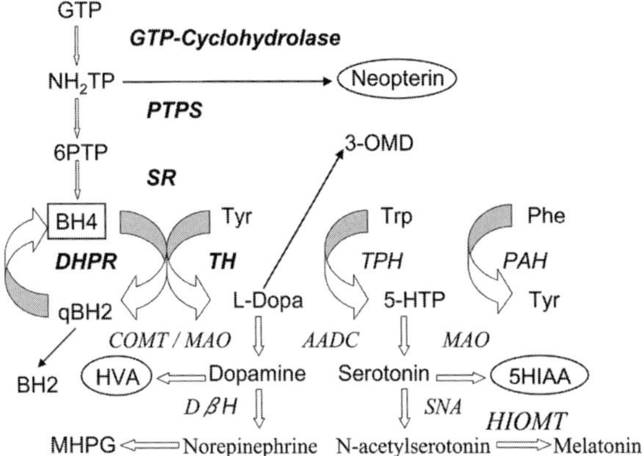


**Figure 2** Inherited defects affecting the synthesis and catabolism of the serotonin and the catecholamines. *Abbreviations*: GTP, guanosine triphosphate; NH2TP, dihydroneopterin triphosphate; PTPS, 6-pyruvoyltetrahydropterin synthase; 6PTP, 6-pyruvoyltetrahydropterin; SR, sepiapterin reductase; BH4, tetrahydrobiopterin; DHPR, dihydropteridine reductase; qBH2, quinonoid dihydrobiopterin; BH2, 7-dihydrobiopterin; Phe, phenylalanine; PAH, phenylalanine hydroxylase; Tyr, tyrosin; Trp, tryptophan; TPH, tryptophan dydroxylase; 5-HTP, 5-hydroxytryptophan; TH, tyrosine hydroxylase; COMT, catechol-O-methyltransferase; 3OMD, 3-O-methyldopa; 5HIAA, 5-hydroxyindoleacetic acid; MAO, monoamine oxidase; HVA, homovanillic acid; MHPG, 3-methoxy-4-hydroxyphenylglycol; SNA, serotonin *N*-acetyltransferase; HIOMT, hydroxyindole-O-methyltransferase; AADC, aromatic L-amino acid decarboxylase. The bars show the position of known inherited defects.

## Recessive GTP Cyclohydrolase I Deficiency

Recessive GTP cyclohydrolase I deficiency is a rare disease among tetrahydropterin deficiencies (93). This disease was initially reported in infants with severe motor and mental retardation, hypotonia of the trunk and the extremities, convulsions, and frequent episodes of hyperthermia without infection (94). These signs suggest severe disturbance of 5HT neurons, and mask the hypertonus caused by DA deficiency. Diagnosis is confirmed by marked decrease of neopterin, biopterin, pterin, isoxanthine, DA, and 5HT in the urine, and decreased CSF HVA, 5-hydroxyindole acetic acid (5-HIAA), neopterin, and biopterin (94). Treatment with L-erythro tetrahydrobiopterin has been demonstrated to be effective, but the D-erythro tetrahydropterin form does not produce clinical benefit (94).

## Recessive Pyruvoyltetrahydropterin Synthase Deficiency

The most common form of $BH_4$ deficiency is 6-pyruvoyltetrahydropterin synthase (PTPS) deficiency (93), and one of the causes of hyperphenylalaninemia (HPA) (95). This disorder is frequently observed in Taiwan Chinese (96).

Symptoms appear in infancy with delay in motor and mental development, hypotonia, abnormal involuntary movements, and seizures. Choreoathetoid movements may not improve, despite good control of HPA (97), and interlimb coordination is poor (98). Limb dystonia becomes apparent later in childhood or in adolescence. Diurnally fluctuating dystonia is also observed in the eyelids, oromandibular region, and trunk (98). In contrast to dominant GCH-I deficiency this fluctuation is observed even in adults over 30 years of age (98). Diagnosis is performed by urine analysis by high-performance liquid chromatography to demonstrate increase of neopterin and decrease of biopterin.

Levodopa with $BH_4$ (97,98) and with $BH_4$5-hydroxytryptophan (5-HTP) (99) produces dramatic and sustained effects. However, Tanaka et al. (100) observed on-off phenomenon in a 10-year-old Japanese girl with oral levodopa (2 mg/kg per day). The motor fluctuations improved after continuous intravenous infusion of levodopa at plasma concentrations in 120 to 150 mg/dL. $BH_4$ supplementation with restriction of high-protein foods reduced HPA, but not improve did motor symptoms. Because 5-HTP is associated with improved cognitive testing (101), early treatment with combination of $BH_4$, levodopa, and 5-HTP is recommended (101).

*Molecular Genetics*

Forty-three mutant alleles associated with deficiency of DA and 5HT, have been identified on chromosome 11q22.3-q23.3 (102). A patient with the homozygous *K219E* allele had transient HPA (103). Upon cotransfection of two *PTPS* alleles, the *N47D* allele had a dominant-negative affect on both the wild-type *PTPS* and the *D116G* mutant, which had around 66% of the mild-type activity with relative reduction to about 20% of control values (104). This suggests the possibility of existence of autosomal-dominant *PTPS* deficiency.

*Pathophysiology*

In PTPS deficiency 5HT and DA demonstrate decreased activity. The 5HT neuron has important roles for development of the central nervous system and modulation of the postural tone and locomotion in early infancy. The decrease in activities of the TH caused by $BH_4$ deficiency is considered to be restricted at the terminal of the NS-DA neuron as observed in AD GCH-I deficiency. With this lesion, DA deficiency does not cause any disturbance of the higher cortical function (HCF) as in AD GCH-I deficiency. The decrease of the DA activity in PTPS deficiency has no effects in development of the mental activity, and mental retardation, hypotonia, and failure in locomotion are results from 5HT deficiency. The 5HT neuron modulating the postural tone and locomotion is involved in the development of the HCF in the later two-third of infancy. Perhaps similar to girls with Rett syndrome, the deficiency of the 5HT neuron which causes postural hypotonia and failure of locomotion leads to the disturbance of the PPN and consequently affects the DA neuron of the substantia nigra (86). These DA defects in the substantia nigra occurred secondarily, which might affect the development of the frontal cortex. Early recognition and treatment for 5HT deficiency are cardinal for preventing the HCF in PTPS deficiency.

## Recessive Sepiapterin Reductase Deficiency

Bonafe et al. (105) reported two patients with progressive early-childhood psychomotor retardation and dystonia associated with severe reduction of 5-HIAA and HVA metabolites and high levels of biopterin and dihydrobiopterin in the CSF. The children also exhibit normal urinary pterines and without HPA. Analysis of skin fibroblast clarified inactive sepiapterin reductase (SR) that was confirmed by mutations in the *SR* gene.

Neville et al. (106) presented additional seven patients with two pairs of siblings from Malta. They presented with motor delay in infancy and severe cognitive impairments and sleep effect became apparent in early childhood. Diurnal variation of motor impairment was clear in all cases. Oculogyric crisis was observed in six of these children. In addition to retrocollis in several of the cases, one exhibited extensor tonic attack of the neck and trunk in infancy without oculogyric crisis. In five cases limb dystonia was observed, two in infancy and three in childhood. Two showed parkinsonian tremor in two to three months and seven months of age, respectively, and the other two had choreic movements in childhood. In three bulbar involvement became apparent in infancy or childhood. One patient shuffled on her bottom until the age of three to four years suggesting abnormalities in locomotion.

Although minor motor problems persisted, levodopa showed dramatic effects on dystonia, tremor, and oculogyric crisis, and six of the seven cases became able to walk. Careful adjustment of the dosage was a need to balance improvement in dystonic against aggravation of chorea. Unfortunately, the progressive intellectual disturbances do not respond to levodopa.

At molecular level, it is due to a single gene defect causing SR deficiency (*IVS-II, 2G*) and the mutation of the second nucleotide in the second exon–intron junction is thought to impair transcription processing and diminish sepiapterin messenger RNA levels [Farrugia R, Scern CA, Montalto SA, et al. Molecular pathology of tetrahydrobiopterin (BH4) deficiency in the Maltese population]. Deficiency of SR affects the alternative pathways of the cofactor $BH_4$ via carbonyl, aldose and dihydrofolate reductases. As a consequence of the low dihydrofolate reductase activity in the brain, dihydrobiopterin intermediately accumulates in the brain and inhibits TH and tryptophan hydroxylase and uncouples nitric oxide synthase leading to deficiency of DA and 5HT and possibly to neuronal cell death (107); while with high dihydrofolate reductase in peripheral tissues, HPA does not occur.

### Recessive Dihydropteridin Reductase Deficiency

Although the incidence of recessive dihydropteridine reductase (R-DHPR) deficiency among $BH_4$ deficiencies are not small (93) case reports of R-DHPR deficiency were rare. A Japanese boy reviewed by Nomura et al. (91) started symptoms at two months of age with dystonic posture in action or taking a certain posture that worsens toward the evening or with longevity of the wakening periods. The boy's motor development was delayed and was able to sit at one year of age. Mental retardation was also observed. Muscle tone at rest remained hypotonic at three years. While anticholinergic drugs aggravated these symptoms, the dystonic movements partially, but transiently, improved with levodopa. Around the age of 14 years, epilepsy developed. Although marked and sustained improvement has been seen with the coadministration of $BH_4$ and levodopa in these patients, there are also reports revealing negative effects of $BH_4$ on DHPR deficiency patients with mutant DHPR molecules (108). Biochemical examination of blood showed moderate HPA and marked increase of plasma biopterin with normal neopterin levels. CSF examination showed below normal neopterin and normal levels of biopterin and marked decrease of HVA and 5HIAA levels.

## RECESSIVE TYROSINE HYDROXYLASE DEFICIENCY

Recessive TH deficiency was first reported by Castaigne et al. (109) and was demarcated as DRD by Rondot et al. (110). Deonna (6) described this disorder as Segawa syndrome with the dominant DRD (3,4). Knappskog et al. (111) demonstrated the mutation of the *TH* gene located on chromosome 15. After the discovery of the gene, a number of phenotypes were described by Hoffmann et al. and failure of intellectual function is emphasized (112).

## Clinical Characteristics

In patients with predominance of motor dysfunction or benign type the first symptoms consist of dystonia and rigidity appearing in infancy to early childhood (110). The dystonia starts in the lower limbs and expands to generalized dystonia (110,113). Tremor is also observed in infancy (110). A girl patient reported by Grattan-Smith et al. (114) developed shaking movements at two months of age that started in the leg spreading to the head, tongue, and arms, and in six months it appeared as tremor. The limb tremor worsened with attempted movements and that of the tibialis anterior muscle showed a frequency of 4 Hz (114). The deep tendon reflexes are brisk and show the feature of spastic paraplegia (115). However, plantar responses are flexion. In some cases, the intensity of the motor disorder is less pronounced in the morning or after a nap and more marked in the evening. However, this feature is not constant and cannot be considered as an essential diagnostic criterion (113). In these patients, academic progress is normal.

An alternative presentation includes severe axial hypotonia, hypokinesia, dystonia, hypomimia, ptosis, and oculogyric crisis (116). Miosis and postural hypotension are also observed, (114) as well as, paroxysmal irritability, sweating, hypersalivation, pyramidal signs, and intellectual impairment. Moreover, these infants exhibit a progressive encephalopathy with seizures and microcephalus (112).

## Diagnosis

Decreased CSF levels of HVA and 3-C, together with normal pterin and CSF tyrosine and 5-HIAA concentrations are the diagnostic hallmarks of TH deficiency. Measurements of HVA, vanillylmandelic acid, or catecholamines in urine are not relevant for diagnosing TH deficiency (117). The diagnosis should be considered in all children with unexplained hypokinesia and other extrapyramidal symptoms (118).

## Treatment

In cases with predominance of dystonia or benign type, levodopa produces favorable and sustained effects (110). Although abnormal movements or dyskinesia are accompanied by an overdose, they regress when the dosage is decreased (113). For a child with severe axial hypotonia and ballistic movement a combination with selegiline, a selective monoamine oxidase-B inhibitor, with low-dose levodopa was effective, though levodopa monotherapy was unsuccessful (119).

## Molecular Biology

Mutation of *TH* gene was firstly detected by Knappskog et al. (111) as a point mutation (*Q138K*) in two siblings who had dystonia responding to levodopa. The residual activity of TH was about 15% of the corresponding wild-type human TH (*hTH*). A girl with severe phenotype had a homozygous point mutation (*L205P*), which has low activity of approximately 1.5% of wild-type *hTH* (120). Three male patients with compound heterozygous for *TH* mutation, two brothers (121), and one isolated case (115) showed dystonia as main symptom and responded well to levodopa. While patients with a blanch site mutation showed severe clinical phenotype (122). At this time 13 separate mutations have been identified, and suggest the grade of decrement of TH activity may be involved in the site of the genotype.

### Pathophysiology

TH catalyzed the rate-limiting step in the biosynthesis of DA, noradrenalin (NA), and adrenaline. Thus, deficiency of TH naturally develops symptoms caused by these catecholamine deficiencies. Grattan-Smith et al. (114) proposed signs of DA deficiency that included tremor, hypersensitivity to levodopa, oculogyric crisis, akinesia, rigidity, and dystonia, while NA deficiency is associated with ptosis, miosis, profuse oropharyngeal secretions, and postural hypotension. Hyperprolactinemia observed in TH deficiency (112) implicates the $D_2$ receptor upward regulation and relates to hypersensitivity to levodopa. Furthermore, NA neurons have important roles for modulation of memory system (123,124), behavior (125), and synaptogenesis of the cortex (126) in the developing brain. Clinically, these are observed in extreme rote memory and aggressive behavior in infantile autism (127) and stagnation of head growth in Rett syndrome (86). The NA neurons also involve postural augmentation and locomotion (128). This clinically appears as postural hypotonia and failure in locomotion and furthermore, this failure in locomotion causes dysfunction of the DA neuron through the PPN that consequently affects development of the frontal cortex (86). Thus, postural hypotonia and mental abnormalities with progressive encephalopathy are considered to be caused by early deficiency of the activities of the NA neurons.

### *DYT14*

Grötzsch et al. (129) report a patient with DRD who had linkage on chromosome 14q13. Clinical symptoms appeared at the age of three years with dystonia of both legs, a peculiar tip toe gait, severe postural instability, and frequent falls. The patient's walking worsened with effort and toward the end of the day. Although the surgical elongation of both of the Achilles tendons showed a transient benefit, dystonia progressed to involve the upper limbs and impaired writing, dressing, eating, and self-caring. The patient required a wheelchair by 12 years of age. At initial movement disorders clinic presentation at the age of 73 years, the patient exhibited a resting tremor on the left leg and a severe rigid akinesia with dystonic posture in all extremities with left-side predominance. Levodopa, at a dosage of 100 mg associated with 25 mg benserazide three times daily, showed dramatic effect. Although walking remained impaired, the patient developed full use of hands, and was stable until she died of cardiopulmonary failure at the age of 77 years.

The autopsy of the brain revealed marked decrease of the melanized neurons both in the substantia nigra pars compacta and in the locus coeruleus without neuronal loss. The substantia nigra was more affected in the lateral part than the medial one and the right side was more affected than the left. There was no glial infiltration or Lewy bodies. These findings were similar to those of dominant *GCH-I* deficiency (52,55).

## JUVENILE PARKINSONISM, PARKINSONISM–DYSTONIA COMPLEX

### Autosomal Recessive Early-Onset Parkinsonism with Diurnal Fluctuation

Autosomal recessive early-onset parkinsonism with diurnal fluctuation (AR-EPDF) (130,131) or autosomal recessive juvenile parkinsonism (ARJP) (132) is a genetic disorder caused by parkin gene located on chromosome 6q25.2-q27 (133). CSF biopterin is reduced markedly but neopterin is within normal range. Neuropathology revealed marked decrease in the pigmented nuclei in the pars compacta of the substantia nigra with glial infiltration in the ventral tier, but there was no Lewy body (131,134). Histochemical examination revealed a decrease in DA and TH activities in both the pars compacta of the substantia nigra and the striatum; in the latter, the decrease of TH was more marked in the putamen than the caudate nucleus and more prominent in its dorsal area than in the ventral area (135). Although the pathophysiology has not been delineated, there is a JP that shows movement-related fatiguability (136,137).

Among cases with AR-EPDF, some developed symptoms before the age of 10 years (138) with diurnal fluctuation of symptoms (130,131,138). However, in contrast to AD GCH-I deficiency, parkinsonian features develop with resting tremor (130,131,138) in the second decade or later and the doses of levodopa need to increase with early development of dopa-induced dyskinesia.

It is sometimes difficult to differentiate AR-EPDF from AD GCH-I D clinically (139). In these cases, evaluation of pteridine metabolites in the CSF and molecular biological studies are necessary, but estimation of voluntary saccade is also valuable because it is preserved in AR-JP. It is important to differentiate AR-EPDF and other JP from AD GCH-I deficiency, because patients with JP develop levodopa-induced dyskinesia early after levodopa and it is often intractable if levodopa is administrated before puberty.

## SUMMARY

AD GCH-I deficiency is an autosomal-dominant DRD caused by heterozygous mutation of the *GCH-I* gene located on 14q22.1-q22.2. Although a number of mutations have been reported, the change remains highly stable within families, and causes decrease of TH protein at the NS-DA neuron terminal. In addition decreased $BH_4$ levels early in the development affect DA receptors age dependently, and produce a spectrum of specific symptoms attributed to neuronal changes traced to processes of the development of the NS-DA neuron, related striatal projection neurons, and the output projection of the basal ganglia (10,140).

Although postural dystonia is the prominent symptom, action dystonia and segmental or focal dystonia may also occur. Moreover, some develop symptoms in adulthood with tremor as a predominant feature but without dystonia and diurnal fluctuation. These clinical symptoms improve completely by levodopa and the effects sustain without any unfavorable side effects, and without any relation to the ages at onset and longevity of the clinical cause before levodopa. These suggest the functional abnormalities of the DA neuron without any neuropathological abnormalities, and may be confirmed by neuroimaging, neuropathological, and neurohistochemical studies.

Recessive disorders of pteridine metabolism also show DRD with similar pathophysiology as AD GCH-I deficiency with loss of DA activity at the terminal of the NS-DA neuron. However, the marked decrease of $BH_4$ in this disorder produces changes in tryptophan hydroxylase and a deficiency of 5HT, producing hypotonia, failure in locomotion, and mental retardation. Although levodopa improves motor symptoms, it does not alter the cognitive abnormalities.

In recessive TH deficiency and in JP, DRD develops age dependently in childhood and early teen and with age it is overcome by parkinsonian symptoms. In recessive TH deficiency $D_2$ receptor is also involved and in JP the DA activities decrease in both the terminal and the perikaryon of the NS-DA neuron. Although the striatal direct projection might be involved in the dystonia, the involvement of the $D_2$ indirect pathway modifies the symptoms.

Existence of *DYT14* suggests the heterogenity of the gene that involves the modulation of the terminal of the NS-DA neuron innervating to the $D_1$ direct pathway connecting to the descending output but does not involve the modulation of the CNS.

## REFERENCES


1. Nygaard TG, Marsden CD, Duvoisin RC. Dopa responsive dystonia. Adv Neurol 1988; 50:377–384.
2. Calne DB. Dopa-responsive dystonia. Ann Neurol 1994; 35:381–382.
3. Segawa M, Ohmi K, Itoh S, et al. Childhood basal ganglia disease with remarkable response to Levodopa, hereditary basal ganglia disease with marked diurnal fluctuation (Japanese). Shinryo (Tokyo) 1971; 24:667–672.
4. Segawa M, Hosaka A, Miyagawa F, et al. Hereditary progressive dystonia with marked diurnal fluctuation. Adv Neurol 1976; 14:215–233.
5. Segawa M. Hereditary progressive dystonia with marked diurnal fluctuation (HPD) (Japanese). Adv Neurol Sci (Tokyo) 1981; 25:73–81.
6. Deonna T. Dopa-responsive progressive dystonia of childhood with fluctuations of symptoms—Segawa's syndrome and possible variants. Neuropediatrics 1986; 17:81–85.
7. Nomura Y, Segawa M. Intrafamilial and interfamilial variations of symptoms of Japanese hereditary progressive dystonia with marked diurnal fluctuation. In: Segawa M, ed. Hereditary Progressive Dystonia with Marked Diurnal Fluctuation. Carnforth: Parthenon, 1993:73–96.
8. Bandmann O, Nygaard TG, Surtees R, et al. Dopa responsive dystonia in British patients: new mutations of the GTP-cyclohydrolase I gene and evidence for genetic heterogeneity. Hum Mol Genet 1996; 5:403–406.
9. Bandmann O, Valene EM, Holmans P, et al. Dopa-responsive dystonia: a clinical and molecular genetic study. Ann Neurol 1998; 44:649–656.
10. Segawa M, Nomura Y, Nishiyama N. Autosomal dominant guanosine triphosphate cyclohydrolase I deficiency (Segawa disease). Ann Neurol 2003; 54:32–45.
11. Segawa M, Hoshino K, Hachimori K, et al. A single gene for dystonia involves both or either of the two striatal pathway. In: Bicholson L, Baull R, eds. The Basal Ganglia VI. New York: Kluwer Academic/Plenum Publishers, 2002:155–163.
12. Furukawa Y, Kish SJ, Bebin EM, et al. Dystonia with motor delay in compound heterozygotes for GTP-cyclohydrolase I gene mutations. Ann Neurol 1998; 44:10–16.
13. Leuzzi V, Carducci C, Carducci C, et al. Autosomal dominant GTP-CH deficiency presenting as a dopa-responsive myoclonus-dystonia syndrome. Neurology 2002; 59: 1241–1243.
14. Segawa M, Nomura Y, Kase M. Diurnally fluctuating hereditary progressive dystonia. In: Vinken PJ, Bruyn GW, eds. Handbook of Clinical Neurology. Extrapyramidal Disorders. Vol. 5. Amsterdam: Elsevier, 491986:529–539.
15. Segawa M, Nomura Y, Yamashita S, et al. Long-term effects of Levodopa on hereditary progressive dystonia with marked diurnal fluctuation. In: Berardelli A, Benecke R, Manfredi M, Marsden CD, eds. Motor Disturbance II. London, New York: Academic Press, 1990:305–318.

16. Segawa M, Nomura Y. Hereditary progressive dystonia with marked diurnal fluctuation and dopa-responsive dystonia: Pathognomonic clinical features. In: Segawa M, Nomura Y, eds. Age-Related Dopamine-Dependent Disorders. Vol. 14. Basel: Karger, 1995:10–24.
17. Segawa M, Nomura Y, Yukishita S, et al. Is phenotypic variation of hereditary progressive dystonia with marked diurnal fluctuation/dopa-responsive dystonia (HPD/DRD) caused by the difference of the locus of mutation on the GTP cyclohydrolase 1 (GCH-1) gene? Adv Neurol 2004; 94:217–223.
18. Furukawa Y, Filiano JJ, Kish SJ. Amantadine for levodopa-induced choreic dyskinesia in compound heterozygotes for GCH1 mutations. Mov Disord 2004; 19: 1256–1258.
19. Nomura K, Negoro T, Takesu E, et al. Bromocriptine therapy in a case of hereditary progressive dystonia with marked diurnal fluctuation. Brain Dev 1987; 9:199.
20. Ibi T, Sahashi K, Watanabe K, et al. Progressive dystonia with marked diurnal fluctuation and tetrahydrobiopterin therapy (Japanese). Neurol Ther (Tokyo) 1991; 8:71–75.
21. Ishida A, Takada G, Kobayashi Y, et al. Involvement of serotonergic neurons in hereditary progressive dystonia; Clinical effects of tetrahydrobiopterin and 5-hydroxytryptophan (Japanese). No-To-Hattatsu (Tokyo) 1988; 20:196–199.
22. Le Witt PA, Miller LP, Newman RP, et al. Pterdine cofactor in dystonia: Pathogenic and therapeutic considerations. Neurology 1983; 33(Suppl 2):161.
23. Le Witt PA, Miller LP, Newman RP, et al. Treatment of dystonia with tetrahydrobiopterin. N Engl J Med 1983; 308:157–158.
24. Le Witt PA, Miller LP, Newman RP, et al. Tetrahydrobiopterin in dystonia: Identification of abnormal metabolism and therapeutic trials. Neurology 1986; 36:760–764.
25. Segawa N, Nomura Y, Takita K, et al. Pallidotomy and thalamotomy on a case with hereditary progressive dystonia with marked diurnal fluctuation. Mov Disord 1998; 13(Suppl 2):S165.
26. Kumamoto I, Nomoto M, Yoshidome M, et al. Five cases of dystonia with marked diurnal fluctuation and special reference to homovanilic acid in CSF (Japanese). Clin Neurol (Tokyo) 1984; 24:697–702.
27. Maekawa N, Hashimoto T, Sasaki M, et al. A study on catecholamine metabolites in CSF in a patient with progressive dystonia with marked diurnal fluctuation (Japanese). Clin Neurol (Tokyo) 1988; 28:1206–1208.
28. Ouvrie RA. Progressive dystonia with marked diurnal fluctuation. Ann Neurol 1978; 4:412–417.
29. Shimoyamada Y, Yoshikawa A, Kashii H, et al. Hereditary progressive dystonia-an observation of the catecholamine metabolism during Levodopa therapy in a nine-year-old girl (Japanese). No-To-Hattatsu (Tokyo) 1986; 18:505–509.
30. Fink JK, Barton N, Cohen W, et al. Dystonia with marked diurnal variation associated with bioperin deficiency. Neurology 1988; 38:707–711.
31. Fujita S, Shintaku H. Etiology and pteridine metabolism abnormality of hereditary progressive dystonia with marked diurnal fluctuation (HPD: Segawa disease). Med J Kushiro City Hosp 1990; 2:64–67.
32. Furukawa Y, Nishi K, Kondo T, et al. CSF biopterin levels and clinical features of patients with juvenile parkinsonism. Adv Neurol 1993; 60:562–567.
33. Takahashi H, Snow B, Nygaard T, et al. Fluorodopa PET scans of juvenile parkinsonism with prominent dystonia in relation to dopa-responsive dystonia. In: Segawa M, Nomura Y, eds. Age-Related Dopamine-Dependent Disorders. Basel: Karger, 1995:86–94.
34. Ichinose H, Ohye T, Takahashi E, et al. Hereditary progressive dystonia with marked diurnal fluctuation caused by mutations in the GTP cyclohydrolase I gene. Nat Genet 1994; 8:236–242.
35. Hyland K, Fryburg JS, Wilson WG. Oral phenylalanine loading in dopa responsive dystonia; a possible diagnostic test. Neurology 1997; 48:1290–1297.

36. Snow BJ, Okada A, Martin WRW, et al. Positron-emission tomography scanning in dopa-responsive dystonia, parkinsonism-dystonia, and young onset parkinsonism. In: Segawa M, ed. Hereditary Progressive Dystonia with Marked Diurnal Fluctuation. Carnforth: Parthenon, 1993:181–186.
37. Sawle GB, Lenders KL, Brooks DJ, et al. Dopa-responsive dystonia: (F-18) Dopa positron emission tomography. Ann Neurol 1991; 30:24–30.
38. Turjanski N, Weeks R, Sawle GV, et al. Positron emission tomography studies of the dopaminergic and opioid function in dopa-responsive dystonia. In: Segawa M, Nomura YM, eds. Age-Related Dopamine-Dependent Disorders. Basel: Karger, 1995:77–86.
39. Okada A, Nakamura K, Snow BJ, et al. PET scan study on the dopaminergic system in a Japanese patient with hereditary progressive dystonia (Segawa's disease): case report. Adv Neurol 1993; 60:591–594.
40. Takahashi H, Levine RA, Galloway MP, et al. Biochemical and fluorodopa positron emission tomographic findings in an asymptomatic carrier of the gene for dopa-responsive dystonia. Ann Neurol 1994; 35:354–356.
41. Leenders KL, Antonini A, Meinck, et al. Striatal dopamine D2 receptors in dopa-responsive dystonia and Parkinson's disease. In: Segawa M, Nomura Y, eds. Age-Related Dopamine-Dependent Disorders. Basel: Karger, 1995:95–100.
42. Kishore A, Nygaard TG, de la Fuente-Fernandez R, et al. Striatal D2 receptors in symptomatic and asymptomatic carriers of dopa-responsive dystonia measured with (11C) raclopride and positron-emission tomography. Neurology 1998; 50:1028–1032.
43. Kunig G, Leenders KL, Antonini A, et al. D2 receptor binding in dopa-responsive dystonia. Ann Neurol 1988; 44:758–762.
44. Jeon BS, Jeong JM, Park SS, et al. Dopamine transporter density measured by (123I) β-CIT single-photon emission computed tomography is normal in dopa-responsive dystonia. Ann Neurol 1998; 43:792–800.
45. Segawa M, Nomura Y, Hikosaka O, et al. Roles of the basal ganglia and related structures in symptoms of dystonia. In: Carpenter MB, Jayaraman A, eds. The Basal Ganglia VI. New York: Kluwer Academic/Plenum Publishers, 2002:489–504.
46. Segawa M, Nomura Y, Tanaka S, et al. Hereditary progressive dystonia with marked diurnal fluctuation: Consideration on its pathophysiology based on the characteristics of clinical and polysomnographical findings. Adv Neurol 1988; 50:367–376.
47. Segawa M, Nomura Y. Hereditary progressive dystonia with marked diurnal fluctuation. Pathophysiological importance of the age of onset. Adv Neurol 1993; 60: 568–576.
48. Segawa M, Nomura Y. Rapid eye movements during stage REM are modulated by nigrostriatal dopamine (NS-DA) neuron? In: Bernardi G, Carpenter MB, Di Chiara G, et al., eds The Basal Ganglia III. New York: Kluwer Academic/Plenum Publishers, 1991:663–671.
49. Hikosaka O, Sakamoto M, Usui S. Functional properties of monkey caudate neurons. I. Activities related to saccadic eye movements. J Neurophysiol 1989; 61:780–798.
50. Hikosaka O, Fukuda H, Kato M, et al. Deficits in saccadic eye movements in hereditary progressive dystonia with marked diurnal fluctuation. In: Segawa M, ed. Hereditary Progressive Dystonia with Marked Diurnal Fluctation. Carnforth: Parthenon, 1993: 159–177.
51. Muller K, Homberg V, Lenard HG. Motor control in child hood onset dopa-responsive dystonia (Segawa syndrome). Neuropediatrics 1989; 20:185–191.
52. Rajput AH, Gibb WRG, Zhong XH, et al. Dopa-responsive dystonia: pathological and biochemical observations in one case. Ann Neurol 1994; 35:396–402.
53. Hornykiewicz O. Striatal dopamine in dopa-responsive dystonia: Comparison with idiopathic Parkinson's disease and other dopamine-dependent disorders. In: Segawa M, Nomura YM, eds. Age-Related Dopamine-Dependent Disorders. Basel: Karger, 1995:101–108.

54. Furukawa Y, Shimadzu M, Rajput AH, et al. GTP-cyclohydrolase I gene mutations in hereditary progressive and dopa responsive dystonia. Ann Neurol 1996; 39:609–617.
55. Furukawa Y, Nygaard TG, Gutlich M, et al. Striatal biopterin and tyrosine hydroxylase protein reduction in dopa-responsive dystonia. Neurology 1999; 53:1032–1041.
56. Furukawa Y, Kapatos G, Haycock JW, et al. Brain biopterin and tyrosine hydroxylase in asymptomatic dopa-responsive dystonia. Ann Neurol 2002; 51:637–641.
57. Nygaad TG, Wihelmsen KC, Risch NJ, et al. Linkage mapping of dopa-responsive dystonia (DRD) to chromosome 14q. Nat Genet 1993; 5:386–391.
58. Nishiyama N, Yukishita S, Hagiwara S, et al. Gene mutation in hereditary progressive dystonia with marked diurnal fluctuation (HPD), strictly defined dopa-responsive dystonia. Brain Dev 2000; 22:102–106.
59. Hirano M, Tamura Y, Nagai Y, et al. Exon skipping caused by a base substitution at a splice site in the GTP cyclohydrolase I gene in a Japanese family with hereditary progressive dystonia/dopa responsive dystonia. Biochem Biphys Res Commun 1995; 213:645–646.
60. Hirano M, Tamaru Y, Ito H, et al. Mutant GTP cyclohydrolase I mRNA levels contribute to dopa-responsive dystonia onset. Ann Neurol 1996; 40:796–798.
61. Nygaad TG, Waran SP, Levine RA, et al. Dopa-responsive dystonia stimulating cerebral palsy. Pediatr Neurol 1994; 44:236–240.
62. Furukawa Y, Kish SJ. Dopa-responsive dystonia: recent advances and remaining issues to be addressed. Mov Disord 1999; 14:709–715.
63. Ichinose H, Ohye T, Segawa M, et al. GTP chclohydrolase I gene in hereditary progressive dystonia with marked diurnal fluctuation. Neurosci Lett 1995; 196:5–8.
64. Furukawa Y, Guttman M, Sparagana SP, et al. Dopa-responsive dystonia due to a large deletion in the GTP cyclohydrolase I gene. Ann Neurol 2000; 47:517–520.
65. Hirano M, Yanagihara T, Ueno S. Dominant negative effect of GTP cyclohydrolase I mutations in dopa-responsive hereditary progressive dystonia. Ann Neurol 1998; 44:365–371.
66. Hwu WL, Chiou YW, Lai SY, et al. Dopa-responsive dystonia is induced by a dominant-negative mechanism. Ann Neurol 2000; 48:609–613.
67. Suzuki T, Ohye T, Inagaki H, et al. Characterization of wild-type and mutants of recombinant human GTP cyclohydrolase I: relationship to etiology of dopa-responsive dystonia. J Neurochem 1999; 73:2510–2516.
68. Ueno S, Hirano M. Missense mutants inactivate guanosine triphosphate cyclohydrolase I in hereditary progressive dystonia. Brain Dev 2000; 22(Suppl 1):S111–S114.
69. Shimoji M, Hirayama K, Hyland K, et al. GTP cyclohydrolase I gene expression in the brains of male and female hph-1 mice. J Neurochem 1999; 72:757–764.
70. Davis MD, Ribeiro P, Tipper J, et al. "7-tetrahydrobiopterin," a naturally occurring analogue of tetrahydrobiopterin, is a cofactor for and a potential inhibitor of the aromatic amino acid hydroxylases. Proc Natl Acad Sci U S A 1992; 89:10109–10113.
71. McGeer EG, McGeer PL. Some characteristics of brain tyrosine hydroxylase. In: Mandel J, ed. New Concepts in Neurotransmitter Regulation. New York, London: Plenum, 1973:53–68.
72. Steinfels FF, Heym J, Strecker R, et al. Behavioral correlates of dopaminergic unit activity in freely moving cats. Brain Res 1983; 25:217–228.
73. Hibiya M, Ichinose H, Ozaki N, et al. Normal values and age-dependent changes in GTP cyclohydrolase I activity in stimulated mononuclear blood cells measured by high-performance liquid chromatography. J Chromatogr B Biomed Sci Appl 2000; 740:35–42.
74. Furukawa Y, Kish SJ. Influence of development and aging on brain biopterin: implications for dopa-responsive dystonia onset. Neurology 1998; 51:632–634.
75. Shintaku H. Early diagnosis of 6-pyruvoyltetrahydropterin synthase deficiency. Pteridines 1994; 5:18–27.
76. Graybiel AM, Ragsdale CW Jr. Histochemically distinct compartments in the striatum of human, monkey and cat demonstrated by acetylthiocholinesterase staining. Proc Natl Acad Sci 1978; 75:5723–5726.

77. Gibb WRG. Selective pathology, disease pathogenesis and function in the basal ganglia. In: Kimura J, Shibasaki H, eds. Recent Advances in Clinical Neurophysiology. Amsterdam: Elsevier, 1996:1009–1015.
78. Segawa M. Development of the nigrostriatal dopamine neuron and the pathways in the basal ganglia. Brain Dev 2000; 22:1–4.
79. Nair VD, Mishra RK. Ontogenic development of dopamine D4 receptor in rat brain. Brain Res Dev Brain Res 1995; 90:180–183.
80. Kreiss DS, Anderson LA, Waters JR. Apomorphine and dopamine D receptor agonists increase the firing rates of subthalamic nucleus neurons. Neuroscience 1996; 72:863–876.
81. Kreiss DS, Mastropietro CW, Rawji SS, et al. The response of subthalamic nucleus neurons to dopamine receptor stimulation in a rodent model of Parkinson's disease. J Neurosci 1997; 17:6807–6819.
82. Nomura Y, Ikeuchi T, Tsuji S, et al. Two phenotypes and anticipation observed in Japanese cases with early-onset torsion dystonia (DYT 1). Brain Dev 2000; 22:92–101.
83. Shima F, Sakata S, Sun SJ, et al. The role of the descending pallido-reticular pathway in movement disorders. In: Segawa M, Nomura Y, eds. Age-Related Dopamine-Dependent Disorders. Basel: Karger, 1995:197–207.
84. Lenz FA, Seike MS, Jaeger CJ, et al. Single unit analysis of thalamus in patients with dystonia. Mov Disord 1992; 7(Suppl 1):126.
85. Segawa M. Progress in Segawa's disease. In: Mizuno Y, Fisher A, Hanin I, eds. Mapping the Progress of Alzheimer's Disease and Parkinson's Disease. New York: Kluwer Academic/Plenum, 2002:353–359.
86. Segawa M. Discussant -pathophysiologies of Rett syndrome. Brain Dev 2001; 23(Suppl 1):S218–S223.
87. Leff SE, Rendahl KG, Spratt SK, et al. In vivo LEVODOPA production by genetically modified primary rat fibroblast or 9L gliosarcoma cell grafts via coexpression of GTPcyclohydrolase I with tyrosine hydroxylase. Exp Neurol 1998; 151:249–264.
88. Sumi-Ichinose C, Urano F, Kuroda R, et al. Catecholamines and serotonin are differently regulated by tetrahydrobiopterin. A study from 6-pyruvoyltetrahydropterin synthase knockout mice. J Biol Chem 2001; 276:41150–41160.
89. Furukawa Y, Lang AE, Trugman JM, et al. Gender-related penetrance and de novo GTP-cyclohydrolase I gene mutations in dopa-responsive dystonia. Neurology 1998; 50:1015–1020.
90. Reisert I, Pilgrim C. Sexual differentiation of monoaminergic neuron genetic epigenetic. Trends Neurosci 1991; 14:468–473.
91. Nomura Y, Uetake K, Yukishita S, et al. Dystonias responding to levodopa and failure in biopterin metabolism. Adv Neurol 1998; 78:253–266.
92. Segawa M. Hereditary progressive dystonia with marked diurnal fluctuation. Brain Dev 2000; 22(Suppl 1):S65–S80.
93. Blau N, Barnes I, Dhondt JL. International database of tetrahydrobiopterin deficiencies. J Inherit Metab Dis 1996; 19:8–14.
94. Niederwieser A, Blau N, Wang M, et al. GTP cyclohydrolase I deficiency, a new enzyme defect causing hyperphenylalaninemia with neopterin, biopterin, dopamine, and serotonin deficiencies and muscular hypotonia. Eur J Pediatr 1984; 141:208–214.
95. Dudesek A, Roschinger W, Muntau AC, et al. Molecular analysis and long-term follow-up of patients with different forms of 6-pyruvoyl-tetrahydropterin synthase deficiency. Eur J Pediatr 2001; 160:267–276.
96. Liu TT, Chang YH, Chiang SH, et al. Identification of three novel 6-pyruvoyl-tetrahydropterin synthase gene mutations (226C > T, IVS3+1G > A, 116–119delTGTT) in Chinese hyperphenylalaninemia caused by tetrahydrobiopterin synthesis deficiency. Hum Mutat 2001; 18:83.
97. Roze E, Vidailhet M, Blau N, et al. Long-term follow-up and adult outcome of 6-pyruvoyl-tetrahydropterin synthase deficiency. Mov Disord 2006; 21:263–266.

98. Hanihara T, Inoue K, Kawanishi C, et al. 6-Pyruvoyl-tetrahydropterin synthase deficiency with generalized dystonia and diurnal fluctuation of symptoms: a clinical and molecular study. Mov Disord 1997; 12:408–411.
99. Demos MK, Waters PJ, Vallance HD, et al. 6-pyruvoyl-tetrahydropterin synthase deficiency with mild hyperphenylalaninemia. Ann Neurol 2005; 58:164–167.
100. Tanaka Y, Matsuo N, Tsuzaki S, et al. On-off phenomenon in a child with tetrahydrobiopterin deficiency due to 6-pyruvoyl tetrahydropterin synthase deficiency (BH4 deficiency). Eur J Pediatr 1989; 148:450–452.
101. Chien YH, Chiang SC, Huang A, et al. Treatment and outcome of Taiwanese patients with 6-pyruvoyltetrahydropterin synthase gene mutations. J Inherit Metab Dis 2001; 24:815–823.
102. Thony B, Blau N. Mutations in the GTP cyclohydrolase I and 6-pyruvoyl-tetrahydropterin synthase genes. Hum Mutat 1997; 10:11–20.
103. Oppliger T, Thony B, Kluge C, et al. Identification of mutations causing 6-pyruvoyl-tetrahydropterin synthase deficiency in four Italian families. Hum Mutat 1997; 10:25–35.
104. Scherer-Oppliger T, Matasovic A, Laufs S, et al. Dominant negative allele (N47D) in a compound heterozygote for a variant of 6-pyruvoyltetrahydropterin synthase deficiency causing transient hyperphenylalaninemia. Hum Mutat 1999; 13:286–289.
105. Bonafe L, Thony B, Penzien JM, et al. Mutations in the sepiapterin reductase gene cause a novel tetrahydrobiopterin-dependent monoamine-neurotransmitter deficiency without hyperphenylalaninemia. Am J Hum Genet 2001; 69:269–277.
106. Neville BG, Parascandalo R, Farrugia R, et al. Sepiapterin reductase deficiency: a congenital dopa-responsive motor and cognitive disorder. Brain 2005; 128:2291–2296.
107. Blau N, Bonafe L, Thony B. Tetrahydrobiopterin deficiencies without hyperphenylalaninemia: diagnosis and genetics of dopa-responsive dystonia and sepiapterin reductase deficiency. Mol Genet Metab 2001; 74:172–185.
108. Cotton RG, Jennings I, Bracco G, et al. Tetrahydrobiopterin non-responsiveness in dihydropteridine reductase deficiency is associated with the presence of mutant protein. J Inherit Metab Dis 1986; 9:239–243.
109. Castaigne P, Rondot P, Ribadeau-Dumas JL, et al. Progressive extra-pyramidal disorder in 2 young brothers. Remarkable effects of treatment with Levodopa (French). Rev Neurol (Paris) 1971; 124:162–166.
110. Rondot P, Ziegler M. Dystonia-Levodopa responsive or juvenile parkinsonism? J Neural Transm Suppl 1983; 19:273–281.
111. Knappskog PM, Flatmark T, Mallet J, et al. Recessively inherited LEVODOPA-responsive dystonia caused by a point mutation (Q381K) in the tyrosine hydroxylase gene. Hum Mol Genet 1995; 4:1209–1212.
112. Hoffmann GF, Assmann B, Brautigam C, et al. Tyrosine hydroxylase deficiency causes progressive encephalopathy and dopa-nonresponsive dystonia. Ann Neurol 2003; 54(Suppl 6):S56–S65.
113. Rondot P, Aicardi J, Goutieres F, et al. Dopa-sensitive dystonia (French). Rev Neurol (Paris) 1992; 148:680–686.
114. Grattan-Smith PJ, Wevers RA, Steenbergen-Spanjers GC, et al. Tyrosine hydroxylase deficiency: clinical manifestations of catecholamine insufficiency in infancy. Mov Disord 2002; 17:354–359.
115. Brautigam C, Steenbergen-Spanjers GC, Hoffmann GF, et al. Biochemical and molecular genetic characteristics of the severe form of tyrosine hydroxylase deficiency. Clin Chem 1999; 45:2073–2078.
116. Brautigam C, Wevers RA, Jansen RJ, et al. Biochemical hallmarks of tyrosine hydroxylase deficiency. Clin Chem 1998; 44:1897–1904.
117. Wevers RA, de Rijk-van Andel JF, Brautigam C, et al. A review of biochemical and molecular genetic aspects of tyrosine hydroxylase deficiency including a novel mutation (291delC). J Inherit Metab Dis 1999; 22:364–373.

118. Dionisi-Vici C, Hoffmann GF, Leuzzi V, et al. Tyrosine hydroxylase deficiency with severe clinical course: clinical and biochemical investigations and optimization of therapy. J Pediatr 2000; 136:560–562.
119. Ludecke B, Knappskog PM, Clayton PT, et al. Recessively inherited LEVODOPA-responsive parkinsonism in infancy caused by a point mutation (L205P) in the tyrosine hydroxylase gene. Hum Mol Genet 1996; 5:1023–1028.
120. Swaans RJ, Rondot P, Renier WO, et al. Four novel mutations in the tyrosine hydroxylase gene in patients with infantile parkinsonism. Ann Hum Genet 2000; 64:25–31.
121. Furukawa Y, Graf WD, Wong H, et al. Dopa-responsive dystonia simulating spastic paraplegia due to tyrosine hydroxylase gene mutations. Neurology 2001; 56:260–263.
122. Janssen RJ, Wevers RA, Haussler M, et al. A branch site mutation leading to aberrant splicing of the human tyrosine hydroxylase gene in a child with a severe extrapyramidal movement disorder. Ann Hum Genet 2000; 64:375–382.
123. Mason ST. Noradrenaline and behaviour. Trends Neurosci 1979; 2:82–84.
124. Tanaka S, Miyagawa F, Imai H, et al. Learning abilities of the rats with lesion in the dorsal noradrenergic bundele (Japanese). Juntendo Med J (Tokyo) 1987; 33:271–272.
125. Valzelli L, Garattini S. Biochemical and behavioural changes induced by isolation in rats. Neuropharmacology 1972; 11:17–22.
126. Brenner E, Mirmiran M, Uylings HB, et al. Impaired growth of the cerebral cortex of rats treated neonatally with 6-hydroxydopamine under different environmental conditions. Neurosci Lett 1983; 42:13–17.
127. Segawa M, Nomura Y. Pathophysiology of Austism: Evaluation of Sleep and locomotion. In: Tuchman R, Rapin I, eds. Autism: a neurological disorder of early brain development. International Review of Child Neurology Series (ICNA). London: Mac Keith Press, 2006:248–264.
128. Mori S, Matsuyama K, Kohyama J, et al. Neuronal constituents of postural and locomotor control systems and their interactions in cats. Brain Dev 1992; 14(Suppl): S109–S120.
129. Grötzsch H, Pizzolato GP, Ghika J, et al. Neuropathology of a case of dopa-responsive dystonia associated with a new genetic locus, DYT14. Neurology 2002; 58(12): 1839–1842.
130. Yamamura Y, Sobue I, Ando K, et al. Paralysis agitans of early onset with marked diurnal fluctuation of symptoms. Neurology 1973; 23:239–244.
131. Yamamura Y, Hamaguchi Y, Uchida M, et al. Parkinsonism of early-onset with diurnal fluctuation. In: Segawa M, ed. Hereditary Progressive Dystonia with Marked Diurnal Fluctation. Carnforth: Parthenon, 1993:51–59.
132. Matsumine M, Saito M, Shimoda-Matsubayashi S, et al. Localization of a gene for an autosomal recessive from of juvenile parkinsonism to chromosome 6q25.2–27. Am J Hum Genet 1997; 60:588–596.
133. Kitada T, Asakawa S, Hattori N, et al. Mutations in the parkin gene cause autosomal recessive juvenile parkinsonism. Nature 1998; 392:605–608.
134. Yokochi M. Clinicopathological identification of juvenile parkinsonism in reference to dopa-responsive disorders. In: Segawa M, ed. Hereditary Progressive Dystonia with Marked Diurnal Fluctuation. Carnforth: Parthenon, 1993:37–47.
135. Kondo T, Mori H, Sugita Y, et al. Juvenile parkinsonian—a clinical, neuropathologic and biochemical study. Mov Disord 1997; 12 (Suppl 1):32.
136. Sunohara N, Mano Y, Ando K, et al. Idiopathic dystonia: parkinsonism with marked diurnal fluctuation of symptoms. Ann Neurol 1985; 17:39–45.
137. Sunohara N, Ikeda K, Tomi H. Idiopathic dystonia-parkinsonism with diurnal fluctuation: a follow-up study and magnetic resonance imaging findings. In: Segawa M, ed. Hereditary Progressive Dystonia with Marked Diurnal Fluctation. Carnforth: Parthenon, 1993:61–70.

138. Yokochi M. Juvenile Parkinsons disease—part I. Clinical aspects (Japanese). Adv Neurol Sci (Tokyo) 1979; 23:1060–1073.
139. Tassin J, Durr A, Bonnet A-M, et al. Levodopa-responsive dystonia: GTP cyclohydrolase I or parkin mutations? Brain 2000; 123:1112–1121.
140. Furukawa Y. Genetics and biochemistry of dopa-responsive dystonia: significance of striatal tyrosine hydroxylase protein loss. Adv Neurol 2003; 91:401–410.

# 16
# Secondary Dystonia

**Arif Dalvi**
*Department of Neurology, University of Chicago, Chicago, Illinois, U.S.A.*

**Kelly E. Lyons and Rajesh Pahwa**
*Department of Neurology, University of Kansas Medical Center, Kansas City, Kansas, U.S.A.*

## INTRODUCTION

Dystonia is a neurological syndrome with sustained muscle contractions producing an abnormal posture, and is usually secondary to central nervous system dysfunction. Dystonia is often classified by etiology, and may be primary (sporadic or familial) or secondary. Secondary causes of dystonia have accompanying neurological deficits or an identifiable structural or metabolic lesion. Classification of dystonia based on etiology has undergone extensive modifications as new genetic bases for some forms of dystonia and other primary neurological diseases have been identified. (Chapters 3 and 8). Secondary dystonia can be further classified into symptomatic dystonia and the dystonia plus syndromes. Symptomatic dystonia is due to an identifiable brain disease, an obvious brain or peripheral insult, or a hereditary or sporadic degeneration of the brain. The dystonia plus syndromes (1) have accompanying neurological signs and/or clinical and laboratory findings suggestive of neurochemical disorders, without evidence of an underlying neurodegenerative process (Table 1).

Careful epidemiologic study of any neurological disorder remains challenging (Chapter 2). Studies evaluating the causes of secondary dystonia are usually done in tertiary movement disorder centers and tend to suffer from referral bias. In a Brazilian study evaluating 46 patients with secondary dystonia, tardive dystonia (34.8%) and perinatal injury (30.4%) were the most common etiologies. Other important causes included stroke (13.0%), encephalitis (6.5%), and Wilson's disease (4.3%) (2). The Movement Disorders Center at Columbia Presbyterian Medical Center reported that 80% of secondary dystonia cases were related to an environmental-exogenous cause, while 13% were psychogenic, 5% were related to inherited diseases, and 2% to 3% were caused by other degenerative diseases (3). The exogenous causes included tardive dystonia (40%), cerebral anoxia (15%), trauma (10%), stroke (5%), encephalitis (4%), tumor or vascular malformation (1%), and other conditions (5%).

**Table 1** Classification of Dystonia

| |
|---|
| **Primary** |
| Hereditary |
| Sporadic |
| **Secondary** |
| ***Symptomatic*** |
| *Acquired* |
| Structural |
| Infectious |
| Metabolic |
| Drugs and toxins |
| *Hereditary syndromes* |
| Autosomal dominant |
| Huntington's disease |
| Dentatorubropallidoluysian atrophy |
| Spinocerebellar syndromes |
| Fahr's disease |
| Autosomal recessive |
| Wilson's disease |
| Juvenile Parkinsonism (PARKIN mutation) |
| Pantothenate kinase-associated neurodegeneration |
| Ataxia–telangiectasia |
| Vitamin E deficiency |
| Metachromatic leukodystrophy |
| Sphingolipidoses |
| Niemann–Pick disease |
| Neuronal ceroid lipofuscinosis |
| Homocystinuria |
| Hartnup disease |
| Organic acidurias |
| Tyrosinemia |
| X-linked |
| Lubag |
| Lesch–Nyhan syndrome |
| Rett syndrome |
| Pelizaeus–Merzbacher disease |
| Dystonia-deafness syndromes |
| Mitochondrial |
| Leber's disease |
| Multiple forms of inheritance |
| Leigh's syndrome |
| Neuroacanthocytosis |
| Neuronal intranuclear inclusion disease |
| Hemochromatosis |
| *Neurodegenerative disorders* |
| Parkinson's disease |
| Progressive supranuclear palsy |
| Multiple system atrophy |
| Corticobasal degeneration |
| Multiple sclerosis |
| ***Dystonia-plus syndromes*** |
| Dopa-responsive dystonia |
| Myoclonus–dystonia |
| Rapid-onset dystonia–parkinsonism |

## CLINICAL FEATURES

A detailed neurological history and examination is helpful in distinguishing primary and secondary dystonia. Unilateral onset and early development of dystonia at rest favors a diagnosis of secondary dystonia. In contrast, primary dystonia is associated with a period of "action dystonia" followed by a period of "overflow dystonia" and finally dystonia at rest. Persistence of dystonia during sleep is more common with secondary dystonia and leads to the consideration of an orthopedic or musculoskeletal cause. Diurnal variation of the severity of the dystonia is suggestive of dopa-responsive dystonia (DRD). Paroxysmal occurrence of dystonia may suggest a paroxysmal kinesogenic or nonkinesogenic dystonia (3).

The presence of other neurologic findings also suggests secondary dystonia. Wilson's disease is associated with tremor, ataxia, parkinsonian features, psychiatric disturbances, and specific signs such as the presence of Kayser–Fleisher rings and signs of hepatic dysfunction. GM1 and GM2 gangliosidoses are associated with cognitive dysfunction and cerebellar signs along with a cherry-red spot on a funduscopic exam. Table 2 offers clues suggestive of the diagnosis of secondary dystonia and Table 3 outlines associated signs and symptoms that are helpful in the differential diagnosis.

## LABORATORY INVESTIGATIONS

The laboratory investigation of dystonia should be focused by clinical presentation. Careful examination collects information concerning distribution of the dystonic spasms, age of onset, and associated neurologic deficits (4). In most adult-onset focal and segmental dystonias, as opposed to progressive or generalized dystonia, work-up is usually not necessary. In general, the extent of imaging, electrophysiological, and

**Table 2** Clinical Clues to Diagnosis of Secondary Dystonia

| |
|---|
| *History* |
| History of etiological factors |
| Head trauma or peripheral trauma |
| Encephalitis or meningitis |
| Exposure to drugs or toxins |
| Perinatal anoxia or kernicterus |
| Associated signs and symptoms (see Table 3) |
| Findings suggestive of psychogenic dystonia (see Chapter 18) |
| *Location* |
| Hemidystonia |
| Reversal of age-related pattern of primary dystonia |
| Cranial onset in a child |
| Leg onset in an adult |
| *Temporal profile* |
| Sudden onset and rapid progression |
| Early speech involvement |
| Onset at rest rather than action |
| *Abnormal brain imaging* |
| *Abnormal laboratory work-up* |

**Table 3** Associated Signs and Symptoms

| |
|---|
| Parkinsonism (tremor, rigidity, and bradykinesia) |
| Parkinson's disease |
| Progressive supranuclear palsy |
| Corticobasal degeneration |
| Hemiatrophy–hemi-parkinsonism syndrome |
| Dopa-responsive dystonia |
| Juvenile parkinsonism |
| Rapid-onset dystonia–parkinsonism |
| Wilson's disease |
| Huntington's disease |
| X-linked parkinsonism–dystonia |
| Machado–Joseph disease (SCA-3) |
| Pantothenate kinase-associated neurodegeneration |
| Ataxia |
| Spinocerebellar ataxias |
| Dentatorubropallidoluysian atrophy |
| Ataxia with vitamin E deficiency |
| Wilson's disease |
| Neuronal ceroid lipofuscinosis |
| Hartnup disease |
| Metachromatic leukodystrophy |
| Gangliosidosis |
| Myoclonus |
| Myoclonus–dystonia syndrome |
| Central pontine myelinolysis |
| Subacute sclerosing panencephalitis |
| X-linked dystonia–parkinsonism |
| Rett syndrome |
| Chorea |
| Huntington's disease |
| Neuroacanthocytosis |
| Oculomotor dysfunction |
| Progressive supranuclear palsy |
| Corticobasal degeneration |
| Spinocerebellar ataxias (especially SCA-3) |
| Niemann–Pick disease |
| Ataxia–telangiectasia |
| Optic/retinal dysfunction |
| Mitochondrial disorders (Leigh's syndrome) |
| Pantothenate kinase-associated neurodegeneration |
| Homocystinuria |
| GM2 gangliosidosis |
| Neuronal ceroid lipofuscinosis |
| Neuropathy |
| Metachromatic leukodystrophy |
| Krabbe's disease |
| Spinocerebellar ataxias (SCA-1 and SCA-3) |
| Mitochondrial disorders |
| Dementia/mental retardation |
| Huntington's disease |
| Dentatorubropallidoluysian atrophy |

(*Continued*)

**Table 3** Associated Signs and Symptoms (*Continued*)

| |
|---|
| Parkinsonian disorders |
| Pantothenate kinase-associated neurodegeneration |
| Niemann–Pick disease |
| Homocystinuria |
| Hartnup disease |
| Lesch–Nyhan Syndrome |
| Metachromatic leukodystrophy |
| Neuronal ceroid lipofuscinosis |
| Rett syndrome (autism) |
| Acute encephalopathy |
| Methylmalonic aciduria |
| Glutaric aciduria |

laboratory study is inversely correlated with age of onset. Imaging may demonstrate a structural abnormality in patients presenting with unilateral symptoms, or in adults with a relatively rapid onset, focal dystonia of a limb, particularly in stances of additional neurological abnormalities, or lack of the action-associated phase typical of idiopathic presentations. In rare instances, electroencephalography may be useful in distinguishing intermittent posturing from focal epilepsy from a paroxysmal dystonia. The development of dystonia, particularly affecting the oromandibular area (sardonic smile) may suggest Wilson's disease. Given the availability of specific treatment for Wilson's disease, young patients should be screened with serum copper, 24-hour urine copper and serum ceruloplasmin testing (5). Confirmatory evidence includes Kayser–Fleisher rings on slit-lamp exam, imaging studies, and abnormal liver biochemistry. Tests for other metabolic disorders should be considered in settings of early childhood presentations, and include serum lactate, pyruvate, uric acid, glutaric acid, methylmalonic acid, and very long chain fatty acids. Tests of urine amino and organic acids, lysosomal analysis, skin biopsy, and electroretinogram may also be helpful. A peripheral blood smear should be examined for acanthocytes, and leukocyte morphology may reveal vacuolation in some storage disorders. A bone marrow biopsy may show sea-blue histiocytes or other features suggestive of a storage disorder (6).

## NEUROIMAGING

Most patients with dystonia should undergo neuroimaging with Computed Tomography or preferably, Magnetic Resonance Imaging (MRI). Neuroimaging is necessary to identify focal structural lesions. In addition, specific patterns on MRI may suggest the etiology of the dystonia. Putamenal and thalamic lesions are associated with limb dystonia (7). Brainstem lesions may occur in cranial dystonia, including oromandibular or facial presentations and blepharospasm (8). Caudate atrophy is associated with Huntington's disease, neuroacanthocytosis, and some GM1 gangliosidoses (9). Generalized brain atrophy may be seen in a number of symptomatic dystonias including pantothenate kinase-associated neurodegeneration (PKAN) (Hallervorden–Spatz disease) in which the "eye-of-the-tiger" sign is characteristic of the disorder (10). Wilson's disease is also associated with putamenal lesions (11) and putamenal and caudate lesions occur in dystonia associated with GM1 gangliosidosis (12). Symmetrical basal ganglia lesions are seen in Leigh's disease (13) and severe neuronal loss especially in the putamen has been seen with glutaric aciduria (14). Basal ganglia calcifications are characteristic of Fahr's disease (15). Postitron Emission Tomography is emphasized in research settings, and is discussed more fully in Chapter 7.

## ETIOLOGY OF SECONDARY DYSTONIA

### Symptomatic Dystonia

*Acquired Dystonia*

**Structural Lesions.** *Focal Lesions.* Focal lesions affecting the basal ganglia, especially those disrupting the striatopallidothalamic projections to the cortex and brainstem can cause secondary dystonia (16). Focal cerebrovascular lesions in adulthood can also lead to dystonia (17). Acute secondary cervical and oromandibular dystonia was identified in 20% of acutely brain-injured patients (18). Cerebral arteriovenous malformations are also associated with dystonia, including hemidystonia and writer's cramp (19,20) (Fig. 1).

*Cerebral Anoxia and Perinatal Insults.* Parkinsonism and dystonia may follow cerebral anoxia. A pyramidal system lacking normal striatal control may be important in this setting (21). Delayed-onset dystonia due to perinatal anoxia is also a consideration in the differential diagnosis of dystonia occurring in childhood (22). The incidence of dystonia in association with perinatal insults may be due to the susceptibility of the striatum during development (23). A dystonic form of cerebral palsy may occur over a backdrop of a static encephalopathy (24).

*Bilateral Striatal Necrosis.* Dystonia and choreoathetosis are also associated with bilateral striatal necrosis. This disorder is often familial and may evolve gradually or in association with a febrile illness (25). Seizures and cognitive impairment are common and the prognosis is poor (26). Progressive generalized dystonia and

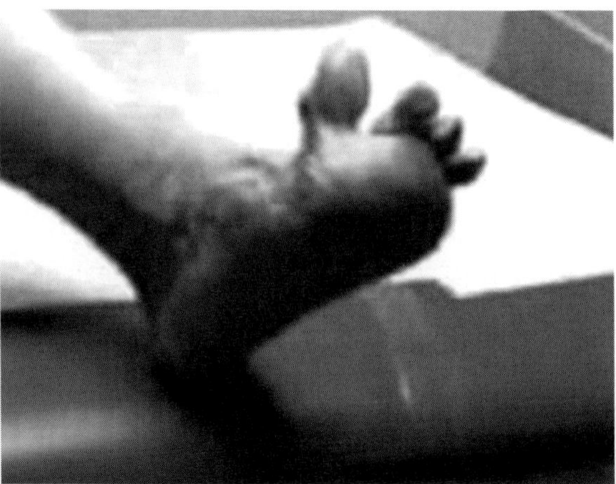

**Figure 1** Limb dystonia after putamenal lacunar infarct. This woman had a long history of hypertensive disease who presented initially to the hospital with weakness of her left side. Although she had a good recovery, over the course of the next several months, she developed this abnormal foot posture.

bilateral striatal necrosis may also occur in association with a mutation (*T14487C*) in the mitochondrial *ND6* gene. Transmitochondrial cell lines harboring 100% mutant mitochondrial DNA (mtDNA) showed a marked decrease in the activity of complex I of the respiratory chain supporting the pathogenic role of *T14487C* (27).

*Peripheral Trauma.* Peripheral injury from a number of causes including trauma, surgery, electrical injury, and entrapment neuropathies has been associated with secondary dystonia (28,29). Fixed dystonia may occur after a peripheral injury and may be associated with a complex regional pain syndrome and, frequently, psychiatric comorbidity (30). Post-traumatic cervical dystonia is recognized as a distinct clinical entity (31,32). The onset is often within hours or a few days of the trauma. Atlantoaxial rotatory subluxation has also been associated with cervical dystonia (33). Cranial dystonia and oromandibular dystonia have been reported within hours to months following a dental procedure or with poorly fitting dentures although a definite causal relationship has not been demonstrated (34,35).

*Central Pontine Myelinolysis.* Extrapontine and central pontine myelinolysis may occur due to excessively rapid correction of hyponatremia. A variety of movement disorders may occur including tremor and myoclonus, followed by a progressive painful dystonia of facial musculature and lower limbs. The dystonia may become generalized and associated with choreoathetosis and parkinsonian features (36). Signal increase in the central pons, thalamus, and striatum on T2-weighted magnetic resonance imaging compatible with central pontine and extrapontine myelinolysis are diagnostic (37).

**Infectious Etiologies.** *Poststreptococcal.* A variety of movement disorders may follow beta-hemolytic streptococcus infection (38), particularly obsessive–compulsive disorders, tic disorders, dystonia, chorea, and dystonic choreoathetosis in children (39). Serological evidence of recent beta-hemolytic streptococcal infection may be found along with the presence of antibasal ganglia antibodies (40). Mycoplasma pneumoniae-associated isolated acute bilateral thalamic necrosis may also result in dystonia (41,42).

*HIV-AIDS.* Movement disorders including dystonia and parkinsonism have been documented with HIV infection (43). Progressive multifocal leukoencephalopathy, and thalamic toxoplasmosis as well as a tardive dystonia syndrome are possible underlying mechanisms (44). A drug interaction with ritonavir, indinavir, and risperidone may lead to a dystonic syndrome (45). Dystonia in association with bilateral striatal lucencies is also seen with HIV infection (46).

*Tuberculosis.* Tubercular meningitis may be associated with tremor, chorea, myoclonus, and dystonia (47). Tuberculomas resulting in focal lesions may also cause dystonia (48).

*Subacute Sclerosing Panencephalitis.* Subacute sclerosing panencephalitis, a postviral syndrome associated with an altered form of the measles virus, may present with frequent paroxysmal dystonic posturing (49). It may also be a cause of myoclonus–dystonia (50).

**Drugs and Toxins.** *Chemical Agents.* A variety of drugs and toxins are associated with secondary dystonia. Carbon monoxide poisoning may cause delayed-onset dystonia and the prognosis in these cases is usually favorable (51). Lamivudine, a drug used to treat chronic hepatitis B infection, may cause acute dystonic reactions (52). Parkinsonism, a bucco-linguo-masticatory syndrome, and dystonia may occur with cinnarizine or flunarizine (53). Cough-suppressant preparations containing dextromethorphan or codeine may cause dystonic reactions in children (54).

*Tardive Dystonia.* With the widespread use of psychotropic agents, drug-induced movement disorders have become increasingly prevalent. Tardive dystonia is one of the most common etiologies of secondary dystonia. Chapter 17 is devoted to a discussion of this disorder.

*Hereditary Syndromes*

**Autosomal-Dominant Inheritance.** *Huntington's Disease.* In adults, Huntington's disease presents with chorea, personality change, and dementia. However, in juvenile Huntington's disease presentations (Westphal variant) bradykinesia, rigidity, dystonia, and epileptic seizures may be the presenting features (55,56) (Fig. 2).

*Spinocerebellar Ataxias and Dentatorubropallidoluysian Atrophy.* Dystonia may be a feature of dominant hereditary ataxias, especially SCA3/Machado–Joseph disease and dentatorubropallidoluysian atrophy (57). A dramatic improvement with levodopa has been seen in some cases (58,59).

*Fahr's Disease.* Fahr's disease or idiopathic basal ganglia calcification is a rare disorder characterized by progressive dystonia, parkinsonism, ataxia, dysphagia, and neuropsychiatric disturbances. While intracerebral calcification is a hallmark, there are no detectable abnormalities of calcium or phosphate metabolism. Imaging reveals calcification predominantly in the globus pallidus, as well as the putamen, caudate,

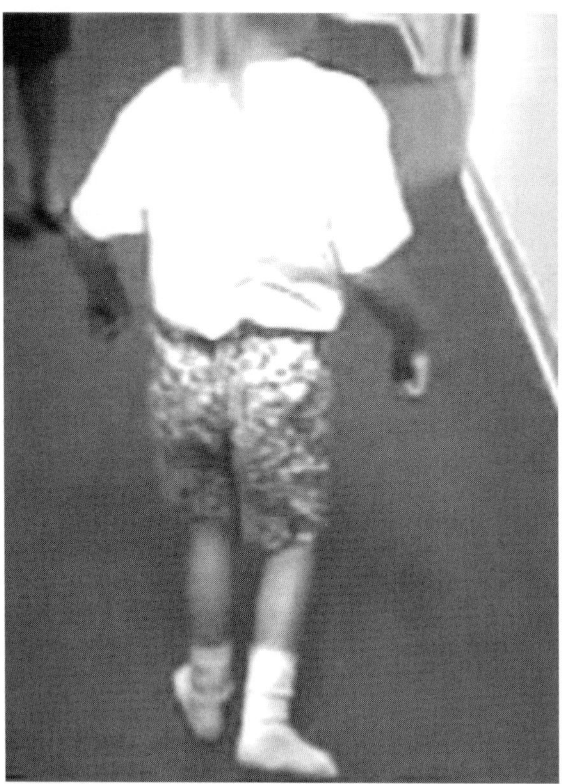

**Figure 2** Juvenile Huntington's disease. This young girl exhibits dystonic posture in her limbs, while walking. She was found to have more than 70 CAG repeats on Huntingon's disease gene testing, and also had generalized seizures, quite refractory to antiepileptic drug therapy.

dentate, thalamus, and cerebral white matter. An autosomal-dominant mode of inheritance has been reported in a few families (60,61).

**Autosomal-Recessive Inheritance.** *Wilson's Disease.* Wilson's disease is a rare autosomal-recessive disease of copper accumulation and copper toxicity, due to mutations in the *ATP7B* gene, which leads to a failure of biliary copper excretion (62). The disease may present with hepatic dysfunction, psychiatric disease, neurological disease, or a combination of these features. The neurological symptoms include abnormalities of speech, tremor, incoordination, and dystonia (Fig. 3). Drooling, risus sardonicus, clumsiness, and cognitive changes may also be seen. The presence of a low serum ceruloplasmin and a 24-hour urine copper excretion of over 100 micrograms are characteristic. Slit-lamp examination may show Kayser–Fleischer rings (63) (Fig. 4). T2- and proton-weighted MRI images may show an increased signal intensity over the thalamus, basal ganglia, and brainstem, especially the midbrain and pons (11) and serial MRI studies may show a gradual resolution of the lesions with chelating therapy (64) (Fig. 5a, b).

*Juvenile Parkinsonism.* The parkin gene (*PRKN*) is the predominant genetic cause of juvenile and early-onset parkinsonism in Japan, Europe, and the United States. In addition to parkinsonian features, the syndrome is characterized by symmetrical foot dystonia at onset, gait disturbance, diurnal change, and very slow progression. Patients with *PRKN* mutations tend to be younger at onset than those without mutations, and require a relatively lower dose of levodopa (65).

*Pantothenate Kinase-Associated Neurodegeneration (Hallervorden–Spatz Disease).* PKAN, formerly Hallervorden–Spatz syndrome, is a rare autosomal-recessive disorder characterized by extrapyramidal dysfunction presenting with dystonia, rigidity, and choreoathetosis. Iron deposition in conjunction with destruction of the globus pallidus gives rise to the characteristic "eye-of-the-tiger" sign on MRI although absence of this finding does not exclude the diagnosis (66). The HARP syndrome, a variant of Hallervorden–Spatz disease, characterized by hypoprebetalipoproteinemia, acanthocytosis, retinitis pigmentosa, and pallidal degeneration is also associated with dystonia (67,68).

*Ataxia with Vitamin E Deficiency.* Ataxia with vitamin E deficiency (AVED) is a rare autosomal-recessive neurodegenerative disease that resembles Friedreich's ataxia and is caused by mutations in the gene for α-tocopherol transfer protein (69).

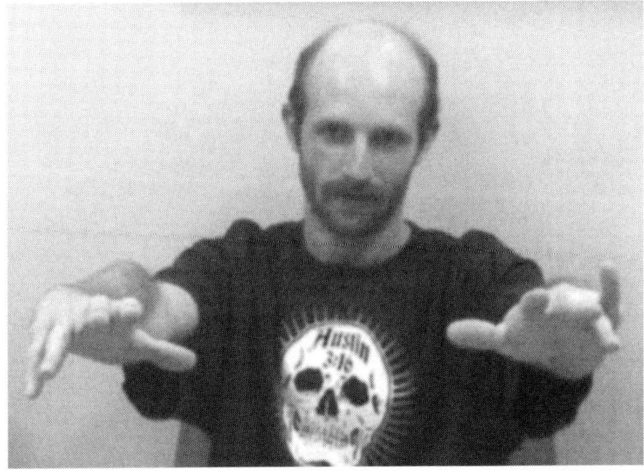

**Figure 3** Dystonic posturing in Wilson's disease.

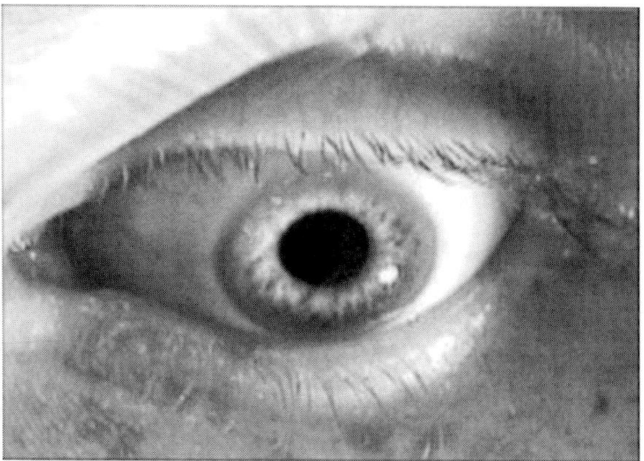

**Figure 4** Kayser-Fleischer ring.

Dystonia may occur in conjunction with AVED and may not respond to vitamin E supplementation (70).

*Niemann–Pick Disease.* Patients with Niemann–Pick disease type C, especially those who survive into adult life, may develop psychosis or other major psychiatric problems. Ataxia and vertical gaze palsy are important clinical clues, and organomegaly is present on the general exam. Increases in plasma chitotriosidase activity helps in the differential diagnosis. The diagnosis is by filipin staining of cultured fibroblasts, as well as cholesterol esterification studies and DNA mutation analysis (71,72).

*Neuronal Ceroid-Lipofuscinosis.* Neuronal ceroid-lipofuscinosis is the most common class of neurodegenerative disease in children and has various subtypes. Clinical features include progressive dementia, ataxia, myoclonic seizures, and retinal changes. Dystonia most commonly occurs in juveniles. Cerebral and cerebellar

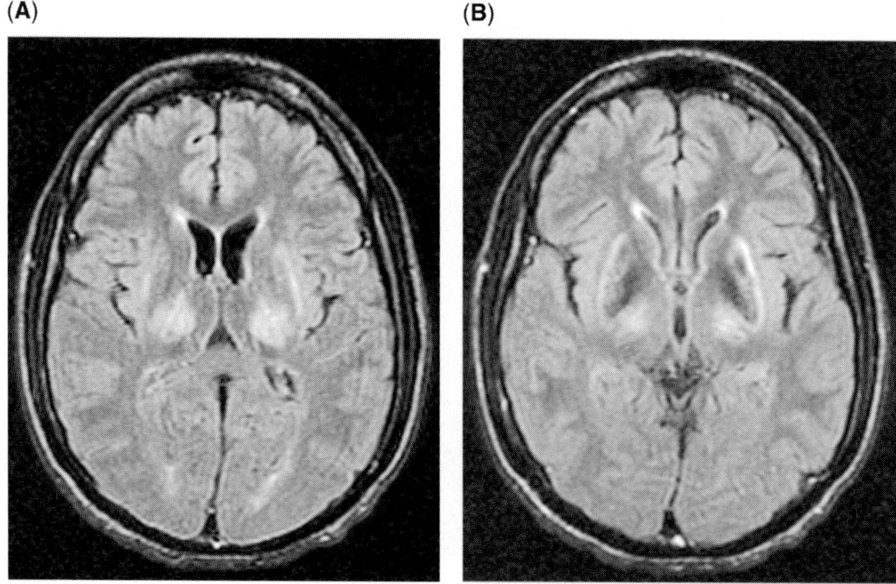


**Figure 5** Wilson's disease. (**A**) Risus thalamic lesions and (**B**) Putaminal changes.

cortical atrophy can be seen on imaging (73). Various tissues including skin, conjunctivae, skeletal muscle, vascular smooth muscle, neurons obtained from rectal biopsy, or peripheral lymphocytes may show characteristic cytoplasmic inclusions, which are periodic acid-Schiff stain positive and sudanophilic when viewed by electron microscopy (74).

*Glutaric Aciduria Type I.* Glutaric aciduria type I is an autosomal-recessive disorder of organic acid metabolism due to glutaryl-coenzyme A dehydrogenase deficiency. Affected infants or children may present with acute dystonia. MRI of the brain with T2-weighted imaging shows bilateral hyperintensity in the caudate and putamen with subtle involvement of the medial frontal lobes and diffusion-weighted images show restricted diffusion bilaterally in the caudate and putamen that is consistent with acute necrosis. Clinical diagnosis of glutaric aciduria type I is confirmed by an elevation of 3-hydroxyglutaric and glutaric acids (75).

*Methylmalonic Aciduria.* Methylmalonic aciduria is a rare inborn error of branched-chain amino acid metabolism. Neurological symptoms include a dystonic syndrome caused by progressive destruction of the basal ganglia, similar to those observed in other organic acid disorders, such as propionic aciduria or glutaric aciduria type I (76).

*Pyruvate Dehydrogenase Deficiency.* Pyruvate dehydrogenase deficiency is a major cause of primary lactic acidosis and neurological dysfunction in infancy and early childhood. Episodic dystonia may occur along with the more common findings of hypotonia and ataxia, and discrete lesions restricted to the globus pallidus, may be seen on imaging studies (77). Cerebrospinal fluid (CSF) lactate is elevated and some cases may respond to levodopa (78).

*Triosephosphate Isomerase Deficiency.* Triosephosphate isomerase deficiency may also feature dystonic movements, tremor, pyramidal tract signs, and evidence of spinal motor neuron involvement. Structures in the basal ganglia, brainstem, and spinal cord seem to be involved in the pathological process, while the cerebral cortex is spared (79).

*GLUT1 Gene Mutation.* Glucose transport protein deficiency due to mutation in *GLUT1* may be associated with movement disorders including ataxia, dystonia, and choreoathetosis, in addition to the characteristic seizure disorder, microcephaly, global developmental delays, and hypoglycorrhachia. A ketogenic diet is helpful for symptomatic relief (80).

*Metachromatic Leukodystrophy.* Metachromatic leukodystrophy may rarely present with dysarthria and dystonia of the neck, spine, and extremities. Diagnostic studies include positive sural nerve biopsies, prolonged nerve conduction times, and a marked deficiency of arylsulfatase A in the urine, leukocytes, and fibroblasts (81,82).

*Krabbe's Disease.* Late-onset globoid cell leukodystrophy (Krabbe's disease) presents with visual failure and severe central pyramidal and extrapyramidal motor disability with spasticity, dystonia, ataxia, and peripheral neuropathy. Neuroimaging is significant for white matter lesions. Nerve conduction velocities are low, and a slowly developing polyneuropathy may be seen. Reduced leukocyte galactosylceramidase activity is diagnostic (83).

*GM1 and GM2 Gangliosidosis.* Deficiency of enzyme acid beta-galactosidase causes GM1 gangliosidosis. Patients with type 3 disease survive into adulthood and develop movement disorders. In these patients, generalized dystonia is a prominent feature and is often associated with akinetic-rigid parkinsonism. Facial dystonia and severe dysarthria are frequent, and eye movements are normal. Bone marrow examination may show Gaucher-like foam cells (12). MRI frequently shows bilateral symmetrical putamenal hyperintensities on T2-weighted and proton density images (84). Diagnosis is confirmed by demonstrating deficiency of beta-galactosidase. GM1 gangliosidosis should be considered in the differential diagnosis of early-onset generalized dystonia, particularly in patients with short stature and skeletal dysplasia (85). A form of juvenile progressive dystonia can also represent a phenotype of GM2 gangliosidosis (86). Dementia, amyotrophy, choreoathetosis, and ataxia may be additional signs (87). Beta-hexosaminidase activity in plasma, leukocytes, and fibroblasts is significantly reduced (88).

*Homocystinuria.* Homocystinuria occurs due to cystathionine beta-synthase. Progressive generalized dystonia can occur secondary to neurochemical changes in the basal ganglia caused by an inherited defect in sulfur amino acid metabolism (89,90).

*Hartnup Disease.* The presentation of Hartnup disease in children includes intermittent dystonic posturing of the lower extremities and eczematous dermatitis without ataxia. Qualitative and quantitative urine amino acid testing help confirm the diagnosis. Spinal fluid hydroxy-indoleacetic acid concentration is low and increases with oral tryptophan loading. Unlike the skin rash, the dystonia may not respond to tryptophan administered alone or with nicotinic acid (91).

*Ataxia–Telangiectasia.* Ataxia–telangiectasia is a rare recessive multisystem disorder characterized by telangiectasia and cerebellar ataxia. Telangiectasias are tiny, red "spider" veins, which appear in the corners of the eyes or on the ears and cheeks. Dystonia and myoclonus may also occur. MRI may show cerebellar atrophy with putamenal lesions (92,93).

**X-Linked Inheritance.** *X-Linked Dystonia–Parkinsonism (Lubag).* X-linked dystonia–Parkinsonism or "Lubag" is an X-linked–recessive disorder that afflicts Filipino men, and in rare cases, women. The clinical features include parkinsonism, dystonia, myoclonus, tremor, and chorea. The dystonia, if present, is usually mild and usually nonprogressive (94).

*Lesch–Nyhan Syndrome.* Lesch–Nyhan syndrome is a rare X-linked–recessive disorder characterized by a near complete deficiency of the purine salvage enzyme hypoxanthine-guanine phosphoribosyltransferase (95). Neurological manifestations include hyperuricemia, mental retardation, spastic cerebral palsy, dystonia, and self-mutilation. The self-mutilatory behavior can be very disabling and botulinum toxin (96) and pallidal deep brain stimulation (97) have been used to control this symptom.

*Mohr–Tranebjaerg Syndrome.* Mohr–Tranebjaerg syndrome is a rare form of deafness associated with dystonia. This recessive neurodegenerative syndrome presents with postlingual progressive sensorineural deafness in early childhood, followed by progressive dystonia, spasticity, dysphagia, mental deterioration, paranoia, and cortical blindness. Mutations in the X-linked deafness-dystonia peptide 1 gene are the underlying cause (98,99).

*Other X-linked Syndromes.* A DRD may occur in Turner's syndrome with bilateral globus pallidus hypointensities on brain MRI (100). X-linked mental retardation in association with dystonia may be caused by a 24 base-pair duplication in ARX. The symptomatology includes mental retardation, infantile spasms (West syndrome), and other less severe forms of seizures along with focal dystonia (101). Extrapyramidal dysfunction in Rett syndrome includes stereotyped movements and bruxism, air–saliva expulsion, self-mutilation, parkinsonian findings, athetosis, myoclonus, and dystonia (Fig. 6). The syndrome is caused by mutations in the *MECP2* gene, which is localized on the X chromosome (102). Pelizaeus–Merzbacher disease is a rare X-linked leukodystrophy caused by a mutation in the gene that

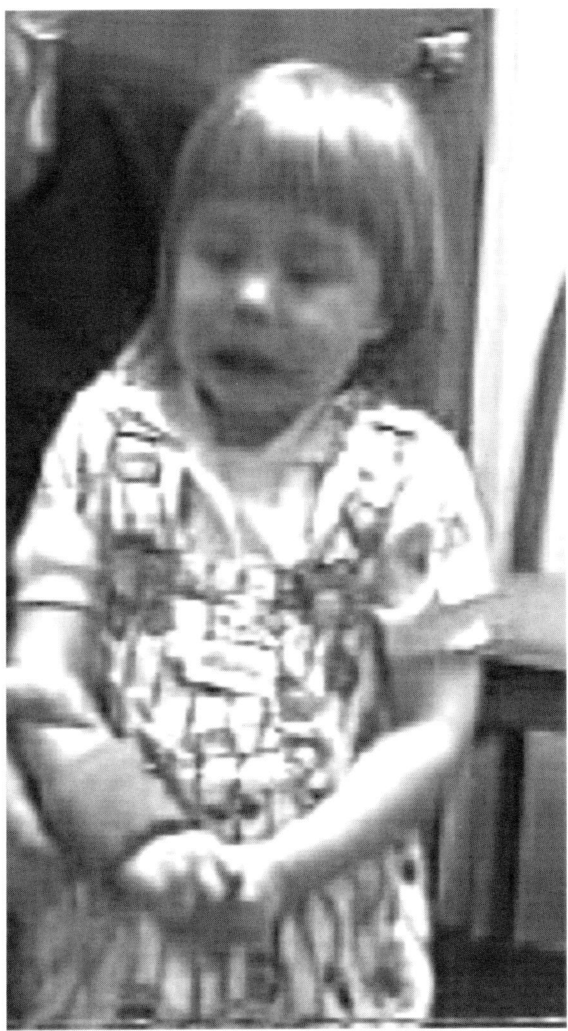

**Figure 6** Rett syndrome. This child exhibits an intermittent dystonic facial expression, quite typical of this disorder. In addition, she has been fitted with a protective wrist band to prevent biting of her right arm. This still photo also demonstrates typical hand-wringing stereotypies.

controls the production of a myelin protein called proteolipid protein. Other clinical findings include progressive psychomotor developmental delay, nystagmus, spastic quadriplegia, dystonia, and cerebellar ataxia (103,104).

**Mitochondrial Inheritance.** *Leber's Hereditary Optic Neuropathy and Other Mitochondrial Disorders.* Leber's hereditary optic neuropathy (LHON) may present with dystonia and a high T2 signal in the putamen bilaterally (105). LHON is associated with a G to A transition at nucleotide position 14459, within the mtDNA-encoded *ND6* gene (106,107).

**Multiple Forms of Inheritance.** *Leigh's Syndrome.* Leigh's syndrome is a form of mitochondrial encephalopathy with mitochondrial or recessive inheritance that presents with impaired mental and/or motor development, and childhood-onset dystonia (108). Optic atrophy, hypotonia, dysphagia, and dysarthria are also common. Imaging studies may show symmetrical bilateral lucencies or calcification in the basal ganglia and blood lactate levels are usually elevated (109).

*Neuronal Intranuclear Inclusion Disease.* Neuronal intranuclear inclusion disease is a rare neurodegenerative disorder with a heterogeneous clinical picture characterized pathologically by eosinophilic intranuclear inclusions in neurons of the peripheral, central, and autonomic nervous systems associated with varying degrees of neuronal loss. Clinical phenomenology may include juvenile parkinsonism or dystonia. A full thickness rectal biopsy is helpful in the diagnosis (110).

*Hereditary Hemochromatosis.* Hereditary hemochromatosis (HH) may be associated with tremor, myoclonus, parkinsonism, and dystonia. The diagnosis of HH is established by iron tests, evidence of a *C282Y* mutation, and liver biopsy. T2-weighted MRI may reveal hyperintensities in hemispheric white matter, and cerebral and cerebellar atrophy (111).

*Neuroacanthocytosis.* Neuroacanthocytosis is a progressive disease characterized by movement disorders, personality changes, cognitive deterioration, axonal neuropathy, and seizures. The neurological abnormalities are associated with speculated, "acanthocytic" red cells in blood thus leading to the term *neuroacanthocytosis* (112). This heterogeneous group of disorders is being redefined due to genetic discoveries. The core neuroacanthocytosis syndromes are autosomal-recessive chorea-acanthocytosis and the X-linked McLeod syndrome. Huntington's disease-like 2 and PKAN are now included in this group of disorders (113). Serum vitamin E and lipoprotein levels are usually normal (although one case of aprebetalipoproteinemia has been reported). Caudate atrophy and increased signal in caudate and lentiform nuclei may be seen on MRI (9).

### *Neurodegenerative Disorders*

**Parkinson's Disease.** One of the most common etiologies for secondary dystonia is Parkinson's disease (PD). Dystonia, particularly when it involves the foot, may be the presenting sign of PD or a parkinsonian syndrome and these disorders should be suspected when adults present with isolated foot dystonia (114). Dystonia is usually an "off-state" symptom although "on-state" dystonia may also occur. In patients with significant motor fluctuations the "dystonia-improvement-dystonia" phenomenon may be observed (115).

**Multiple System Atrophy.** Although a mild stooped posture is common in PD, extreme forward flexion of the trunk is unusual. This phenomenon called camptocormia or the Pisa syndrome may be seen in multiple system atrophy (116). Primary dystonia and Tourette syndrome are also associated with such posturing (117).

**Progressive Supranuclear Palsy and Corticobasal Degeneration.** Dystonia is a common feature of progressive supranuclear palsy and corticobasal degeneration. Cervical dystonia and blepharospasm with eyelid apraxia associated with these conditions may respond to botulinum toxin treatment (118) (Fig. 7).

**Multiple Sclerosis and Autoimmune Disorders.** While tremor is a common presentation of multiple sclerosis (MS), dystonia or chorea may also occur during clinical exacerbation of MS and may respond to steroid therapy (119). Paroxysmal dystonia in MS may be associated with a demyelinating lesion of the thalamus (120). Rasmussen's encephalitis, a rare autoimmune disorder characterized by intractable epilepsy and progressive hemispheric dysfunction can present with foot dystonia, arm athetosis, and epilepsia partialis continua. There may be a transient response to intravenous immunoglobulin (121). A complex regional pain syndrome with progression toward

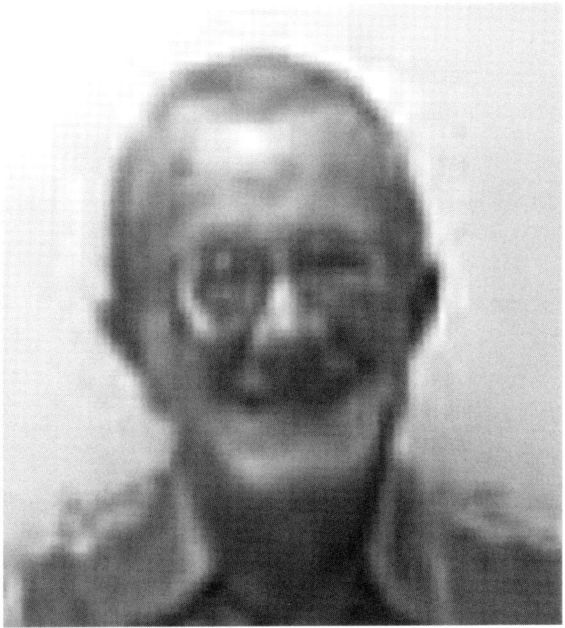

**Figure 7** Progressive supranuclear palsy (PSP). This subject exhibits typical astonished facial expression associated with PSP.

a multifocal or generalized tonic dystonia has been described in association with significant elevation of *HLA-DR13*. The dystonia began distally, involved mainly flexor muscles, and was associated with sensory and autonomic symptoms (122). Meige syndrome may occur in the setting of thyroid autoimmune disease (123).

**Dystonia-Plus Syndromes.** *Dopa-Responsive Dystonia.* Autosomal-dominant guanosine triphosphate cyclohydrolase I (GCH-I) deficiency (Segawa disease) is a DRD caused by mutation of the *GCH-I* gene located on 14q22.1-q22.2. DRD has an excellent response to levodopa (124,125). DRD is discussed in detail in chapter 15.

*Other Biopterin Deficiencies.* Another form of DRD may be seen in patients with 6-pyruvoyl-tetrahydropterin synthase (PTPS) deficiency (126). Symptoms include hypotonia, dystonia, choreoathetosis, mental retardation, behavioral disturbances, and incomplete puberty due to PTPS deficiency. Progressive hypotonia and choreoathetoid movements may occur despite good control of hyperphenylalaninemia. There is an excellent long-term response to levodopa.

Sepiapterin reductase deficiency may also result in a dystonia that responds to levodopa. The patients show a novel mutation in the tetrahydrobiopterin pathway involving sepiapterin reductase, and no abnormality in the gene encoding GCH-I. The disorder is autosomal recessive and oculogyric crises and parkinsonism are also seen (127).

*Myoclonus–Dystonia Syndrome.* Myoclonus–Dystonia Syndrome (MDS) is an autosomal-dominant disorder characterized by bilateral myoclonic jerks in association with dystonic posturing. Electromyogram (EMG) studies of the "myoclonic" movements reveal prolonged EMG bursts typical of dystonia rather than the short-duration EMG bursts more typical of myoclonus (128). The epsilon-sarcoglycan gene (*SGCE*) on chromosome 7q21 has been reported to be a major locus for inherited myoclonus–dystonia (129,130). However, autosomal-dominant MDS may also occur without an *SGCE* mutation suggesting genetic heterogeneity (131). MDS has also been reported in association with vitamin E deficiency with mutation in the tocopherol transfer protein alleles (132). Patients may show a significant improvement with alcohol and sodium oxybate (133,134).

*Rapid-Onset Dystonia–Parkinsonism.* Rapid-onset dystonia–parkinsonism (135) may also occur with a missense mutation in the Na/K-ATPase alpha3 subunit (*ATP1A3*). Asymmetrical parkinsonian symptoms may be seen at onset followed by a sudden-onset oromandibular dystonia and worsening parkinsonian symptoms (136).

## TREATMENT

Treatment of secondary dystonia is guided by the underlying etiology and the topographical presentation of the dystonia. Focal lesions such as tumors, arteriovenous malformations, subdural hematomas, and abscesses may be amenable to surgical resection. However, dystonia may occasionally arise as a complication of such resections. Infectious etiologies such as tuberculosis, syphilis, viral encephalitis, AIDS, and toxoplasmosis are treated by therapy targeting the specific organism. Control of the underlying infectious cause may result in improvement in the dystonic posturing. Treatment in Wilson's disease is aimed at eliminating copper using chelating agents such as D-penicillamine and triethylamine or reducing copper absorption with zinc gluconate. Chelating therapy may result in initial worsening of neurological deficits, while sodium thiomolybdate is an experimental therapy less associated with this risk (63,64). The "off state" dystonia in PD may respond to optimizing dopaminergic therapy. Pallidotomy or deep brain stimulation of the globus pallidus or subthalamic nucleus may be indicated in more advanced cases (137,138). Surgical treatment is also a consideration in secondary dystonia with deep brain stimulation being preferred to lesioning techniques. However, secondary dystonia tends to be less responsive than primary dystonia (139). Symptomatic treatment of dystonia is discussed in Chapters 20–26.

## REFERENCES


1. Fahn S. Concept and classification of dystonia. Adv Neurol 1988; 50:1–8.
2. Ferraz HB, Andrade LA. Symptomatic dystonia: clinical profile of 46 Brazilian patients. Can J Neurol Sci 1992; 19(4):504–507.
3. Fahn S, Greene P, Ford B, Bressman S. Secondary dystonias. In: Fahn S, Greene P, Ford B, Bressman S, eds. Handbook of Movement Disorders. Philadelphia: Current Medicine Inc., 1997:51–71.
4. Marsden CD, Fahn S. Dystonia 3. Summary and conclusions. Adv Neurol 1998; 78: 359–364.
5. El-Youssef M. Wilson disease. Mayo Clin Proc 2003; 78(9):1126–1136.
6. Bressman SB. Dystonia genotypes, phenotypes, and classification. Adv Neurol 2004; 94:101–107.
7. Fross RD, Martin WR, Li D, et al. Lesions of the putamen: their relevance to dystonia. Neurology 1987; 37(7):1125–1129.
8. Kostic VS, Stojanovic-Svetel M, Kacar A. Symptomatic dystonias associated with structural brain lesions: report of 16 cases. Can J Neurol Sci 1996; 23(1):53–56.
9. Kutcher JS, Kahn MJ, Andersson HC, Foundas AL. Neuroacanthocytosis masquerading as Huntington's disease: CT/MRI findings. J Neuroimaging 1999; 9(3):187–189.

10. Hayflick SJ, Westaway SK, Levinson B, et al. Genetic, clinical, and radiographic delineation of Hallervorden-Spatz syndrome. N Engl J Med 2003; 348(1):33–40.
11. Kozic D, Svetel M, Petrovic B, Dragasevic N, Semnic R, Kostic VS. MR imaging of the brain in patients with hepatic form of Wilson's disease. Eur J Neurol 2003; 10(5):587–592.
12. Muthane U, Chickabasaviah Y, Kaneski C, et al. Clinical features of adult GM1 gangliosidosis: report of three Indian patients and review of 40 cases. Mov Disord 2004; 19(11):1334–1341.
13. Rossi A, Biancheri R, Bruno C, et al. Leigh Syndrome with COX deficiency and SURF1 gene mutations: MR imaging findings. AJNR Am J Neuroradiol 2003; 24(6):1188–1191.
14. Oguz KK, Ozturk A, Cila A. Diffusion-weighted MR imaging and MR spectroscopy in glutaric aciduria type 1. Neuroradiology 2005; 47(3):229–234.
15. Wimberger D, Prayer L, Kramer J, Binder H, Imhof H. MRI in basal ganglia diseases. J Neural Transm Suppl 1991; 33:133–140.
16. Lorenzana L, Cabezudo JM, Porras LF, Polaina M, Rodriguez-Sanchez JA, Garcia-Yague LM. Focal dystonia secondary to cavernous angioma of the basal ganglia: case report and review of the literature. Neurosurgery 1992; 31(6):1108–1111; discussion 1111–1102.
17. Burton K, Farrell K, Li D, Calne DB. Lesions of the putamen and dystonia: CT and magnetic resonance imaging. Neurology 1984; 34(7):962–965.
18. Lo SE, Rosengart AJ, Novakovic RL, et al. Identification and treatment of cervical and oromandibular dystonia in acutely brain-injured patients. Neurocrit Care 2005; 3(2):139–145.
19. Krauss JK, Kiriyanthan GD, Borremans JJ. Cerebral arteriovenous malformations and movement disorders. Clin Neurol Neurosurg 1999; 101(2):92–99.
20. Kurita H, Sasaki T, Suzuki I, Kirino T. Basal ganglia arteriovenous malformation presenting as "writer's cramp". Childs Nerv Syst 1998; 14(6):285–287.
21. Boylan KB, Chin JH, DeArmond SJ. Progressive dystonia following resuscitation from cardiac arrest. Neurology 1990; 40(9):1458–1461.
22. Burke RE, Fahn S, Gold AP. Delayed-onset dystonia in patients with "static" encephalopathy. J Neurol Neurosurg Psychiatry 1980; 43(9):789–797.
23. Giladi N, Burke RE, Kostic V, et al. Hemiparkinsonism-hemiatrophy syndrome: clinical and neuroradiologic features. Neurology 1990; 40(11):1731–1734.
24. Treves T, Korczyn AD. Progressive dystonia and paraparesis in cerebral palsy. Eur Neurol 1986; 25(2):148–153.
25. Craver RD, Duncan MC, Nelson JS. Familial dystonia and choreoathetosis in three generations associated with bilateral striatal necrosis. J Child Neurol 1996; 11(3):185–188.
26. Roig M, Calopa M, Rovira A, Macaya A, Riudor E, Losada M. Bilateral striatal lesions in childhood. Pediatr Neurol 1993; 9(5):349–358.
27. Solano A, Roig M, Vives-Bauza C, et al. Bilateral striatal necrosis associated with a novel mutation in the mitochondrial ND6 gene. Ann Neurol 2003; 54(4):527–530.
28. Jankovic J. Post-traumatic movement disorders: central and peripheral mechanisms. Neurology 1994; 44(11):2006–2014.
29. Tarsy D, Sudarsky L, Charness ME. Limb dystonia following electrical injury. Mov Disord 1994; 9(2):230–232.
30. Schrag A, Trimble M, Quinn N, Bhatia K. The syndrome of fixed dystonia: an evaluation of 103 patients. Brain 2004; 127(Pt 10):2360–2372.
31. O'Riordan S, Hutchinson M. Cervical dystonia following peripheral trauma-a case-control study. J Neurol 2004; 251(2):150–155.
32. Truong DD, Dubinsky R, Hermanowicz N, Olson WL, Silverman B, Koller WC. Posttraumatic torticollis. Arch Neurol 1991; 48(2):221–223.
33. Crook TB, Eynon CA. Traumatic atlantoaxial rotatory subluxation. Emerg Med J 2005; 22(9):671–672.
34. Schrag A, Bhatia KP, Quinn NP, Marsden CD. Atypical and typical cranial dystonia following dental procedures. Mov Disord 1999; 14(3):492–496.
35. Sankhla C, Lai EC, Jankovic J. Peripherally induced oromandibular dystonia. J Neurol Neurosurg Psychiatry 1998; 65(5):722–728.

36. Seah AB, Chan LL, Wong MC, Tan EK. Evolving spectrum of movement disorders in extrapontine and central pontine myelinolysis. Parkinsonism Relat Disord 2002; 9(2):117–119.
37. Yoshida Y, Akanuma J, Tochikubo S, et al. Slowly progressive dystonia following central pontine and extrapontine myelinolysis. Intern Med 2000; 39(11):956–960.
38. Dale RC, Heyman I, Surtees RA, et al. Dyskinesias and associated psychiatric disorders following streptococcal infections. Arch Dis Child 2004; 89(7):604–610.
39. Hahn RG, Knox LM, Forman TA. Evaluation of poststreptococcal illness. Am Fam Physician 2005; 71(10):1949–1954.
40. Dale RC, Church AJ, Benton S, et al. Post-streptococcal autoimmune dystonia with isolated bilateral striatal necrosis. Dev Med Child Neurol 2002; 44(7):485–489.
41. Ashtekar CS, Jaspan T, Thomas D, Weston V, Gayatri NA, Whitehouse WP. Acute bilateral thalamic necrosis in a child with Mycoplasma pneumoniae. Dev Med Child Neurol 2003; 45(9):634–637.
42. Green C, Riley DE. Treatment of dystonia in striatal necrosis caused by Mycoplasma pneumoniae. Pediatr Neurol 2002; 26(4):318–320.
43. Tse W, Cersosimo MG, Gracies JM, Morgello S, Olanow CW, Koller W. Movement disorders and AIDS: a review. Parkinsonism Relat Disord 2004; 10(6):323–334.
44. Factor SA, Troche-Panetto M, Weaver SA. Dystonia in AIDS: report of four cases. Mov Disord 2003; 18(12):1492–1498.
45. Kelly DV, Beique LC, Bowmer MI. Extrapyramidal symptoms with ritonavir/indinavir plus risperidone. Ann Pharmacother 2002; 36(5):827–830.
46. Abbruzzese G, Rizzo F, Dall'Agata D, Morandi N, Favale E. Generalized dystonia with bilateral striatal computed-tomographic lucencies in a patient with human immunodeficiency virus infection. Eur Neurol 1990; 30(5):271–273.
47. Alarcon F, Tolosa E, Munoz E. Focal limb dystonia in a patient with a cerebellar mass. Arch Neurol 2001; 58(7):1125–1127.
48. Tey HL, Seet RC, Lim EC. Tuberculomas causing cervical dystonia. Intern Med J 2005; 35(4):261–262.
49. Ondo WG, Verma A. Physiological assessment of paroxysmal dystonia secondary to subacute sclerosing panencephalitis. Mov Disord 2002; 17(1):154–157.
50. Oga T, Ikeda A, Nagamine T, et al. Implication of sensorimotor integration in the generation of periodic dystonic myoclonus in subacute sclerosing panencephalitis (SSPE). Mov Disord 2000; 15(6):1173–1183.
51. Choi IS, Cheon HY. Delayed movement disorders after carbon monoxide poisoning. Eur Neurol 1999; 42(3):141–144.
52. Song X, Hu Z, Zhang H. Acute dystonia induced by Lamivudine. Clin Neuropharmacol 2005; 28(4):193–194.
53. Fabiani G, Pastro PC, Froehner C. Parkinsonism and other movement disorders in outpatients in chronic use of cinnarizine and flunarizine. Arq Neuropsiquiatr 2004; 62(3B):784–788.
54. Polizzi A, Incorpora G, Ruggieri M. Dystonia as acute adverse reaction to cough suppressant in a 3-year-old girl. Eur J Paediatr Neurol 2001; 5(4):167–168.
55. Louis ED, Anderson KE, Moskowitz C, Thorne DZ, Marder K. Dystonia-predominant adult-onset Huntington disease: association between motor phenotype and age of onset in adults. Arch Neurol 2000; 57(9):1326–1330.
56. Vargas AP, Carod-Artal FJ, Bomfim D, Vazquez-Cabrera C, Dantas-Barbosa C. Unusual early-onset Huntingtons disease. J Child Neurol 2003; 18(6):429–432.
57. Garcia Ruiz PJ, Mayo D, Hernandez J, Cantarero S, Ayuso C. Movement disorders in hereditary ataxias. J Neurol Sci 2002; 202(1–2):59–64.
58. Nandagopal R, Moorthy SG. Dramatic levodopa responsiveness of dystonia in a sporadic case of spinocerebellar ataxia type 3. Postgrad Med J 2004; 80(944):363–365.
59. Wilder-Smith E, Tan EK, Law HY, Zhao Y, Ng I, Wong MC. Spinocerebellar ataxia type 3 presenting as an L-DOPA responsive dystonia phenotype in a Chinese family. J Neurol Sci 2003; 213(1–2):25–28.

60. Manyam BV, Walters AS, Narla KR. Bilateral striopallidodentate calcinosis: clinical characteristics of patients seen in a registry. Mov Disord 2001; 16(2):258–264.
61. Geschwind DH, Loginov M, Stern JM. Identification of a locus on chromosome 14q for idiopathic basal ganglia calcification (Fahr disease). Am J Hum Genet 1999; 65(3):764–772.
62. Brewer GJ. Neurologically presenting Wilson's disease: epidemiology, pathophysiology and treatment. CNS Drugs 2005; 19(3):185–192.
63. Roberts EA, Schilsky ML. A practice guideline on Wilson disease. Hepatology 2003; 37(6):1475–1492.
64. Huang CC, Chu NS. Wilson's disease: resolution of MRI lesions following long-term oral zinc therapy. Acta Neurol Scand 1996; 93(2–3):215–218.
65. Wu RM, Bounds R, Lincoln S, et al. Parkin mutations and early-onset parkinsonism in a Taiwanese cohort. Arch Neurol 2005; 62(1):82–87.
66. Baumeister FA, Auer DP, Hortnagel K, Freisinger P, Meitinger T. The eye-of-the-tiger sign is not a reliable disease marker for Hallervorden-Spatz syndrome. Neuropediatrics 2005; 36(3):221–222.
67. Orrell RW, Amrolia PJ, Heald A, et al. Acanthocytosis, retinitis pigmentosa, and pallidal degeneration: a report of three patients, including the second reported case with hypoprebetalipoproteinemia (HARP syndrome). Neurology 1995; 45(3 Pt 1):487–492.
68. Higgins JJ, Patterson MC, Papadopoulos NM, Brady RO, Pentchev PG, Barton NW. Hypoprebetalipoproteinemia, acanthocytosis, retinitis pigmentosa, and pallidal degeneration (HARP syndrome). Neurology 1992; 42(1):194–198.
69. Cavalier L, Ouahchi K, Kayden HJ, et al. Ataxia with isolated vitamin E deficiency: heterogeneity of mutations and phenotypic variability in a large number of families. Am J Hum Genet 1998; 62(2):301–310.
70. Roubertie A, Biolsi B, Rivier F, Humbertclaude V, Cheminal R, Echenne B. Ataxia with vitamin E deficiency and severe dystonia: report of a case. Brain Dev 2003; 25(6): 442–445.
71. Imrie J, Vijayaraghaven S, Whitehouse C, et al. Niemann-Pick disease type C in adults. J Inherit Metab Dis 2002; 25(6):491–500.
72. Uc EY, Wenger DA, Jankovic J. Niemann-Pick disease type C: two cases and an update. Mov Disord 2000; 15(6):1199–1203.
73. Boustany RM, Alroy J, Kolodny EH. Clinical classification of neuronal ceroid-lipofuscinosis subtypes. Am J Med Genet Suppl 1988; 5:47–58.
74. Goebel HH, Wisniewski KE. Current state of clinical and morphological features in human NCL. Brain Pathol 2004; 14(1):61–69.
75. Santos CC, Roach ES. Glutaric aciduria type I: a neuroimaging diagnosis?. J Child Neurol 2005; 20(7):588–590.
76. Horster F, Hoffmann GF. Pathophysiology, diagnosis, and treatment of methylmalonic aciduria-recent advances and new challenges. Pediatr Nephrol 2004; 19(10):1071–1074.
77. Head RA, de Goede CG, Newton RW, et al. Pyruvate dehydrogenase deficiency presenting as dystonia in childhood. Dev Med Child Neurol 2004; 46(10):710–712.
78. Neubauer D, Frelih J, Zupancic N, Kopac S, Cindro-Heberle L. 'Pyruvate dehydrogenase deficiency presenting as dystonia and responding to levodopa'. Dev Med Child Neurol 2005; 47(7):504.
79. Poll-The BT, Aicardi J, Girot R, Rosa R. Neurological findings in triosephosphate isomerase deficiency. Ann Neurol 1985; 17(5):439–443.
80. Friedman JR, Thiele EA, Wang D, et al. A typical GLUT1 deficiency with prominent movement disorder responsive to ketogenic diet. Mov Disord 2005. In press.
81. Yatziv S, Russell A. An unusual form of metachromatic leukodystrophy in three siblings. Clin Genet 1981; 19(4):222–227.
82. Baumann N, Turpin JC, Lefevre M, Colsch B. Motor and psycho-cognitive clinical types in adult metachromatic leukodystrophy: genotype/phenotype relationships?. J Physiol Paris 2002; 96(3–4):301–306.

83. Arvidsson J, Hagberg B, Mansson JE, Svennerholm L. Late onset globoid cell leukodystrophy (Krabbe's disease)-Swedish case with 15 years of follow-up. Acta Paediatr 1995; 84(2):218–221.
84. Uyama E, Terasaki T, Watanabe S, et al. Type 3 GM1 gangliosidosis: characteristic MRI findings correlated with dystonia. Acta Neurol Scand 1992; 86(6):609–615.
85. Roze E, Paschke E, Lopez N, et al. Dystonia and parkinsonism in GM1 type 3 gangliosidosis. Mov Disord 2005; 20(10):1366–1369.
86. Meek D, Wolfe LS, Andermann E, Andermann F. Juvenile progressive dystonia: a new phenotype of GM2 gangliosidosis. Ann Neurol 1984; 15(4):348–352.
87. Oates CE, Bosch EP, Hart MN. Movement disorders associated with chronic GM2 gangliosidosis. Case report and review of the literature. Eur Neurol 1986; 25(2):154–159.
88. Nardocci N, Bertagnolio B, Rumi V, Angelini L. Progressive dystonia symptomatic of juvenile GM2 gangliosidosis. Mov Disord 1992; 7(1):64–67.
89. Kempster PA, Brenton DP, Gale AN, Stern GM. Dystonia in homocystinuria. J Neurol Neurosurg Psychiatry 1988; 51(6):859–862.
90. Ekinci B, Apaydin H, Vural M, Ozekmekci S. Two siblings with homocystinuria presenting with dystonia and parkinsonism. Mov Disord 2004; 19(8):962–964.
91. Darras BT, Ampola MG, Dietz WH, Gilmore HE. Intermittent dystonia in Hartnup disease. Pediatr Neurol 1989; 5(2):118–120.
92. Goyal V, Behari M. Dystonia as presenting manifestation of ataxia telangiectasia : a case report. Neurol India 2002; 50(2):187–189.
93. Koepp M, Schelosky L, Cordes I, Cordes M, Poewe W. Dystonia in ataxia telangiectasia: report of a case with putaminal lesions and decreased striatal [123I]iodobenzamide binding. Mov Disord 1994; 9(4):455–459.
94. Evidente VG, Nolte D, Niemann S, et al. Phenotypic and molecular analyses of X-linked dystonia-parkinsonism ("lubag") in women. Arch Neurol 2004; 61(12):1956–1959.
95. Neychev VK, Mitev VI. The biochemical basis of the neurobehavioral abnormalities in the Lesch-Nyhan syndrome: a hypothesis. Med Hypotheses 2004; 63(1):131–134.
96. Dabrowski E, Smathers SA, Ralstrom CS, Nigro MA, Leleszi JP. Botulinum toxin as a novel treatment for self-mutilation in Lesch-Nyhan syndrome. Dev Med Child Neurol 2005; 47(9):636–639.
97. Taira T, Kobayashi T, Hori T. Disappearance of self-mutilating behavior in a patient with lesch-nyhan syndrome after bilateral chronic stimulation of the globus pallidus internus. Case report. J Neurosurg 2003; 98(2):414–416.
98. Jin H, May M, Tranebjaerg L, et al. A novel X-linked gene, DDP, shows mutations in families with deafness (DFN-1), dystonia, mental deficiency and blindness. Nat Genet 1996; 14(2):177–180.
99. Tranebjaerg L, Schwartz C, Eriksen H, et al. A new X linked recessive deafness syndrome with blindness, dystonia, fractures, and mental deficiency is linked to Xq22. J Med Genet 1995; 32(4):257–263.
100. Nitschke M, Steinberger D, Heberlein I, Otto V, Muller U, Vieregge P. Dopa responsive dystonia with Turner's syndrome: clinical, genetic, and neuropsychological studies in a family with a new mutation in the GTP-cyclohydrolase I gene. J Neurol Neurosurg Psychiatry 1998; 64(6):806–808.
101. Partington MW, Turner G, Boyle J, Gecz J. Three new families with X-linked mental retardation caused by the 428–451dup(24bp) mutation in ARX. Clin Genet 2004; 66(1):39–45.
102. FitzGerald PM, Jankovic J, Percy AK. Rett syndrome and associated movement disorders. Mov Disord 1990; 5(3):195–202.
103. Lee ES, Moon HK, Park YH, Garbern J, Hobson GM. A case of complicated spastic paraplegia 2 due to a point mutation in the proteolipid protein 1 gene. J Neurol Sci 2004; 224(1–2):83–87.
104. Berger J, Moser HW, Forss-Petter S. Leukodystrophies: recent developments in genetics, molecular biology, pathogenesis and treatment. Curr Opin Neurol 2001; 14(3):305–312.

105. Inglese M, Rovaris M, Bianchi S, et al. Magnetic resonance imaging, magnetisation transfer imaging, and diffusion weighted imaging correlates of optic nerve, brain, and cervical cord damage in Leber's hereditary optic neuropathy. J Neurol Neurosurg Psychiatry 2001; 70(4):444–449.
106. Gropman A, Chen TJ, Perng CL, et al. Variable clinical manifestation of homoplasmic G14459A mitochondrial DNA mutation. Am J Med Genet A 2004; 124(4):377–382.
107. Tarnopolsky MA, Baker SK, Myint T, Maxner CE, Robitaille J, Robinson BH. Clinical variability in maternally inherited leber hereditary optic neuropathy with the G14459A mutation. Am J Med Genet A 2004; 124(4):372–376.
108. Macaya A, Munell F, Burke RE, De Vivo DC. Disorders of movement in Leigh syndrome. Neuropediatrics 1993; 24(2):60–67.
109. Lera G, Bhatia K, Marsden CD. Dystonia as the major manifestation of Leigh's syndrome. Mov Disord 1994; 9(6):642–649.
110. Paviour DC, revesz T, Holton JL, Evans A, Olsson JE, Lees AJ. Neuronal intranuclear inclusion disease: report on a case originally diagnosed as dopa-responsive dystonia with Lewy bodies. Mov Disord 2005; 20(10):1345–1349.
111. Demarquay G, Setiey A, Morel Y, Trepo C, Chazot G, Broussolle E. Clinical report of three patients with hereditary hemochromatosis and movement disorders. Mov Disord 2000; 15(6):1204–1209.
112. Rampoldi L, Danek A, Monaco AP. Clinical features and molecular bases of neuroacanthocytosis. J Mol Med 2002; 80(8):475–491.
113. Danek A, Jung HH, Melone MA, Rampoldi L, Broccoli V, Walker RH. Neuroacanthocytosis: new developments in a neglected group of dementing disorders. J Neurol Sci 2005; 229–230:171–186.
114. Jankovic J, Tintner R. Dystonia and parkinsonism. Parkinsonism Relat Disord 2001; 8(2):109–121.
115. Muenter MD, Sharpless NS, Tyce GM, Darley FL. Patterns of dystonia ("I-D-I" and "D-I-D-") in response to l-dopa therapy for Parkinson's disease. Mayo Clin Proc 1977; 52(3):163–174.
116. Slawek J, Derejko M, Lass P, Dubaniewicz M. Camptocormia or Pisa syndrome in multiple system atrophy. Clin Neurol Neurosurg 2005. In press.
117. Azher SN, Jankovic J. Camptocormia: pathogenesis, classification, and response to therapy. Neurology 2005; 65(3):355–359.
118. Lang AE. Treatment of progressive supranuclear palsy and corticobasal degeneration. Mov Disord 2005; 20(Suppl 12):S83–S91.
119. Minagar A, Sheremata WA, Weiner WJ. Transient movement disorders and multiple sclerosis. Parkinsonism Relat Disord 2002; 9(2):111–113.
120. Zenzola A, De Mari M, De Blasi R, Carella A, Lamberti P. Paroxysmal dystonia with thalamic lesion in multiple sclerosis. Neurol Sci 2001; 22(5):391–394.
121. Frucht S. Dystonia, athetosis, and epilepsia partialis continua in a patient with late-onset Rasmussen's encephalitis. Mov Disord 2002; 17(3):609–612.
122. van Hilten JJ, van de Beek WJ, Roep BO. Multifocal or generalized tonic dystonia of complex regional pain syndrome: a distinct clinical entity associated with HLA-DR13. Ann Neurol 2000; 48(1):113–116.
123. Lang AE. Familial Meige syndrome and thyroid dysfunction. Neurology 1985; 35(1):138.
124. Segawa M, Nomura Y, Nishiyama N. Autosomal dominant guanosine triphosphate cyclohydrolase I deficiency (Segawa disease). Ann Neurol 2003; 54(suppl 6):S32–S45.
125. Nygaard TG, Marsden CD, Duvoisin RC. Dopa-responsive dystonia. Adv Neurol 1988; 50:377–384.
126. Roze E, Vidailhet M, Blau N, et al. Long-term follow-up and adult outcome of 6-pyruvoyl-tetrahydropterin synthase deficiency. Mov Disord 2005. In press.
127. Neville BG, Parascandalo R, Farrugia R, Felice A. Sepiapterin reductase deficiency: a congenital dopa-responsive motor and cognitive disorder. Brain 2005; 128(Pt 10): 2291–2296.

128. Obeso JA, Rothwell JC, Lang AE, Marsden CD. Myoclonic dystonia. Neurology 1983; 33(7):825–830.
129. Valente EM, Misbahuddin A, Brancati F, et al. Analysis of the epsilon-sarcoglycan gene in familial and sporadic myoclonus-dystonia: evidence for genetic heterogeneity. Mov Disord 2003; 18(9):1047–1051.
130. Klein C, Gurvich N, Sena-Esteves M, et al. Evaluation of the role of the D2 dopamine receptor in myoclonus dystonia. Ann Neurol 2000; 47(3):369–373.
131. Kock N, Kasten M, Schule B, et al. Clinical and genetic features of myoclonus-dystonia in 3 cases: a video presentation. Mov Disord 2004; 19(2):231–234.
132. Angelini L, Erba A, Mariotti C, Gellera C, Ciano C, Nardocci N. Myoclonic dystonia as unique presentation of isolated vitamin E deficiency in a young patient. Mov Disord 2002; 17(3):612–614.
133. Quinn NP, Rothwell JC, Thompson PD, Marsden CD. Hereditary myoclonic dystonia, hereditary torsion dystonia and hereditary essential myoclonus: an area of confusion. Adv Neurol 1988; 50:391–401.
134. Frucht SJ, Bordelon Y, Houghton WH, Reardan D. A pilot tolerability and efficacy trial of sodium oxybate in ethanol-responsive movement disorders. Mov Disord 2005; 20(10):1330–1337.
135. Dobyns WB, Ozelius LJ, Kramer PL, et al. Rapid-onset dystonia-parkinsonism. Neurology 1993; 43(12):2596–2602.
136. Kamphuis DJ, Koelman H, Lees AJ, Tijssen MA. Sporadic rapid-onset dystonia-parkinsonism presenting as Parkinson's disease. Mov Disord 2005; 21(1):118–119.
137. Dalvi A, Winfield L, Yu Q, Cote L, Goodman RR, Pullman SL. Stereotactic posteroventral pallidotomy: clinical methods and results at 1-year follow up. Mov Disord 1999; 14(2):256–261.
138. Rodriguez-Oroz MC, Obeso JA, Lang AE, et al. Bilateral deep brain stimulation in Parkinson's disease: a multicentre study with 4 years follow-up. Brain 2005; 128(Pt 10): 2240–2249.
139. Toda H, Hamani C, Lozano A. Deep brain stimulation in the treatment of dyskinesia and dystonia. Neurosurg Focus 2004; 17(1):E2.

# 17
# Drug-Induced Dystonia

**Francisco Cardoso**
*Department of Internal Medicine, Movement Disorders Clinic, Neurology Service, The Federal University of Minas Gerais, Brazil*

## INTRODUCTION

The aim of this chapter is to provide a review of the dystonias related to drugs with emphasis on phenomenology and management. Although epidemiology data are lacking, it is probable that levodopa-induced dystonia in patients with Parkinson's disease is the most common form of drug-induced dystonia seen by movement disorders specialists. However, it is not within the scope of this chapter to discuss levodopa-induced dyskinesias. The discussion will be focused on acute dystonic reaction and tardive dystonia. It also includes descriptions of dystonia occurring in association with recreational use of illicit drugs (1,2). In virtually all instances, these patients have a pre-existent movement disorder that is exacerbated by use of the drug. As discussed later in this chapter, previous use of cocaine has also been described as a risk factor for development of acute dystonic reaction after exposure to neuroleptic drugs.

## ACUTE DYSTONIC REACTION

This term describes dystonia following acute exposure to dopamine receptor blocking agents (DRBA), a phenomenon observed since the introduction of neuroleptic agents or DRBA in clinical practice in the 1950s. Typically, the patients present with a painful cranial–cervical dystonia with oculogyric crisis (tonic conjugate, often upward, eye deviation) and prominent trismus. If the patient remains exposed to the offending agent, the severity of the dystonia increases, becoming more widespread. Conversely, discontinuation of the drug leads to spontaneous remission of the dystonia. Most subjects with acute dystonic reaction become quite anxious. In 90% of the instances, the onset of the movement disorder is in the first three days of introduction of the drug or after the increase of its dosage (3). There is a direct relationship between the affinity for D2 dopamine receptor and the likelihood of a given drug to induce this type of dystonia (4). It is not surprising that typical neuroleptic drugs, such as traditional antipsychotic medications or antiemetic medications (prochlorperazine), are the most common drugs related to acute dystonic reaction.

In fact, in the preatypical neuroleptic era, at least 5% of the patients treated with dopamine receptor blocking drugs developed this side effect (5). A more recent study describes the occurrence of acute dystonic reaction in 2.1% of 1559 patients treated with neuroleptic medications (6). There are, however, reports of this movement disorder induced by use of risperidone, olanzapine, quetiapine, and clozapine (7–9). Tetrabenazine, a presynaptic monoamine-depleting agent with a weak dopamine receptor blocking action (10), has also been described as inducing acute dystonic reaction (11). Even nonneuroleptic agents (e.g., modified benzamides such as metoclopramide) also have the potential to cause acute dystonic reaction (12). Other risk factors for acute dystonic reaction include dosage of the neuroleptic, male gender, lower age, and previous use of cocaine (4). The pathogenesis of acute dystonic reaction remains largely unknown. Because of the relationship with anti-D2 potency, it has been proposed that this form of dystonia is caused by abrupt decrease of dopamine levels in the basal ganglia. It has also been speculated that it represents an acute imbalance between dopamine and acetylcholine in the brain. This theory is derived from the clinical observation that anticholinergic agents are highly effective to treat acute dystonic reaction (5). Management of this form of dystonia involves immediate discontinuation of the offending agent and use of medications to alleviate the movement disorder. Parenteral anticholinergic drugs (e.g., biperiden 5 mg intramuscularly or diphenhydramine 25–50 mg intravenously), benzodiazepines or antihistamines, usually provide rapid relief of the acute dystonic symptoms. A final observation of practical importance: Once one patient has developed acute dystonic reaction with a given agent, this side effect will be observed whenever the drug is used at the same dosage. There is also a high probability that this reaction will occur with another drug of similar or higher anti-D2 effect. The physician should attempt, thus, to prescribe an agent of smaller dopamine receptor blocking potency.

## TARDIVE DYSTONIA

The first reports of occurrence of dystonia in patients under chronic treatment with neuroleptic medications emerged in the early 1980s (13,14). In the original description of a cohort of patients with tardive dystonia, Burke et al. drew attention to two core features of this condition: onset usually after long-term exposure to DRBA and tendency for persistence even after discontinuation of the offending agent (14). These findings distinguished the then newly described phenomenon from acute dystonic reactions and justified its nosological classification under the umbrella of tardive syndromes. After the original description, there was a steady increase of the number of reports on tardive dystonia. More recently, coinciding with the increasing use of atypical antipsychotic drugs, there has been a decline in number of publications dealing with this form of dystonia. Nevertheless, because of its frequency, chronic nature, and difficulties in management, tardive dystonia remains an important clinical problem to physicians who prescribe DRBA and those interested in movement disorders. The aim of this section is to provide an overview of epidemiology, causative agents, pathogenesis, clinical findings, principles of management, and natural history of tardive dystonia.

### Epidemiology

There are few epidemiological studies of tardive dystonia, and the findings from these reports vary widely. The discrepancies most likely reflect differences in the methodology and characteristics of the studied population. Studies of chronic hospitalized patients, cohort of subjects treated with typical neuroleptic drugs, investigations performed by movement disorders specialists, and use of standardized rating scales for movement disorders are associated with higher prevalence figures. In a study of 351 inpatients, Yassa et al. (15) found a prevalence of 2% of tardive dystonia. Another investigation of chronic hospitalized psychiatric patients, this time conducted by neurologists, reported a similar figure, 1.5% (16). In contrast, another group, describing a cohort of 125 chronic psychiatric inpatients, reported a frequency of 21.6%. This high figure likely reflects the use of a detailed and systematic examination, and increased clinician sensitivity in detecting mild forms of tardive dystonia (17). A similar approach examining all psychiatric inpatients (194) in the Netherland Antiles with rating scales specific for movement disorders also found a high prevalence of tardive dystonia at 13.4% (18). Epidemiological studies have also identified presence of risk factors for development of this complication: younger age, male gender, African-American ethnicity, history of previous acute dystonic reaction, mental retardation, and prior electroconvulsive therapy (16,19–23). These findings must be interpreted with caution because most conclusions are based on noncontrolled, retrospective studies. In particular, the association with ethnicity is controversial. It is well known that the nature of the care provided to patients may vary according to the ethnic background of the patient (24). Based on this premise, one may reason that a particular ethnic group may be exposed to agents more likely implicated in the development of tardive dystonia.

### Causative Agents

Traditional antipsychotic agents are the drugs classically associated with the development of tardive dystonia. There are, however, reports of the association of this side effect with exposure to atypical agents such as sulpiride, risperidone, and olanzapine (25–27). Modified benzamides (particularly metoclopramide), drugs often used as antinausea therapy and to treat other gastrointestinal problems, are also unequivocally implicated in the development of tardive dystonia (12,28). Cinnarizine and flunarizine, calcium-channel blockers widely used in many areas of the world for treatment of vertigo and prophylaxis of migraine, have been associated with the development of tardive dystonia and other forms of tardive dyskinesia (29,30). There are reports, mostly noncontrolled studies or single-case reports, describing the development of tardive dystonia in association with drugs such as lithium, buspirone, fluoxetine, and others (31–35). These findings must be viewed with caution due to the methodological limitations of some of the studies.

### Pathogenesis

The mechanism underlying the development of tardive dystonia and other forms of tardive dyskinesia remains to be determined. An obvious candidate to account for the relationship with the exposure to neuroleptic agents is the theory that chronic blockade of the D2 dopamine receptor leads to denervation hypersensitivity with upregulation of these receptors (36). However, there are little or no experimental data to support this hypothesis (37,38). Other theory, also involving the dopaminergic system of the basal ganglia, proposes that there is an imbalance between D1 and D2 families of receptors in the basal ganglia (39). More recently, investigators have suggested that stimulation of D3 receptors is related to development of tardive dystonia (40). Others have submitted that long-term use of DRBA leads to hyperactivity of the indirect pathway connecting the striatum with the medial portion of the globus pallidum and pars reticulata of the substantia nigra. Ultimately, this abnormality results in disinhibition of the ventrolateral thalamus with hyperexcitability of motor areas of the cerebral cortex (41). Changes in GABAergic systems in the brain have also been implicated as playing a role in the pathogenesis of tardive dyskinesia (42). There is no explanation for the relatively low frequency of subjects exposed to DRBA who develop tardive dystonia. Attempts to identify genetic markers to account for the vulnerability of some patients have failed. Loci and polymorphisms eliminated as risk factors for tardive dystonia include *DYT1* (43) and polymorphisms of cytochrome P4502D6, dopamine D2 and D3 receptors (44,45).

## Clinical Findings

The onset of the dystonia usually coincides with use of the offending drug but may also develop after discontinuation of the medication (withdrawal dyskinesia) (13). In most series, tardive dystonia appears after long-term treatment with DRBA. In one British series of 107 patients, for instance, the median time of exposure to the offending drugs was five years. However, in some patients development of dystonia was associated with use of medication for as little time as four days (22). Another study of a series of 67 patients with tardive dystonia confirms that there is no safe period of use of drugs with the potential to induce this complication; 21% of these patients developed the tardive syndrome within one year of exposure to these agents (46). In most series of patients reported in literature, tardive dystonia occurs more often in younger males (16,20–23) but there are exceptions. Tan and Jankovic (47), for instance, reported that tardive oromandibular dystonia is more common among women.

Tardive dystonia can fully mimic the clinical picture of any form of idiopathic dystonia, rendering impossible a distinction from idiopathic forms exclusively based on phenomenology (22). However, very often there are findings suggesting the role of DRBA in the development of the movement disorder. Many patients present with prominent axial involvement and opisthotonic posturing, often associated with repetitive arm extension and pronation (Fig. 1) (37). In a careful clinical evaluation of 100 patients with different forms of tardive dyskinesia, Stacy et al. (28) found that in the vast majority of subjects, dystonia coexisted with other phenomena, particularly stereotypies. Tan and Jankovic, comparing 24 patients with tardive and 92 subjects with idiopathic oromandibular dystonia, confirmed the findings of Stacy et al. (28). In this study, orofacial–lingual stereotypies, stereotypic movements in the limbs, akathisia, and respiratory dyskinesias were significantly more frequent in the tardive than the idiopathic group. On the other hand, patients with idiopathic OMD, there is often coexistent cervical dystonia. Molho et al. (48) compared the clinical features of 102 patients with idiopathic and 20 patients with tardive cervical dystonia. The presence of extracervical involvement, retrocollis, and spasmodic head movements were individually found to be predictive of tardive cervical dystonia. Conversely, head tremor (42.2%) and family history of dystonia (9.8%) were present only in the idiopathic group, whereas torticollis, laterocollis, and presence of sensory tricks were predictive of idiopathic cervical dystonia. Less usual and more infrequent features have been reported in association with tardive dystonia. In some patients, the dystonic movements can be so severe that they cause rib and even spine fractures (49,50). In others, the dystonia can be task specific, as in one patient with oromandibular dystonia exclusively triggered by eating (51). Nonmotor features often

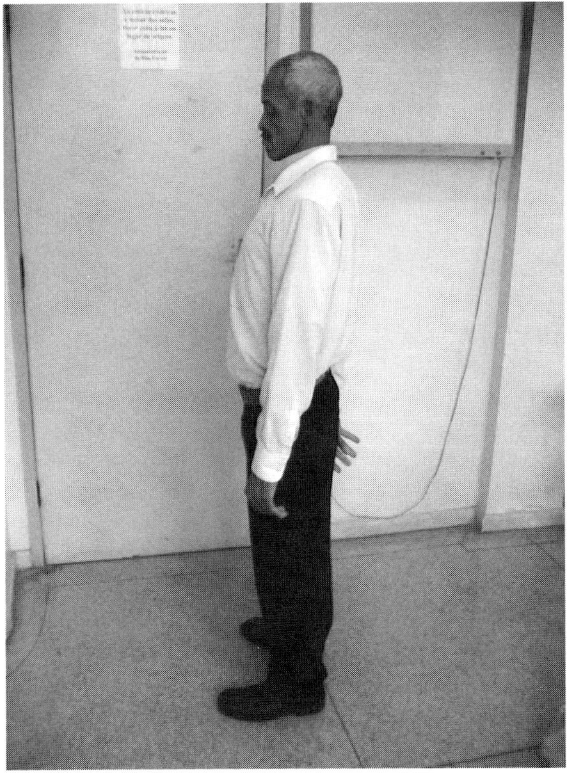

**Figure 1** This man exhibits the typical opisthotonic posture associated with dopamine receptor blocking agents exposure. In addition, he also exhibits dystonic features involving the face and neck.

coexist with dystonia in these patients. Stacy et al. (28) reported on the frequent association between tardive dystonia and akathisia. Green et al. (52) described the presence of oral and/or genital severe pain in a series of 11 patients with tardive dyskinesia.

## Management

In the absence of treatment data collected from well-designed trials, therapeutic recommendations are at best based on extensive anecdotal, but open-label experience. First, as soon as the dystonia is detected, the clinician must attempt to discontinue the offending agent. Second, in the case where there is need of use of DRBA for symptoms of psychosis, seemingly safe drugs include quetiapine and clozapine. In addition, there are no reports on the existence of tardive dystonia in association with sertindole, aripiprazole, ziprasidone, and other new agents. Nevertheless, caution should be employed when prescribing these drugs because of the limited clinical exposure.

The symptomatic management of tardive dystonia is often challenging, with many patients being left with significant disability despite the use of different medications and interventions (22). Anticholinergic agents can alleviate the severity of dystonia (37,46). There are several studies suggesting the efficacy of tetrabenazine to treat tardive dystonia (10,46,53). However, all of these reports are based on open-label, noncontrolled trials. Additionally, tetrabenazine is not devoid of side effects, such as parkinsonism and depression, and its availability is limited in the United States. Clinical experience indicates that this drug is more effective for stereotypies, and patients with tardive dystonia tend to be less responsive. There are reports indicating the usefulness of risperidone and olanzapine to treat dystonia in the context of tardive dyskinesia (54,55). These studies should be viewed with great caution in the light of articles demonstrating that these agents can induce tardive dystonia (26,27). It is possible that the ameliorating effect described in the reports reflect masking of the tardive dystonia by the anti-D2 property of these agents. The situation is different with quetiapine and clozapine (56–59). Although there is a need of placebo-controlled trials, it is more likely that these two atypical antipsychotic agents have a beneficial effect on tardive dystonia. What remains to be determined is whether quetiapine and, particularly, clozapine do not worsen the movement disorder or accelerate the rate of remission of tardive dystonia. A report of improvement of nontardive dystonia with clozapine (60) suggests that the latter possibility may be true. Because patients with tardive dystonia have a low response rate to treatment with oral agents, alternative therapeutic agents have been tried. The scarce data available in the literature suggest that botulinum toxin type A or B are effective in improving focal problems (oromandibular, cervical, and axial dystonia) in patients with tardive dystonia (47,48,61–63). Dressler et al. (64) reported positive benefit with use of intrathecal baclofen in one patient with severe axial tardive dystonia refractory to other treatments. There is more interest in the role of use of surgical treatment of tardive dystonia with deep brain stimulation of the medial globus pallidum. Although this surgical technique appears to be more effective for idiopathic dystonias (65), many reports suggest that patients with otherwise intractable tardive dystonias may benefit from it. Another study indicates that pallidal stimulation may improve patients with this condition (66). Indeed, a recent open-label study of five patients with tardive dystonia refractory to medical treatment showed that this surgical treatment resulted in 87% improvement of the scores of the motor section of the Burke–Fahn–Marsden section (67) [Chapter 24].

## Natural History

In the original description of tardive dystonia, Burke et al. (13,14) had already recognized the tendency of this condition not to undergo remission with or without treatment. Later studies confirmed this characteristic of tardive dystonia. The Columbia group reported that withdrawal of the neuroleptic increased the chance of remission (46). Still the results were quite modest because not more than five of the 42 patients, where withdrawal of offending agents was possible, underwent remission of the tardive dystonia. This concept of poor prognosis of tardive dystonia was confirmed in the British series of 104 patients, where Kiriakakis et al. (22) found that only 14% of our patients had a remission over a mean follow-up period of 8.5 years. In those patients where DRBA could be discontinued, remission occurred 5.2 years after withdrawal of the medications. Confirming the importance of early recognition of the casual relationship between dystonia and neuroleptic therapy, discontinuation of these drugs increased the chances of remission fourfold. Moreover, patients with 10 years or less on antipsychotic drugs had a five times greater chance of remission than those with more than 10 years of treatment.

## REFERENCES

1. Cardoso F, Jankovic J. Movement disorders. Neurol Clin 1993; 11(3):625–638.
2. Cardoso FE, Jankovic J. Cocaine-related movement disorders. Mov Disord 1993; 8(2): 175–178.
3. Keepers GA, Clappison VJ, Casey DE. Initial anticholinergic prophylaxis for neuroleptic-induced extrapyramidal syndromes. Arch Gen Psychiatry 1983; 40:1113–1117.
4. Keepers GA, Casey DE. Prediction of neuroleptic-induced dystonia. J Clin Psychopharmacol 1987; 7:342–344.
5. Marsden CD, Jenner P. The pathophysiology of extrapyramidal side-effects of neuroleptic drugs. Psychol Med 1980; 10:55–72.
6. Muscettola G, Barbato G, Pampallona S, et al. Extrapyramidal syndromes in neuroleptic-treated patients: prevalence, risk factors, and association with tardive dyskinesia. J Clin Psychopharmacol 1999; 19(3):203–208.
7. Alevizos B, Papageorgiou C, Christodoulou GN. Acute dystonia caused by low dosage of olanzapine. J Neuropsychiatry Clin Neurosci 2003; 15(2):241.
8. Coffey GL, Botts SR, de Leon J. High vulnerability to acute dystonic reactions: a case of antipsychotic exposure and uncontrolled seizure activity. Prog Neuropsychopharmacol Biol Psychiatry 2005; 29(5):770–774.
9. Kastrup O, Gastpar M, Schwarz M. Acute dystonia due to clozapine. J Neurol Neurosurg Psychiatry 1994; 57:119.
10. Jankovic J. Treatment of hyperkinetic movement disorders with tetrabenazine: a double-blind crossover study. Ann Neurol 1982; 11:41–47.
11. Burke RE, Reches A, Traub MM, et al. Tetrabenazine induces acute dystonic reactions. Ann Neurol 1985; 17(2):200–202.
12. Ganzini L, Casey DE, Hoffman WF, McCall AL. The prevalence of metoclopramide-induced tardive dyskinesia and acute extrapyramidal movement disorders. Arch Intern Med 1993; 153(12):1469–1475.
13. Burke RE, Fahn S, Jankovic J, et al. Tardive dystonia and inappropriate use of neuroleptic drugs. Lancet 1982;1(8284):1299.
14. Burke RE, Fahn S, Jankovic J, et al. Tardive dystonia: late-onset and persistent dystonia caused by antipsychotic drugs. Neurology 1982; 32(12):1335–1346.
15. Yassa R, Nair V, Dimitry R. Prevalence of tardive dystonia. Acta Psychiatr Scand 1986; 73(6):629–633.
16. Friedman JH, Kucharski LT, Wagner RL. Tardive dystonia in a psychiatric hospital. J Neurol Neurosurg Psychiatry 1987; 50(6):801–803.
17. Sethi KD, Hess DC, Harp RJ. Prevalence of dystonia in veterans on chronic antipsychotic therapy. Mov Disord 1990; 5(4):319–321.
18. van Harten PN, Matroos GE, Hoek HW, Kahn RS. The prevalence of tardive dystonia, tardive dyskinesia, parkinsonism and akathisia the curacao extrapyramidal syndromes study: I. Schizophr Res 1996; 19(2–3):195–203.
19. Gimenez-Roldan S, Mateo D, Bartolome P. Tardive dystonia and severe tardive dyskinesia. A comparison of risk factors and prognosis. Acta Psychiatr Scand 1985; 71(5):488–494.
20. Sachdev P. Risk factors for tardive dystonia: a case-control comparison with tardive dyskinesia. Acta Psychiatr Scand 1993; 88(2):98–103.
21. Raja M, Azzoni A. Tardive dystonia. Prevalence, risk factors and clinical features. Ital J Neurol Sci 1996; 17(6):409–418.
22. Kiriakakis V, Bhatia KP, Quinn NP, Marsden CD. The natural history of tardive dystonia. A long-term follow-up study of 107 cases. Brain 1998; 121(Pt 11):2053–2066.
23. Wonodi I, Adami HM, Cassady SL, et al. Ethnicity and the course of tardive dyskinesia in outpatients presenting to the motor disorders clinic at the Maryland psychiatric research center. J Clin Psychopharmacol 2004; 24(6):592–598.
24. Clark LT. Issues in minority health: atherosclerosis and coronary heart disease in African Americans. Med Clin North Am 2005; 89(5):977–1001.

25. Miller LG, Jankovic J. Sulpiride-induced tardive dystonia. Mov Disord 1990; 5(1):83–84.
26. Vercueil L, Foucher J. Risperidone-induced tardive dystonia and psychosis. Lancet 1999; 20353(9157):981.
27. Dunayevich E, Strakowski SM. Olanzapine-induced tardive dystonia. Am J Psychiatry 1999; 156(10):1662.
28. Stacy M, Cardoso F, Jankovic J. Tardive stereotypy and other movement disorders in tardive dyskinesias. Neurology 1993; 43(5):937–941.
29. Chouza C, Scaramelli A, Caamano JL, et al. Parkinsonism, tardive dyskinesia, akathisia, and depression induced by flunarizine. Lancet 1986; 1(8493):1303–1304.
30. Barbosa MT, Caramelli P, Maia DP, et al. Parkinsonism and Parkinson's disease in the elderly: a community-based survey in Brazil (The Bambuí study). Mov Disord 2006; 21(6):800–808.
31. LeWitt PA, Walters A, Hening W, McHale D. Persistent movement disorders induced by buspirone. Mov Disord 1993; 8(3):331–334.
32. Ghadirian AM, Annable L, Belanger MC, Chouinard G. A cross-sectional study of parkinsonism and tardive dyskinesia in lithium-treated affective disordered patients. J Clin Psychiatry 1996; 57(1):22–28.
33. Chakrabarti S, Chand PK. Lithium - induced tardive dystonia. Neurol India 2002; 50(4): 473–475.
34. Leo RJ. Movement disorders associated with the serotonin selective reuptake inhibitors. J Clin Psychiatry 1996; 57(10):449–454.
35. Vandel P, Bonin B, Leveque E, et al. Tricyclic antidepressant-induced extrapyramidal side effects. Eur Neuropsychopharmacol 1997; 7(3):207–212.
36. Calabresi P, De Murtas M, Mercuri NB, et al. Chronic neuroleptic treatment: D2 dopamine receptor supersensitivity and striatal glutamatergic transmission. Ann Neurol 1992; 31:366–373.
37. Cardoso F, Jankovic J. Dystonia and dyskinesia. Psychiatr Clin North America 1997; 20(4):821–838.
38. Cross AJ, Crow TJ, Ferrier IN, et al. Chemical and structural changes in the brain in patients with movement disorder. In: Casey DE, Chase TN, Chritine AV, Gerlach J, eds. Dyskinesia: Research and Treatment. New York: Springer-Verlag, 1985:104–110.
39. Gerlach J. Current views on tardive dyskinesia. Pharmacopsychiatry 1991; 27:47–48.
40. Casey DE. Pathophysiology of antipsychotic drug-induced movement disorders. J Clin Psychiatry 2004; 65(Suppl 9):25–28.
41. Mitchell IJ, Crossman AR, Liminga U, et al. Regional changes in 2-deoxyglucose uptake associated with neurleptic-induced tardive dyskinesia in the Cebus monkey. Mov Disord 1992; 7:32–37.
42. Gunne LM, Haggstrom JE, Sjoquist B. Association with persistent neuroleptic-induced dyskinesia of regional changes in brain GABA synthesis. Nature 1984; 309:347–349.
43. Bressman SB, de Leon D, Raymond D, et al. Secondary dystonia and the DYTI gene. Neurology 1997; 48(6):1571–1577.
44. Mihara K, Kondo T, Higuchi H, et al. Tardive dystonia and genetic polymorphisms of cytochrome P4502D6 and dopamine D2 and D3 receptors: a preliminary finding. Am J Med Genet 2002; 114(6):693–695.
45. Kaiser R, Tremblay PB, Klufmoller F, Roots I, Brockmoller J. Relationship between adverse effects of antipsychotic treatment and dopamine D(2) receptor polymorphisms in patients with schizophrenia. Mol Psychiatry 2002; 7(7):695–705.
46. Kang UJ, Burke RE, Fahn S. Natural history and treatment of tardive dystonia. Mov Disord 1986; 1(3):193–208.
47. Tan EK, Jankovic J. Tardive and idiopathic oromandibular dystonia: a clinical comparison. J Neurol Neurosurg Psychiatry 2000; 68(2):186–190.
48. Molho ES, Feustel PJ, Factor SA. Clinical comparison of tardive and idiopathic cervical dystonia. Mov Disord 1998; 13(3):486–489.

49. Konrad C, Vollmer-Haase J, Gaubitz M, et al. Fracture of the odontoid process complicating tardive dystonia. Mov Disord 2004; 19(8):983–985.
50. Hacking D, Werring DJ. Bilateral first rib fractures due to tardive dystonia. J Neurol Neurosurg Psychiatry 2005; 76(7):983.
51. Achiron A, Melamed E. Tardive eating dystonia. Mov Disord 1990; 5(4):331–333.
52. Ford B, Greene P, Fahn S. Oral and genital tardive pain syndromes. Neurology 1994; 44(11):2115–2119.
53. Paleacu D, Giladi N, Moore O, et al. Tetrabenazine treatment in movement disorders. Clin Neuropharmacol 2004; 27(5):230–233.
54. Lucetti C, Bellini G, Nuti A, et al. Treatment of patients with tardive dystonia with olanzapine. Clin Neuropharmacol 2002; 25(2):71–74.
55. Bai YM, Yu SC, Chen JY, et al. Risperidone for pre-existing severe tardive dyskinesia: a 48-week prospective follow-up study. Int Clin Psychopharmacol 2005; 20(2):79–85.
56. Gourzis P, Polychronopoulos P, Papapetropoulos S, et al. Quetiapine in the treatment of focal tardive dystonia induced by other atypical antipsychotics: A report of 2 cases. Clin Neuropharmacol 2005; 28(4):195–196.
57. Friedman JH. Clozapine treatment of psychosis in patients with tardive dystonia: report of three cases. Mov Disord 1994; 9(3):321–324.
58. Trugman JM, Leadbetter R, Zalis ME, et al. Treatment of severe axial tardive dystonia with clozapine: case report and hypothesis. Mov Disord 1994; 9(4):441–446.
59. Adityanjee, Estrera AB. Successful treatment of tardive dystonia with clozapine. Biol Psychiatry 1996; 39(12):1064–1065.
60. Karp BI, Goldstein SR, Chen R, et al. An open trial of clozapine for dystonia. Mov Disord 1999; 14(4):652–657.
61. Brashear A, Ambrosius WT, Eckert GJ, Siemers ER. Comparison of treatment of tardive dystonia and idiopathic cervical dystonia with botulinum toxin type A. Mov Disord 1998; 13(1):158–161.
62. Comella CL, Shannon KM, Jaglin J. Extensor truncal dystonia: successful treatment with botulinum toxin injections. Mov Disord 1998; 13(3):552–555.
63. Cardoso F. Botulinum toxin type B in the management of dystonia non-responsive to botulinum toxin type A. Arq Neuropsiquiatr 2003; 61(3A):607–610.
64. Dressler D, Oeljeschlager RO, Ruther E. Severe tardive dystonia: treatment with continuous intrathecal baclofen administration. Mov Disord 1997; 12(4):585–587.
65. Krause M, Fogel W, Kloss M, et al. Pallidal stimulation for dystonia. Neurosurgery 2004; 55(6):1361–1368.
66. Starr PA, Turner RS, Rau G, et al. Microelectrode-guided implantation of deep brain stimulators into the globus pallidus internus for dystonia: techniques, electrode locations, and outcomes. Neurosurg Focus 2004; 17(1):E4.
67. Trottenberg T, Volkmann J, Deuschl G, et al. Treatment of severe tardive dystonia with pallidal deep brain stimulation. Neurology 2005; 64(2):344–346.

# 18
# Psychogenic Dystonia

**Anette Schrag**
*University Department of Clinical Neurosciences, Royal Free and University College Medical School, London, U.K.*

**Anthony E. Lang**
*Movement Disorders Unit, Toronto Western Hospital, and University of Toronto, Ontario, Canada*

## INTRODUCTION

Dystonia due to a psychogenic cause represents a relatively small proportion of cases seen in movement disorder clinics. However, this can be an extremely difficult diagnosis to make and one that is probably still often over- as well as underdiagnosed.

Historically, idiopathic torsion dystonia was often thought to be a consequence of a psychological problem (1) although, even in some of the early descriptions (2,3), it was considered to be due to an organic cause. Particularly between the 1940s and 1970s, the psychiatric interpretation of idiopathic torsion dystonia prevailed and resulted in unnecessary and unhelpful treatments and considerable psychological consequences for many patients and their families. It then became once again recognized as a neurological disorder particularly through the work of Marsden (4) and Fahn (5), and in the last decades a plethora of studies on its phenomenology, genetics, pathophysiology, and treatment have been published. An understandable reluctance by modern neurologists and psychiatrists alike to make a diagnosis of psychogenic dystonia may have pushed the pendulum too far to the other extreme and has probably led to an underdiagnosis of psychogenic dystonia, although neurologically determined dystonia is still occasionally misdiagnosed as a psychogenic disorder. A misdiagnosis either way may subject a patient to potentially harmful diagnostic procedures and treatments or deny the patient potentially effective treatments. In addition, possible association with work-related injuries may result in major legal issues. At the same time, biological markers for the diagnosis of neurologically determined dystonia are still lacking, and the diagnosis remains largely clinical.

For the purpose of this chapter, we will refer to the perhaps overly simplified classification into "psychogenic" contrasting with "organic" dystonia, which has been used in the literature to distinguish such patients from those with neurological disorders. However, we recognize that this is somewhat controversial, implying a psychological causation that cannot always be demonstrated.

## EPIDEMIOLOGY

Overall, psychogenic dystonia is a rare cause of dystonia and represents only approximately 1% to 5% of patients with dystonia (6,7), but among psychogenic movement disorders dystonia accounts for approximately 20% to 50% of cases (8–11).

## DIAGNOSIS

The definition of dystonia is descriptive (12) and clearly encompasses psychogenic dystonia as the cause for abnormal muscle contraction. Within the classification system of dystonia by Fahn and others (12), psychogenic dystonia is classified as a secondary dystonia due to a symptomatic cause. The diagnosis relies almost entirely on clinical history, examination, and clinical judgment. There is no biological marker or pathognomonic sign that in isolation allows an unequivocal diagnosis of psychogenic dystonia, and, conversely, with the exception of a few available genetic tests for some types of dystonia, there is no biological marker for primary dystonia. Even for secondary dystonia a cause cannot always be found, and in at least two-thirds of patients with organic dystonia investigations are normal. Without doubt, an organic condition causing secondary dystonia must always be excluded by appropriate investigations, but the diagnosis of dystonia in the majority of cases remains clinical. As organic and psychogenic dystonia both have a wide and overlapping spectrum of presentations, which often includes bizarre and unusual presentations that may appear inconsistent and be unique to individual patients, it is important that the diagnosis of psychogenic dystonia is only made by a clinician with extensive experience with the wide spectrum of presentations of dystonia. Organic and psychogenic dystonia can also occur together, and a psychogenic dystonia may have developed superimposed on an organic condition. Although this co-occurrence is probably not as frequent as the co-occurrence of epileptic and nonepileptic attacks [which is estimated to be up to 25% (13)], functional overlay in an underlying organic condition should be considered.

Despite these caveats, a diagnosis of psychogenic dystonia is possible and can be made when (i) appropriate investigations have been negative, (ii) positive findings allow a diagnosis based on standardized diagnostic criteria (see below).

### Characteristics of Dystonia

The often bizarre or apparently inconsistent nature of dystonia has often contributed to the confusion between organic and psychogenic dystonia. However, the characteristic patterns of primary dystonia, which is the main area of diagnostic difficulty, help in the differentiation of primary from psychogenic dystonia: action-specific dystonia will occur reliably during the specific action, be consistent over time with little change in its distribution and phenotype (although it may progress and spread), and follow characteristic patterns in distribution and progression, e.g., lower-limb onset of dystonia in childhood with slow spread, absence of pain (with the exception of cervical dystonia), and mobility of dystonia until very late stages of advanced disease. Only with rare exceptions are these criteria not met, e.g., in secondary dystonia or the autosomal dominant disorder of rapid-onset dystonia–parkinsonism (14). However, history, examination, and investigations will identify these exceptions. The most helpful features in making a diagnosis of psychogenic dystonia are those that do not fit with these recognized patterns of primary dystonia, and that are therefore incongruent with primary dystonia. In particular, in psychogenic dystonia, attempted voluntary movement to command in the opposite direction of the dystonic posturing may activate antagonists with little apparent action in agonist muscles, startle may elicit marked response, and dystonic posturing may be suggestible or distractible. Paroxysmal primary nonkinesigenic dystonia does occur, but psychogenic dystonia is a more common cause of this presentation (15). A list of features suggestive of psychogenic dystonia is listed in Table 1. However, none of the signs are specific for psychogenic dystonia, particularly as many can occur in other secondary dystonias, which must be excluded before a diagnosis of psychogenic dystonia is made.

## Medical History

The past medical history may also be revealing, e.g., for episodes of a different movement disorder in the same or another limb (with complete or partial remissions) or for nonepileptic seizures or other somatizations, putting the current presentation in the context of a wider somatoform illness. Previous somatizations may include other "functional" syndromes, such as fibromyalgia, atypical chest pain, or irritable bowel syndrome (16), or other medically unexplained symptoms, which may have resulted in a number of investigations and treatments, including operations (17) with no clear final diagnosis. While patients with somatoform illness often report a number of previous diagnoses or complaints, their somatoform nature often only becomes apparent when specifically sought in questions about the outcome of investigations to the patients or their general practitioner (18).

The history may also be informative in other respects, e.g., revealing abnormal illness behavior such as noncompliance with treatment, "splitting" behavior among the health professionals involved in their care, or "doctor shopping." Litigation or a compensation claim may represent a maintaining factor or there may be obvious secondary gain. There may also have been an obvious psychological stressor before the onset of the psychogenic dystonia, suggesting a diagnosis of conversion disorder or psychological trauma in the past history. However, an obvious trigger may be missing and, on the other hand, its presence may be misleading, as psychological conflicts are common in the population, and the coincidence between past psychological trauma and the presentation may be spurious.

## Examination

Four aspects of the physical examination are important in the diagnosis of psychogenic dystonia:

1. Absence of 'hard' neurological signs (such as an extensor plantar response): However, as mentioned above, psychogenic overlay may exist comorbidly with an underlying organic illness. This may have a variety of reasons, including the patients' wish to demonstrate the extent of their problem, e.g., in patients referred for stereotactic surgery for undoubted Parkinson's disease, or when patients have had previous experience with doctors who were unconvinced of the seriousness of their problem. In addition, secondary physical changes may have occurred following a long-standing psychogenic dystonia with prolonged immobilization,

(*Text continues p. 281*)

**Table 1** Differences Between Primary Dystonia and Psychogenic Dystonia

| | Features typical of primary dystonia | Features that may be seen in psychogenic dystonia |
|---|---|---|
| Past medical history | Unremarkable for age | Previous somatizations |
| History of dystonia | Onset after injury rare | Onset after minor injury/operation common |
| | Often positive family history | No family history |
| | No clear association with psychological stressors | Psychological stressor before onset |
| | Onset in childhood (generalized dystonia) | Onset in adolescence or adulthood |
| | Gradual onset | Abrupt onset |
| | Spread slow | Rapid progression |
| | Leg onset only in childhood | Onset in legs common |
| | No or little fluctuation over time | Marked fluctuations in severity and exacerbations |
| | Pattern consistent over time | Movement disorder often changed over time |
| | No pain (exception cervical dystonia and secondary pain) | Severe pain |
| | May have sleep benefit | No sleep benefit |
| | Remissions rare | Remissions common |
| Examinations | Consistently action-specific | Inconsistent activation pattern |
| | Disability predictable from dystonia pattern (including task specific movement disorders) | Discrepancy between dystonia pattern/examination and reported disability |
| | Recognized pattern of dystonia (can be deceptive) | Pattern incongruent with organic dystonia |
| | Mobile dystonia | Fixed dystonic posture |
| | Geste antagonists | Sensory tricks rare |
| | No startle | Startle response |
| | Rarely modifiable | Distractibility/increase with attention/trigger points/ suggestibility |
| | Neurological examination otherwise normal | Nonorganic signs and/or other psychogenic movement disorders (often paroxysmal) |
| | No or only mild or transient response to placebo, suggestion, or psychotherapy | Marked or persistent response to placebo, suggestion or psychotherapy possible but not uniform |
| | – | Scars indicating self-harm or previous somatisations |
| Psychiatric assessment | Mild depression or anxiety may coexist | Significant psychopathology, particularly depression, anxiety, personality disorders |
| | – | Past history of abuse |
| | – | Secondary gain |
| | – | Compensation claim, litigation |
| | – | Abnormal illness behavior |

including wasting, trophic changes, or even osteoporosis. Furthermore, pseudoneurological signs are not uncommon, including pseudoclonus, abnormal reflexes in a rigidly held limb, or a pseudo-Babinski response (often as a delayed, prolonged plantar extension), which can mislead the examiner. Although the interpretation of such findings is difficult, the recognition of the possibility of a pseudoneurological sign facilitates the recognition of a psychogenic disorder.

2. The presence of other nonorganic signs and findings (such as nonorganic weakness, nonanatomical sensory loss, resistance to passive movements, bouts of whole body shaking, or an excessive startle response): There may be extreme slowness that, unlike bradykinesia, is not fatiguing and without a decrement in the amplitude of the movement. There may be consistent past-pointing in an otherwise normal (sometimes excessively slow) finger–nose test, and other tasks may simply not be completed, e.g., repeatedly stopping two inches short of the target on the finger–nose test. The most useful sign is probably Hoover's sign, which has been shown to quantitatively differentiate organic and nonorganic weakness (19). However, caveats apply to all nonorganic signs. For example, give-way weakness may be seen if the movement causes pain, and nonspecific sensory symptoms not following a nerve or radicular distribution are common in Parkinson's disease and often predate the onset of motor symptoms. In addition, classical signs such as midline splitting, splitting of vibration sense (reporting a difference in the sensation of a tuning fork placed over the left compared to the right side of the sternum), and la belle indifference have poor specificity and are, therefore, of limited value in assessing these patients (20). There may also be a discrepancy of objective signs and disability (e.g., patients with mild unilateral weakness who are bed—or wheelchair-bound or, conversely, patients with no use of both arms who manage at home on their own). Similarly, there may be a discrepancy of subjectively reported symptoms and investigations that exclude a pathophysiological correlate, e.g., normal sensory-evoked potentials in a patient reporting total loss of sensation in a limb.
3. Features of a psychogenic movement disorder: There are a number of specific, positive features, which suggest the diagnosis of a psychogenic movement disorder, including psychogenic dystonia. These include fluctuations during the examination, particularly an increase of the dystonia with attention and suggestion and a decrease with distraction; a changing frequency, amplitude, or pattern; the ability to trigger movements with unusual or nonphysiological interventions (e.g., trigger points on the body, passive movements of another limb); and the character of the dystonia may be incongruous with the features of organic dystonia. The most reliable feature allowing a confident diagnosis of a psychogenic dystonia (or other psychogenic movement disorder), however, is a marked and persistent improvement with psychotherapy, placebo, or suggestion. It is important that this response is significant and sustained, as placebo effects are well recognized to improve movement disorders transiently up to 30% (21).
4. Scars from multiple operations or self-inflicted injuries: The physical examination may reveal multiple scars from multiple previous operations, which may be due to previous abnormal illness behavior or somatization, or self-inflicted injury, suggesting an underlying psychiatric disturbance.

## Psychiatric Assessment

There are few studies assessing psychiatric aspects specifically in psychogenic dystonia. However, psychiatric aspects of psychogenic movement disorders in general also apply to psychogenic dystonia. Thus, "psychogenic movement disorders" from a psychiatric point of view are comprised of a mixture of conversion disorders, somatoform disorders, factitious disorders, and malingering in the framework of the Diagnostic and Statistical Manual of Mental Disorders 4th Edition-Revised (22). While the diagnosis of conversion disorder requires an acute stressor before the onset of the motor or sensory dysfunction, this may not always be evident when a diagnosis of a psychogenic dystonia is made. In somatoform disorders in general, other somatizations are commonly present. Factitious disorders and malingering as a cause of psychogenic dystonia are probably rare but have been reported (23).

Many patients with psychogenic dystonia report an entirely normal mental state and are often reluctant to see a psychiatrist. However, comorbidity between conversion disorder and both Axis I (clinical disorders) and Axis II (personality disorders) is significant. Most patients with conversion disorder have at least one comorbid Axis I diagnosis, with rates of depression ranging from 26% to 71%, and anxiety disorder present in 7% to 38% (8,10,11,24–26). Personality disorders are diagnosed in 42% to 67% of patients and include a variety of personality subtypes (with dependent and borderline personality of higher frequency). Thus, psychiatric assessment can provide useful, often critical, information and potentially allows underlying psychological causes to be addressed. In addition, previous episodes of psychiatric illness, behavioral abnormalities, and self-harm may be revealed, psychological stressors as precipitating or maintaining factors identified and addressed, or a history of psychological trauma, including childhood sexual, physical, or emotional abuse, uncovered. Whilst these features may support a diagnosis of a psychogenic problem, none of them is specific for this and may be coincidental. In addition, many neurological disorders such as myoclonic dystonia (27), stiff person syndrome (28), or idiopathic torsion dystonia (29) have psychiatric manifestations including depression, anxiety (including phobia), psychosis, or behavioral disorders. Nevertheless, addressing these issues may improve patients' overall quality of life and lead to improvement of the physical presentation of a psychogenic dystonia in a proportion of patients.

## Diagnostic Criteria for Psychogenic Dystonias

None of the features listed above is specific for psychogenic dystonia. Not only does psychiatric comorbidity, a history of psychological stressors, or childhood abuse occur in a high proportion of people with "true" neurological illness or the general population but also psychogenic signs may occur in organic illness and single episodes of somatization occur in a high proportion of people without reaching the diagnostic criteria for somatization disorder (30). However, some of these features of psychogenic dystonia and psychogenic movement disorders in general are more suggestive of this diagnosis than others, and the presence of several of these features increases the likelihood of this diagnosis. Based on these features, the diagnostic classification of psychogenic movement disorders, which reflects the degree of diagnostic certainty of this diagnosis (documented, clinically established, probable, or possible), was modified for psychogenic dystonia (6) (Table 2).

**Table 2** Diagnostic Criteria for Psychogenic Dystonia

| | |
|---|---|
| Documented[a] | Persistent relief by psychotherapy, suggestion, or placebo has been demonstrated, which may be helped by physiotherapy, or the patients were seen without the dystonia when believing themselves unobserved |
| Clinically established[a] | The dystonia is incongruent with classical dystonia, or there are inconsistencies in the examination, plus at least one of the following three: other psychogenic signs, multiple somatizations, or an obvious psychiatric disturbance |
| Probable | The dystonia is incongruent or inconsistent with typical dystonia, or there are psychogenic signs or multiple somatizations |
| Possible | Evidence of an emotional disturbance |

[a]As only the first two categories provide a clinically useful degree of diagnostic certainty, they have been combined to one category of "clinically definite." *Source*: From Ref. 10.

### Investigations

Other than excluding causes for secondary dystonia, there are a few specific investigations that may contribute to the diagnosis of dystonia. Several abnormalities in spinal and motor cortical circuits have been reported in patients with dystonia, which include abnormalities of intracortical inhibition and of the cortical silent period (31), reduced reciprocal inhibition of H-reflexes in the forearm muscles (32), evidence of broad peak synchronization of motor units in antagonist muscles (33), and evidence for a new low-frequency drive that is absent in controls but present in cervical dystonia (34). In addition, several imaging studies have demonstrated abnormal function on functional magnetic resonance imaging (35) or positron emission tomography (36). However, while all of these have helped the understanding of dystonia on a group level, the sensitivity and specificity of these investigations are unknown, particularly compared to those with a limb permanently held in an abnormal position, and it is not clear how useful these techniques are on an individual basis. There is preliminary evidence to support the possibility that many of these electrophysiological abnormalities, indicating altered cortical and spinal inhibition and thought to be characteristic for "organic" dystonia, can also be seen in patients with clinically established psychogenic dystonia (37). In addition, these tests are only available in specialized centers and are not available in routine clinical practice. Therefore, these tests, at present, do not appear useful in the diagnosis of individual patients in clinical practice. Further studies are urgently needed to determine the sensitivity and specificity of these tests in distinguishing psychogenic and organic dystonia and to establish the effects of simply maintaining the muscles of the body in question tonically contracted for prolonged periods (in a dystonic-like posture). In a similar way, functional imaging studies have not evaluated whether changes that may be seen in patients with dystonia (36,38,39) are also present in individuals with psychogenic dystonia or with voluntary abnormal posturing of body parts.

## COURSE OF ILLNESS

As mentioned above, many patients with psychogenic dystonia have a history of previous somatizations or other psychogenic movement disorders, which may have remitted spontaneously or with treatment. There may also have been paroxysmal exacerbations and remissions, but in others no fluctuations occur and the disorder remains stable over years. The prognosis of psychogenic motor disorders is generally poor, with the majority of patients suffering long-term disability, requiring a wheel chair, assistance with self-care, and loss of ability to work or participate in many social activities. However, outcome varies considerably and psychogenic dystonia may remain stable, be replaced by other psychogenic movement disorders or by a mental disorder, or symptoms may completely remit (9,10,40). The chance of remission of psychogenic movement disorders appears higher in those case series that included patients with a short disease duration, with up to 60% remissions if the history was less than three months (41). In most case series from movement disorders centers, where disease duration is generally longer, remissions only occurred in 10% to 30% of cases (10,25,26). Sudden onset, new psychiatric diagnosis coinciding with the unexplained motor symptom has been reported to predict a better course, whereas receipt of financial benefits and pending litigation appears to be associated with worse prognosis (25,26).

## MANAGEMENT

Patients with psychogenic dystonia should be thoroughly investigated at the initial presentation to exclude an organic diagnosis and to reassure the patient. Continued further investigations, however, lead to reinforcement of illness beliefs, and unnecessary investigations and treatments after a diagnosis of psychogenic dystonia has been made carry the danger of iatrogenic illness. Whilst controversial, the use of placebo or suggestion can be used to relieve movements and, thus, may provide further diagnostic information and reassure patients of the intactness of their bodily function. Some patients with recent onset symptoms require little further treatment than an explanation of possible mechanisms of psychological influences on physical symptoms. In those with longer duration of symptoms, involvement of a psychiatrist, if acceptable to the patient, may reveal underlying psychopathology or psychological stressors. If an underlying psychological cause can be addressed using psychotherapy, physical therapy, and psychopharmacologic therapy, this may lead to resolution of symptoms. Good results have been claimed for admission to an inpatient ward for diagnosis and treatment (10), but the lack of availability of such facilities limits this approach. At present, there are no randomized controlled trials to establish the most successful treatment. Such trials are particularly difficult to undertake, given the heterogeneity of underlying psychiatric diagnoses and stressors. Cognitive-behavioral therapy is a practical approach that has been reported to have good results in patients with conversion disorders (42,43), but patients with more complex and long-standing psychological problems may require different types of therapy, including interpersonal therapy, family therapy, or dynamic psychotherapy. Collaboration among neurologist, primary care physician, psychiatrist, psychologist, and therapist is crucial, and regular follow-up may limit the development of new symptoms prompting further investigations.

## POSTTRAUMATIC DYSTONIA

A controversial area overlapping with psychogenic dystonia is that of dystonia following peripheral trauma ("posttraumatic dystonia") (44), which differs from idiopathic torsion dystonia triggered by a peripheral trauma. The features of posttraumatic dystonia overlap with many aspects of psychogenic dystonia, including abrupt onset, often with a fixed posture from the beginning, rapid progression to maximum disability, severe pain, lack of a "geste antagoniste," and onset in the lower limbs in adults (44–46). In addition, minor trauma is a typical precipitant for the development of psychogenic motor disturbances (40). One study (47) reported that all of their followed patients with complex regional pain syndrome (CRPS) and abnormal movements exhibited nonorganic signs, and in some cases malingering was documented. Another recent study (48) reported that most patients with posttraumatic cervical dystonia had nonorganic signs, features suggestive of a psychogenic movement disorder; were involved in litigation (49); responded with improvement of posture and/or pain to intravenous sodium-amytal tests; and had psychological conflicts on psychological testing. In another series of 103 patients with fixed (usually limb) dystonia, of which the majority occurred after a minor injury, a large proportion fulfilled strict criteria for psychogenic dystonia or for somatization disorder, particularly when this history was specifically sought (50). Patients with a posttraumatic dystonia in whom psychogenic dystonia was proven have been reported (23,47,51). However, others disagree and have disputed an association between posttraumatic dystonia, which overlaps with CRPS type I, and psychological disorders (52–56). In patients with CRPS type I and dystonic postures, abnormalities similar to those seen in primary dystonia, including impaired reciprocal inhibition of H-reflexes (57–59) and abnormal stretch reflexes (58,60), have been reported, and one group reported genetic susceptibilities related to the human leukocyte antigen system (61,62). In addition, changes in contralateral thalamic perfusion on Iodine-123-labelled single-photon emission computed tomography imaging in cases of CRPS (56) have suggested that central adaptation mechanisms occur in CRPS. However, abnormalities of regional cerebral blood flow in the contralateral thalamus and basal ganglia, which resolve after recovery, have also been described in patients with psychogenic, unilateral sensorimotor loss (63), and the neurophysiological abnormalities can also been seen in psychogenic dystonia (37). It is therefore currently unknown whether the reported central changes on electrophysiological and functional imaging studies are primary or secondary to the clinical changes, and the controversy regarding the etiology of posttraumatic dystonia currently remains unresolved (52,64). We believe that psychogenic dystonia is an important cause of abnormal postures associated with posttraumatic dystonia, with or without features of CRPS.

## CONCLUSION

Psychogenic dystonia is a rare but important consideration in the differential diagnosis of dystonia. Exclusion of secondary dystonia at the initial presentation is important, but the diagnosis is not simply a diagnosis of exclusion. Instead, it can be made based on positive diagnostic features using the classification system of diagnostic certainty. It requires considerable experience with the presentations of dystonia, which may appear bizarre and inconsistent. Studies to examine the pathophysiology and diagnostic usefulness of specific neuroimaging and electrophysiological tests to differentiate psychogenic from neurologically determined dystonia are urgently needed. While it is clear that minor trauma can be a precipitant for the onset of a psychogenic movement disorder, the classification of posttraumatic dystonia remains controversial. Management rests on a firm diagnosis following appropriate investigations and a sympathetic and multidisciplinary approach to the patient, with appropriate follow-up following diagnosis. The prognosis of psychogenic dystonia is very poor, and so carefully designed and controlled studies are critically needed to establish the best approach for the management of this complicated disorder.

## REFERENCES


1. Schwalbe W. aug Diss, ed. Eine eigentumliche tonische Krampfform mit hysterischen Symptomen. Berlin: Schade G, 1908.
2. Oppenheim H. Über eine eigenartige Krampfkrankheit des kindlichen und jugendlichen alters (dysbasia lordotica progressiva dystonia musculorum deformans). Neurol Zentralblatt 1911; 30:1090–1107.
3. Flatau E, Sterling W. Progressiver Torsionsspasmus bei Kindern. Neurol Psychiatr 2004: 586–612.
4. Marsden CD. Dystonia: The spectrum of the disease. In: Yahr MD, ed. The Basal Ganglia. New York: Raven Press, 1976:351–367.
5. Fahn S, Eldridge R. Definition of dystonia and classification of the dystonic states. Adv Neurol 1976; 14:1–5.
6. Fahn S, Williams DT. Psychogenic dystonia. Adv Neurol 1988; 50:431–455.
7. Marsden CD. Psychogenic problems associated with dystonia. Adv Neurol 1995; 65: 319–326.
8. Miyasaki JM, Sa DS, Galvez-Jimenez N, Lang AE. Psychogenic movement disorders. Can J Neurol Sci 2003; 30(Suppl 1):S94–S100.
9. Pringsheim T, Lang AE. Psychogenic dystonia. Rev Neurol (Paris) 2003; 159:885–891.
10. Williams DT, Ford B, Fahn S. Phenomenology and psychopathology related to psychogenic movement disorders. Adv Neurol 1995; 65:231–257.
11. Factor SA, Podskalny GD, Molho ES. Psychogenic movement disorders: frequency, clinical profile, and characteristics. J Neurol Neurosurg Psychiatry 1995; 59:406–412.
12. Fahn S, Bressman SB, Marsden CD. Classification of dystonia. Adv Neurol 1998; 78: 1–10.
13. Francis P, Baker GA. Non-epileptic attack disorder (NEAD): a comprehensive review. Seizure 1999; 8:53–61.
14. Dobyns WB, Ozelius LJ, Kramer PL, et al. Rapid-onset dystonia-parkinsonism. Neurology 1993; 43:2596–2602.
15. Bressman SB, Fahn S, Burke RE. Paroxysmal non-kinesigenic dystonia. Adv Neurol 1988; 50:403–413.
16. Wessely S, Nimnuan C, Sharpe M. Functional somatic syndromes: one or many? Lancet 1999; 354:936–939.
17. Cohen ME, Robins E, Cohen ME, Purtell JJ, Altmann MW, Reid DE. Excessive surgery in hysteria; study of surgical procedures in 50 women with hysteria and 190 controls. J Am Med Assoc 1953; 151:977–986.
18. Schrag A, Brown R, Trimble M. The reliability of self-reported diagnoses in patients with neurologically unexplained symptoms. J Neurol Neurosurg Psychiatry 2004; 75:608–611.
19. Ziv I, Djaldetti R, Zoldan Y, Avraham M, Melamed E. Diagnosis of "non-organic" limb paresis by a novel objective motor assessment: the quantitative Hoover's test. J Neurol 1998; 245:797–802.
20. Stone J, Zeman A, Sharpe M. Functional weakness and sensory disturbance. J Neurol Neurosurg Psychiatry 2002; 73:241–245.
21. Goetz CG, Leurgans S, Raman R. Placebo-associated improvements in motor function: comparison of subjective and objective sections of the UPDRS in early Parkinson's disease. Mov Disord 2002; 17:283–288.
22. American Psychiatric Association. Diagnostic and Statistical Manual of Mental Disorders. 4th (DSM IV-R) ed. Washington, DC: American Psychiatric Association, 2000.

23. Kurlan R, Brin MF, Fahn S. Movement disorder in reflex sympathetic dystrophy: a case proven to be psychogenic by surveillance video monitoring. Mov Disord 1997; 12: 243–245.
24. Binzer M, Eisemann M. Childhood experiences and personality traits in patients with motor conversion symptoms. Acta Psychiatr Scand 1998; 98:288–295.
25. Feinstein A, Stergiopoulos V, Fine J, Lang AE. Psychiatric outcome in patients with a psychogenic movement disorder: a prospective study. Neuropsychiatry Neuropsychol Behav Neurol 2001; 14:169–176.
26. Crimlisk HL, Bhatia K, Cope H, David A, Marsden CD, Ron MA. Slater revisited: 6 year follow up study of patients with medically unexplained motor symptoms. BMJ 1998; 316:582–586.
27. Saunders-Pullman R, Shriberg J, Heiman G, et al. Myoclonus dystonia: possible association with obsessive-compulsive disorder and alcohol dependence. Neurology 2002; 58: 242–245.
28. Henningsen P, Meinck HM. Specific phobia is a frequent non-motor feature in stiff man syndrome. J Neurol Neurosurg Psychiatry 2003; 74:462–465.
29. Wenzel T, Schnider P, Wimmer A, Steinhoff N, Moraru E, Auff E. Psychiatric comorbidity in patients with spasmodic torticollis. J Psychosom Res 1998; 44:687–690.
30. Rief W, Hessel A, Braehler E. Somatization symptoms and hypochondriacal features in the general population. Psychosom Med 2001; 63:595–602.
31. Edwards MJ, Huang YZ, Wood NW, Rothwell JC, Bhatia KP. Different patterns of electrophysiological deficits in manifesting and non-manifesting carriers of the DYT1 gene mutation. Brain 2003; 126:2074–2080.
32. Panizza M, Lelli S, Nilsson J, Hallett M. H-reflex recovery curve and reciprocal inhibition of H-reflex in different kinds of dystonia. Neurology 1990; 40:824–828.
33. Farmer SF, Sheean GL, Mayston MJ, et al. Abnormal motor unit synchronization of antagonist muscles underlies pathological co-contraction in upper limb dystonia. Brain 1998; 121 (Pt 5):801–814.
34. Tijssen MA, Marsden JF, Brown P. Frequency analysis of EMG activity in patients with idiopathic torticollis. Brain 2000; 123(Pt 4):677–686.
35. Filipovic SR, Siebner HR, Rowe JB, et al. Modulation of cortical activity by repetitive transcranial magnetic stimulation (rTMS): a review of functional imaging studies and the potential use in dystonia. Adv Neurol 2004; 94:45–52.
36. Eidelberg D, Moeller JR, Antonini A, et al. Functional brain networks in DYT1 dystonia. Ann Neurol 1998; 44:303–312.
37. Espay AJ, Morgante F, Gunraj CA, Lang AE, Chen R. Abnormal Cortical inhibition in Psychogenic Dystonia. 64th ed. 2005.
38. Ceballos-Baumann AO, Passingham RE, Warner T, Playford ED, Marsden CD, Brooks DJ. Overactive prefrontal and underactive motor cortical areas in idiopathic dystonia. Ann Neurol 1995; 37:363–372.
39. Hutchinson M, Nakamura T, Moeller JR, et al. The metabolic topography of essential blepharospasm: a focal dystonia with general implications. Neurology 2000; 55: 673–677.
40. Lang AE. Psychogenic dystonia: a review of 18 cases. Can J Neurol Sci 1995; 22:136–143.
41. Binzer M, Kullgren G. Motor conversion disorder. A prospective 2- to 5-year follow-up study. Psychosomatics 1998; 39:519–527.
42. Bleichhardt G, Timmer B, Rief W. Cognitive-behavioural therapy for patients with multiple somatoform symptoms-a randomised controlled trial in tertiary care. J Psychosom Res 2004; 56:449–454.
43. Kroenke K, Swindle R. Cognitive-behavioral therapy for somatization and symptom syndromes: a critical review of controlled clinical trials. Psychother Psychosom 2000; 69: 205–215.
44. Jankovic J. Post-traumatic movement disorders: central and peripheral mechanisms. Neurology 1994; 44:2006–2014.

45. Truong DD, Dubinsky R, Hermanowicz N, Olson WL, Silverman B, Koller WC. Posttraumatic torticollis. Arch Neurol 1991; 48:221–223.
46. Goldman S, Ahlskog JE. Posttraumatic cervical dystonia. Mayo Clin Proc 1993; 68: 443–448.
47. Verdugo RJ, Ochoa JL. Abnormal movements in complex regional pain syndrome: assessment of their nature. Muscle Nerve 2000; 23:198–205.
48. Sa DS, Mailis-Gagnon A, Nicholson K, Lang AE. Posttraumatic painful torticollis. Mov Disord 2003; 18:1482–1491.
49. O'Riordan S, Hutchinson M. Cervical dystonia following peripheral trauma-a case-control study. J Neurol 2004; 251:150–155.
50. Schrag A, Trimble M, Quinn N, Bhatia K. The syndrome of fixed dystonia: an evaluation of 103 patients. Brain 2004.
51. Stone J, Carson A, Sharpe M. Functional symptoms in neurology: management. J Neurol Neurosurg Psychiatry 2005; 76(Suppl 1):i13–i21.
52. Jankovic J. Can peripheral trauma induce dystonia and other movement disorders? Yes! Mov Disord 2001; 16:7–12.
53. Ciccone DS, Bandilla EB, Wu W. Psychological dysfunction in patients with reflex sympathetic dystrophy. Pain 1997; 71:323–333.
54. Lynch ME. Psychological aspects of reflex sympathetic dystrophy: a review of the adult and paediatric literature. Pain 1992; 49:337–347.
55. Birklein F, Riedl B, Sieweke N, Weber M, Neundorfer B. Neurological findings in complex regional pain syndromes-analysis of 145 cases. Acta Neurol Scand 2000; 101:262–269.
56. Fukumoto M, Ushida T, Zinchuk VS, Yamamoto H, Yoshida S. Contralateral thalamic perfusion in patients with reflex sympathetic dystrophy syndrome. Lancet 1999; 354: 1790–1791.
57. Koelman JH, Hilgevoord AA, Bour LJ, Speelman JD, Ongerboer d V. Soleus H-reflex tests in causalgia-dystonia compared with dystonia and mimicked dystonic posture. Neurology 1999; 53:2196–2198.
58. van de Beek WJ, Vein A, Hilgevoord AA, van Dijk JG, van Hilten BJ. Neurophysiologic aspects of patients with generalized or multifocal tonic dystonia of reflex sympathetic dystrophy. J Clin Neurophysiol 2002; 19:77–83.
59. van de Beek WJ, Schwartzman RJ, van Nes SI, Delhaas EM, van Hilten JJ. Diagnostic criteria used in studies of reflex sympathetic dystrophy. Neurology 2002; 58:522–526.
60. van Hilten JJ, van de Beek WJ, Vein AA, van Dijk JG, Middelkoop HA. Clinical aspects of multifocal or generalized tonic dystonia in reflex sympathetic dystrophy. Neurology 2001; 56:1762–1765.
61. van de Beek WJ, Roep BO, van der Slik AR, Giphart MJ, van Hilten BJ. Susceptibility loci for complex regional pain syndrome. Pain 2003; 103:93–97.
62. van Hilten JJ, van de Beek WJ, Roep BO. Multifocal or generalized tonic dystonia of complex regional pain syndrome: a distinct clinical entity associated with HLA-DR13. Ann Neurol 2000; 48:113–116.
63. Vuilleumier P, Chicherio C, Assal F, Schwartz S, Slosman D, Landis T. Functional neuroanatomical correlates of hysterical sensorimotor loss. Brain 2001; 124:1077–1090.
64. Weiner WJ. Can peripheral trauma induce dystonia? No! Mov Disord 2001; 16:13–22.

# 19
# Nonmotor Symptoms in Dystonia

**Joanne Green and Stewart A. Factor**
*Department of Neurology, Emory University School of Medicine, Wesley Woods Health Center, Atlanta, Georgia, U.S.A.*

## INTRODUCTION

Nonmotor symptoms are increasingly recognized in Parkinson's disease (PD), and have a significant impact on quality of life (QOL). The presence of such symptoms as cognitive dysfunction, psychiatric symptoms (psychosis, depression, anxiety, apathy, and poor impulse control), sensory symptoms (pain, restless leg syndrome, and akathisia), fatigue, and autonomic dysfunction has dominated the literature and led to the development of a nonmotor-unified PD rating scale. The occurrence of nonmotor features has not been as well established or studied in dystonia. While both disorders are due to abnormalities in the basal ganglia, they differ in that PD is neurodegenerative while dystonia is not. This may explain, at least partially, why nonmotor phenomena are less emphasized in dystonia. Nevertheless, it is clear that the basal ganglia govern the development of nonmotor symptoms through connections with sensory cortex, thalamus, limbic structures, and other regions. Although sensory and psychological symptoms are reported, a search of the dystonia literature identifies few, if any, references on dementia, autonomic features, and fatigue. This chapter will review what has been examined with regard to psychiatric symptoms, sleep disorders, pain, and the nonmotor hallmark of dystonia, sensory tricks.

## NEUROPSYCHOLOGICAL AND PSYCHIATRIC CHANGES

### Physiological Basis for Change

Consideration of the pathophysiology of primary dystonia provides one basis for predicting that this disorder may be accompanied by cognitive and psychiatric symptoms. Normal control of movement is heavily dependent upon a system of parallel, segregated neural circuits connecting the basal ganglia, thalamus, and cortex. Several of these neural circuits include areas within the frontal lobe, notably the orbitofrontal and dorsolateral prefrontal regions, and modulate cognitive "executive abilities." These abilities are important to working memory, problem solving, establishing and switching cognitive strategies and response sets, and response inhibition. Other circuits within this system implicate limbic regions important for modulating mood and affect.

Disruption in cognitive and limbic neuronal activity from altered subcortical basal ganglia and thalamic input may be one basis for executive and mood dysfunction associated with PD, Huntington's disease (HD), and, perhaps, dystonia. It has been hypothesized that, in dystonia, inhibition within the motor system is reduced, possibly caused by underactive inhibitory output from the internal globus pallidus to the thalamus (1). Consistent with this, in patients with generalized or focal limb dystonia, abnormally increased activation of the dorsolateral prefrontal cortex has been observed on positron emission tomography scanning during joystick movements (2). Similarly, even asymptomatic individuals who carry the *DYT1* gene for primary dystonia show prefrontal activation during motor sequence learning (3). Thus, the pathophysiology of dystonia provides one basis for predicting that patients with primary dystonia will exhibit cognitive and mood changes.

Another basis for predicting neuropsychological changes derives from possible medication side effects. Treatment of dystonia often involves use of anticholinergic medication, most commonly trihexyphenidyl (Artane) and benztropine (Cogentin). Cholinergic transmission is fundamental to memory and attention, and disruption of cholinergic systems is an important basis for memory deficits seen in neurodegenerative disorders such as Alzheimer's disease and PD. In normal, healthy individuals, administration of anticholinergic agents such as scopolamine induces memory deficits, particularly in initial learning and memory encoding. Thus, use of anticholinergic medication in patients with dystonia can potentially disrupt neuropsychological abilities, particularly memory and attention.

## Neuropsychological Studies

Given these bases for neuropsychological change, existing research suggests that cognitive changes observed in patients with primary dystonia are selective and subtle, and that medication effects may play a significant role (4,5). In one well-controlled study (5), 20 subjects with idiopathic dystonia untreated with anticholinergic medications for at least two years were compared with 25 age- and education-matched controls. The two groups did not differ at baseline on measures of explicit memory, procedural learning, verbal and conditional associate learning, visuospatial function, or executive functions, suggesting that dystonia alone was not associated with significant cognitive deficits. To more closely examine the effect of medication on cognition, 12 of the patients and 20 control subjects were retested after at least two months of high-dose trihexyphenidyl therapy. Direct statistical comparisons of the controls and patients indicated that the patients showed weaker performance on only a few measures dependent upon mental speed, including a test of immediate and delayed verbal memory (Wechsler Memory Scale Logical Memory) and an executive function test of response inhibition (the Stroop Test). Older patients were more affected than younger patients. It was hypothesized that the anticholinergic medication slowed the rate of information processing, thus affecting initial memory encoding in conditions more dependent upon speeded processing.

There are only a few other studies examining neuropsychological deficits in dystonia, and these do not involve large patient samples or control for possible medication side effects. One study of 14 patients with primary dystonia used a computer-based battery of executive functions, spatial working memory, and attentional vigilance from the CANTAB as well as standard neuropsychological tests (6). The quality of patient performance was assessed relative to published, normative data obtained from large samples of healthy control subjects. As a whole, the patient group was impaired only on measures derived from a test of intra-extra-dimensional (IED) set shifting. Ten of the 14 patients exhibited a selective deficit on this measure, a task dependent upon frontal lobe integrity. The interpretation of these findings are complicated by the presence of several, possibly confounding variables. It appears that the 14 patients who exhibited the IED deficit were taking more medications and that they had had lower intelligence quotient (IQ) scores (estimated IQ = 102) than the patients without the deficit (estimated IQ = 118).

Another relevant study compared 10 patients with primary dystonia to 12 matched control subjects on a test battery focusing on frontal lobe function. Applying a stringent criterion for statistical significance ($p < .002$) that controlled for the number of comparisons, the two groups did not differ on any of the neuropsychological measures. Even when a less stringent criterion was considered ($p < .05$), only a few subtle differences (in semantic fluency and dual motor performance) were observed.

Thus, the existing literature suggests that the pathophysiology of dystonia itself is unlikely to be associated with significant cognitive dysfunction except, perhaps, in subtle aspects of response set shifting. These deficits are unlikely to have a major impact on the patient's everyday functioning. However, there is evidence that anticholinergic medications used to relieve the symptoms of the disease are associated with subtle cognitive deficits. Thus, the use of anticholinergic drugs must be carefully considered in patients of older age or who are taking other anticholinergic medications. One question left unanswered is whether the long-term use of anticholinergic therapy may have even more detrimental effects on information processing speed and memory.

## Psychiatric Changes

The bulk of the research on psychiatric correlates of dystonia focuses on the incidence of depression and the potential of premorbid personality or psychiatric disorder. In several studies, patients with focal hand dystonia (writer's cramp) or cervical dystonia (CD) did not have elevated rates of psychopathology or personality disorder prior to or during the course of their illness (7–9). A study comparing 201 CD patients with 135 control subjects with spine pain observed elevated rates of depression among the CD patients as assessed by the depression scale on the Minnesota Multiphasic Personality Inventory (4). In a study comparing 85 CD patients to 49 patients with cervical stenosis, although the two groups did not differ in their premorbid history of depression, the CD patients had a higher level of depression as assessed by the Beck Depression Inventory (BDI) (9). The CD patients more frequently endorsed BDI items that were negatively self-referring (self-blame, self-accusation, sense of punishment, suicidal ideation, and attempt). Thirty-nine percent of these patients, but only 4% of the cervical stenosis patients, endorsed an item reflecting that they had a negative body image.

In a follow-up study (10), self-depreciation was observed to be a major predictor of depression, and negative body concept resulting from postural abnormality was a major variable accounting for the level of self-depreciation. Longitudinal changes in the clinical status of the patient's CD had a significant effect on body concept, depression, and functional disability. Moreover, among 22 of 26 patients who received benefits from treatment with botulinum neurotoxin, type A, there were significant posttreatment improvements in depression and disability. Finally, self-consciousness was reported by 80% of patients to aggravate motor features of CD (11).

In one study examining the issues of QOL in CD, 289 patients completed the SF-36 by mail. The strongest predictors of physical and mental QOL scores were anxiety and depression (12). These authors suggested that treatment should not only focus on the motor components but also psychological well-being as well. The work was followed by the development of a disease-specific QOL measure for CD. The result was a 24-item version craniocervical dystonia questionnaire with five subscales including emotional well-being (13).

The finding of a negative self-view among CD patients has implications for the origin and treatment of depression in dystonia in general. If depression is partly in reaction to a negative self-concept, then cognitive behavior therapy aimed at adjusting the negative self-concept, particularly body concept, may be an important adjunct to medication treatment of depression. Given that the relief of dystonic symptoms is often temporary and variable even when treatment is effective, it is probably important for cognitive behavioral strategies to be practiced repetitively and on a routine basis in order to develop a stable, improved body concept.

### Conclusions

Existing research suggests that patients with primary dystonia experience subtle difficulty in response set shifting and slowness in the rate of information processing that may disrupt initial memory encoding. These patients may also experience elevated rates of depression, perhaps in part related to their self-perception of a negative body image. Cognitive behavior therapy may be helpful in adjusting this perception.

There are clearly areas where additional research would be useful, including large-scale studies examining the impact of factors such as disease duration, duration of anticholinergic treatment, patient age, and possible variation in neuropsychological and psychiatric symptoms as a function of the type of primary dystonia (focal vs. multifocal, generalized vs. hemidystonic). Additional research might also differentiate more specifically the type of basal ganglia-thalamocortical system disruption associated with primary dystonia, in which neuropsychological and psychiatric changes appear to be largely subtle, from that associated with other movement disorders, such as PD and HD, where such changes are more pronounced, often leading to dementia.

## SLEEP DISORDERS

Sleep research in dystonia began over two decades ago in an effort to show that it is an "organic psychomotor syndrome" (14). These authors reported difficulty with sleep initiation, maintenance, and an abnormality of rapid eye movement (REM) sleep in patients with dystonia musculorum deformans. What followed were several polysomnographic studies that demonstrated increases in stage two sleep, latency to sleep, and reduced sleep efficiency with increased number of awakenings in patients with generalized torsion dystonia (15–17). These abnormalities correlated with dystonia severity.

These authors suggested that changes in sleep spindle activity may be associated with generalized dystonia. In a review of nine patients, sleep spindle activity was pronounced, high amplitude, and continuous in nature for all of stage two and portions of stage three in the severe cases (as opposed to the short trains seen in normals) (17), but diminished in mildly dystonic patients. These authors also report little change in the declining spindle activity, normally seen with advancing age in dystonic patients (17). This same group reported a dystonia patient whose sleep physiology abnormalities normalized after thalamotomy (18), although some patients in a prior study had high spindle activity despite treatment with thalamotomy (17). Although these discrepancies are somewhat difficult to resolve, sleep evaluation in another lab also noted these spindle changes in both generalized and CD (14), and that similarities in nearly 30 cases from several studies suggested that sleep spindle abnormalities may be a specific feature of dystonia (16,17). On the other hand, sleep analysis in 24 dystonia patients, 10 control subjects, and 39 subjects with other neurological disorders found increased sleep spindles in only a minority of dystonic patients (4 patients) and an abnormal amplitude in only one case, suggesting that spindle changes are probably not of clinical significance (19). One patient with a previous thalamotomy had an increase in spindle number and amplitude.

Few studies have examined sleep in focal dystonias, but an assessment of 10 patients with blepharospasm-oromandibular dystonia demonstrated impaired sleep efficiency and reduced slow-wave and REM sleep that correlated with disease severity (20). Interestingly, these authors reported that the dystonic movements decreased with deeper sleep but did not completely disappear. In a controlled study of nine CD patients and nine age-matched controls, polysomnography demonstrated normal sleep organization and no difference in subjective sleep complaints (21). The only difference between groups was a larger variance in sleep latency in the CD group, a finding, perhaps, related to continued cervical muscle spasm associated with head positioning. However, most patients had a significant decrease in abnormal muscle activity with lying down, and muscle activity was normal during sleep. One other study demonstrated that some CD patients developed brief bursts of cervical muscle activity during REM sleep leading to arousals (22). Lastly, some dystonia patients report symptom benefit after sleep, but this clinical phenomenon has not been evaluated in the neurophysiology laboratory.

## PAIN

Pain is an important feature of dystonia and may lead to an increase in disability or decline in QOL (23). While the frequency of pain ranges from 68% to 80% in large series of CD (24–26), reviews of idiopathic torsion dystonia find almost no mention of pain as a disease symptom. It is probably much less prevalent in other forms of dystonia although this has not been studied systematically. Most authors believe that the pain of CD increases over time, emanates from muscle, experienced along the contours of muscles, and correlates with constant severe muscle spasm (24,27,28). The pain has been described as widespread and diffuse over the neck and shoulders with some radiation toward the side of deviation. The intensity is highly variable but many patients require analgesia. Ten percent of patients have pain before the onset of obvious dystonic movements. Sleep alleviates pain leading to a diurnal pattern (21). There is some benefit from such treatments as biofeedback, relaxation therapies, and physiotherapies but more so with botulinum toxin (types A and B). The improvement of pain parallels the motor response to botulinum toxin, but about 25% of patients may fail to have an improvement in pain with individual doses (29). In addition, pain alleviation from therapeutic injection may wane over time (30,31).

There has been one systematic study of pain in dystonia and that was in 39 patients with CD (32). A semistructured interview determined that pain was present in 26 of the subjects. Visual analog measures in subjects with this symptom reported current pain severity at 30 and severity over the prior five days to be 47. The

Finnish Pain Questionnaire assessed several descriptive terms for the pain, the 10 most common included tiring, unilateral, radiating, continuous, tugging, aching, exhausted, tender, deep, and pricking. These terms are common to description of other forms of muscular pain as well. A pain drawing found that the pain was mostly ipsilateral to the rotation, included the arm and upper chest, and tended to radiate up the head and down the trunk. Pain in lower trunk and back was not ipsilateral but equally distributed to sides. Muscle palpation and algometer measures did not demonstrate differences in painful and nonpainful CD. The trapezius was usually the most tender of the muscles. The Tsui scale for CD severity found no difference in severity between painful and nonpainful groups. Finally, radiological examination of the neck was also not different between painful and nonpainful CD, suggesting that arthritic change was not a primary source of pain. The authors suggested that altered central nervous system processing might play a role, be it spinal cord or basal ganglia. One other study (33) examined pain pressure thresholds in nine CD patients versus five controls and found a much lower (2x) threshold to pain in CD. Thresholds were also higher at maximal voluntary contraction than at rest.

Pain is less commonly associated with cranial dystonia, but periorbital eye pain and eye irritation have been reported in blepharospasm patients (34). In a series of 11 consecutive patients, pain, discomfort, distortion of sensory modalities, and phantom kinetic or postural sensations preceded the dystonia of the face by weeks to months, and then disappeared when the dystonia occurred (35). The location of the sensory phenomenon preceded and correlated with later developing dystonic symptoms. These authors suggest that the sensory component may have been the earliest manifestation of an evolving process. Initial voluntary movement relieved the sensation and when involuntary facial movements developed the sensory component resolved in the same way. Lower facial pain has been studied in one patient who developed perioral and jaw pain which was initially diagnosed as atypical facial pain (36). Prior to developing blepharospasm, the patient, being misdiagnosed was treated with dissection of the zygomatico-temporal branch of the facial nerve, multiple sinus surgeries, extraction of all upper jaw teeth, psychotherapy, and treatment with many medications including dopamine receptor blocking drugs. While there was no clinically obvious perioral spasm, electromyography (EMG) demonstrated its presence and botulinum toxin relieved the pain for two months (36). Other, more straightforward, facial pain syndromes appear to be misdiagnosed frequently. Pain is also not uncommon in association with jaw dystonia, jaw opening, closing, or deviation types. Here, the pain is located in the temporomandibular joint and frequently misdiagnosed as temporomandibular joint (TMJ) syndrome if the dystonia is not obvious (34). Some patients undergo surgery for this problem before the correct diagnosis is made. Here too injection of botulinum toxin into the appropriate pterygoid muscles generally relieves the pain. One other focal dystonia associated with muscle pain is writer's cramp. While in the act of writing, many patients complain of aches in the hand forearm or upper arm. One study demonstrated prominent writing pain in 11 of 19 cases, with pain resolution at rest (37).

## SENSORY TRICKS

Patients with dystonic disorders, particularly the focal forms, often discover ways to suppress their movements using an interesting array of "tricks." These usually consist of postural alterations or counterpressure maneuvers that are often tactile or

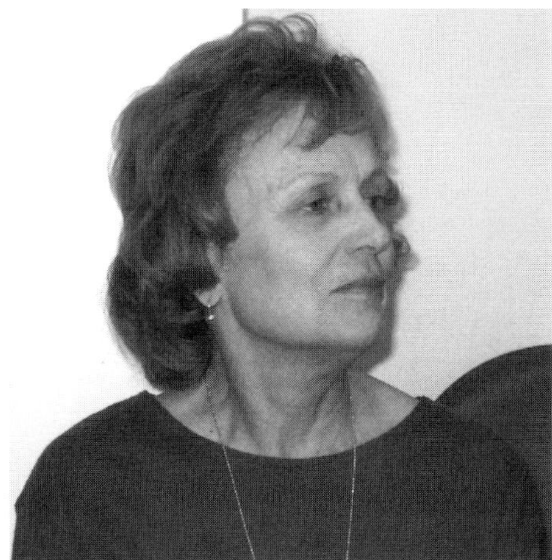

**Figure 1** Cervical dystonia with rotation left, mild retrocollis, and hypertrophy of the sternocleidomastoid.

proprioceptive in nature (38,39). This has been reported in the medical literature since 1901 (40), but despite that the unusual characteristics of this phenomenon has often led physicians to diagnose dystonic patients as psychogenic. The best-known example of a sensory trick is the classical "geste antagonistique (GA)," where a finger placed lightly on the chin, either ipsilateral or contralateral to the side of turning, will neutralize neck turning in CD (Figs. 1 and 2). Others include touching an eyebrow in blepharospasm, which leads to eye opening, touching the chin to control oromandibular dystonia, touching the roof of the mouth with the tongue or holding a toothpick in the mouth to prevent tongue protrusion, and sensation applied to the arm to prevent writer's cramp (see Table 1 for a detailed list). The

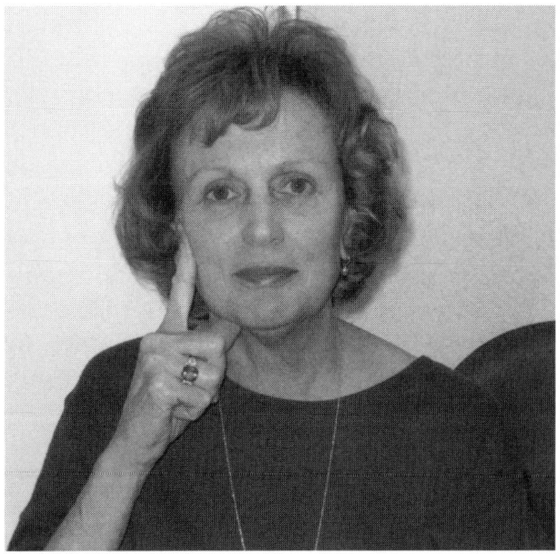

**Figure 2** Cervical dystonia patient demonstrating the "geste antagonistique." She has placed two fingers on the cheek and jaw on the side contralateral to the turning. This demonstrates that the trick is a sensory maneuver that corrects the turning and not a pressure maneuver pushing the head to the correct position.

**Table 1** Tricks for Various Dystonia

| | |
|---|---|
| Blepharospasm | Finger on eyebrow |
| | Whistling |
| | Mouth opening |
| | Wearing sunglasses |
| | Using an eyelid crutch |
| | Talking |
| | Singing |
| Cervical dystonia | Finger on chin, cheek, or forehead |
| | Hand on top of head or back of neck |
| | Leaning occiput against a wall or headrest |
| | Yawning |
| Oromandibular dystonia | Touching chin |
| | Tooth pick, straw, cigarette holder held in mouth |
| | Touching roof of mouth with tongue |
| | Chewing gum |
| | Using a dental appliance |
| Upper Limb dystonia | Touching wrist or forearm |
| | Changing posture of hand in writers cramp |
| | Using a writing appliance |
| | Changing size of the writing implement |
| | Writing upside down |
| Lower limb | Walking backwards |
| | Running |
| Axial dystonia | Jumping jacks |
| | Dancing |
| | Walking backwards |

pathophysiology of dystonic movements and behind the usefulness of tricks remains a mystery. Other sensory phenomena include bright light worsening blepharospasm, vibration triggering limb dystonia, and lidocaine injection abolishing writer's cramp. Furthermore, CD patients have poor proprioception with regard to head and neck position, and abnormal finger representation has been reported in the sensorimotor cortex in patients with hand dystonia and in nonhuman primates performing joystick tasks in an overuse model. Together, these observations point to an abnormality of central sensory processing on a background of lack of inhibition in dystonia (40–43). More recent imaging and physiological study has lead some investigators to suggest that dystonia may be a sensory disorder (40,44,45). The focus on sensory input may represent an over simplification of the mechanisms associated with tricks because motor phenomenon also exist, such as walking backward and running for lower limb dystonia, dancing for truncal dystonia, whistling for blepharospasm (46). In addition, it has been demonstrated that dystonia can improve if the subject simply imagines the trick without actually performing it (38).

Several studies have examined the clinical nature of the GA. This phenomenon was reportedly present in approximately 80% of CD patients in several clinics (25,26). Filipovic et al. (47) distributed a questionnaire to 102 subjects with CD from two clinics to assess demographics, clinical effects, and phenomenology, and found GA in 64% of subjects. Most CD patients with GA reported a significantly earlier age of onset than those without the GA, and that 60% discovered the trick at onset of CD and most of the other 40% discovered it within five years of disease. In a majority of patients, the effectiveness remained; however, there was some loss of effectiveness with time. Although 30% of subjects responding well to botulinum toxin reported the disappearence of the need for the trick, 53% felt that there was no impact on the GA, but 13% thought that toxin injections made the GA less effective. The geste itself improved the symptoms (position, movements, and pain) by at least 50%, although responsiveness to it was somewhat variable in a majority of patients. The GA seemed to improve position and head movement more than pain. There was less of an effect on head tremor, although it has been shown by others that the use of tricks is one way to distinguish essential head tremor from CD with tremor (48). There was no influence of direction or complexity of CD on the effectiveness of the trick.

Muller and colleagues (49,50) completed a similar study in 50 patients aware of a GA, but, in addition to a questionnaire, also completed a motor exam, the Tsui scale; quantified clinical effects of the GA on videotape; and performed EMG with polygraphy. Ninety-two percent were unaware of a delay between onset of CD and discovery of the geste and were unaware of a specific time of discovery. The remainder discovered their geste later when actively searching for relief. The geste effects, while still present, decreased in magnitude of effect over time, possibly due to progression of dystonia. In some patients, this loss of effect was restored after botulinum toxin therapy. Laterality of the movement or the facial target was unimportant, a finding that argues against the tricks simply being a counterpressure maneuver. More than half demonstrated multiple tricks, and the chin and occiput were the most common targets. Several other tricks were discovered other than touching the face or head. Deviation of the head improved by a mean of 60% with the most effective geste; this was often greater than the maximum effect of botulinum toxin. Of course, the effectiveness of the trick is brief while the effect of botulinum toxin is prolonged for months. Complexity of CD did not appear to influence the magnitude of effect from the trick. Finally, the EMG demonstrated two very interesting findings. First, some patients demonstrated a decreased recruitment density and amplitude (this was seen in the majority of patients), while others demonstrated an increase of tonic muscle activation. The latter was seen in those with phasic CD in essence changing it from phasic to tonic CD. Second, approximately half the patients demonstrated the reduction in neck muscle activity during arm movement without actually touching the face, while the other half demonstrated that change only with touching the face. The GA features were identical for both groups. These variations suggest that several physiological mechanisms may be in play, including one that involves movement-related alteration in the sensorimotor cortex and another involving changes due to sensory input, both of which may alter neuronal activity in the basal ganglia-thalamocortical circuitry. The addition of those patients who improve with imagining the trick (38) clearly points to the complexity of these phenomena. The discovery of the effectiveness of sensory tricks has lead to the use of various techniques that simulate sensory tricks, selective sensory stimulation, and transcranial magnetic stimulation for treatment of CD, and pilot studies have demonstrated potential effectiveness (51,52).

## CONCLUSION

The importance of nonmotor phenomena is increasingly recognized in PD and HD, however cognitive and psychiatric features, pain, and sensory tricks may not receive adequate attention in the study and treatment of dystonia. While cognitive disturbances appear to be more an effect of medical therapy, the potential of basal ganglia influence on orbitofrontal and dorsolateral prefrontal pathways may provide insight into the nature of the physiological changes seen in dystonia, especially when considering applications for functional magnetic resonance imaging. It is also important to realize that depression in dystonia, particularly CD, is influenced greatly by patient self-perception, and suggests that biofeedback and psychological counseling may be important. While pain may be a direct or indirect effect of muscle spasm in dystonia, treatment remains an issue in patients, especially those with CD. Lastly, the sensory trick remains a fascinating and poorly understood phenomenon in dystonia, and it is highly likely that this sensory-linked clinical finding may provide insight into the abnormalities in the afferent basal ganglia pathways.

## ACKNOWLEDGMENTS

This work was supported by the Emory Parkinson's Research and Professorship fund.

## REFERENCES

1. Berardelli A, Rothwell JC, Hallett M, et al. The pathophysiology of primary dystonia. Brain 1998; 121 (Pt 7):1195–1212.
2. Ceballos-Baumann AO, Passingham RE, Warner T, et al. Overactive prefrontal and underactive motor cortical areas in idiopathic dystonia. Ann Neurol 1995; 37(5):363–372.
3. Eidelberg D, Moeller JR, Antonini A, et al. Functional brain networks in DYT1 dystonia. Ann Neurol 1998; 44(3):303–312.
4. Duane DD, Vermilion KJ. Cognition and affect in patients with cervical dystonia with and without tremor, in Dystonia 4: Advances in Neurology. Fahn S, Hallett M, DeLong M, eds. Philadelphia: Lippincott Williams & Wilkins, 2004:179–189.
5. Taylor AE, Lang AE, Saint-Cyr JA, et al. Cognitive processes in idiopathic dystonia treated with high-dose anticholinergic therapy: implications for treatment strategies. Clin Neuropharmacol 1991; 14(1):62–77.
6. Scott RB, Gregory R, Wilson J, et al. Executive cognitive deficits in primary dystonia. Mov Disord 2003; 18(3):539–550.
7. Grafman J, Cohen LG, Hallett M. Is focal hand dystonia associated with psychopathology? Mov Disord 1991; 6(1):29–35.
8. Jahanshahi M, Marsden CD. Personality in torticollis: a controlled study. Psychol Med 1988; 18(2):375–387.
9. Jahanshahi M, Marsden CD. Depression in torticollis: a controlled study. Psychol Med 1988; 18(4):925–933.
10. Jahanshahi M. Psychosocial factors and depression in torticollis. J Psychosom Res 1991; 35(4–5):493–507.
11. Jahanshahi M. Factors that ameliorate or aggravate spasmodic torticollis. J Neurol Neurosurg Psychiatry 2000; 68(2):227–229.
12. Ben-Shlomo Y, Camfield L, Warner T. What are the determinants of quality of life in people with cervical dystonia?. J Neurol Neurosurg Psychiatry 2002; 72(5):608–614.
13. Muller J, Wissel J, Kemmler G, et al. Craniocervical dystonia questionnaire (CDQ-24): development and validation of a disease-specific quality of life instrument. J Neurol Neurosurg Psychiatry 2004; 75(5):749–753.
14. Wein A, Golubev V. Polygraphic analysis of sleep in dystonia musculorum deformans. Waking Sleeping 1979; 3(1):41–50.

15. Fahn S, Bressman SB, Marsden CD. Classification of dystonia. Adv Neurol 1998; 78:1–10.
16. Jankel WR, Allen RP, Niedermeyer E, et al. Polysomnographic findings in dystonia musculorum deformans. Sleep 1983; 6(3):281–285.
17. Jankel WR, Niedermeyer E, Graf M, et al. Polysomnography of torsion dystonia. Arch Neurol 1984; 41(10):1081–1083.
18. Jankel WR, Niedermeyer E, Graf M, et al. Case report: polysomnographic effects of thalamotomy for torsion dystonia. Neurosurgery 1984; 14(4):495–498.
19. Fish DR, Allen PJ, Sawyers D, et al. Sleep spindles in torsion dystonia. Arch Neurol 1990; 47(2):216–218.
20. Sforza E, Montagna P, Defazio G, et al. Sleep and cranial dystonia. Electroencephalogr Clin Neurophysiol 1991; 79(3):166–169.
21. Lobbezoo F, Thu Thon M, Remillard G, et al. Relationship between sleep, neck muscle activity, and pain in cervical dystonia. Can J Neurol Sci 1996; 23(4):285–290.
22. Forgach L, Eisen A, Fleetham J, Calne DB. Studies on dystonic torticollis during sleep. Neurology 1986; 36 (Suppl 1):120.
23. Muller J, Kemmler G, Wissel J, et al. The impact of blepharospasm and cervical dystonia on health-related quality of life and depression. J Neurol 2002; 249(7):842–846.
24. Chan J, Brin MF, Fahn S. Idiopathic cervical dystonia: clinical characteristics. Mov Disord 1991; 6(2):119–126.
25. Jankovic J, Leder S, Warner D, et al. Cervical dystonia: clinical findings and associated movement disorders. Neurology 1991; 41(7):1088–1091.
26. Molho ES, Feustel PJ, Factor SA. Clinical comparison of tardive and idiopathic cervical dystonia. Mov Disord 1998; 13(3):486–489.
27. Jahanshahi M, Marion MH, Marsden CD. Natural history of adult-onset idiopathic torticollis. Arch Neurol 1990; 47(5):548–552.
28. Lowenstein DH, Aminoff MJ. The clinical course of spasmodic torticollis. Neurology 1988; 38(4):530–532.
29. Blackie JD, Lees AJ. Botulinum toxin treatment in spasmodic torticollis. J Neurol Neurosurg Psychiatry 1990; 53(8):640–643.
30. Comella CL, Jankovic J, Shannon KM, et al. Comparison of botulinum toxin serotypes A and B for the treatment of cervical dystonia. Neurology 2005; 65(9):1423–1429.
31. Factor SA, Molho ES, Evans S, et al. Efficacy and safety of repeated doses of botulinum toxin type B in type A resistant and responsive cervical dystonia. Mov Disord 2005; 20(9):1152–1160.
32. Kutvonen O, Dastidar P, Nurmikko T. Pain in spasmodic torticollis. Pain 1997; 69(3): 279–286.
33. Lobbezoo F, Tanguay R, Thon MT, et al. Pain perception in idiopathic cervical dystonia (spasmodic torticollis). Pain 1996; 67(2–3):483–491.
34. Jankovic J, Ford J. Blepharospasm and orofacial-cervical dystonia: clinical and pharmacological findings in 100 patients. Ann Neurol 1983; 13(4):402–411.
35. Ghika J, Regli F, Growdon JH. Sensory symptoms in cranial dystonia: a potential role in the etiology?. J Neurol Sci 1993; 116(2):142–147.
36. Kunig G, Pogarell O, Oertel WH. Facial pain in a case of cranial dystonia: a case report. Cephalalgia 1998; 18(10):709–711.
37. Cohen LG, Hallett M. Hand cramps: clinical features and electromyographic patterns in a focal dystonia. Neurology 1988; 38(7):1005–1012.
38. Greene PE, Bressman S. Exteroceptive and interoceptive stimuli in dystonia. Mov Disord 1998; 13(3):549–551.
39. Weiner WJ, Nora LM. "Trick" movements in facial dystonia. J Clin Psychiatry 1984; 45(12):519–521.
40. Kaji R, Murase N, Urushihara R, et al. Sensory deficits in dystonia and their significance. Adv Neurol 2004; 94:11–17.

41. Hallett M. Physiology of dystonia. Adv Neurol 1998; 78:11–18.
42. Bara-Jimenez W, Catalan MJ, Hallett M, et al. Abnormal somatosensory homunculus in dystonia of the hand. Ann Neurol 1998; 44(5):828–831.
43. Bara-Jimenez W, Shelton P, Hallett M. Spatial discrimination is abnormal in focal hand dystonia. Neurology 2000; 55(12):1869–1873.
44. Hallett M. Is dystonia a sensory disorder?. Ann Neurol 1995; 38(2):139–140.
45. Naumann M, Magyar-Lehmann S, Reiners K, et al. Sensory tricks in cervical dystonia: perceptual dysbalance of parietal cortex modulates frontal motor programming. Ann Neurol 2000; 47(3):322–328.
46. Molho ES, Factor SA, Podskalny GD, et al. The effect of dancing on dystonia. Mov Disord 1996; 11(2):225–227.
47. Filipovic SR, Jahanshahi M, Viswanathan R, et al. Clinical features of the geste antagoniste in cervical dystonia. Adv Neurol 2004; 94:191–201.
48. Masuhr F, Wissel J, Muller J, et al. Quantification of sensory trick impact on tremor amplitude and frequency in 60 patients with head tremor. Mov Disord 2000; 15(5): 960–964.
49. Muller J, Wissel J, Masuhr F, et al. Clinical characteristics of the geste antagoniste in cervical dystonia. J Neurol 2001; 248(6):478–482.
50. Wissel J, Muller J, Ebersbach G, et al. Trick maneuvers in cervical dystonia: investigation of movement- and touch-related changes in polymyographic activity. Mov Disord 1999; 14(6):994–999.
51. Leis AA, Dimitrijevic MR, Delapasse JS, et al. Modification of cervical dystonia by selective sensory stimulation. J Neurol Sci 1992; 110(1–2):79–89.
52. Bhidayasiri R, Bronstein JM. Improvement of cervical dystonia: possible role of transcranial magnetic stimulation simulating sensory tricks effect. Med Hypotheses 2005; 64(5): 941–945.

# 20
# Medical Therapy for Dystonia

**Roongroj Bhidayasiri**
*Division of Neurology, Chulalongkorn University Hospital, Bangkok, Thailand, and Department of Neurology, David Geffen School of Medicine at UCLA, Los Angeles, California, U.S.A.*

**Daniel Tarsy**
*Department of Neurology, Beth Israel Deaconess Medical Center, Harvard Medical School, Boston, Massachusetts, U.S.A.*

## INTRODUCTION

Currently, several therapeutic options are available for the management of dystonia, including pharmacologic therapy, botulinum toxin injections (BTX), and stereotactic surgery. While botulinum toxin and functional neurosurgery have gained popularity in recent years for the treatment of both generalized and focal dystonia, medical therapy still plays a significant role, particularly for alleviation of pain and dystonic spasms. With the exception of dopa-responsive dystonia (DRD) and Wilson's disease, where specific therapies are available, the treatment of dystonia is largely symptomatic with the goal of reducing pain, decreasing abnormal movements, preventing contractures, and restoring functional abilities while minimizing side effects of the treatment.

The selection of a therapy is partly guided by personal clinical experience and empirical trials, but the patient's age, the anatomical distribution of the dystonia, and the potential risk of adverse effects are also important determinants of the choice of therapy. Identification of a specific cause of dystonia, such as DRD, Wilson's disease, or drug-induced dystonia, may lead to a treatment targeted to the particular etiology. Therefore, it is prudent to search for the cause of dystonia, particularly when atypical features are present. For patients with early onset primary torsion dystonia (PTD), particularly if presenting with segmental or generalized dystonia, oral medication is usually the mainstay of therapy. For those with adult-onset PTD in which the dystonia tends to be focal, botulinum toxin therapy is generally considered to be the treatment of choice. Symptomatic or secondary dystonias tend to respond less well to pharmacotherapy.

A large number of drugs with a variety of pharmacologic actions have been reported to ameliorate dystonia. These medications include anticholinergic agents, dopaminergic agents, benzodiazepines, dopamine depleting drugs, dopamine antagonists, and others. However, most of these reports are anecdotal, and the efficacy of these drugs is often difficult to assess for several reasons: trials have often been conducted in small samples of patients; there are limited available data from double-blind, placebo-controlled studies; the spontaneous evolution of the dystonia with occasional transient remissions may interfere with clinical results of the trials. Furthermore, a large placebo effect has been demonstrated in clinical trials of dystonia (1). Therefore, the medical strategy is usually based on anecdotal and personal experience together with empirical use over many years, rather than evidence-based scientific data (2,3). Until 10 years ago, reports of major drug trials in dystonia were rare. Since then, there have been a number of fairly large clinical trials. Furthermore, enough experience has accumulated concerning some drugs to summarize these findings and to draw some general conclusions. In general, when initiating an oral medication, it is important to begin at a relatively low dose, and slowly titrate to minimize side effects and to use the lowest effective dose. All drugs should be given in divided doses throughout the day. It is also important to reassure patients of a possible delayed response and that they need to be patient while awaiting this.

Medical therapy of dystonia could be discussed in terms of therapy for specific focal dystonias, such as blepharospasm, cervical dystonia, or writer's cramp, varieties of segmental dystonia, or generalized dystonia. However, there is insufficient evidence to determine whether pharmacologic differences exist among the various focal, segmental, and generalized dystonias. Therefore, this chapter considers pharmacotherapy of all types of dystonia organized by drug class.

## DOPAMINERGIC THERAPY

By contrast with Parkinson's disease in which therapy with levodopa is based on the known depletion of dopamine in the brains of parkinsonian animals and humans, current knowledge of biochemical alterations in idiopathic dystonia is still lacking. An important exception is DRD, where biochemical and genetic mechanisms have been demonstrated in several postmortem, molecular DNA, and biochemical studies. DRD is usually a childhood-onset dystonia, characterized by dystonia of the lower limbs progressively evolving into generalized dystonia and parkinsonism, diurnal variations with worsening toward the evening, and female predominance (4). Nygaard et al. estimated that 5% to 10% of patients with childhood-onset dystonia have DRD (5). DRD is a true biochemical disorder because of a mutation in the guanosine triphosphate cyclohydrolase I gene on chromosome 14q, which indirectly regulates the production of tetrahydrobiopterin, a cofactor of tyrosine hydroxylase, the rate-limiting enzyme in the synthesis of dopamine. There is no evidence of nigrostriatal neurodegeneration (6,7). Therefore, patients with DRD typically exhibit dramatic responses to levodopa within days to a few weeks, even with relatively small doses of levodopa such as 100 mg of levodopa with 25 mg of decarboxylase inhibitor three times daily. Many patients return to nearly or completely fully functional levels. In some surveys, the daily dosage of levodopa has been 100 to 3000 mg/day, with an average of 500 to 1000 mg/day (5).

In the usual clinical setting, a trial of levodopa up to doses of 600 mg/day is the most useful method for diagnosis in DRD because it provides dramatic improvement with virtual elimination of symptoms. The benefits are usually sustained in typical cases (8–10). However, a frequent error is to expect an immediate and dramatic response in every patient with DRD, as the response is sometimes moderate in adults when symptoms have been longstanding or in patients with compound heterozygous mutations. Moreover, progressive improvement can continue to occur over several years. Therefore, it is important that patients with suspected DRD continued on a sufficiently high dose of levodopa for a reasonable period of time. Some authors recommend that a sufficient trial in adults should include 400 mg/day of levodopa/carbidopa for the first four weeks and 600 mg/day for the second four weeks (11). In children, the starting dose should be 1 mg/k (11). Although a dramatic response to levodopa supports the diagnosis of DRD, this test cannot distinguish DRD from early-onset parkinsonism due to parkin mutations where a dramatic response can also occur. The absence of marked levodopa-induced dyskinesias and motor fluctuations after sustained treatment helps to differentiate DRD from dystonia due to parkin mutations (12,13). This difference is explained by the absence of dopaminergic cell loss in the substantia nigra in DRD, where the mutation causes only neuronal dysfunction, as opposed to parkin mutations that cause marked dopaminergic cell loss in the substantia nigra.

Because of the exquisite response to levodopa and the varied phenotypes in DRD including focal and more generalized dystonia, parkinsonism, and spastic paraplegia, a therapeutic trial of levodopa should be considered in all patients with childhood-onset dystonia with or without classic features of DRD (14,15). Patients with DRD may also respond to low-dosage anticholinergic drugs and dopamine agonists (9,16). Tetrahydrobiopterin, a cofactor for hydroxylation of tyrosine, has also been shown to have a mild-to-moderate effect in patients with progressive dystonia and diurnal variation in two uncontrolled studies (17,18). In general, if no clinically evident improvement is observed after one to three months of levodopa therapy, DRD is probably not present and alternative medications should be considered.

Surprisingly, patients with idiopathic or symptomatic dystonia, not of the DRD phenotype, have responded to levodopa but usually require higher dosages. Because these early uncontrolled attempts to treat generalized dystonia with levodopa reached contradictory conclusions, its potential for a placebo effect must not be discounted (19). Some studies reported improvement in dystonia, while others found that levodopa may exacerbate dystonia (20–26). There are numerous problems with interpretation in early studies of dopaminergic agents in dystonia. From the outset, response measurement may be compromised because at that time DRD was not distinguished from other forms of idiopathic dystonia. In addition, dopamine agonists used in later studies may have other pharmacologic properties. Among these agents are lisuride, a dopamine agonist with additional serotonergic agonist activity, and apomorphine, a dopamine agonist that at low dosages may act presynaptically, resulting in a net decrease of dopamine release (27,28). Furthermore, there have been no reports concerning the same patients comparing different dopamine agonists. In a large review of dopaminergic agents in the treatment of generalized and focal dystonia, an attempt was made to exclude cases with diurnal variation and parkinsonism that may have had DRD (23). It appeared that about 35% of patients with generalized dystonia improved with levodopa in open trials, but the improvement was rarely dramatic (23). In addition, 19% of patients became worse. Open trials with apomorphine, bromocriptine, and lisuride in small numbers of patients with focal and generalized dystonia also did not yield dramatic benefit (29–33). Given these data, a reasonable algorithmic approach for treating dystonia is that, after excluding patients with diurnal dystonia, a trial and error approach has been suggested for the use of dopaminergic drugs in treating dystonia (23). Greene et al. reported that many patients who had failed previous trials of levodopa responded to anticholinergic therapy (25). Thus, although there is no head-to-head comparison between anticholinergic drugs and dopaminergic agents, it appears fairly consistent that a lower percentage of patients respond favorably to dopaminergic therapy compared to anticholinergic drugs.

Most patients with dystonia tolerate dopaminergic agents quite well. Major side effects are uncommon and include nausea, light-headedness, sedation, confusion, or visual hallucinations. In cases where there is worsening of dystonia with dopaminergic agents, this increase in symptoms will resolve when the medications are discontinued.

## Anticholinergic Drugs

Historically, the first patient who received an anticholinergic drug for treatment of dystonia was Wolf Lewin, a member of the family reported in the first paper on idiopathic dystonia by Schwalbe in 1908 (34). In the modern era, Fahn reported that high-dose anticholinergic therapy was beneficial in patients with dystonia (35,36). Other studies have replicated these results in both open-label and controlled, double-blind trials (24,25,37–40). Trihexiphenidyl is the only anticholinergic agent shown to be effective in a double-blind, randomized, placebo-controlled trial for the symptomatic treatment of segmental and generalized dystonia in young patients, but not in adults (19,38). In these studies, approximately 50% of children and 40% of adults with idiopathic dystonia demonstrate moderate-to-dramatic benefit. In addition, a similar benefit of 31% of patients with secondary dystonia, including those with dystonia after birth injury and tardive dystonia, are reported to have a good response to anticholinergic agents (24,41). The best clinical effect was achieved when treatment was initiated within five years after symptom onset (25,35). In general, children enjoy more frequent and dramatic improvement with fewer side effects than adults. The difference between response rates in children and adults may be due, at least in part, to the ability of children to tolerate much higher doses of these agents. Dose-limiting side effects with anticholinergic agents are their peripheral and central adverse effects. Peripheral side effects such as dry mouth and blurred vision are common. Coadministration of a peripherally acting anticholinesterase such as pyridostigmine, synthetic saliva, and eye drops of pilocarpine, a muscarinic agonist, can ameliorate these symptoms. In contrast, central side effects such as forgetfulness, visual hallucinations, confusion, and behavioral changes are usually dose limiting (42). Despite these acute adverse effects, no long-term sequelae have been reported.

Although anticholinergic agents are accepted as the most common systemic agents in the treatment of dystonia, the mechanism of action is not well understood (24,43). Trihexiphenidyl and benztropine are the two most commonly used anticholinergic agents. Trihexiphenidyl works through direct inhibition of the parasympathetic nervous system. Therefore, it has a relaxing effect on smooth muscles. Benztropine has both anticholinergic and antihistaminic effects. Anticholinergic therapy is better tolerated if the dose is increased slowly. For trihexiphenidyl, the treatment should be started at 1 mg/day at bedtime and increased by 2 mg/week up to the maximum tolerated dose. In one study, the average daily dose achieved was 41 mg/day, with a dosage range of 8 to 80 mg/day (24,25). Some patients may require up to 120 mg/day, but may experience dose-related drowsiness, confusion, or memory difficulty. Although most patients require high doses of anticholinergic drugs before improvement occurs, the anticholinergic dose should be kept as low as possible so as to maintain physical independence, rather than increasing the dose to its limits in the hope of abolishing all dystonic spasms. Paradoxical worsening of symptoms with anticholinergic drugs is rarely observed although some patients worsen at a low dose followed by improvement at higher doses (35).

In patients with primary dystonia, following a trial with levodopa, anticholinergic agents are usually considered the next pharmacologic agent (3,19,44). Some patients who fail to respond to dopaminergic agents may improve with anticholinergic therapy (24). However, in many cases of focal dystonia, botulinum toxin type A has replaced trihexiphenidyl as the treatment of choice. One controlled trial comparing botulinum toxin type A to trihexiphenidyl demonstrated the superiority for focal injections in the treatment of cervical dystonia (45).

Diphenhydramine, a histamine $H_1$ antagonist with anticholinergic and sedative properties, has been reported to have an antidystonic effect in three of five patients with idiopathic dystonia (46), and many patients with blepharospasm use this agent during times of increased visual difficulties. In the three subjects carefully studied in prospective fashion, the jerky and clonic components in their dystonia markedly improved. Although diphenhydramine has anticholinergic properties, the authors claimed that its anticholinergic effect was unlikely to account for the remarkable improvement because some patients had failed to respond to prior treatment with anticholinergic therapy at high doses (46).

*Baclofen*

Baclofen is a derivative of gamma aminobutyric acid (GABA) that reduces spinal cord interneuron and motor neuron excitability, possibly via activation of the presynaptic $GABA_B$ receptor (47). In the spinal cord, it impedes the release of excitatory neurotransmitters such as glutamate. In the brain, baclofen has been shown to increase serotonin in the basal ganglia, decrease dopamine release in the striatum, produce neuronal hyperpolarization in the substantia nigra, and inhibit noradrenergic neurons in the locus coeruleus (48–50). While several actions at many sites in the nervous system have been described, the exact mechanism by which baclofen affects dystonia is still unknown, but may be related to its activity as a GABA agonist at both spinal cord and cortical levels.

There have been no controlled studies of baclofen in the treatment of dystonia, but it has been shown to be effective in a number of case reports and retrospective trials, particularly in children and adolescents (51–56). Significant improvement in dystonic symptoms, especially gait, was found in 30% of 31 children with primary idiopathic dystonia at doses ranging from 40 to 180 mg daily (51). In this trial, the average daily dose of baclofen in clinically responsive patients was 79 mg daily. Furthermore, in children with, *DYT1* dystonia, baclofen improved leg dystonia and gait in 14 of 33 patients with a dosage above 50 mg daily, and nine patients reported prolonged and stable benefit (56). Patients with milder dystonia at the start of therapy tended to have a better clinical response. On the other hand, the response to baclofen in adults with focal dystonias was less impressive, ranging from minimal improvement to no benefit (25,57). Marsden and Fahn observed no improvement in seven adults with torticollis and six with writer's cramp who were treated with baclofen (58). A combination of baclofen and valproate has been suggested to be of benefit in a small number of patients with various forms of focal dystonias (53–55). Side effects of baclofen include lethargy, drowsiness, dizziness, dry mouth, and urinary urgency, which can prevent treatment with the high doses of baclofen necessary to improve dystonic symptoms. A rapid decrease or abrupt discontinuation of baclofen may precipitate psychosis or seizures so that slow tapering of this agent is recommended.

Baclofen is absorbed into the bloodstream rapidly. However, because of the blood–brain barrier, corresponding cerebrospinal fluid (CSF) levels are usually significantly lower than expected (59). This observation may, in part, explain the limited efficacy of oral baclofen therapy. Narayan et al. suggested that intrathecal baclofen (ITB) was effective for treatment of dystonia in an 18-year-old man with severe cervical and truncal dystonia refractory to all oral therapy and to large doses of paraspinal BTX (60). Within a few hours after administration of ITB infusion, his dystonia markedly improved. Subsequent studies confirmed the benefits of ITB in dystonia and spasticity, including segmental or generalized dystonias, dystonic cerebral palsy, stroke, head injury, tardive dystonia, Friedreich's ataxia, pantothenate kinase-associated neurodegeneration, parkinsonism, and reflex sympathetic dystrophy, but not conclusively in primary generalized dystonia (61–72). Significant benefits were demonstrated as a reduction in tone and spasticity and improved quality of life, activities of daily living, level of function, and cost effectiveness (73–75). However, it is presently unclear whether ITB can induce lasting remissions in patients with dystonia. Ford et al. failed to demonstrate a predictable or consistently significant difference in dystonia and disability score following ITB (76). However, these results may have been due to the small sample size, failure to optimize the dose of baclofen, or insensitivity of the rating scale that was used (77).

In the past, the usual indication for ITB in some centers has been severe, generalized dystonia refractory to oral medications, although currently stereotactic globus pallidus deep brain stimulation is increasingly considered in this setting. ITB has also been shown to be effective in patients with hemidystonia or segmental dystonia (66,71). More specific indications include increased comfort, enhanced function, and greater ease of positioning or care. ITB is particularly helpful for patients with dystonia when accompanied by spasticity, such as in stroke, head injury, or cerebral palsy (69,71,78). Patient reliability and compliance are also critical for the success of ITB therapy because they must return for periodic pump refills and dose adjustments. Despite limited and preliminary results, the American Academy for Cerebral Palsy and Developmental Medicine published a systematic review of the use of ITB for spastic and dystonic cerebral palsy, supporting the benefit of ITB in reducing spasticity and dystonia, particularly in the lower extremities (79).

ITB is administered via an implanted pump connected to an intrathecal catheter (Fig. 1). Before a pump is implanted for long-term therapy, responsiveness to ITB should be tested in one of two ways: by bolus injection or by continuous infusion. The purpose of screening is to identify patients whose dystonia is likely to respond to ITB infusion. Although there is no clear accepted standard regarding a clinically significant response to ITB trial in dystonia, most specialists accept a significant (for example 25%) reduction in the Barry–Albright dystonia or Burke–Fahn–Marsden scores during two consecutive time intervals (77). After implantation for dystonia, improvement typically occurs in two to three days, which is the time required for the medication to get up over the cerebral convexities (not within two to four hours as it does in spasticity). After intrathecal infusion, the concentration of baclofen within the cervical region and brain has been shown to be less than that within the lumbar region (80). The mean baclofen dose at the time of response was 485 μg/day (66). Dystonia also requires higher doses than spasticity, as more medication is probably needed to achieve therapeutic concentrations at a cortical level (81). Approximately 10% of patients with severe generalized dystonia lose their responsiveness to ITB over time. This may occur as early as during the first year of therapy.

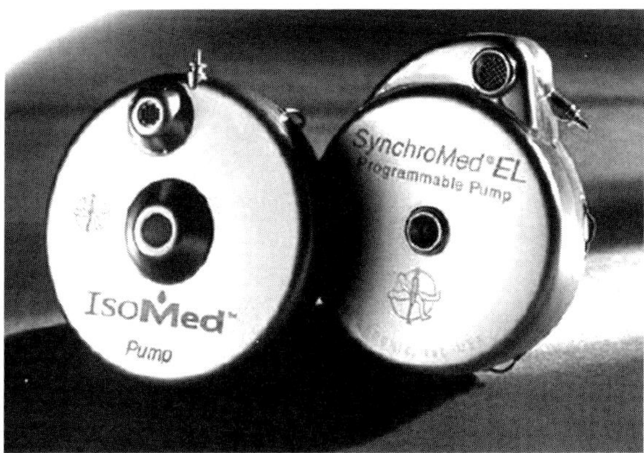


**Figure 1** Synchromed® infusion system for intrathecal baclofen therapy. *Source*: Courtesy of Medtronic Inc., Minneapolis, U.S.A.

Whether the lack of response is due to development of tolerance or progression of symptoms is uncertain. Other side effects, which may occur in about 25% of patients, include constipation, infection, CSF leaks, or catheter malfunction. Lastly, worsening dystonia has been reported after ITB, speculated to be a result of a reduction in spasticity (82).

## Antidopaminergic Drugs

There appears to be a group of patients with dystonia who respond favorably to dopaminergic agents and others who improve with the oppositely acting dopamine antagonist drugs [dopamine receptor blocking agents (DRBAs) and dopamine depletors]. The effect of DRBAs is paradoxical because they cause both acute and tardive dystonia in some patients (83). While positive effects have been observed in several case reports and case series with DRBAs, most clinical trials have produced mixed results (24,25). In addition, undesirable side effects, including sedation, parkinsonism, and tardive dyskinesia, are common. Therefore, the use of DRBAs, particularly traditional typical neuroleptic drugs, for the treatment of dystonia is discouraged. However, notable exceptions have been reported with clozapine and risperidone (both atypical DRBAs) in a small number of open trials. While the mechanism of clozapine is unclear in both psychosis and dystonia, it has a high affinity for several receptor types, including $H_1$, muscarinic, 5-hydroxytryptophan (5-HT2), and α1-adrenergic receptor with moderate affinity for D1, D2, D5, and ∝2 adrenergic receptors. Clozapine has been reported to be moderately effective in the treatment of segmental, axial, and generalized dystonia but with conflicting results in patients with spasmodic torticollis (84–87). Clozapine should be initiated at a low dose of 12.5 mg/day with slow increments of 12.5 to 25 mg/week until clinical improvement or side effects are observed. While subjective improvement has been reported in patients with cervical dystonia with a dose ranging between 37 and 100 mg/day, a much higher dose (450–900 mg/day) is usually required in patients with axial, truncal, or generalized dystonia (85,87). Although these results are promising, its efficacy has not been verified in a controlled trial setting. A further advantage of clozapine is that it does not cause tardive dyskinesia and rare, acute extrapyramidal side effects commonly associated with conventional DRBAs. Clozapine has, in fact, been used to treat tardive dyskinesia in some patients and may be effective in tardive dystonia (88–90). Any use of clozapine needs to be closely monitored for agranulocytosis, and the dose should be maintained at the lowest effective dose to minimize side effects. Risperidone (a D2 receptor blocking agent with a high affinity for 5-HT2 receptors), at a dose between 1.5 and 3 mg/day, has been shown in one trial to decrease duration and amplitude of involuntary movements in segmental and generalized dystonia (91). Other DRBAs, such as the phenothiazines, haloperidol, and pimozide, are of variable efficacy in dystonia and have fallen out of favor in recent years because of concerns for tardive dyskinesia.

Tetrabenazine (TBZ) has the advantage over DRBAs in that it rarely causes dystonic reactions and to date there has been no documented case of tardive dyskinesia secondary to TBZ (92). It acts as a reversible high-affinity inhibitor of monoamine uptake into granular vesicles of presynaptic neurons and secondary depletion at low doses, as well as a weak D2 postsynaptic receptor blocker in high doses (93). TBZ has been shown to be effective in various forms of generalized and focal dystonia in small double-blind crossover studies, large open studies, and retrospective data analysis (92,94–96). Furthermore, TBZ has been proven to be moderately effective in a large variety of hyperkinetic movement disorders, particularly in chorea and facial dystonia/dyskinesias (92,95,96). The effects of TBZ can be further modulated by lithium, either by augmenting the therapeutic efficacy of TBZ or by allowing a reduction in daily dose of TBZ in patients who had already experienced side effects without loss of therapeutic benefits (95,97,98). Some patients with idiopathic dystonia reported a favorable response on lithium alone (25,99,100). Moreover, in some patients, TBZ may be combined with levodopa to ameliorate side effects of parkinsonism (101). Among various forms of dystonia, TBZ resulted in marked improvement in 80.5% of patients with tardive dystonia and 62.9% with idiopathic dystonia, including oromandibular dystonia (92,102). The average maximum dose of TBZ was around 100 mg daily, ranging from 12.5 to 400 mg. Long-term benefits have been reported up to 180 months (average 28.9 months) (92). Common side effects of TBZ include drowsiness, parkinsonism, depression, insomnia, nervousness, anxiety, and akathisia, which improve with reduction in dosage (92). Reversal of TBZ-induced depression has been reported with a number of antidepressants (103). Overall, TBZ is considered to be an effective and safe drug for the treatment of dystonia. Unfortunately, it is not available in the United States, but can be obtained from the United Kingdom or Canada under the trade names Nitoman or Xenazine (25).

### *Benzodiazepines*

Although benzodiazepines are frequently used to treat dystonia, no large controlled trials have been conducted to evaluate their efficacy. In an open study, Greene et al. reported that clonazepam and other benzodiazepines were effective in 15% of 177 patients with idiopathic dystonia (25). In a double-blind study of 11 patients with cranial dystonia, 1 mg of clonazepam given intravenously improved symptoms in 82% (9 of 11) of patients, but the difference between active drug and placebo for the group did not reach statistical significance (104). Since then, a number of open and retrospective studies followed, which demonstrated improvement of blepharospasm, dystonic choreoathetosis, cervical dystonia, and secondary dystonia with benzodiazepines, particularly clonazepam (3,25,105,106). While in these trials only

6% to 23% of patients with generalized or focal dystonia had a good clinical response, clonazepam may be particularly effective in myoclonic dystonia (25,107). Dosages of clonazepam range from 1 to 4 mg daily and dose increases may be limited by sedation. Benefits may derive from decreased anxiety, spasm, and pain. Intravenous diazepam was reportedly effective in the treatment of spasmodic torticollis (108). Currently, there is no evidence for superiority of any particular benzodiazepine. It is important to be aware that clonazepam or other benzodiazepines should be gradually tapered in case of discontinuation because abrupt withdrawal can cause seizures and other withdrawal symptoms.

## Other Pharmacologic Agents

Many patients with dystonia require a combination of several medications for effective treatment. In fact, Marsden et al. proposed a triple therapy ("the Marsden cocktail"), consisting of a dopamine depletor (reserpine or TBZ), a dopamine receptor blocker (pimozide), and an anticholinergic drug (benzhexol) for treatment of severe dystonia (39). In addition to the medications already discussed, there are scattered, largely open-label reports concerning the efficacy of a variety of other miscellaneous drugs in the treatment of dystonia. Initial enthusiastic reports on the efficacy of carbamazepine were not replicated in subsequent larger studies that showed minimal efficacy (109–111). Currently, anticonvulsants are more commonly used in paroxysmal kinesigenic dystonia. Mexiletine, an antiarrhythmic drug related to lidocaine, has been shown in a small case series to improve blepharospasm and cervical dystonia for three to six months (112,113). In another study, test doses of intravenous lidocaine produced transient and rapid decreased muscle contractions, and in an open-label study of mexilitene in cervical and generalized dystonia, six patients showed significant improvement in severity of dystonia as assessed by rating scales and videotapes (114). Although these results seem encouraging, the total number of patients treated is too small to confirm the role of mexilitene in dystonia therapy.

Alcohol is effective in patients with autosomal dominant dystonia with lightning jerks, currently known as myoclonus–dystonia (115). An intravenous infusion of alcohol decreased dystonic scores in five of seven patients with cervical dystonia, but had no effect in patients with Meige's syndrome, tardive dystonia, and generalized torsion dystonia (116). Gamma-hydroxybutyric acid has been reported to be helpful in patients with severe myoclonus and dystonia, particularly when the disorder is alcohol sensitive (117). Clonidine has been evaluated in patients with torticollis and generalized dystonia (25,118). However, the results were inconsistent and only a small number of patients obtained partial relief. Riluzole has also been considered as a potential agent for treatment of spasmodic torticollis refractory to other therapies (119).

Tizanidine is a centrally acting muscle relaxant that works through agonistic activity at noradrenergic $\alpha$-2 receptors (120). Tizanidine has primarily been used to control spasticity in pyramidal disorders, and its efficacy in the treatment of dystonia has not been extensively studied (121). An open-label, single-blind placebo study in patients with cranial dystonia showed inconclusive results with a large dropout rate (5 out of 11 patients) (122). Because in practice tizanidine is commonly used to treat dystonia with uncertain results, a controlled trial is needed to determine its efficacy. Side effects of tizanidine are similar to baclofen and include sedation, confusion, light-headedness, weakness, and hepatotoxicity (121).

### Treatment of Dystonic Storm

Dystonic storm, also known as status dystonicus, refers to an acute worsening of primary or secondary dystonia, comprised of severe episodes of generalized dystonia and rigidity, severe enough to be associated with bulbar and ventilatory compromise (123). Complications may be caused by metabolic derangement, renal failure, hyperpyrexia, and respiratory distress. Precipitating factors that have been reported include infection, postoperative stress, introduction of clonazepam, and reduction of lithium (60,123). Although the condition is rare, it can be life threatening. Patients with dystonic storm should be managed in an intensive care unit with aggressive respiratory and hemodynamic support. It is often necessary to institute paralysis, ventilation, and sedation in order to avert bulbar and respiratory complications. In addition to supportive measures, the Marsden cocktail (benzhexol, TBZ, and pimozide) or ITB may be therapeutically helpful and should be considered (39). Stereotactic surgical intervention (pallidal deep brain stimulation) may be indicated in extreme drug-resistant cases.

## CONCLUSION

As reviewed in this chapter, options for effective medical therapy for dystonia are very limited. The goal of treatment is largely symptomatic in order to improve posture, function, and relieve associated pain. The majority of patients with dystonia require a combination of different pharmacologic agents in order to obtain adequate relief. As discussed, many drugs have been reported to be of some benefit in variable numbers of patients with various forms of dystonia, but a strong claim cannot be made for any single drug (monotherapy) except for the special case of levodopa in DRD. Therefore, the selection and order of introducing drugs in a given patient is still largely individualized and guided by personal clinical experience and empirical trials. However, based on the current evidence, it is recommended to begin therapy with a short course of levodopa to rule in or rule out the remote possibility of DRD (Fig. 2). Once a levodopa trial has been performed, the next drug to be considered

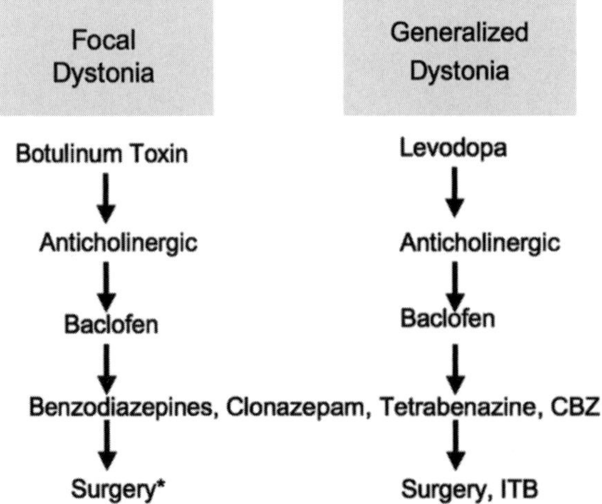


**Figure 2** Treatment algorithm of dystonia. *Denotes only in selected cases. *Source*: From Ref. 3.

should be an anticholinergic agent because they are effective in the highest percentage of patients. To minimize adverse effects, one should start with a low dose and titrate slowly until benefit appears or intolerable side effects occur. If further drugs are needed, baclofen or benzodiazepines can be considered because persistent side effects are rarely encountered. Baclofen can sometimes produce dramatic results, especially ITB in patients with combined dystonia and spasticity affecting the lower extremities. Antidopaminergic therapy, including dopamine depletors such as TBZ, can later be considered as an "add-on" if dystonic symptoms still persist. Despite the numerous medications to be considered, patient education and supportive care, including physical and occupational therapy, should not be overlooked. Well-fitted braces may improve posture, prevent contractures, and may serve as a "sensory trick" in some patients. Treating dystonia in children or adults requires persistence and patience on the part of the patient, family, and physician. Although deep brain stimulation surgery and BTX are increasingly available, medical therapy still plays an important role, particularly in patients with generalized dystonia or as a useful adjunct to BTX in patients with focal or segmental dystonia.

## ACKNOWLEDGMENT

Roongroj Bhidayasiri, MD, is supported by Lilian Schorr Postdoctoral Fellowship of Parkinson's Disease Foundation.

## REFERENCES

1. Lindeboom R, de Haan RJ, Brans JWM, et al. Treatment outcomes in cervical dystonia: a clinimetric study. Mov Disord 1996; 11:371–376.
2. Goldman JG, Comella CL. Treatment of dystonia. Clin Neuropharmacol 2003; 26: 102–108.
3. Jankovic J. Dystonia: medical therapy and botulinum toxin. Adv Neurol 2004; 94: 275–286.
4. Segawa M, Ohmi K, Itoh S, et al. Childhood basal ganglia disease with remarkable response to L-dopa: hereditary basal ganglia disease with marked diurnal fluctuation (in Japanese). Shinryo, Tokyo 1971; 24:667–672.
5. Nygaard TG, Marsden CD, Duvoisin RC. Dopa-responsive dystonia. Adv Neurol 1988; 50:377–384.
6. Ichinose H, Ohye T, Takahashi E, M, et al. Hereditary progressive dystonia with marked diurnal fluctuation caused by mutations in the GTP cyclohydrolase I gene. Nat Genet 1994; 8:236–242.
7. Ichinose H, Suzuki T, Inagaki H, Ohye T, Nagatsu T. Molecular genetics of dopa-responsive dystonia. Biol Chem 1999; 380:1355–1364.
8. Nygaard TG, Takahashi H, Heiman G, Snow B, Fahn S, Calne D. Long-term treatment response and fluorodopa positron emission tomographic scanning of parkinsonism in a family with dopa-responsive dystonia. Ann Neurol 1992; 32:603–608.
9. Nygaard TG, Marsden CD, Fahn S. Dopa-responsive dystonia: long-term treatment response and prognosis. Neurology 1991; 41:174–181.
10. Dewey RB, Muenter MD, Kishore A, Snow BJ. Long-term follow-up of levodopa responsiveness in generalized dystonia. Arch Neurol 1998; 55:1320–1323.
11. Bandmann O, Nygaard TG, Surtees R, Marsden CD, Wood NW, Harding AE. Dopa-responsive dystonia in British patients: new mutations of the GTP-cyclohydrolase I gene and evidence for genetic heterogeneity. Hum Mol Genet 1996; 5:403–406.

12. Paviour DC, Surtees RAH, Lees AJ. Diagnostic considerations in juvenile parkinsonism. Mov Disord 2004; 19:123–135.
13. Tassin J, Durr A, Bonnet AM, et al. Levodopa-responsive dystonia. GTP cyclohydrolase I or parkin mutations? Brain 2000; 123:1112–1121.
14. Nygaard TG, Trugman JM, de Yebenes JG, Fahn S. Dopa-responsive dystonia: the spectrum of clinical manifestations in a large North American family. Neurology 1990; 40:66–69.
15. Bandmann O, Marsden CD, Wood NW. Atypical presentations of dopa-responsive dystonia. Adv Neurol 1998; 78:283–290.
16. Nomura K, Yamamoto N, Takahashi I, et al. (Bromocriptine and L-dopa therapy: comparison in a case of hereditary progressive dystonia with marked diurnal fluctuation). No To Hattatsu 1987; 19:244–248.
17. LeWitt PA, Miller LP, Levine RA, et al. Tetrahydrobiopterin in dystonia: identification of abnormal metabolism and therapeutic trials. Neurology 1986; 36:760–764.
18. Fink JK, Ravin P, Argoff CE, et al. Tetrahydrobiopterin administration in biopterin-deficient progressive dystonia with diurnal variation. Neurology 1989; 39:1393–1395.
19. Balash Y, Giladi N. Efficacy of pharmacological treatment of dystonia: evidence-based review including meta-analysis of the effect of botulinum toxin and other cure options. Eur J Neurol 2004; 11:361–370.
20. Hongladarom T. Levodopa in dystonia musculorum deformans. Lancet 1973; 1:1114.
21. Cooper IS. Levodopa-induced dystonia. Lancet 1972; 2:1317–1318.
22. Rajput AH. Levodopa in dystonia musculorum deformans. Lancet 1973; 1:432.
23. Lang AE. Dopamine agonists in the treatment of dystonia. Clin Neuropharmacol 1985; 8:38–57.
24. Greene P, Shale H, Fahn S. Experience with high dosages of anticholinergic and other drugs in the treatment of torsion dystonia. Adv Neurol 1988; 50:547–556.
25. Greene P, Shale H, Fahn S. Analysis of open-label trials in torsion dystonia using high dosages of anticholinergics and other drugs. Mov Disord 1988; 3:46–60.
26. Defazio G, Lamberti P, Lepore V, et al. Facial dystonia: clinical features, prognosis and pharmacology in 31 patients. Ital J Neurol Sci 1989; 10:553–560.
27. Silbergeld EK, Hruska RE. Lisuride and LSD: dopaminergic and serotonergic interactions in the "serotonin syndrome". Psychopharmacology (Berl) 1979; 65:233–237.
28. Tolosa ES. Modification of tardive dyskinesia and spasmodic torticollis by apomorphine. Arch Neurol 1978; 35:459–462.
29. Obeso JA, Luquin MR. Bromocriptine and lisuride in dystonias. Neurology 1984; 34:135–136.
30. Nutt JG, Hammerstad JP, Carter JH, deGarmo PL. Lisuride treatment of focal dystonias. Neurology 1985; 35:1242–1243.
31. Quinn NP, Lang AE, Sheehy MP, Marsden CD. Lisuride in dystonia. Neurology 1985; 35:766–769.
32. Lees A, Shaw KM, Stern GM. Bromocriptine and spasmodic torticollis. Br Med J 1976; 1:1343.
33. Stahl SM, Berger PA. Bromocriptine, physostigmine, and neurotransmitter mechanisms in the dystonias. Neurology 1982; 32:889–892.
34. Truong DD, Fahn S. An early description of dystonia: translation of Schwalbe's thesis and information on his life. Adv Neurol 1988; 50:651–664.
35. Fahn S. High dosage anticholinergic therapy in dystonia. Neurology 1983; 33:1255–1261.
36. Fahn S. Treatment of dystonia with high-dose anticholinergic medication. Neurology (NY) 1979; 29:605.
37. Burke RE, Fahn S. Double-blind evaluation of trihexyphenidyl in dystonia. Adv Neurol 1983; 37:189–192.
38. Burke RE, Fahn S, Marsden CD. Torsion dystonia: a double-blind, prospective trial of high-dosage trihexyphenidyl. Neurology 1986; 36:160–164.

39. Marsden CD, Marion MH, Quinn N. The treatment of severe dystonia in children and adults. J Neurol Neurosurg Psychiatry 1984; 47:1166–1173.
40. Lang AE. High dose anticholinergic therapy in adult dystonia. Can J Neurol Sci 1986; 13:42–46.
41. Kang UJ, Burke RE, Fahn S. Natural history and treatment of tardive dystonia. Mov Disord 1986; 1:193–208.
42. Taylor AE, Lang AE, Saint-Cyr JA, Riley DE, Ranawaya R. Cognitive processes in idiopathic dystonia treated with high-dose anticholinergic therapy: implications for treatment strategies. Clin Neuropharmacol 1991; 14:62–77.
43. Tanner CM, Goetz CS, Weiner WJ, Nausieda PA, Wilson R, Klawans HL. The role of cholinergic mechanisms in spasmodic torticollis. Neurology 1979; 29:604–605.
44. Roubertie A, Echenne B, Cif L, Vayssiere N, Hemm S, Coubes P. Treatment of early-onset dystonia: update and a new perspective. Childs Nerv Syst 2000; 16:334–340.
45. Brans JW, Lindeboom R, Snoek JW, et al. Botulinum toxin versus trihexyphenidyl in cervical dystonia: a prospective, randomized, double-blind controlled trial. Neurology 1996; 46:1066–1072.
46. Truong DD, Sandroni P, van den Noort S, Matsumoto RR. Diphenhydramine is effective in the treatment of idiopathic dystonia. Arch Neurol 1995; 52:405–407.
47. Davidoff RA. Antispasticity drugs: mechanisms of action. Ann Neurol 1985; 17(2): 107–116.
48. Bowery NG, Hill DR, Hudson AL, et al. Baclofen decreases neurotransmitter release in the mammalian CNS by an action at a novel GABA receptor. Nature 1980; 283:92–94.
49. Seabrook GR, Howson W, Lacey MG. Electrophysiological characterization of potent agonists and antagonists at pre- and postsynaptic GABAB receptors on neurones in rat brain slices. Br J Pharmacol 1990; 101:949–957.
50. Guyenet PG, Aghajanian GK. ACh, substance P and met-enkephalin in the locus coeruleus: pharmacological evidence for independent sites of action. Eur J Pharmacol 1979; 53:319–328.
51. Greene P. Baclofen in the treatment of dystonia. Clin Neuropharmacol 1992; 15: 276–288.
52. Greene PE, Fahn S. Baclofen in the treatment of idiopathic dystonia in children. Mov Disord 1992; 7:48–52.
53. Sandyk R. Blepharospasm–successful treatment with baclofen and sodium valproate. A case report. S Afr Med J 1983; 64:955–956.
54. Sandyk R. Treatment of writer's cramp with sodium valproate and baclofen. A case report. S Afr Med J 1983; 63:702–703.
55. Brennan MJ, Ruff P, Sandyk R. Efficacy of a combination of sodium valproate and baclofen in Meige's disease (idiopathic orofacial dystonia). Br Med J (Clin Res Ed) 1982; 285:853.
56. Anca MH, Zaccai TF, Badarna S, Lozano AM, Lang AE, Giladi N. Natural history of Oppenheim's dystonia (DYT1) in Israel. J Child Neurol 2003; 18:325–330.
57. Arthurs B, Flanders M, Codere F, Gauthier S, Dresner S, Stone L. Treatment of blepharospasm with medication, surgery and type A botulinum toxin. Can J Ophthalmol 1987; 22:24–28.
58. Marsden CD, Fahn S. Movement Disorders 3. Oxford: Butterworth-Heinemann, 1994.
59. Knutsson E, Lindblom U, Martensson A. Plasma and cerebrospinal fluid levels of baclofen (Lioresal) at optimal therapeutic responses in spastic paresis. J Neurol Sci 1974; 23:473–484.
60. Narayan RK, Loubser PG, Jankovic J, Donovan WH, Bontke CF. Intrathecal baclofen for intractable axial dystonia. Neurology 1991; 41:1141–1142.
61. Rawicki B. Treatment of cerebral origin spasticity with continuous intrathecal baclofen delivered via an implantable pump: long-term follow-up review of 18 patients. J Neurosurg 1999; 91:733–736.

62. Hou JG, Ondo W, Jankovic J. Intrathecal baclofen for dystonia. Mov Disord 2001; 16:1201–1202.
63. van Hilten JJ, Hoff JI, Thang MC, van de Meerakker MM, Voormolen JH, Delhaas EM. Clinimetric issues of screening for responsiveness to intrathecal baclofen in dystonia. J Neural Transm 1999; 106:931–941.
64. van Hilten BJ, van de Beek WJ, Hoff JI, Voormolen JH, Delhaas EM. Intrathecal baclofen for the treatment of dystonia in patients with reflex sympathetic dystrophy. N Engl J Med 2000; 343:625–630.
65. Albright AL, Barry MJ, Shafton DH, Ferson SS. Intrathecal baclofen for generalized dystonia. Dev Med Child Neurol 2001; 43:652–657.
66. Walker RH, Danisi FO, Swope DM, Goodman RR, Germano IM, Brin MF. Intrathecal baclofen for dystonia: benefits and complications during six years of experience. Mov Disord 2000; 15:1242–1247.
67. Albright AL, Barry MJ, Fasick P, Barron W, Shultz B. Continuous intrathecal baclofen infusion for symptomatic generalized dystonia. Neurosurgery 1996; 38:934–938; discussion 938–939.
68. Penn RD, Gianino JM, York MM. Intrathecal baclofen for motor disorders. Mov Disord 1995; 10:675–677.
69. Albright AL, Barry MJ, Painter MJ, et al. Infusion of intrathecal baclofen for generalized dystonia in cerebral palsy. J Neurosurg 1998; 88:73–76.
70. Dressler D, Oeljeschlager RO, Ruther E. Severe tardive dystonia: treatment with continuous intrathecal baclofen administration. Mov Disord 1997; 12:585–587.
71. Meythaler JM, Guin-Renfroe S, Hadley MN. Continuously infused intrathecal baclofen for spastic/dystonic hemiplegia: a preliminary report. Am J Phys Med Rehabil 1999; 78:247–254.
72. Paret G, Tirosh R, Ben Zeev B, Vardi A, Brandt N, Barzilay Z. Intrathecal baclofen for severe torsion dystonia in a child. Acta Paediatr 1996; 85:635–637.
73. Nance P, Schryvers O, Schmidt B, Dubo H, Loveridge B, Fewer D. Intrathecal baclofen therapy for adults with spinal spasticity: therapeutic efficacy and effect on hospital admissions. Can J Neurol Sci 1995; 22:22–29.
74. Becker WJ, Harris CJ, Long ML, Ablett DP, Klein GM, DeForge DA. Long-term intrathecal baclofen therapy in patients with intractable spasticity. Can J Neurol Sci 1995; 22:208–217.
75. Gianino JM, York MM, Paice JA, Shott S. Quality of life: effect of reduced spasticity from intrathecal baclofen. J Neurosci Nurs 1998; 30:47–54.
76. Ford B, Greene P, Louis ED, et al. Use of intrathecal baclofen in the treatment of patients with dystonia. Arch Neurol 1996; 53:1241–1246.
77. Burke RE, Fahn S, Marsden CD, Bressman SB, Moskowitz C, Friedman J. Validity and reliability of a rating scale for the primary torsion dystonias. Neurology 1985; 35: 73–77.
78. Meythaler JM, Guin-Renfroe S, Grabb P, et al. Long-term continuously infused intrathecal baclofen for spastic-dystonic hypertonia in traumatic brain injury: 1-year experience. Arch Phys Med Rehabil 1999; 80:13–19.
79. Butler C, Campbell S. AACPDM Treatment outcomes committe review panel: evidence of the effects of intrathecal baclofen for spastic and dystonic cerebral palsy. Dev Med Child Neurol 2000; 42:634–645.
80. Penn RD, Savoy SM, Corcos DM, et al. Intrathecal baclofen for severe spinal spasticity. N Engl J Med 1989; 320:1517–1521.
81. Kroin JS, Ali A, York M, Penn RD. The distribution of medication along the spinal canal after chronic intrathecal administration. Neurosurgery 1993; 33:226–230; discussion 230.
82. Silbert PL, Stewart-Wynne EG. Increased dystonia after intrathecal baclofen. Neurology 1992; 42:1639–1640.
83. Jimenez-Jimenez FJ, Garcia-Ruiz PJ, Molina JA. Drug-induced movement disorders. Drug Saf 1997; 16:180–204.

84. Karp BI, Goldstein SR, Chen R, Samii A, Bara-Jimenez W, Hallett M. An open trial of clozapine for dystonia. Mov Disord 1999; 14:652–657.
85. Wolf ME, Mosnaim AD. Improvement of axial dystonia with the administration of clozapine. Int J Clin Pharmacol Ther 1994; 32:282–283.
86. Thiel A, Dressler D, Kistel C, Ruther E. Clozapine treatment of spasmodic torticollis. Neurology 1994; 44:957–958.
87. Burbaud P, Guehl D, Lagueny A, et al. A pilot trial of clozapine in the treatment of cervical dystonia. J Neurol 1998; 245:329–331.
88. VanHarten PN, Kamphuis DJ, Matroos GE. Use of clozapine in tardive dystonia. Prog Neuropsychopharmacol Biol Psychiatry 1996; 20:263–274.
89. Trugman JM, Leadbetter R, Zalis ME, Burgdorf O, Wooten GF. Treatment of severe axial tardive dystonia with clozapine: case report and hypothesis. Mov Disord 1994; 9:441–446.
90. Raja M, Maisto G, Altavista MC, Albanese A. Tardive lingual dystonia treated with clozapine. Mov Disord 1996; 11:585–586.
91. Zuddas A, Cianchetti C. Efficacy of risperidone in idiopathic segmental dystonia. Lancet 1996; 347:127–128.
92. Jankovic J, Beach J. Long-term effects of tetrabenazine in hyperkinetic movement disorders. Neurology 1997; 48:358–362.
93. Pettibone DJ, Totaro JA, Pflueger AB. Tetrabenazine-induced depletion of brain monoamines: characterization and interaction with selected antidepressants. Eur J Pharmacol 1984; 20:425–430.
94. Jankovic J. Treatment of hyperkinetic movement disorders with tetrabenazine: a double-blind crossover study. Ann Neurol 1982; 11:41–47.
95. Jankovic J, Orman J. Tetrabenazine therapy of dystonia, chorea, tics, and other dyskinesias. Neurology 1988; 38:391–394.
96. Paleacu D, Giladi N, Moore O, Stern A, Honigman S, Badarny S. Tetrabenazine treatment in movement disorders. Clin Neuropharmacol 2004; 27:230–233.
97. Furukawa T, Ushizima I, Ono N. Modifications by lithium of behavioral responses to methamphetamine and tetrabenazine. Psychopharmacologia 1975; 42:243–248.
98. Reches A, Hassan MN, Jackson VR, Fahn S. Lithium attenuates dopamine depleting effects of reserpine and tetrabenazine but not of alpha methyl-p-tyrosine. Life Sci 1983; 33:157–160.
99. Jankovic J, Ford B. Blepharospasm and orofacial-cervical dystonia: clinical and pharmacological findings in 100 patients. Ann Neurol 1988; 13:402–411.
100. Marti-Masso JF, Obeso JA, Carrera N, Astudillo W, Martinez Lage JM. Lithium therapy in torsion dystonia. Ann Neurol 1982; 11:106–107.
101. Giladi N, Melamed E. Levodopa therapy can ameliorate tetrabenazine-induced parkinsonism. Mov Disord 1999; 14:158–159.
102. Pekkenberg H, Fog R. Spontaneous oral dyskinesia. Results of treatment with tetrabenazine, pimozide, or both. Arch Neurol 1974; 31:352–353.
103. Schreiber W, Krieg JC, Eichhorn T. Reversal of tetrabenazine-induced depression by selective noradrenaline (norepinephrine) reuptake inhibition. J Neurol Neurosurg Psychiatry 1999; 67:550.
104. Gimenez-Roldan S, Mateo D, Orbe M, Munoz-Blanco JL, Hipola D. Acute pharmacologic tests in cranial dystonia. Adv Neurol 1988; 49:451–466.
105. Hughes AJ, Lees AJ, Marsden CD. Paroxysmal dystonic head tremor. Mov Disord 1991; 6:85–86.
106. Marino Junior R, Benabou R, Benabou S. Therapeutic effects of flunitrazepam in dystonias and torticollis. Preliminary communication. Arq Neuropsiquiatr 1993; 51:285–286.
107. Obeso JA, Rothwell JC, Lang AE, et al. Myoclonic dystonia. Neurology 1983; 33: 825–830.
108. Ahmad S, Meeran MK. Treatment of spasmodic torticollis with diazepam. Br Med J 1979; 1:127.

109. Geller M, Kaplan B, Christoff N. Treatment of dystonia symptoms with carbamazepine. Adv Neurol 1976; 14:403–410.
110. Isgreen WP, Fahn S, Barrett RE, Snider SR, Chutorian AM. Carbamazepine in torsion dystonia. Adv Neurol 1976; 14:411–416.
111. Garg BP. Dystonia musculorum deformans: implications of therapeutic response to levodopa and carbamazepine. Arch Neurol 1982; 39:376–377.
112. Ohara S, Hayashi R. Mexiletine in the treatment of spasmodic torticollis. Mov Disord 1998; 13:934–940.
113. Ohara S, Tsuyuzaki J, Hayashi R. Mexiletine in the treatment of blepharospasm: experience with the first three patients. Mov Disord 1999; 14:173–175.
114. Lucetti C, Nuti A, Gambaccini G, et al. Mexiletine in the treatment of torticollis and generalized dystonia. Clin Neuropharmacol 2000; 23:186–189.
115. Quinn NP, Rothwell JC, Thompson PD, Marsden CD. Hereditary myoclonic dystonia, hereditary torsion dystonia and hereditary essential myoclonus: an area of confusion. Adv Neurol 1988; 50:391–401.
116. Biary N, Koller W. Effect of alcohol on dystonia. Neurology 1985; 35:239–240.
117. Priori A, Bertolasi L, Pesenti A, Cappellari A, Barbieri S. Gamma hydroxybutyric acid for alcohol-sensitive myoclonus with dystonia. Neurology 2000; 54:1706–1708.
118. Riker DK, Hurtig H, Lake CR, Copeland P, Roth R. Open trial of clonidine in dystonia musculorum deformans. Abstr Soc Neurosci 1982; 8:563.
119. Muller J, Wenning GK, Wissel J, et al. Riluzole therapy in cervical dystonia. Mov Disord 2002; 17:198–200.
120. Coward DM. Tizanidine: neuropharmacology and mechanism of action. Neurology 1994; 11(Suppl 9):S6–S10.
121. Wagstaff AJ, Bryson HM. Tizanidine: a review of its pharmacology, clinical efficacy and tolerability in the management of spasticity associated with cerebral and spinal disorders. Drugs 1997; 53:435–452.
122. Lang AE, Riley DE. Tizanidine in cranial dystonia. Clin Neuropharmacol 1992; 15: 142–147.
123. Manji H, Howard RS, Miller DH, et al. Status dystonicus: the syndrome and its management. Brain 1998; 121:243–252.

# 21

# Anatomic Principles for Botulinum Toxin Injection

**Richard L. Barbano**
*Department of Neurology, University of Rochester, Rochester, New York, U.S.A.*

Successful treatment with botulinum toxin (BoTN) is critically dependent on the appropriate localization of the intended target muscles. Clearly, one needs to identify the muscle or muscles producing the abnormal movement, be it dystonic, spastic, or even secondary to ephatic transmission, as in hemifacial spasm. The initial and most important step in this process is the physical exam, and as such, a thorough knowledge of muscles and their action is necessary. This chapter will address a systematic approach to determine appropriate muscles for BoTN injection, electrophysiologic tools to improve therapeutic success, and specific sites for injecting the more commonly involved muscles in primary and focal dystonia. While it is beyond the scope of this chapter to document all the structures that could be potentially injured while injecting with BoTN, care must be taken with every procedure and frequent reference to an anatomy atlas is recommended (1,2).

## OVERVIEW OF ANATOMIC LOCALIZATION

Localization of dystonic muscles can be divided into two broad categories: clinical examination and supplemental guiding techniques. Clinical examination initially requires careful observation of the abnormal position or movement. The patient should be examined both at rest and while performing any movement or activity that might provoke the dystonic posture. In addition, some patients, continually accustomed to countering the involuntary muscle pull, may also require distraction to ensure the active muscles, rather than the compensating muscles, are identified.

Once the abnormal position or movement has been visually determined, confirmation is achieved with muscle palpation for muscle hypertrophy or asymmetry, and both passive and active movement toward and away from the dystonic posture. While patient report of areas of tightness or pain is sometimes helpful, given that symptoms of pain may arise from "compensatory" muscles constantly struggling to return the head or limb to the "normal" position or from other soft or bony tissue inflammation, some caution is suggested.

Supplemental guiding techniques [e.g., electromyography (EMG), electrical stimulation, and motor point localization] are useful for confirming anatomic localization of nonsuperficial muscles as well as smaller muscles, such as in hand dystonias. To increase benefit, these tools must correlate with the clinical activity observed; "compensatory" muscles may also be active as patients consciously or unconsciously attempt to counteract the abnormal position or movement. Motor point localization with surface stimulation is more often used in studies of spasticity rather than dystonia and will not be covered in this chapter. Direct visual guidance techniques with ultrasound and fluoroscopy have also been described for deep, otherwise difficult to assess muscles such as the iliopsoas, but are rarely used in treating dystonia (3).

The decision to use supplemental techniques ultimately depends on multiple factors. If the appropriate muscles are superficial and readily accessible, direct injection without supplemental guiding techniques may be appropriate depending on the experience of the injector. However, several studies have reported that even experienced injectors may not be as accurate as one might predict (4). The ability to accurately localize a dystonic muscle depends on its size and depth. Hypertrophied superficial muscles such as the sternocleidomastoid in cervical dystonia or large superficial muscles such as the deltoid or biceps do not usually require EMG confirmation. However, deeper muscles involved in cervical dystonia, such as longissimus capitus or even the levator scapulae are not as readily assessed by palpation alone. Limb dystonias, especially of the hand and arm, are further complicated by the close proximity of dystonic muscles to unaffected muscles. Accurate injection in such cases is critical to satisfactory outcome.

## THE IMPORTANCE OF ACCURACY

Obviously, the ability to deliver BoTN into the appropriate muscle or muscles is tantamount to clinical success. After clinical observation and exam, once a target muscle is chosen, the injection needle must be placed into the muscle itself. Earlier studies have shown that BoTN can diffuse across fascia to distances up to 4 cm with injected doses of 10 IU (5). Muscle fascia can reduce the spread of BoTN by about 20% in experimental animal models, although even low doses are able to cross this potential barrier (6). Additional toxin outside of the intended target muscle increases the risk of local and distant unwanted side effects. Local side effect include weakness of contiguous or nearby muscles. Other side effects include dysphagia with neck injection or ptosis after eyelid injection. Additionally, some nearby muscles may have opposing actions to the intended muscles and weakening them may exacerbate the abnormal position (for example, flexor carpi ulnaris and extensor carpi ulnaris). Distant side effects are dose dependent and likely a result of toxin entering the circulatory or lymphatic system. Systemic effects have been shown to occur even in relatively low total dose injections; increased jitter has been found in distant muscles after injections for blepharospasm (7). Therefore, delivering the least effective amount of toxin in the most accurate manner decreases the risk of unwanted local and distant side effects as well as the risk of the development of neutralizing antibodies.

The area of paralysis within a muscle increases with the dose of toxin delivered, although there is a plateau effect if sufficient toxin is given to paralyze the cross-sectional area of the muscle (8). BoTN diffusion within a muscle is dependent on several factors. Borodic et al. showed that BoTN diffuses within a muscle proportional to its concentration and dilution (9). The study demonstrated that there is linear spread of biologic effect within a muscle as a function of the dose administered, and that the biological effect spreads to contiguous muscles when larger doses are used. Although BoTN diffusion is dependent on volume of injection, the dose seems to be the more potent factor. In an animal study, a 25-fold increase in dose with constant volume resulted in a doubling of paralysis, whereas a 100-fold increase in volume with constant dose was needed to produce the same effect (8). Even with maximal accuracy, toxin diffuses to local nearby muscles, as noted in a study using single injections per muscle (10). These results might favor multiple injections of smaller doses per muscle over a single larger dose injection in order to minimize diffusion side effect, but this would need to be balanced against the potential for creating multiple punctures in the fascia through which there is the potential for medication "leakage." Decreased spread with smaller-volume injections had been demonstrated by earlier works in animals (11). Single-site, larger-volume injections versus multiple-site, smaller-volume injections was evaluated in humans with cervical dystonia (12). Although the multiple injections per muscle group appeared superior in terms of the treatment of pain, posture, and range of motion, no analysis of side effect reflecting diffusion was reported.

The above discussion pertains to the importance of accurately injecting the appropriate muscle. Additionally, there is at least theoretical advantage to injecting certain regions *within* the desired muscle. This is a situation where electrophysiologic guidance might play a role and is discussed below.

## ELECTROPHYSIOLOGIC GUIDANCE

EMG has long been used to aid in the localization of dystonic muscles. The procedure is adjunctive to the physical exam (13). Because BoTN works at the neuromuscular junction and diffuses within a muscle proportional to the dose and volume, delivering the toxin directly to this site should be the most efficient way to produce paralysis. In spasticity, and likely in dystonia as well, there is good theoretical reason to specifically target the neuromuscular junction (motor end plate) within the muscle (14). In an animal study, the targeting of the end plate with EMG guidance produced more effective force reduction when compared to non-EMG–guided mid-belly multiple site injections intended to maximize spread within the muscle (15). In clinical practice, however, this effect has been harder to demonstrate. A prospective study of injections of the gastrocnemius in spasticity comparing mid-belly (and presumably closer to the end plates) versus a proximal motor point region failed to show any clinical difference between the two injection sites, although as pointed out by the authors, several limitations in the study may have confounded the results (16).

Motor end plates may be concentrated in a single band at the mid-belly of the muscle, localized in several bands, or diffusely scattered throughout the muscle. Spindle-shaped muscles are typical muscles with a single innervation band at mid-belly. Most limb muscles have such a band, found roughly half-way between tendon insertions (mid-belly); notable exceptions being the gastrocnemius, deltoid, forearm flexors and extensors, and rectus femoris (17).

Finding the neuromuscular junction via EMG in patients with dystonia may be problematic, however. Finding the "seashell noise" and end-plate spikes characteristic of neuromuscular junction is difficult in a muscle that has persistent activity; it is also more uncomfortable for the patient as this area is more painful to probe.

EMG guidance might also be useful given that dystonic muscle activity, at least in torticollis, may change patterns after BoTN injections (18,19). Brans et al. showed that not only can activity switch from one most active muscle to another but also noninjected muscles can increase in activity (20). This phenomenon was not specifically related to treatment with BoTN, as it occurred after treatment with trihexyphenidyl as well. Such switching may occur even as the neck resumes its pretreatment position. In some individuals, muscle activity patterns might change spontaneously despite constant head position. In a small study of 17 patients with BoTN treatment "failure" who were undergoing evaluation for surgical denervation, nine had spontaneously changing muscle activation patterns despite a stable dystonic position over a 10-minute evaluation (21). Therefore, should similar injection patterns and doses fail to produce the desired response, one must consider the possibility that other muscles might have increased activity. This possibility could be explored with EMG prior to testing for immunoresistance (19).

Finally, most injectors who use EMG have noted that on repeat injection cycles there are certain regions within the cross-section of a muscle that are more active than other regions within the same muscle. It is not known whether this represents incomplete diffusion of the toxin on the prior injection, or an earlier region of reinnervation. At least in theory, targeting the most active region of a muscle might lead to a more effective decrease in force production, although this has not been demonstrated.

## Electromyography

One of the most important aspects of EMG for guided injections is the interference pattern. When a patient is not attempting to self-correct a dystonic posture, dystonic muscles usually display a full or near-full interference pattern. This is readily contrasted with nondystonic muscles that will only display such a density of activity with strong voluntary activation. This interference pattern can either be persistent (tonic, with sustained posture) or intermittent and bursting (tremor or "spasm"). In patients with associated dystonic tremor, the phasic tremor activity can be seen and heard electrophysiologically, often timed to the clinical tremor. It must be remembered that this activity should be found with the patient relaxed and not performing voluntary activity in order to be certain that the muscle sampled is contributing to the involuntary action. Confirming that the needle is in the target muscle can be further accomplished by having the patient voluntarily activate the muscle to reproduce the dystonic position (remembering however that different sets of muscles may produce identical neck positions) this may be especially important in the limb dystonias where dynamic EMG studies are technically difficult. If the patient is unable to voluntarily activate the muscle of interest, passive movement of the limb or finger by the examiner may be detected by the EMG, and confirm localization. Otherwise electrical stimulation might be considered.

Research criteria for dystonic EMG activity have included consistent tonic or phasic patterns of discharge; amplitude of discharge of 50% or more the amplitude during maximal voluntary activation; and the EMG discharge occurring in the presence of the patient's abnormal posture (4). Others have used the amplitude of the motor units while recording in the dystonic position, with amplitudes greater than 100 microvolts considered diagnostic for involvement of the recorded muscle in producing the posture (20). It must be remembered that such EMG is not specific to dystonia. It is also important to take into consideration that muscle activity may be "compensatory," that is, a conscious or unconscious attempt by the patient to counteract the abnormal dystonic position or to relieve pain. Additionally, there is frequently cocontraction of antagonistic pairs of muscles, a physiologic hallmark of dystonia (22). Thus, clinical correlation must always be considered prior to injection, rather than making that decision based solely on the electrophysiological recording.

It is important that the EMG activity be "crisp" sounding, with rapid rise times ($< 500\,\mu$sec from baseline to peak) and with appropriate motor unit amplitudes. All these will indicate that the recording tip of the needle electrode is close to the muscles producing the activity. Dull or "thuddy" sounding units are still at some distance to the recording tip. Distant units also have less rapid rise time and are often of smaller amplitudes. A rapid change in the "crispness" of the auditory signal is heard when the muscle membrane is pierced. With experience, the injector will be able to use the change in auditory frequency of firing units to guide the position of the needle into active muscles, or even the most active part of a particular muscle.

Surface recording electrodes have been used in some studies but their recordings are limited to superficial muscles. Fine-wire electrodes have also been used, mainly for simultaneous recordings of several muscles. Both of these EMG techniques are more appropriate in the research setting. In the clinical setting, the most useful electrode type is the hollow monopolar electrode. Hollow monopolar electrodes are available with Teflon coating and in a range of lengths and gauges. These needle electrodes allow for simultaneous analysis of activity and injection of BoTN without requiring a change in the needle or the needle position. As in all monopolar EMG analysis, a surface reference electrode is also needed. For the most accurate motor unit action potential waveform analysis, the surface reference electrode is placed on the skin as close to the recording electrode as practical. In the clinical practice of delivering intramuscular BoTN, however, proximate reference location is not as critical and it is usually unnecessary to change locations of the surface electrode for each muscle. Placing the surface electrode in a central location will usually suffice for all ipsilateral muscles.

## Electrical Stimulation

An alternative to the use of EMG to localize dystonic muscles is to use electrical stimulation (10). The same hollow monopolar electrodes used for EMG can be used for electrical stimulation. A surface reference electrode is also needed; in electrical stimulation technique, however, the placement of this electrode is more important and should be as close as possible to the target muscle. Most EMG machines are able to provide low current stimulation directly to muscle by using the stimulators available for nerve conduction studies. Portable stimulators are also available and are relatively inexpensive. Low current (1–5 mA) applied directly into muscle results in visible contraction of the muscle. Keeping current low is important to avoid injuring the muscle as well as for patient comfort. Furthermore, keeping the current to the minimum necessary also allows the stimulation to be isolated to the desired muscle by preventing costimulation of adjacent muscles. Once visible twitch of the desired muscle is observed, the stimulation can be slowly decreased with repositioning of the needle tip so that the minimum stimulation continues to produce the maximum twitch. This assures that the needle tip is in the desired muscle or even into individual fascicles within a muscle (for example, stimulation of a particular digit within flexor digitorum superficialis). Electrical stimulation can be especially useful for patients who may have limited ability to voluntarily activate a particular muscle due to either physical or cognitive disability. Results with electrical stimulation appear to be comparable to EMG localization (23).

## Electrophysiological Guidance in Specific Conditions

In dystonias where the active muscles are superficial and not lying in close proximity to antagonistic muscles, EMG is rarely needed. Such is the case for blepharospasm (as well as hemifacial spasm) and in many jaw-closing dystonias. On the other hand, when the dystonic muscles are small and not readily accessible to palpation, EMG is very useful if not critical. This would be the case for spasmodic dysphonia and jaw-opening dystonia. EMG is also extremely useful when small dystonic muscles are in close proximity to nondystonic muscles, such as in hand and foot dystonias.

Controversy exists in the need for EMG guidance in cervical dystonia (24,25). Certainly, EMG guidance aids in the localization of muscle. As has been noted, there may still be botulinum-induced atrophy of muscle at the time of repeat injection. When the muscles known to produce a specific dystonic position have been injected and are still atrophic, and the head has returned to its dystonic position, there are either areas of the injected muscles that remain active, or other muscles are involved. These other active muscles may have been dystonic initially or may have assumed new activity as noted in the above section (18,20). Such circumstances would benefit from EMG exploration.

BoTN-induced atrophy can make palpation of dystonic muscles more difficult. However, even without such atrophy, given the complexity of the cervical musculature, it can be difficult for even experienced injectors to be sure that their needle is in the intended muscle. An earlier study demonstrated that the needle was not in the target muscle in 17% to 53% of injections, leading the authors to conclude that EMG guidance was necessary for accuracy (26). Other investigators reported that EMG guidance limited neck weakness and dysphagia when compared to prior experience with non-EMG–guided injections (27), and allowed for lower injection doses with similar clinical benefit (28). In a study involving four experienced injectors, localization of the muscle was poorly predicted (4). The vector(s) of the abnormal head position, presence or absence of shoulder elevation, and muscle hypertrophy were evaluated after which the examiners predicted the presence of dystonic activity in six pairs of predetermined muscles. EMG mapping showed that the clinical examination had a sensitivity of only 59% and a specificity of 75%; therefore, without EMG guidance 41% of dystonic muscles would not be recognized and inactive muscles would have been misinjected in 25% of encounters. Brans et al. studied 420 muscles in 42 patients with CD before and after BoTN treatment (20). They found that the physical exam for all neck muscles in aggregate had a sensitivity of only 0.35, a specificity of 0.74, a positive predictive value of 0.77, and a negative predictive value of 0.31 for the detection of involved muscles. The sensitivity was highest for the sternocleidomastoid (0.42) and splenius capitis (0.44) and lowest for trapezius (0.24) and scalenes (0.16).

Although questions regarding the clinical benefit of EMG guidance remain, there are few studies addressing this question. Comella et al. carried out an evaluation of 52 patients with cervical dystonia, prospectively randomized to receive BoTN therapy either with or without EMG guidance (29). Although there was no difference in the number of patients showing improvement, patients in the EMG group showed greater response. This was especially notable in patients with retrocollis, head tilt and shoulder elevation; postures typically involving the deeper cervical muscles. There was no significant difference in adverse events between the groups. Conversely, there are a number of large published series of patients with cervical dystonia treated with BoTN without EMG guidance demonstrating comparable outcomes to

EMG-guided therapy (30,31). More recently, a post hoc analysis comparing the outcome measures of subjects who received BoTN with EMG guidance versus those who received BoTN without EMG guidance failed to show any significant difference between the groups (32). The study, however, was not designed or powered to look at such an effect and so must be interpreted cautiously.

## SPECIFIC GUIDE FOR INJECTIONS

As noted in the introduction, subcutaneous and intramuscular injections of medications have inherent risks. There are many potential structures that can be injured including blood vessels and nerves; some, but not all, will be listed below.

### Blepharospasm and Hemifacial Spasm

BoTN therapy is the treatment of choice for blepharospasm (33). Blepharospasm involves the *orbicularis oculi* muscle, and may be divided into two major concentric sections: the *palpebral and the orbital portions* (Figs. 1 and 2). The palpebral portion closes the eyelid gently as in blinking; the orbital portion closes the eye more forcefully as in attempting to wink with one eye. The muscle lies immediately beneath the skin and is readily accessible with a 30 gauge, half-inch needle. Subcutaneous injections will readily spread into the underlying orbicularis muscle. This is especially true for the lower lateral and lateral canthus injections of the orbicularis oculus. Toxin in these locations can diffuse inferiorly and affect the *zygomaticus major and minor* and result in an asymmetric nasolabial fold and smile. Care must be taken not to pierce through the interior side of the muscle as deeper diffusion can lead to weakness of

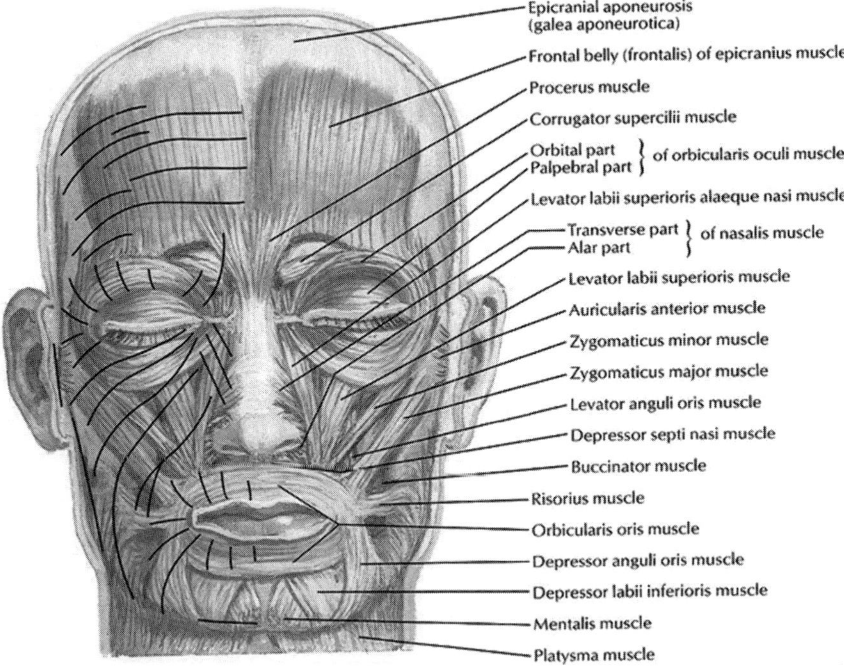


**Figure 1** Superficial facial muscles, anterior view.

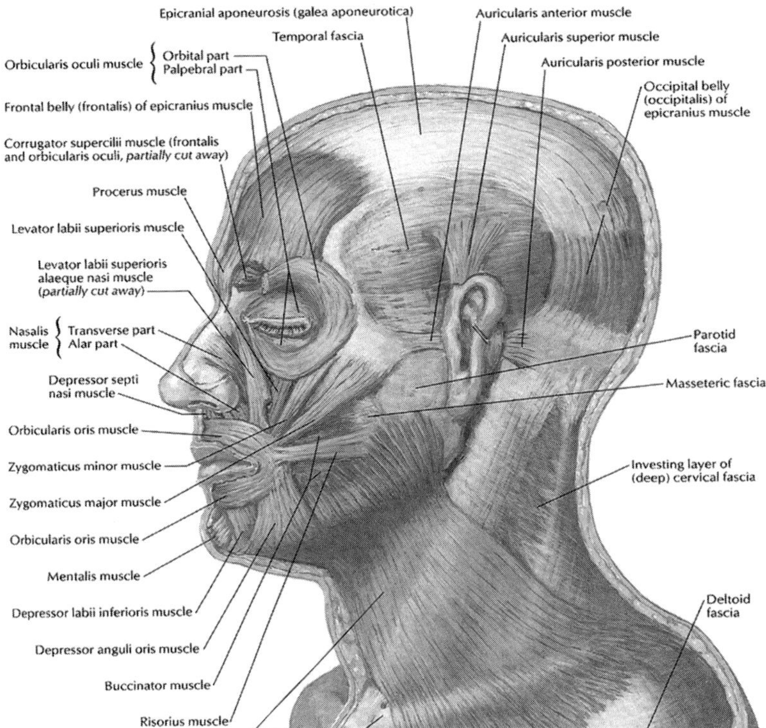


**Figure 2** Facial muscles, lateral view.

the extraocular muscles resulting in diplopia. This most commonly involves the inferior oblique muscle, since it lies just inside the inferior orbital rim and may be affected by medial lower lid injections. In addition to diplopia, another undesirable side effect is ptosis, resulting from weakness of the levator palpebra. In order to minimize the risk of ptosis, injections should be avoided near the center of the superior portion of the orbicularis oculus. Injections in the lower lid should also avoid the medial segment near the medial palpebral ligament, as damage to the lacrimal duct can result in epiphora (tears running down cheek).

Other facial muscles may be involved in blepharospasm. Muscles associated with "squinting" include the *corrugators*, *procerus*, and *nasalis* muscles (Figs. 1 and 2). The *corrugators* draw the eyebrow "medially" and downward. This muscle lies below the fibers of the frontalis and orbicularis oculus and requires somewhat deeper injections than most other facial muscles. The *procerus* muscle produces transverse wrinkling over the bridge of the nose. The *nasalis* muscle has two parts: the *transverse part* and the *alar part*. The *transverse part* serves as a compressor or sphincter of the nostril. The *alar part* flares the nostrils by drawing the ala of the nose downward and laterally. Injections of the *nasalis* muscles have the potential to spread to the *levator labii superioris* muscle, which, as the name implies, could cause some weakness in raising the upper lip (Figs. 1 and 2).

The *frontalis* (technically the frontal portion of the *occipitofrontalis* muscle) muscle may be voluntarily activated in blepharospasm, but usually to counteract the involuntary forced eye closure. Given the action of this muscle, care must be maintained if it is injected for symptoms of blepharospasm, and, even then, the needle should be inserted quite inferiorly, just above the lateral margins of the eyebrows.

The *frontalis*, as well as lower facial muscles that might be involved in blepharospasm or cranial dystonias will be discussed below with hemifacial spasm.

*Hemifacial spasm*

Hemifacial spasm can involve any muscle innervated by the facial nerve. The facial nerve innervates the muscles of facial expression including the muscles of the scalp; muscles surrounding the apertures of the eyes, nose, mouth, and ears; as well as the *platysma, stapedius, stylohyoid*, and *posterior belly of the digastric*. Hemifacial spasm may be accompanied by mild underlying muscular weakness and as such, starting doses of BoTN are less than those required for blepharospasm or other cranial dystonias.

The *frontalis* muscle is connected over the top of the head with its occipital portion and as such draws the scalp back. In doing so, it raises the eyebrows as in an expression of surprise or horror and results in the familiar transverse wrinkles of the forehead (Figs. 1 and 2). In younger patients, the skin over the frontalis may be tight and the muscle quite thin; pinching the skin may help decrease the discomfort of needle insertion and also decrease the risk of hitting the sensitive periosteum. Injections should be kept well above the brow ( > 2.5 cm) in order to avoid sagging of the eyebrow (brow ptosis).

Not surprisingly, given their importance in vocalization and expression, there are many muscles activating the mouth and lips (Figs. 1 and 2). The *orbicularis oris* is a large circumferential muscle at least partially derived from surrounding muscles inserting into the lips. It has many functions including closing the lips, pressing the lips together in a purse string motion as in blowing a kiss, and pressing the lips against the teeth. Portions of this muscle can be seen to be active in hemifacial spasm, although this may be due in part to the fibers of other muscles (e.g., *risorius*) passing into the *orbicularis oris* to insert at the lip. Care must be taken when injecting the *orbicularis oris*: not only is it particularly sensitive to the needle, weakness can produce an inability to form a tight seal around the lips resulting in dribbling of liquids when drinking.

The *zygomatic major and minor muscles* are powerful elevators of the upper lip. These muscles can lie some distance below the skin surface underneath the fat pad of the cheek, coming more superficial near their origin at the zygomatic bone. They can be affected by injections of the lower lateral *orbicularis oculus*. The *zygomatic major* pulls the angle of the mouth upward and backward and is important in laughing; overweakness of this muscle can result in a cosmetically unsatisfactory asymmetric smile and starting at low doses and increasing at subsequent injections to the desired effect is strongly recommended. The *zygomaticus minor* muscle elevates the upper lip and, along with the *levator anguli oris*, which raises the angle of the mouth, forms the nasolabial fold. The same caveat regarding "start low, go slow" can apply here as well. Some have even advocated treating the unaffected contralateral side of the face with low-dose BoTN to produce more symmetry; symmetric weakness may be more cosmetically acceptable (34). However, reduction of the dosage to prevent weakness seems much more appropriate.

The other muscle attaching to the upper lip is the *levator labii superioris*, which has its origin at the inferior margin of the orbit, where it lies deep to the *orbicularis oculus*. As it courses toward the upper lip, a small slip of muscle (the *alaque nasi*) inserts on the nasal alar cartilage and helps dilate the nostril. The main body inserts in the lateral upper lip and raises it.

Several muscles insert into the angle of the mouth and lower lip. The *buccinator* is the deepest of the muscles and forms the inner musculature of the cheek (Figs. 2 and 3). It serves to compress the cheeks in order to keep food between the molars

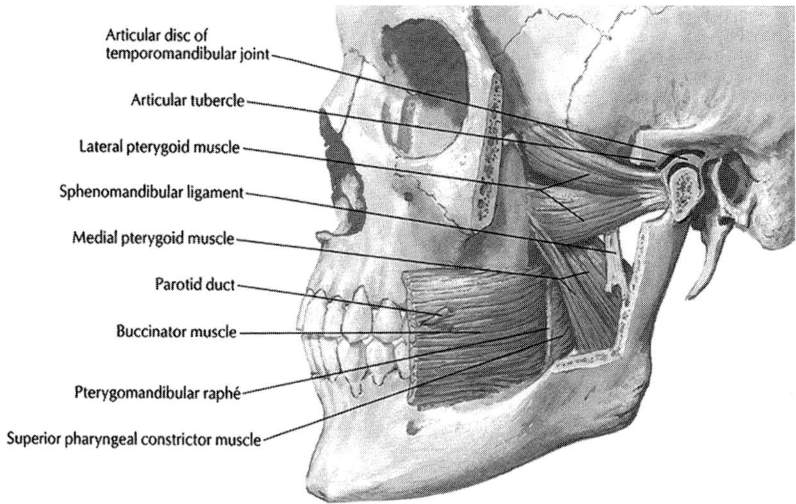


**Figure 3** Deep muscles of jaw and cheek.

while chewing, and also to forcibly bring air into the mouth while sucking and blow air out while whistling or playing a wind instrument. To inject this muscle, one would need to go deeper than the usual subcutaneous injections, although this muscle rarely needs to be treated. Treatment should be cautious as well because lack of control of this muscle can sometimes result in the patient biting the inside of the mouth. Also, the parotid duct pierces this muscle opposite the third molar and should be avoided during injection.

The *risorius* muscle inserts into the angle of the mouth (Figs. 1 and 2). It pulls the corner of the mouth laterally as in grinning.

Three major muscles act on the lower lip in addition to the orbicularis oris (Figs. 1 and 2). The *depressor anguli oris* inserts at the angle of the mouth and pulls the angle downward and laterally as in the expression of grief. Occasionally, it is helpful to treat this muscle with a low dose of medication if treatment of the *zygomaticus* leaves the latter muscle weak. In that situation, unopposed action of the depressors can have the cosmetically undesirable effect of having the patient appear sad. The *depressor labii inferioris* pulls the lower lip downward. The deepest and most medial muscle is the *mentalis* muscle. This muscle wrinkles the chin, and raises and protrudes the lower lip as in an expression of doubt or disdain.

Finally, although not officially classified as a muscle of the circum-oral group, the *platysma* can be active in an expression of fear, drawing down the lower lip, especially at the angle of the mouth (Fig. 2). This broad muscle is innervated by the cervical branch of the facial nerve, originating at the lower border of the parotid gland. It is quite thin and when activated exhibits a "corded" appearance. Injections for this muscle should be performed subcutaneously, as it is easy to inadvertently pierce the muscle, and should be spread out over multiple sites to get adequate spread.

## Oromandibular Dystonia

Oromandibular dystonia may occur alone or as part of a regional dystonia, and is often associated with temporomandibular joint dysfunction or bruxism (35). The abnormal spasm or persistent activity can involve the lingual, masticatory, facial

**Table 1** Muscles Involved in Jaw Movement

| Jaw opening | Jaw closing | Lateral deviation | Protrusion |
|---|---|---|---|
| Lateral pterygoid<br>Suprahyoid muscles<br>Digastric, mylohyoid, geniohyoid | Masseter<br>Medial pterygoid<br>Temporalis (anterior fibers) | Cocontraction of Contralateral lateral and medial pterygoids | Cocontraction of Bilateral lateral and medial pterygoids |

muscles of expression, and pharyngeal muscles (36). This activity results in several functional subtypes; jaw opening, jaw closing, jaw deviation, and a combination of these movements (Table 1). Alternating activity of the laterally deviating muscles will produce a grinding action.

### *Jaw-Closing Dystonia*

Jaw-closing dystonia mostly involves the *masseter* and the anterior fibers of the *temporalis* muscles, but the *medial pterygoid* may also contribute to jaw closing and would need to be considered if jaw closing persists despite adequate treatment of the masseters and temporali (Fig. 4).

The *masseter* muscle is superficial and readily located over the posterior third and ramus of the mandible (Figs. 2 and 4). The posterior-most part lies deep to the parotid gland. The anterior fibers of the *temporalis* are most involved with jaw closing (the posterior fibers tending to pull the jaw backwards, or retrusion). These are best located two or so fingerbreadths superior and anterior to the ear and can be palpated on forceful jaw closure.

The *medial pterygoid* muscle also participates in jaw closure (Fig. 3). This muscle is most often approached from the inside of the mouth and injections are more technically difficult than many of the other muscles. This area is highly vascular, and thus at higher risk for bleeding complications, and there is also a higher risk of dysphagia than with externally approached injections.

### *Jaw-Opening Dystonia*

Jaw opening is accomplished primarily by the *lateral pterygoid* muscles aided by the muscles collectively called the suprahyoid musculature (37). The *lateral pterygoid* is the major force producer for this action, with the *digastric* muscle assisting. The *geniohyoid* and *mylohyoid* are weak depressors of the mandible.

Injection of the *lateral pterygoid* muscle requires EMG guidance (Fig. 3). With the jaw in the open position, the notch between the condylar and the coronoid processes in the ramus of the mandible will be palpable just anterior to the temporomandibular joint and inferior to the zygomatic arch. The needle is inserted at this notch, passing through the superior part of the parotid gland, then the masseter muscle, over the mandible, and into the lateral pterygoid muscle. With the jaw voluntarily opened, and the EMG on, one can see and hear the needle approach and the familiar motor unit activity will verify the needle placement when the muscle fascia is penetrated. Caution must be taken with any patient on anticoagulants as this area is very vascular.

The *digastric* muscle can be located for injection approximately one fingerbreadth behind the posterior edge of the mental tubercle (chin bone) and one fingerbreadth on either side of the midline (both sides should be injected) (Fig. 4).

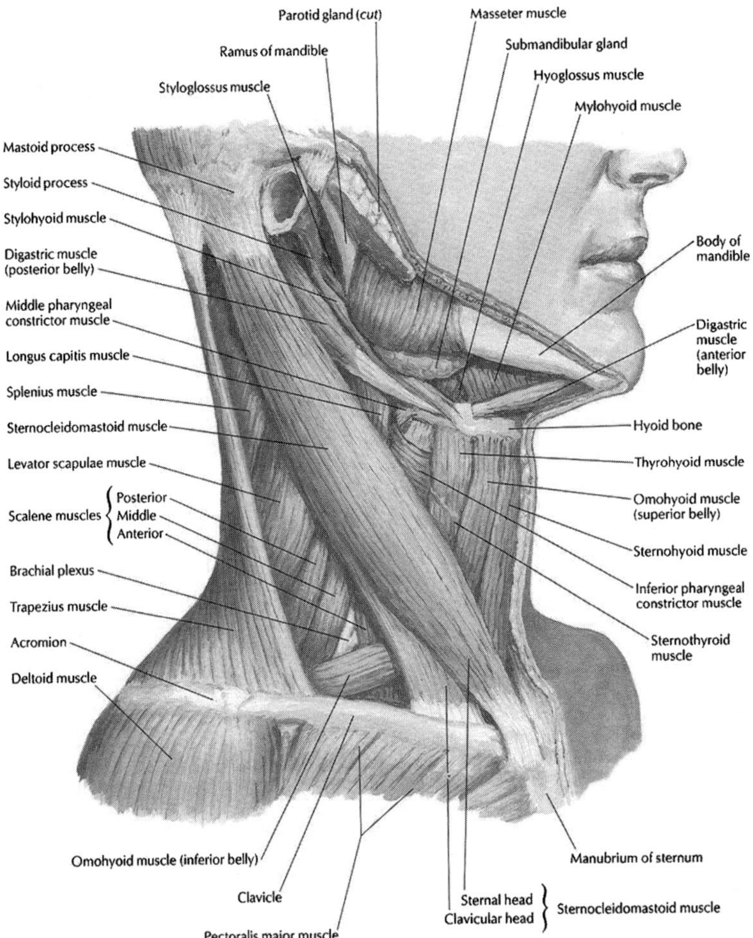


**Figure 4** Cervical muscles, superficial, anterolateral view.

Again, using EMG and advancing the needle with the amplifier on, this muscle is readily found when the jaw is actively opened.

The *mylohyoid* muscles are broad and flat forming a muscular diaphragm that serves as the inferior-most layer of the floor of the mouth (Fig. 4). The *geniohyoid* muscles are paired midline muscles just superior to the mylohyoid.

Jaw opening can also be treated by injection into the "submental complex" alone (nonspecific treatment of the *digastric, geniohyoid, and mylohyoid*) with injections given in the midline, 1 cm posterior to and under the tip of the mandible (38).

### *Tongue Protrusion*

Tongue protrusion is accomplished by muscles in the floor of the mouth, superior to the mylohyoid. The *genioglossus* muscle is the dominant tongue protruder; the *hyoglossus* assists by keeping the tongue depressed during protrusion (Fig. 5).

The *genioglossus* is a large muscle underneath the intrinsic musculature of the tongue. It can be accessed through the submental approach. The needle can be placed two fingerbreadths behind the mandible, one fingerbreadth lateral to midline,

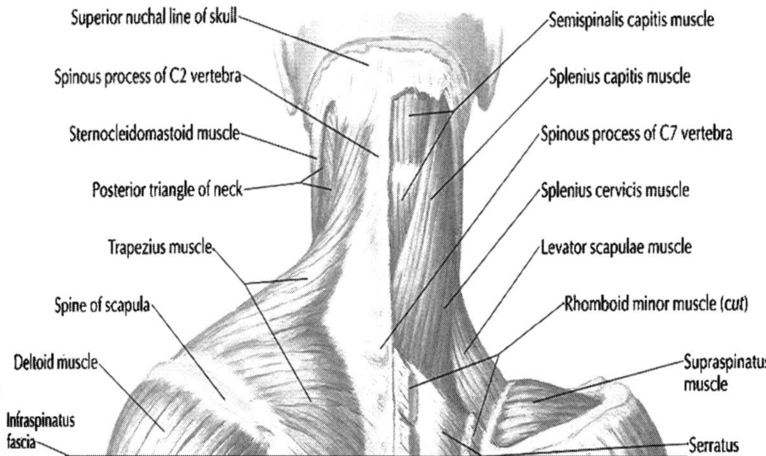


**Figure 5** Cervical muscles, superficial and first layer; posterior view.

and will pass through the *digastric*, *mylohyoid*, and *geniohyoid* muscles. Because these latter three muscles aid in jaw opening, localization in the *genioglossus* can be confirmed by sharp EMG activity while the patient keeps the jaw closed and pushes the tongue forward against the teeth.

## Cervical Dystonia

Cervical dystonia can produce almost any abnormal head position with or without superimposed tremor activity. For purposes of anatomical description as well as evaluation for rating scales, the primary abnormal positions are described as follows: rotation (torticollis), flexion (anterocollis), extension (retrocollis), tilt (laterocollis), and translation (shift). Translation is the abnormal positioning of the head off of the central axis with the head otherwise remaining upright in all other planes. Translation can occur in any horizontal plane (anterior–posterior and laterocollis). In clinical practice, many patients will exhibit some combination of these primary abnormal positions, sometimes referred to as a "complex" pattern. The tremor associated with dystonia is often irregular in amplitude with the amplitude increasing as the head position is moved further away from the primary dystonic (null) position. Tremor frequency is less regular than other organic tremors and the direction may not follow a single plane of motion, although direction preponderance may be seen (39).

The patient should be examined in several positions, but initially, while sitting comfortably without the head resting against or touching anything and without the use of a sensory trick. She or he should be instructed to not try to correct the involuntary position. Having the patient shut their eyes may help in this matter. Range of motion exam can add information regarding muscles that may be restricting full excursion. If a dystonic tremor is present, finding a null position with the smallest amplitude tremor may also help categorize the underlying dystonic posture. The patient should also be examined while walking as well as doing any other activity that he or she identifies as provoking the symptoms.

There are 23 muscle pairs connecting the skull to the spine, and it has been shown in normal subjects that combinations of different muscle activities can produce the same head position (40). The same ultimate head vector might be produced by different muscle combinations depending on the task (for example, if the head position were obtained by a stationary subject following a moving object or vice versa), suggesting that the central nervous system programs the neck muscles to respond to specific task-induced orientations rather than generating an infinite variety of muscle patterns (41). Certain muscles and combinations appear to be more commonly involved in cervical dystonia, or are at least more commonly injected with good clinical effect. These include the *splenius capitis*, *semispinalis capitis*, *sternocleidomastoid*, and *scalene* muscles (28,40,42) (Table 2).

The anatomy of the neck is complex and replete with critical structures to be avoided when injecting BoTN. The neck is often conceptually divided into anatomic regions by readily identified landmarks. Although the relative depths of muscles will be pointed out (see also appropriate figures), needle depths are often not designated as they can vary greatly with the girth of patient's necks.

The *anterior triangle* is bordered superiorly by the jaw and laterally by the anterior border of the *sternocleidomastoid* (Fig. 4). It is covered superficially by the *platysma*, which is not usually involved in cervical dystonia. Deeper in this triangle are the pharynx and esophagus, which if weakened by BoTN can produce dysphagia and changes in voice volume or enunciation. Fortunately, the anterior triangle almost never needs to be penetrated in cervical dystonia.

The *sternocleidomastoid* muscle (SCM) is readily localized with contralateral rotation and it may be hypertrophied in contralateral torticollis; providing resistance will accentuate it further (Figs. 4–6). The SCM has its two familiar heads, one originating from the manubrium of the sternum and the other from the medial third of

**Table 2** Muscles Producing Abnormal Postures in Cervical Dystonia

| | | |
|---|---|---|
| Rotation | Contralateral | Sternocleidomastoid muscle, anterior, and middle scalenes, trapezius, semispinalis capitis and cervicis, multifidus |
| | Ipsilateral | Splenius capitis and cervicis, levator scapulae, longissimus capitis and cervicis, rectus capitis posterior major, Obliquus capitis inferior |
| Flexion | Midsagittal flexion if muscles are bilaterally active; otherwise unilateral activity will cause deviation off midline | Sternocleidomastoid, scalenes, longus capitis and colli, rectus capitis anterior |
| Extension | Midsagittal extension if muscles are bilateral active; otherwise unilateral activity will pull head off midsagittal plane | Levator scapulae, splenius capitis and cervicis, longissimus capitis and cervicis, spinalis capitis and cervicis, semispinalis capitis and cervicis, rectus capitis posterior major and minor, obliquus capitis superior |
| Tilt | Ipsilateral | Sternocleidomastoid, scalenes, trapezius, splenius capitis and cervicis, longissimus capitis and cervicis, multifidus, obliquus capitis superior |
| Shoulder elevation | Ipsilateral | Levator scapulae, trapezius |

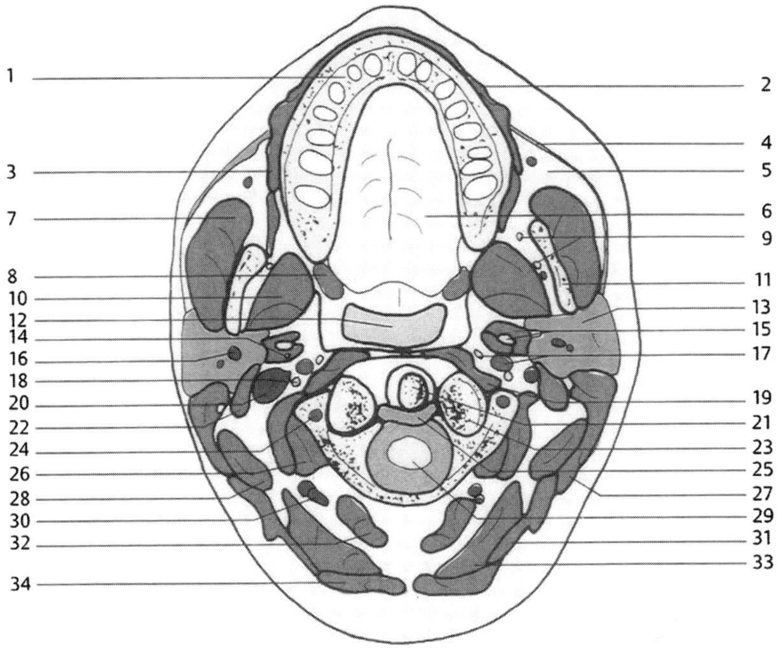


1 Maxilla (alveolar process)
2 Orbicularis oris muscle
3 Depressor anguli oris muscle
4 Parotid duct
5 Retromolar fossa
6 Hard palate
7 Masseter muscle
8 Palatine tonsil, superior pharyngeal constrictor muscle
9 Inferior alveolar nerve, lingual nerve
10 Medial pterygoid muscle
11 Mandible
12 Nasopharynx
13 Parotid gland
14 Cranial nerve XI
15 Styloid process and styloid muscles
16 Retromandibular vein
17 Internal carotid artery and cranial nerve XII
18 Cranial nerves IX and X
19 Longus capitis muscle
20 Internal jugular vein
21 Dens of axis
22 Digastric muscle (posterior belly)
23 Atlas (lateral mass)
24 Vertebral artery
25 Cruciform ligament of atlas
26 Obliquus capitis inferior and superior muscles
27 Sternocleidomastoid muscle
28 Longissimus capitis muscle
29 Spinal cord
30 Deep cervical vein
31 Splenius capitis muscle
32 Rectus capitis posterior muscle (major)
33 Semispinalis capitis muscle
34 Trapezius muscle

**Figure 6** Cervical muscles, cross sectional view at the level of the atlas/upper jaw.

the clavicle, which join to form the bulk of the muscle before inserting at the mastoid process. Activity of the SCM is responsible for contralateral rotation as well as ipsilateral tilt. If both SCMs are active, neck flexion occurs. Experienced injectors differ in approach to this muscle, with some injecting in the upper half of the muscle, after the two heads have joined, and others distributing the toxin to the clavicular and sternal components of the muscle, inferiorly. The latter approach may allow for more focused treatment for anterocollis (clavicular muscle) versus torticollis (sternal muscle). Because anterior cervical musculature is anatomically closer to the pharyngeal muscles, care must be taken to keep the toxin within the muscle; also, smaller-volume injections as well as limiting the dose will likely decrease the risk of dysphagia (5).

The same caution would hold true for injections into the scalene muscles, which can be involved in anterocollis, torticollis, laterocollis, and shift.

The *external jugular vein* crosses over the SCM and can be visible enough to be avoided. The *great auricular nerve* and the *lesser occipital nerve* exit the posterior triangle and pass superficial to the SCM on the upper half of the muscle, a typical injection area. If the needle passes very near, or touches these nerves, the patient may complain of dysesthesias radiating to the back of the ear or mastoid area, respectively.

Posterior to the SCM is the *posterior triangle* (Figs. 4 and 7). This anatomic region is demarcated anteriorly by the posterior edge of the SCM; posteriorly by the anterior edge of the trapezius; and inferiorly by the clavicle. The posterior triangle contains muscles, which may need injection as well as structures that need to be avoided. These include the *brachial plexus*, discussed below, and the *inferior belly of the omohyoid* that lies just above and deep to the clavicle. Leakage of toxin onto (or direct injection into) this omohyoid has the potential to cause a sensation of difficulty in swallowing, as these muscles depresses the hyoid after it is raised during swallowing.

The muscles of interest in the posterior triangle include the *scalenes* anterior and inferior, and moving posterior and superiorly, the *levator*, the *splenius capitis*, and at its uppermost margin, a small, lateral portion of the *semispinalis capitis*.

The *anterior scalene* muscle is deep to the SCM and attaches the anterior surfaces of the transverse processes of C3 to C6 to the first rib (Figs. 4 and 8). The *middle scalene* is the largest of the three scalenes and can be palpated in the posterior triangle when it is activated either voluntarily or in dystonia. Both anterior and posterior scalenes elevate the first rib, or if the rib is fixed, will flex and tilt the cervical spine; they will also contribute to contralateral rotation. The middle scalene can be injected approximately two fingerbreadths anterior to the edge of the trapezius; staying approximately two fingerbreadths above the clavicle will lessen the odds of hitting the brachial plexus. The *brachial plexus* passes posterior to the anterior scalene, between it and the middle scalene. Care should be taken to avoid injuring the plexus. If the needle is advanced slowly, patients will complain of dysesthesias if the needle comes to touch the plexus. The *posterior scalene* is the deepest of the three, arising from the posterior aspect of the transverse processes of C4 to C6 and inserting on the second rib. It elevates the rib, or alternatively, will flex and tilt the neck.

The *levator scapulae* may be palpated immediately anterior to the anterior edge of the trapezius, at the angle of the neck (Figs. 4,8–10). Although a superficial muscle, the electrically active parts may be at some depth, occasionally up to 3 cm. The levator can also be accessed through the trapezius (about two fingerbreadths

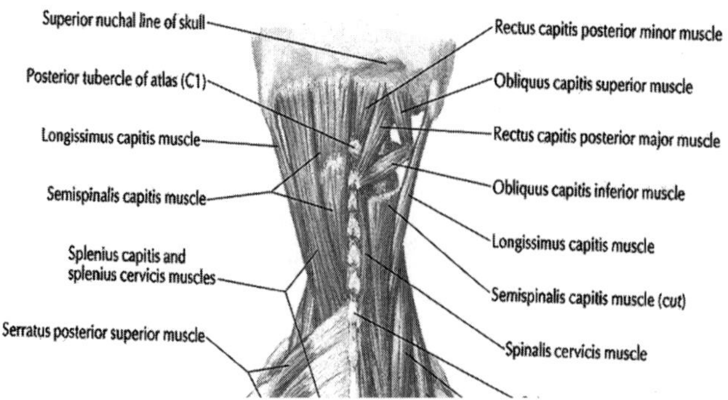


**Figure 7** Cervical muscles, middle layer, posterior view.

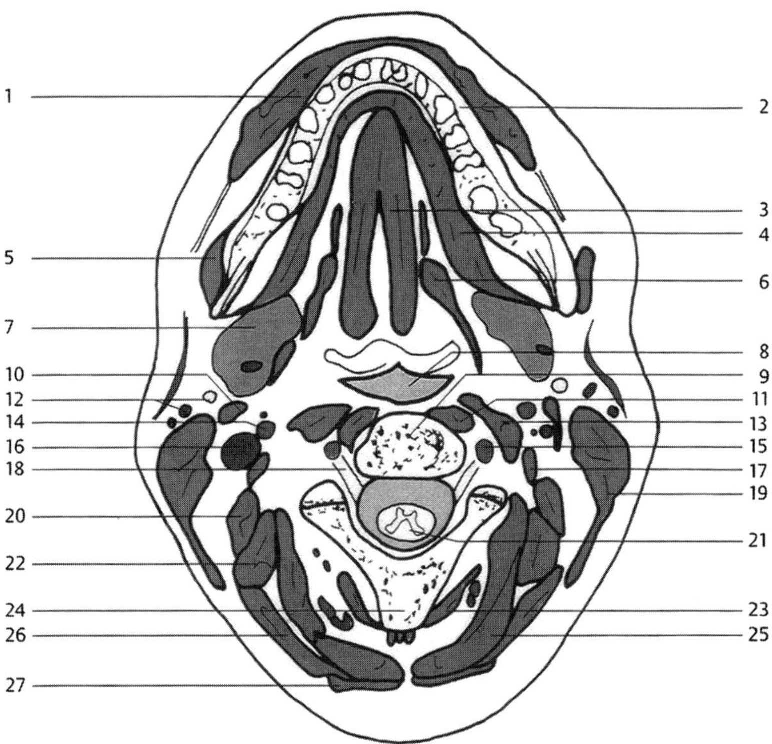


**1** Depressor anguli oris muscle
**2** Mandible (body)
**3** Genioglossus muscle
**4** Mylohyoid muscle
**5** Masseter muscle
**6** Hyoglossus muscle
**7** Submandibular gland
**8** Oropharynx
**9** Axis (body)
**10** Digastric muscle (posterior belly)
**11** Longus colli muscle
**12** Auriculotemporal nerve (branch) and retromandibular vein
**13** Longus capitis muscle
**14** Internal carotid artery
**15** Vertebral artery
**16** Internal jugular vein
**17** Splenius cervicis muscle
**18** Nerve root of C3
**19** Sternocleidomastoid muscle
**20** Levator scapulae muscle
**21** Spinal cord (cervical)
**22** Longissimus cervicis muscle
**23** Inferior oblique muscle
**24** Spinous process
**25** Semispinalis capitis muscle
**26** Splenius capitis muscle
**27** Trapezius muscle

**Figure 8** Cervical muscles, cross sectional view at the level of C3/angle of mandible.

posterior to its lateral edge) at the angle of the neck. The levator primarily elevates the scapula in conjunction with the trapezius, but can also extend the neck and rotate the head to the same side.

Just superior to the levator in the posterior triangle, the *splenius capitis* will be the most superficial muscle, although a large part of the muscle will lie beneath the trapezius (Figs. 4–6,9–12). The splenius arises from the spinous processes of C7 to T4 and inserts on the lateral 1/3 of the nuchal line and the mastoid process. At its inferior portion, the *splenius cervicis* muscle meshes with the capitis and is difficult to distinguish (Figs. 8,9,11). When active unilaterally, the *splenius capitis* ipsilaterally rotates and tilts the head; bilateral activation extends the neck. This muscle is frequently involved in horizontally predominant dystonic tremor.

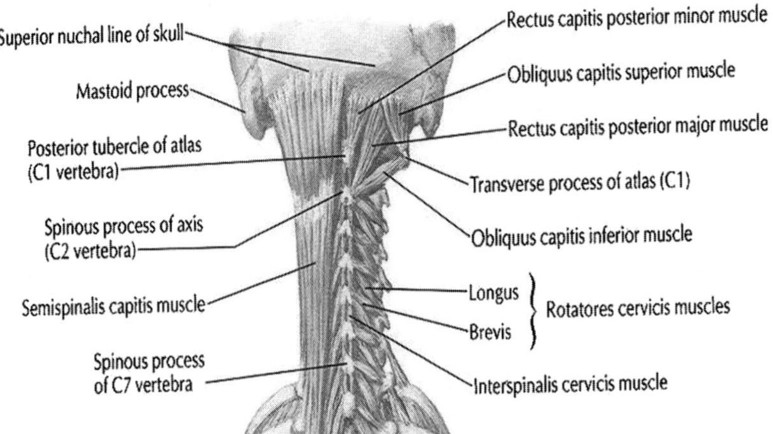


**Figure 9** Cervical muscles, deep layer, posterior view.

Finally, deep behind the posterior triangle lies the group of muscles that flex the head: the *longus colli, longus capitis*, and *rectus capitis anterior* (Figs. 5,6,12). The *longus colli* has three parts, all of which essentially originate on the anterior surface of the transverse processes or the anterior surface of the bodies of C3 through T3 and insert on the anterior surfaces of higher cervical vertebrae or the anterior arch of the atlas. The *longus capitis* originates on the transverse processes of C3 through C6 and inserts on the basilar part of the occipital bone. The *rectus capitis anterior* joins the anterior surface of the atlas with the jugular process of the occipital bone. It functions to flex the head and stabilize the atlanto-occipital joint. These muscles can be approached with the injection needle by starting at the posterior border of the SCM (at approximately the C5 level—for longus colli) or actually through the SCM (at C4 level—for longus capitis) and directing toward the anterior surface of the vertebral body. Extreme caution must be taken as the needle will pass close to the carotid artery and the internal jugular vein. Additionally, these muscles are very close to the pharyngeal muscles and the risk of dysphagia is quite high.

Leaving the posterior triangle and following around laterally, lays the superficial and relatively thin *trapezius* muscle (Figs. 4 and 12). The trapezius is the most superficial muscle encountered in the majority of the back of the neck and is easy to inject at a depth of about 1 cm, depending on the amount of subcutaneous tissue in the individual. Because of its breadth, the trapezius will likely require several injection sites for adequate spread, although the fibers come together superior to C6 allowing for more efficient use of toxin. The superior portion of the *trapezius* is more likely to cause cervical dystonic posturing. The *trapezius* serves to control the position of the scapula and elevate the shoulder; it also can rotate the head and neck to the contralateral side. Just below the level of the nuchal line, the *greater occipital nerve* pierces the trapezius to run superficially up to the occipital region. Injections to the trapezius greater than two fingerbreadths below the nuchal line should avoid hitting this nerve. If the nerve is touched by the needle, the patient will experience a Tinel sign radiating to the ipsilateral occipital region.

The layer of muscles deep to the trapezius, sometimes referred to as the second layer, include the levator and the splenius capitis. The deep layer is collectively called the *erector spinae* group, a largely vertically oriented group, and from lateral to medial, includes the *iliocostalis cervicis*, the *longissimi*, the *semispinali*, and the *spinali*

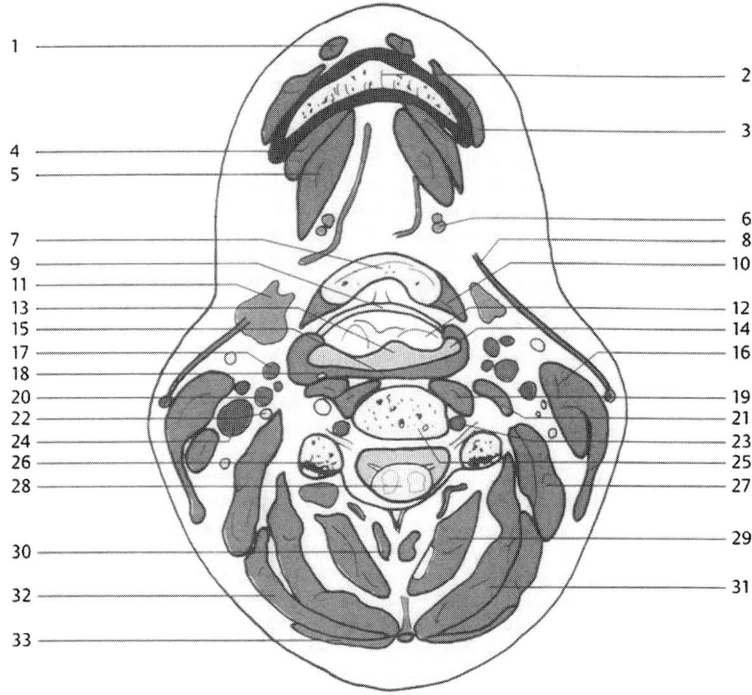

**1** Mentalis muscle
**2** Mandible
**3** Depressor anguli oris muscle
**4** Mylohyoid muscle
**5** Geniohyoid muscle
**6** Sublingual gland
**7** Hyoid bone
**8** Platysma
**9** Epiglottis
**10** Infrahyoid muscles
**11** Submandibular gland
**12** Aryepiglottic fold
**13** Larynx
**14** Piriform sinus
**15** Inferior pharyngeal constrictor muscle and retropharyngeal space
**16** Sternocleidomastoid muscle
**17** External carotid artery
**18** Sympathetic trunk
**19** Longus colli muscle
**20** Internal carotid artery
**21** Anterior scalene muscle
**22** Vagus nerve
**23** Vertebral artery
**24** Internal jugular vein
**25** Body of C4 vertebra
**26** C3/C4 facet joint
**27** Levator scapulae and longissimus capitis muscles
**28** Spinal cord (cervical)
**29** Semispinalis cervicis muscle
**30** Multifidus muscles
**31** Semispinalis capitis muscle
**32** Splenius capitis muscle
**33** Trapezius muscle

**Figure 10** Cervical muscles, cross sectional view at the level of C4/chin.

muscles. The latter three pairs consist of both *cervicis* and *capitis* muscles, depending on whether they insert onto the cervical spine or skull, respectively. All of these muscles will serve to extend the neck and head (Figs. 5,6,8,10–13).

The *iliocostalis* muscle is lateral most of the erector spinae that originates at the angles of the third through sixth ribs and inserts on the transverse process of C4 through C6. In addition to extension, this muscle serves to laterally flex the neck to the same side.

The *longissimus cervicis and capitis* run together and are medial to the *iliocostalis*. They originate on the transverse processes from T1 to T4 and articular

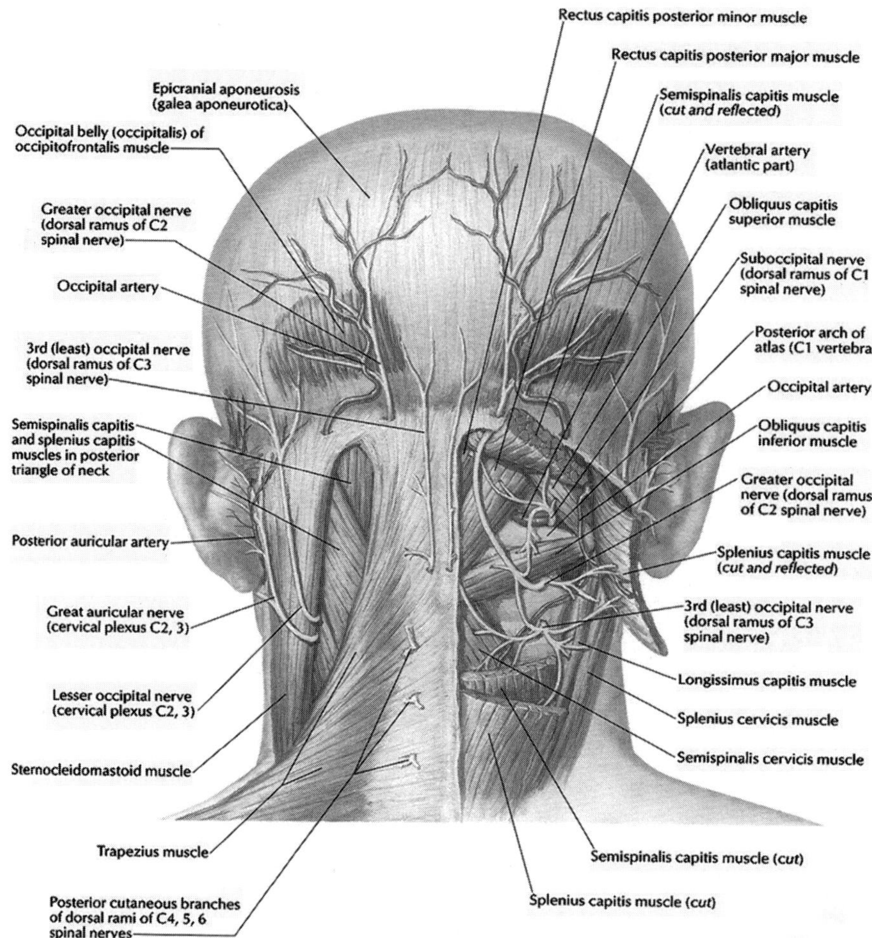


**Figure 11** Cranio-occipital junction, superficial and deep muscles.

processes of C5 to C7 and insert into the transverse processes of C2 to C6 (*longissimus cervicis*) or the mastoid process (*longissimus capitis*). As with all muscles of the erector spinae group, bilateral activity will produce extension of the neck and head. Unilateral activity causes ipsilateral rotation and tilt and brings the face toward the shoulder. The *longissimus capitis* can be injected by directing the needle parallel to the spinous processes (perpendicular to the shoulder) about two fingerbreadths below the lower palpable border of the skull, and about three fingerbreadths lateral to midline. This will be aiming just medial to the mastoid process. The depth will be about 2 cm (as always, depending on the "thickness" of the patient's neck) or at least enough to pass through the *splenius capitis*.

The *semispinali* muscles run longitudinally along the vertebral column, medial to the longissimus. These muscles originate from the transverse processes of C4 through T6. The *semispinalis cervicis* inserts on the spinous processes of the axis to C5, while the *semispinalis capitis* inserts on the occipital bone between the superior and the inferior nuchal lines. These muscles are not only involved in retrocollis, as would be predicted, but are also frequently involved in rotation (28). This rotation is contralateral, turning the face to the opposite side. The *semispinalis* muscle can

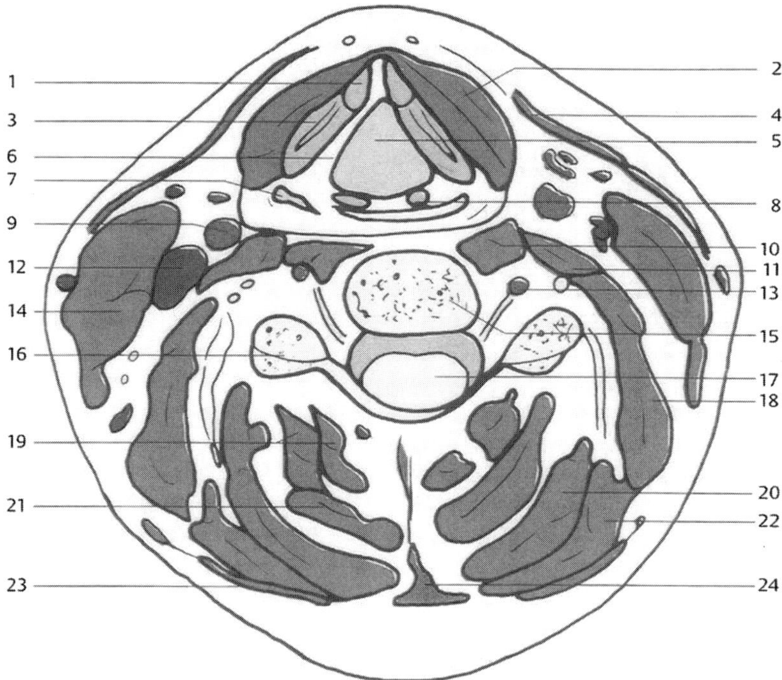


**1** Thyroid cartilage (lamina)
**2** Infrahyoid muscles (sternothyroid, omohyoid)
**3** Thyroid cartilage
**4** Platysma
**5** Larynx (vestibule)
**6** Vestibular fold
**7** Piriform sinus
**8** Arytenoid cartilage
**9** Common carotid artery
**10** Anterior scalene muscle
**11** Longus colli muscle
**12** Jugular vein
**13** Vertebral artery
**14** Sternocleidomastoid muscle
**15** Body of C5 vertebra
**16** C5/C6 facet joint
**17** Spinal cord
**18** Levator scapulae muscle
**19** Multifidus muscles
**20** Semispinalis capitis muscle
**21** Semispinalis cervicis muscle
**22** Splenius capitis muscle
**23** Trapezius muscle
**24** Nuchal ligament

**Figure 12** Cervical muscles, cross sectional view at the level of C5/thyroid cartilage.

be found and injected two fingerbreadths lateral to the midline, passing through the *trapezius* when injecting higher on the neck, approximately two fingerbreadths below the occipital protuberance (posterior to the atlas—C2). Inferior to this point, the needle will pass through *trapezius* and *splenius capitis*, at a depth of about 3 to 4 cm, again depending on the obesity and/or muscularity of the patient's neck. Because the overlying *splenius capitis* is an ipsilateral rotator, and the *semispinalis* a contralateral rotator, EMG activity can help in determining the necessary depth of the needle.

The *spinali* muscle is most medial of the group, running vertically and just alongside the vertebral spinous processes. The *spinali* muscles originate on the spinous processes and ligament flavum of T2 through the lower cervical levels and insert on the axis through C4 (*spinalis cervicis*) and between the inferior and the superior nuchal line of the occipital bone (*spinalis capitis*)—all very close to midline. These muscles extend the neck and head, and may be injected by placing the needle deep along the midline, just lateral to the cervical spinous processes.

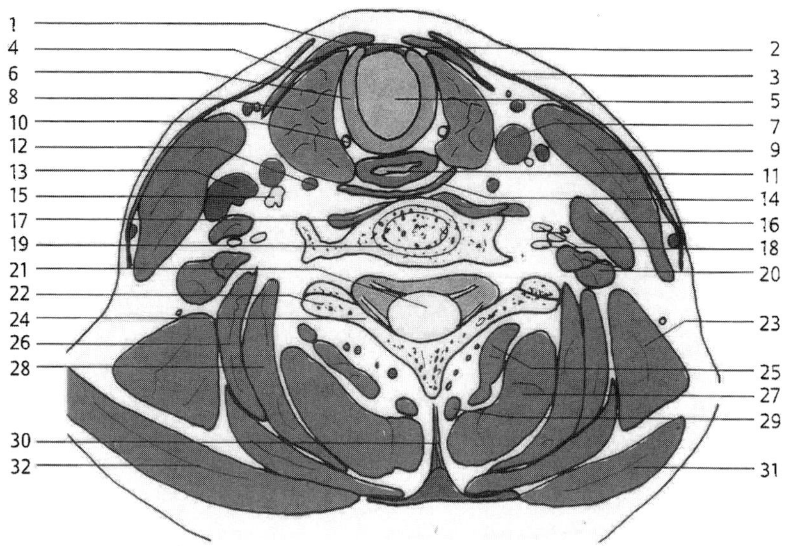


1 Sternohyoid muscle
2 Cricothyroid ligament
3 Platysma
4 Sternothyroid muscle
5 Infraglottic space
6 Cricoid cartilage
7 Common carotid artery
8 Thyroid gland
9 Sternocleidomastoid muscle
10 Thyroid cartilage, inferior cornu
11 Esophagus
12 Vertebral artery
13 Internal jugular vein
14 Inferior pharyngeal constrictor muscle
15 Vagus nerve
16 Anterior scalene muscle
17 Longus colli muscle
18 Brachial plexus
19 Body of C7 vertebr
20 Medial and posteri muscles
21 Spinal cord (cervic
22 Facet joint
23 Levator scapulae muscle
24 Arch of C7 vertebra
25 Multifidus muscles
26 Iliocostalis cervicis muscle
27 Semispinalis muscle
28 Longissimus muscle
29 Spinalis muscle
30 Nuchal ligament
31 Splenius cervicis and capitis muscles
32 Trapezius muscle

**Figure 13** Cervical muscles, cross sectional view at the level of C7.

The *multifidus* muscles are rarely treated with BoTN, but are a series of small muscles, deep to the *semispinalis*, originating essentially from the transverse or articular processes and running diagonally along the spine to insert on the spinous processes of superior vertebrae, two to four levels higher (Figs. 8,10,12). When active, the *cervical multifidi* will cause ipsilateral tilt of the neck and rotate the neck contralaterally, and due to the depth of these muscles, injection will require longer needles.

The *suboccipital triangle* is just inferior to the occipital protuberance and deep; its muscles lie posterior to the atlas and axis (Figs. 5–7). Although small in size and, when active, produce only short excursions, these muscles are in a strategic position to cause notable discomfort to patients, both in deep pain and in loss of fine control of head movements. Muscles in the region include the *rectus capitis posterior major and minor* and the *obliquus capitis superior and inferior*. It should also be noted that the *vertebral artery* crosses the lateral floor of the triangle, about two to three fingerbreadths from midline and deep to these muscles. The suboccipital nerve as well as the greater occipital nerve and the nerve of C3 pass here. The latter two nerves supply sensation to the posterior scalp and neck and if contacted can cause dysesthesias to these regions. The nerve of C3 is more medial and passes over *rectus capitis posterior minor*; the greater occipital nerve is lateral to that, passing over *obliquus capitis inferior* and *rectus capitis posterior major*.

The *rectus capitis posterior major and minor* are the most medial and deep of the group. The *rectus capitis posterior major* muscle originates on the spinous process of the axis and inserts on the lateral part of the inferior nuchal line of the occipital bone, and extends and ipsilaterally rotates the neck. It can be found about one fingerbreadth below the palpable base of the skull (essentially behind the atlas) and two fingerbreadths off midline. The *rectus capitis posterior minor* muscle extends the head, and is medial to the major, about one fingerbreadth off the midline.

The *obliquus capitis superior* is found in the same axial plane as the *rectus capitis* muscles (behind the atlas), but slightly more lateral. It originates on the transverse process of the atlas and inserts on the occipital bone serving to extend and ipsilaterally rotate the head. The *obliquus capitis inferior*, another ipsilateral rotator of the head, lies at the level of the axis; its origin is on the spinous process of the axis and it inserts onto the transverse process of the atlas. These muscles may be reached by starting approximately 45° between the spinous and the transverse processes (at the level of the atlas for the superior or axis for the inferior) and advancing the needle toward the vertebral bodies until the appropriate electrical activity is found.

## Limb Dystonias

Dystonia may involve both the upper and the lower limbs. Therapeutic BoTN injections have become a first-line treatment for the focal limb dystonias, with focal upper limb dystonia being the much more common entity, frequently starting as a task-specific or "occupational" cramp (43).

Because limb dystonias, especially of the hands, vary greatly from patient to patient, almost any muscle or combination of muscles may be involved. This requires careful examination and evaluation of the patient, often while performing the specific activity, associated with the dystonic posture. Videotaping the patient both at rest and with movements may allow the examiner systematic assessment of the dystonic posture that often changes rapidly. Another useful technique is to observe the contralateral hand for any "mirror" movements while the specific activity is performed or ask the patient to attempt to perform the activity with the contralateral limb (44).

Adult-onset focal dystonia of the foot is rare entity (45). This most often involves foot inversion and toe flexion, although as with other limb dystonias almost any combination of muscles can be involved. When foot inversion is a significant problem, injection into the posterior tibialis is frequently helpful; with a component of ankle plantar flexion, injection into the medial gastrocnemius may be added.

Limb dystonias, however, provide a perfect situation where electrophysiological guidance can make a significant difference. For example, the finger flexors, *flexor digitorum profundus*, and *flexor digitorum superficialus* are the most commonly injected muscles in task-specific arm dystonias (46). Within these muscles there are fascicles to the individual fingers. Electrical stimulation is particularly helpful for identifying individual fascicles within the finger flexors. Alternatively, EMG recording with the patient attempting to isolate individual finger movements can also allow localization of these fascicles. Accuracy is of utmost importance to minimize spread to adjacent muscles that can limit satisfactory results (10).

## CONCLUSION

Successful treatment with BoTN of the dystonic patient begins with careful observation of the dystonic posturing or activity. Coupled with a thorough knowledge of the pertinent anatomy and the adjunctive use of electrophysiological techniques when appropriate, focal treatment with BoTN injections has become the most satisfactory treatment for most if not all focal dystonias.

## REFERENCES


1. Clemente CD. Anatomy: a regional atlas of the human body. 4th ed. Baltimore: Williams & Wilkins, 1997.
2. Cutter NC, Kevorkian CG, eds. Handbook of Manual Muscle Testing. New York: McGraw-Hill, 1999.
3. Berweck S, Wissel J. Sonographic imaging for guiding BoTN injections in limb muscles. ACNR 2004; 4:28–31.
4. Van Gerpen JA, Matsumoto JY, Ahlskog E, et al. Utility of an EMG mapping study in trating cervical dystonia. Muscle Nerve 2000; 23:1752–1756.
5. Borodic GE, Joseph M, Fay L, et al. BoTN A for the treatment of spasmodic torticollis: dysphagia and regional toxin spread. Head Neck 1990; 12:392–398.
6. Shaari CM, George E, Wu BL, et al. Quantifying the spread of BoTN through muscle fascia. Laryngoscope 1991; 101:960–964.
7. Sanders DB, Massey EW, Buckley ER. BoTN for blepharospasm: single fiber EMG studies. Neurology 1985; 35:271–272.
8. Shaari CM, Sanders I. Quantifying how location and dose of BoTN injections affect muscle paralysis. Muscle Nerve 1993; 16:964–969.
9. Borodic GE, Ferrante R, Pearce B, et al. Histologic assessment of dose-related diffusion and muscle fiber response after therapeutic botulinum A toxin injections. Mov Disord 1994; 9:31–39.
10. Ross MH, Charness ME, Sudarsky L, et al. Treatment of occupational cramp with BoTN: diffusion of toxin to adjacent noninjected muscles. Muscle Nerve 1997; 20:593–598.
11. Scott A. BoTN injection of eye muscles to correct strabismus. Trans Am Ophthalmol Soc 1981; 79:734–770.
12. Borodic GE, Pearce LB, Smith K, Joseph M. Botulinum A toxin for spasmodic torticollis: multiple vs single injection points per muscle. Head Neck 1992; 14:33–37.
13. Leis AA, Trapani VC. Atlas of Electromyography. New York: Oxford University Press, 2000.
14. Childers MK. Rationale for localized injection of BoTN type A in spasticity. Eur J Neurol 1997:S37–S40.
15. Childers MK, Kornegay JN, Aoki R, et al. Evaluating motor end-plate-targeted injectins of BoTN type A in a canine model. Muscle Nerve 1998; 21:653–655.
16. Childers MK, Stacy M, Cooke DL, et al. Comparison of two injection techniques using BoTN in spastic hemiplegia. Am J Phys Med Rehabil 1996; 75:462–469.
17. Childers MK. Targeting the neuromuscular junction in skeletal muscles. Am J Phys Med Rehabil 2004; 83(suppl):S38–S44.
18. Gelb DJ, Yoshimura DM, Olney RK, et al. Change in pattern of muscle activity following BoTN injections for torticollis. Ann Neurol 1991; 29:370–376.
19. Kanovsky D, Dufck J, Halackova H, et al. Change in pattern of cervical dystonia might be the cause of benefit loss during BoTN treatment. Eur J Neurol 1997; 4:79–84.
20. Brans JW, Aramideh M, Koelman JH, et al. Electromyography in cervical dystonia: changes after botulinum and trihexyphenidyl. Neurology 1998; 51:815–819.
21. Munchau A, Filipovic SR, Oester-Barkey A, et al. Spontaneously changing muscular activation pattern in patients with cervical dystonia. Mov Disord 2001; 16:1091–1097.

22. Dubinsky RM. Anatomy and neurophysiology of neck muscles. In: Jankovic J, Hallett M, eds. Therapy With BoTN. New York: Marcel Dekker, 1994:307–321.
23. Geenan C, Consky E, Ashby P. Localizing muscles for BoTN treatment of focal hand dystonia. Can J Neurol Sci 1996; 23:194–197.
24. Barbano RL. Needle EMG guidance for injection of BoTN: Needle EMG guidance is useful. Muscle Nerve 2001; 24:1567–1568.
25. Jankovic J. Needle EMG guidance for injection of BoTN: Needle EMG guidance is rarely required. Muscle Nerve 2001; 24:1568–1570.
26. Speelman JD, Brans JWM. Cervical dystonia and botulinum treatment: is electromyographic guidance necessary?. Mov Disord 1995; 10:802.
27. Dubinsky RM, Gray CS, Vetere-Overfield B, et al. Electromyographic guidance of BoTN treatment in cervical dystonia. Clin Neuropharmacol 1991; 14:262–267.
28. Brans JWM, de Boer IP, Aramideh M, et al. BoTN in cervical dystonia: low dosage with electromyographic guidance. J Neurol 1995; 242:529–534.
29. Comella CL, Buchman AS, Tanner CM, et al. BoTN injection for spasmodic torticollis: increased magnitude of benefit with Electromyographic assistance. Neurology 1992; 42:878–882.
30. Jankovic J, Schwartz K. BoTN injections for cervical dystonia. Neurology 1990; 40: 277–280.
31. Borodic GE, Mills L, Joseph M. Botulinum A toxin for the treatment of adult-onset spasmodic torticollis. Plast Reconstr Surg 1991; 87:285–289.
32. Barbano R, Comella C, Fan W, et al. Utility of Adjunct Electromyography in BoTN Injection for Cervical Dystonia. 9th International Movement Disorders Society Meeting, New Orleans, LA: 2005.
33. Jankovic J, Brin MF. Drug Therapy: Therapeutic uses of BoTN. N Engl J Med 1991; 324:1186–1194.
34. Borodic GE. Hemifacial spasm: evaluation and management, with emphasis on BoTN therapy. In: Jankovic J, Hallett M, eds. Therapy With BoTN. New York: Marcel Dekker, 1994:331–351.
35. Wooten-Watts M, Tan EK, Jankovic J. Bruxism and cranial-cervical dystonia: is there a relationship? Cranio 1999; 17:1–6.
36. Cardoso F, Jankovic J. Oromandibular dystonia. In: Tsui JK, Caine DB, eds. Handbook of Dystonia. New York: Marcel Dekker, 1995:181–190.
37. Berkovitz BKB, Moxham BJ. A Textbook of Head and Neck Anatomy. London: Year Book Medical Publishers, Inc, 1988:171–189.
38. Tan EK, Jankovic J. BoTN A in patients with oromandibular dystonia. Long-term follow-up. Neurology 1999; 53(9):2102–2107.
39. Rivest J, Marsden CD. Trunk and head tremor as isolated manifestations of dystonia. Mov Disord 1990; 5:60–65.
40. Keshner EA, Campbell D, Katz RT, et al. Neck muscle activation patterns in humans during isometric head stabilization. Exp Brain Res 1989; 75:335–344.
41. Keshner EA, Peterson BW. Motor control strategies underlying head stabilization and voluntary movements in humans and cats. Prog Brain Res 1988; 76:329–339.
42. Deuschl G, Heinen F, Kleedorfer B, et al. Clinical and polymyographic investigation of spasmodic torticollis. J Neurol 1992; 239:9–15.
43. Pullman S. Limb dystonia: treatment with BoTN. In: Jankovic J, Hallett M, eds. Therapy with BoTN. New York: Marcel Dekker, 1994:307–321.
44. Karp BI. BoTN treatmentfo occupational and focal hand dystonia. Mov Disord 2004; 19(suppl 8):S116–S119.
45. Singer C, Papapetropoulos S. Adult-onset primary focal foot dystonia. Parkinsonism Relat Disord 2005; 12:1–4.
46. Karp BI. The role of BoTN type A in the management of occupational dystonia and writer's cramp. In: Brin MF, Hallett M, Jankovic J, eds. Scientific and Therapeutic Aspects of BoTN. Philadelphia: Lippincott, Williams and Wilkins, 2002:251–258.

# 22
# Botulinum Toxin: From Molecule to Clinic

**Nicole Calakos**
*Departments of Medicine/Neurology and Neurobiology, Center for Translational Neuroscience, Duke University, Durham, North Carolina, U.S.A.*

## INTRODUCTION

Treatment with botulinum toxin has fast become the mainstay for the management of focal dystonias. Its wide utility lies in the fact that, by harnessing the chemical denervation properties of this toxin, one can functionally weaken the endpoint of dystonia irrespective of its etiology. The goal of this chapter is to summarize the molecular and cellular mechanisms of botulinum toxin, highlighting areas in need of further investigation and practical treatment issues in need of optimization. Such an understanding of the principles of botulinum toxin action is paramount to developing the next generation of therapeutic agents.

## THE CLOSTRIDIAL NEUROTOXINS

The Clostridial bacteria are the source of a number of medically important toxins. Of these, tetanus and botulinum toxins, produced by "Clostridium tetani" and "Clostridium botulinum," respectively, are the two that produce major neurological syndromes. Both types of toxins cause a blockade of neurotransmitter release presynaptically. Minor differences in their cellular transport result in clinically distinct syndromes (Fig. 1) (2). Botulinum poisoning characteristically produces a flaccid paralysis due to blockade of acetylcholine release by the lower motor neuron at the neuromuscular junction (NMJ). In contrast, tetanus intoxication causes a spastic paralysis with profound, painful episodic spasms. These strikingly different presentations are due to the retrograde transport of the tetanus toxin through the motor neuron without activity, followed by release and uptake trans-synaptically by inhibitory interneurons of the spinal cord.

There are seven distinct serotypes of botulinum toxin (A through G) and a single tetanus toxin, each with slightly different activities. The Clostridial neurotoxins share a common protein structure mediating their activities (Fig. 2) (4). The toxins are initially synthesized as a single polypeptide chain of approximately 150 kDa that is subsequently cleaved ("nicked") to its active form yielding two

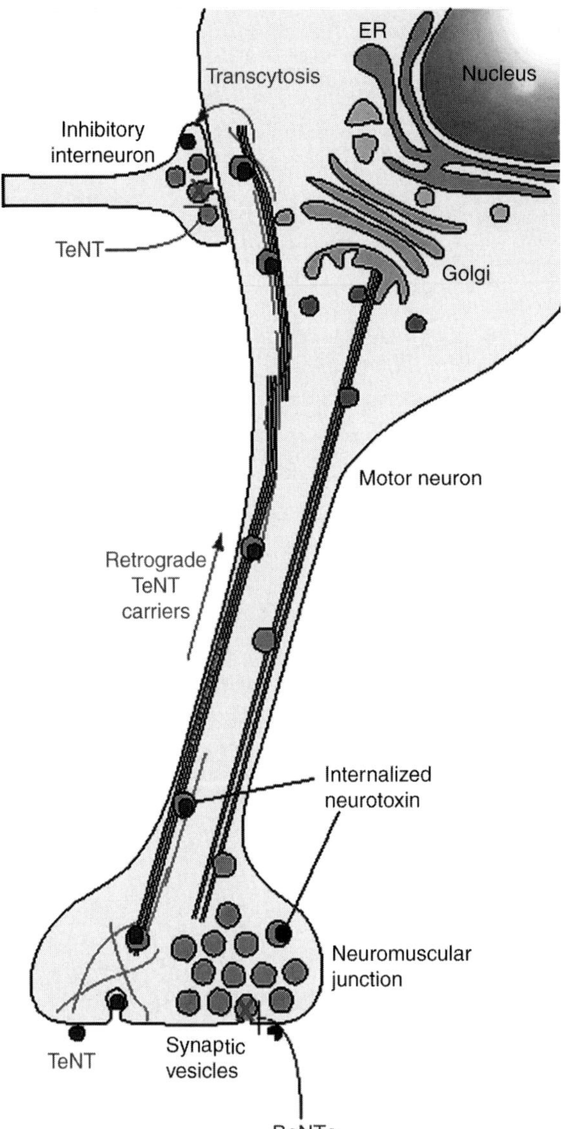


**Figure 1** Cellular trafficking of Clostridial neurotoxins. Botulinum toxins are endocytosed and act locally at the neuromuscular junction to block neurotransmitter release by cleaving SNARE proteins. Tetanus toxin is endocytosed by a distinct vesicular carrier and transported retrogradely up the motor neuron axon. Ultimately, it is transcytosed at spinal cord inhibitory interneuronal synapses and blocks neurotransmitter release in the presynaptic terminal. *Abbreviation*: SNARE: soluble *N*-ethylmaleimide-sensitive fusion protein attachment receptor. *Source*: From Ref. 12.

polypeptide chains linked together by a disulfide bond. The "heavy chain" (HC) of 100 kDa has two functional domains carried by the amino (Hn domain) and carboxy (Hc domain) terminal regions of the polypeptide, respectively. The Hc domain determines cellular uptake specificity by binding to extracellular receptors (Fig. 3). The Hn domain mediates translocation through the lipid bilayer to the cytosol, once

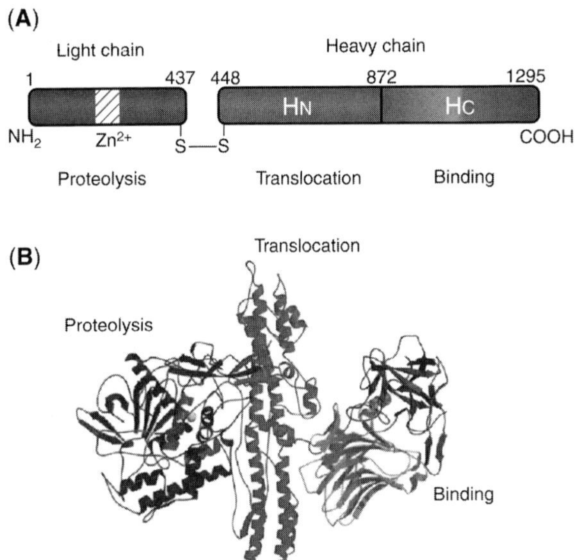


**Figure 2** Protein domain structure of the Clostridial neurotoxins. (**A**) Linear representation of key features, $Zn^{2+}$ indicates zinc coordination site of protease, S–S indicates disulfide bond. (**B**) Secondary structure of botulinum toxin A. *Source*: (**B**) From Ref. 33.

the toxin has been endocytosed (Fig. 3). The "light chain" (LC) of 50 kDa is a zinc-dependent endoprotease. The targets of the protease are a family of presynaptic proteins called "soluble *N*-ethylmaleimide-sensitive fusion protein attachment receptor (SNARE)" proteins that are critical for the exocytosis of synaptic vesicles (Fig. 3).

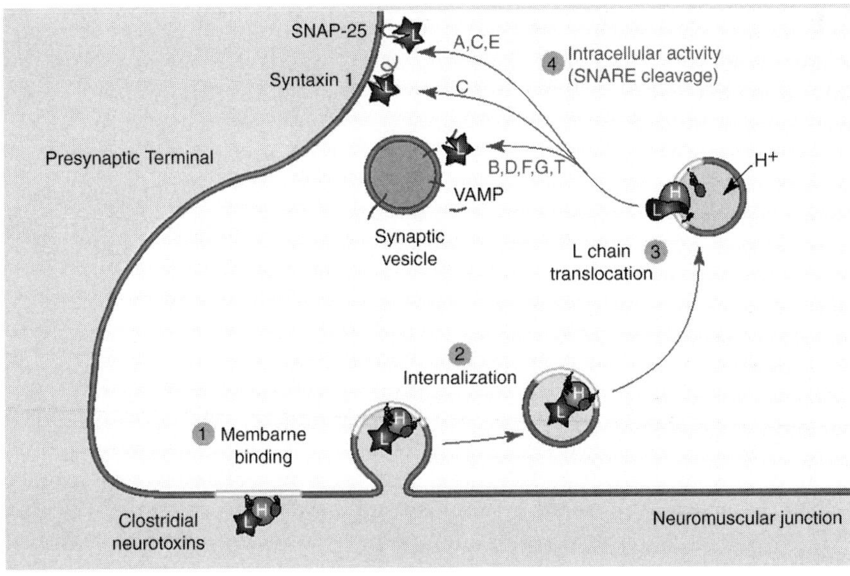


**Figure 3** Intrasynaptic trafficking of Clostridial neurotoxins. H, heavy chain; L, light chain; T, tetanus toxin, A, B, C, D, E, F, and G indicate botulinum toxin serotypes. *Source*: From Ref. 12.

## CELLULAR UPTAKE AND SPECIFICITY

To date, identification of a simple ligand–receptor interaction has eluded biochemists attempting to identify the receptors for the Clostridial neurotoxins. Rather, it appears that multiple components of the cell surface mediate a complex interaction with the toxin resulting in its uptake via endocytosis (5). The current view is that both proteinaceous and nonproteinaceous components participate. The nonproteinaceous "coreceptors" appear to be polygangliosides, in particular the GQ1b, GT1b, and Gd1b subtypes (6–9). A proteinaceous component is also required for both tetanus and botulinum toxin binding. Botulinum toxins have been shown to bind the synaptic vesicle proteins, Synaptotagmins I and II (8,10,11), while tetanus toxin interacts with the Thy-1 protein (12,13).

At the NMJ, binding of botulinum toxin but not tetanus toxin may be related to synaptic vesicle release and endocytosis (1,4). Tetanus toxin, however, appears to be endocytosed into a distinct subcellular organelle, which is nonacidic and retrogradely transits through the motor neuron to ultimately be released and taken up trans-synaptically by inhibitory interneurons. The identity of the retrograde transport vesicle is uncertain, but may be the vesicle that also transports the p75/NGF (nerve growth factor) complex (14). Similarly, little is known about the mechanism of uptake of tetanus toxin by the inhibitory interneurons. It may be similar to that of botulinum toxin uptake at the NMJ via synaptic vesicles. As comparison of the pathways of these two toxins indicates, the Hc domain can determine markedly different cell uptake and transport patterns (Fig. 1). Identifying the receptors and ligand domains that determine this specificity would be powerful for directing the delivery of toxins to cell types of choice.

## CYTOSOLIC TRANSLOCATION

Once the toxin is intracellular following endocytic uptake of the plasma membrane, the toxin is still sequestered in a membranous organelle without access to the cytoplasm, where its targets reside. Translocation of the LC through the lipid bilayer into the cytoplasm is mediated by the Hn domain (15). Upon acidification, the Hn domain undergoes a conformational change that exposes a hydrophobic domain (4). The Hn domain is then able to facilitate passage of the LC through the lipid bilayer, perhaps in a manner analogous to the protein conducting channels of the endoplasmic reticulum and mitochondria (16). Lastly, the disulfide bond between the H and L chains must be cleaved in order to free the L chain into the cytosolic compartment.

## PROTEOLYTIC CLEAVAGE OF NEURONAL SNAREs

Of all the steps in the intoxication by the Clostridial neurotoxins, the proteolytic cleavage of its substrates is the best understood. The targets of the neurotoxin proteases are the neuron-specific isoforms of a family of proteins called SNAREs (Fig. 4). These proteins are required for intracellular vesicular membrane trafficking and widely expressed in all cell types from yeast to humans (17). The neuronal isoforms targeted by the Clostridial neurotoxins are critical for synaptic vesicle-mediated release of neurotransmitter. Historically, it was known for many decades through electrophysiological and electron microscopic studies that botulism and

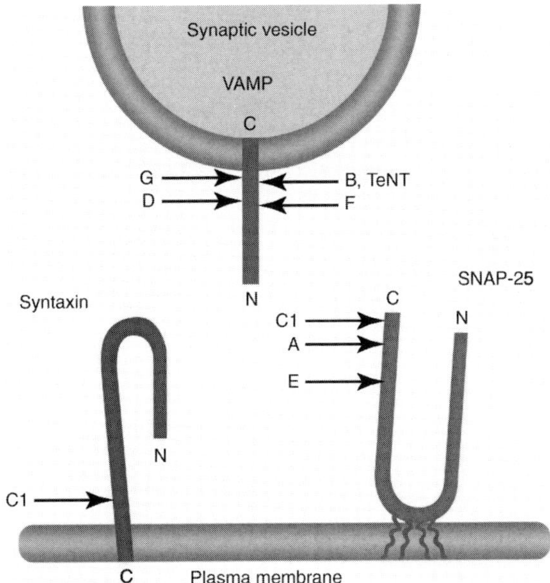


**Figure 4** Relative locations of proteolytic cleavage sites of SNARE proteins by Clostridial neurotoxins. A, B, C1, D, E, F, and G indicate botulinum neurotoxin serotypes. *Abbreviation*: TeNT, tetanus neurotoxin.

tetanus were caused by a presynaptic blockade of neurotransmitter release. However, the molecular targets for this blockade eluded identification until the early 1990s, when a functional role in neurotransmitter release was proposed for the presynaptic proteins—vesicle associated membrane protein (VAMP)/Synaptobrevin, Syntaxin, and SNAP-25 (18–20). Using antibodies specific to these proteins, investigators were then able to evaluate Clostridial neurotoxin-intoxicated synapses and find evidence for their cleavage (21).

SNARE proteins form an α-helical coiled-coil complex between SNARE proteins residing on the vesicular and target membranes for fusion. Vesicular or v-SNAREs involved in synaptic vesicle fusion are VAMPs (also known as Synaptobrevins) 1 and 2. Target membrane or t-SNAREs residing on the nerve terminal plasma membrane are Syntaxin 1 and SNAP-25. VAMP and Syntaxin each provide two proteins, each one has domain participating one α-helical domain, whereas SNAP-25 provides two, ultimately forming a coiled-coil bundle of four α-helices. This complex is critical for neurotransmitter release and an abundance of evidence indicates that this complex acts at the vesicle fusion step (22–26). However, controversy exists over whether the complex might act at other steps in the synaptic vesicle pathway. In particular, observations from botulism and tetanus intoxication contribute to these arguments because of the ability to partially rescue neurotransmission by increasing extracellular calcium. Elegant experiments have recently shed light on this controversy and indicate that both SNAP-25 and VAMP have properties that reduce the calcium sensitivity of release (but not the stoichiometry) when cleaved by the toxins (27). Cleavage of SNAP-25 alters the calcium sensitivity of neurotransmitter release even when excess calcium is available intracellularly. Cleavage of VAMP, however, appears to decrease release sensitivity only by impairing the availability of calcium from extracellular, voltage-dependent sources, possibly by coordinating the localization of calcium channels with the fusion apparatus (27–31).

The eight Clostridial neurotoxins all target components of the SNARE complex, although with distinct cleavage sites (Fig. 4). Tetanus toxin and botulinum toxins B, D, F, and G target VAMP/Synaptobrevin 1 and 2. Botulinum toxins A, C1, and E target SNAP-25, again at differing sites (except for tetanus toxin and botulinum toxin B that share a common cleavage site). Botulinum toxin C1 targets Syntaxin 1 in addition to SNAP-25. Crystal structures for LC of botulinum toxin serotype A bound to SNAP-25 and tetanus toxin and botulinum B toxin bound to VAMP 2 have been solved, providing a great resource to make predictions about structural determinants of substrate specificity (3,32–35). Although, a nine amino acid motif SNARE secondary recognition, is common to cleavage sites (36–39), structural studies indicate that much larger regions are required for specific interaction with the L chain protease (40). Conflicting studies using the toxins to poison synapses have raised the issue of whether SNARE proteins in varying conformational states are equally accessible to the toxins. However, for the time course of action of the proteases this is not much of a practical issue for dystonia treatment because the SNARE proteins would be predicted to cycle through all of their conformational states in a matter of minutes.

## LONGEVITY OF PARALYTIC ACTIVITY

An area of immense clinical importance is the determinants for duration of toxin effect. Data from animal and human studies indicate that the relative duration of paralytic activity for botulinum serotypes is A > C1 > B > F > E (41–44). Many factors could potentially influence this duration. These include (i) toxin protease half-life, (ii) target SNARE protein turnover, (iii) SNARE cleavage product activity, and (iv) synaptic remodeling time course. Knowing the relative contribution of each of these factors and their underlying molecular basis will greatly facilitate the rational design of toxins with prolonged activity.

Duration of protease activity in the nerve terminal appears to be a significant determinant for longevity of clinical effect. Proteases with the longest activity in cultured cerebellar neurons correlated with those serotypes having the longest paralytic effect in mice, namely serotypes A, B, and C1 (43,45). Several factors that may underlie, a toxin's duration of activity have been identified. Resistance to degradation by cellular exoproteases may contribute to the stability of botulinum A toxin (46). Subcellular localization may also contribute (47,48). Lastly, modification by host signaling molecules such as tyrosine kinases can influence protease stability (49,50).

The rate of replacement of cleaved SNARE proteins with newly synthesized protein can also contribute to the duration of clinical effect. In vitro studies in cerebellar neurons revealed half-lives on the order of one to two days for VAMP and SNAP-25 and six days for Syntaxin (43). SNARE protein turnover is likely to be rate limiting in the case of botulinum E and F toxins, given the relatively short duration of protease activity for these serotypes (43). In a similar fashion, the activity of the cleavage products may also influence recovery of function. For example, the SNAP-25 cleavage product of Botulinum A toxin is itself inhibitory to the vesicle fusion reaction (51). In this instance, the rate of clearance of this cleavage product will also contribute to duration of activity. Lastly, in the case of Botulinum C1 toxin, the duration of effect may be combinatorial, reflecting contributions of both protease half-life and the relatively slower turnover of Syntaxin as compared to the other SNAREs.

A final potential determinant of paralysis duration is the time course for the recovery of functional synapses. The properties of the NMJ in response to denervation have been well characterized. Two important features are that the postsynaptic acetylcholine receptors quickly disperse upon loss of presynaptic neurotransmitter release and that despite the dispersal of postsynaptic receptors, key markers of the original NMJ persist (such as agrin), allowing the synapse to reform at its original site should neurotransmitter release be restored (52). In the case of synaptic remodeling following chemical denervation by botulinum toxin, the most informative study to date has used time lapse imaging in combination with styryl dyes that indicate actively cycling synaptic vesicles (53). Two important findings were that (i) upon denervation, collateral axonal sprouts formed nascent synapses that initially restored activity to the NMJ and (ii) ultimately neurotransmitter release was recovered at the original NMJ site and was followed by retraction of the newly formed collateral synapses. At least at the gross light microscopic level, these findings showed that the original NMJ architecture was restored to baseline. However, as discussed in the following section, whether the NMJ is functionally identical in physiologic criteria and to what extent the cycle of denervation/reinnervation can repeat with perfect restorative fidelity is presently uncertain.

## MECHANISMS OF RESISTANCE

At least for the most commonly used serotype, it is clear that over time many patients may require more toxin for a similar clinical effect and some may become resistant altogether to its effect. Resistance due to the presence of circulating, antitoxin antibodies has been demonstrated and is currently believed to be the dominant mechanism for resistance. Secondly, it is widely held that mitigation of humoral resistance can be achieved by decreasing toxin doses and frequency. While both of these observations may be true in certain cases, for the purposes of discussion, additional theoretical possibilities will be presented for consideration.

The likelihood of developing function-blocking antibodies is likely to be multifactorial and includes genetic host factors (54). Besides the absolute quantity of protein delivered, toxin immunogenicity may also be influenced by whether a given toxin possesses highly antigenic epitopes. The issue of antigenicity is an important one because custom toxins can be designed with minimally antigenic epitopes if a solid understanding of the dominant antigenic epitopes is gained. Current work in both human and animal models will be critical for the design of both minimally antigenic toxins and vaccines (55–57). There is also evidence that besides the Botulinum A neurotoxin protein, associated neurotoxin complex proteins (in particular, hemagglutinin-33) may be significant contributors to the immunogenic response (58,59). In light of this, developing commercial preparations with as few associated neurotoxin complex proteins may be one mechanism to decrease function-blocking antibody responses (60).

Besides function-blocking antibodies, there may be other as yet unidentified mechanisms for toxin resistance. For example, while there is evidence that restoration of the original, denervated NMJ and retraction of collateral synapses occur in response to a single intoxication, it is not known whether over repeated toxin exposures the physiological fidelity of the motor unit is perfectly preserved (61). One can imagine that if collateral synapses were not completely retracted, over time an increase in synapse number and density could contribute to toxin resistance.

Secondly, the remodeling process itself may activate host signaling factors that influence toxin stability or upregulate the synthesis of "resistant SNAREs," perhaps via alternative mRNA splicing.

## DESIGNING THE NEXT GENERATION OF TOXINS

Harnessing the activity of the normally harmful Clostridial neurotoxins to be useful for the treatment of clinical disorders has had enormous significance for the management of dystonia. The resultant stimulation of interest and research into the mechanisms of the Clostridial neurotoxins has also yielded important insights to normal synaptic function as well as disease pathogenesis and vaccine production. While great strides in our understanding of the molecular basis of botulinum toxin activity have been made, the potential for many exciting developments in the future still exists.

Rational manipulation of each step in the pathway of Clostridial neurotoxins can result in improved therapeutic applications (Fig. 5). Obviating the need for toxin injection by creating transdermal applications would greatly simplify the lives of many patients, potentially reduce costs, and increase the application of this therapy to a wider patient population (Fig. 5) (62,63). Manipulating the receptor-binding properties of the toxin would allow both targeting different "cargo" to the lower

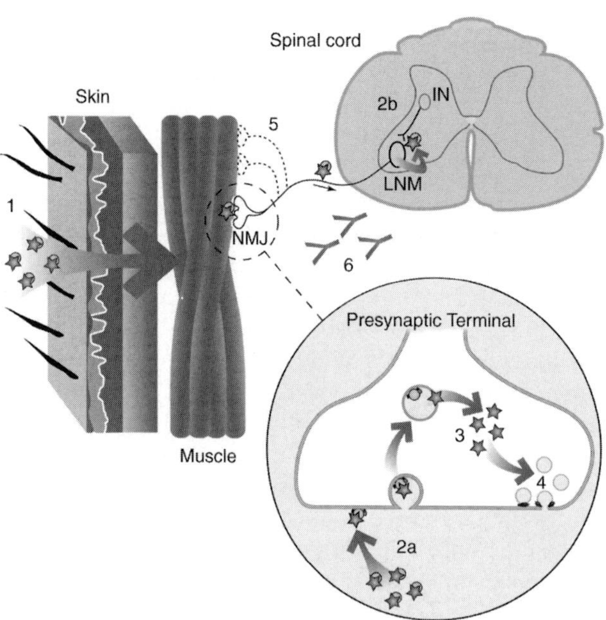


**Figure 5** Future directions in Clostridial neurotoxin research. (**1**) Creating transdermal application technologies, (**2**) customizing protein delivery to NMJ or IN by manipulating Hc domain/surface receptor interactions, (**3**) improving toxin stability in the presynaptic terminal, (**4**) modifying target SNARE cleavage sites, (**5**) understanding long-term consequences of repeated denervation/reinnervation cycles, and (**6**) overcoming issues of toxin resistance. *Abbreviations*: NMJ, neuromuscular junction, IN, inhibitory interneuron, LMN, lower motor neuron.

motor neuron and directing cargo to different cell types (Fig. 5). Chimeric protein complexes with the L and Hn domains of botulinum toxin have been used effectively for this purpose (64,65). Harnessing the retrograde, trans-synaptic transport properties of the tetanus toxin Hc domain could facilitate delivery of a wide range of molecules to the central nervous system via peripheral NMJ access. Such an application could be especially powerful for delivering modulators of inflammation and regeneration. Through a more detailed understanding of the factors resulting in prolonged toxin stability and activity at the synapse, targeted modifications of other toxin serotypes could increase the number of toxins useful in clinical practice (Fig. 5). In special circumstances, the expression of toxin-resistant SNAREs could be useful in limiting the duration or extent of toxin effect (Fig. 5) (45,66). Strategies targeted at SNARE cleavage site specificity of the L chain could potentially lengthen the duration of Botulinum A toxin activity by selecting for a target SNARE with the lowest turnover and avoiding active cleavage products. The routine application of botulinum toxin therapeutically is still a relatively recent development. It would thus be prudent to continue to investigate the long-term sequelae of such treatment, especially in regards to the process of continued cycles of denervation and reinnervation (Fig. 5). Additionally, such studies are likely to yield insights useful for regenerative therapies in a wide range of neurological diseases. Finally, the issue of toxin resistance is an important clinical limitation (Fig. 5). It is imperative to understand whether the development of function-blocking antibodies is the complete explanation for resistance, and, if so, to develop effective strategies to overcome this obstacle.

## CONCLUSION

In summary, the Clostridial neurotoxins represent a family of proteases that have targeted discrete components of the synaptic vesicle release machinery. As such, they provide therapeutic opportunities wherever long-lasting inhibition of neurotransmitter release is desirable. Dystonia management is an important illustration of the power of this approach. The treatment of this etiologically heterogeneous condition has benefited greatly by botulinum toxins because the toxins target the final common output, muscle contraction. Yet, as is often the case, with success comes the realization of limitations as well as opportunities for even greater achievements. In this chapter, a summary of our current understanding of toxin mechanisms and therapeutic issues has been presented, highlighting areas of uncertainty and in need of improvement. Through careful studies of the mechanisms of the Clostridial neurotoxins, significant advances in the field are likely to be realized in the decade ahead. Such advances may improve not only the lives of our patients with dystonia but also those with other neurological conditions as well.

## REFERENCES

1. Goonetilleke A, Harris JB. Clostridial neurotoxins. J Neurol Neurosurg Psychiatry 2004; 75(suppl 3):iii35–iii39.
2. Grumelli C et al. Internalization and mechanism of action of Clostridial toxins in neurons. Neurotoxicology 2005; 26(5):761–767.
3. Montecucco C, Rossetto O, Schiavo G. Presynaptic receptor arrays for Clostridial neurotoxins. Trends Microbiol 2004; 12(10):442–446.

4. Habermann E, Dreyer F. Clostridial neurotoxins: handling and action at the cellular and molecular level. Curr Top Microbiol Immunol 1986; 129:93–179.
5. Halpern JL, Loftus A. Characterization of the receptor-binding domain of tetanus toxin. J Biol Chem 1993; 268(15):11188–11192.
6. Nishiki T et al. The high-affinity binding of Clostridium botulinum type B neurotoxin to synaptotagmin II associated with gangliosides GT1b/GD1a. FEBS Lett 1996; 378(3): 253–257.
7. Halpern JL, Neale EA. Neurospecific binding, internalization, and retrograde axonal transport. Curr Top Microbiol Immunol 1995; 195:221–241.
8. Li L, Singh BR. Isolation of synaptotagmin as a receptor for types A and E botulinum neurotoxin and analysis of their comparative binding using a new microtiter plate assay. J Nat Toxins 1998; 7(3):215–226.
9. Nishiki T et al. Identification of protein receptor for Clostridium botulinum type B neurotoxin in rat brain synaptosomes. J Biol Chem 1994; 269(14):10498–10503.
10. Herreros J, Ng T, Schiavo G. Lipid rafts act as specialized domains for tetanus toxin binding and internalization into neurons. Mol Biol Cell 2001; 12(10):2947–2960.
11. Herreros J et al. Tetanus toxin fragment C binds to a protein present in neuronal cell lines and motoneurons. J Neurochem 2000; 74(5):1941–1950.
12. Lalli G et al. The journey of tetanus and botulinum neurotoxins in neurons. Trends Microbiol 2003; 11(9):431–437.
13. Lalli G, Schiavo G. Analysis of retrograde transport in motor neurons reveals common endocytic carriers for tetanus toxin and neurotrophin receptor p75NTR. J Cell Biol 2002; 156(2):233–239.
14. Shone CC, Hambleton P, Melling J. A 50-kDa fragment from the NH2-terminus of the heavy subunit of Clostridium botulinum type A neurotoxin forms channels in lipid vesicles. Eur J Biochem 1987; 167(1):175–180.
15. Koriazova LK, Montal M. Translocation of botulinum neurotoxin light chain protease through the heavy chain channel. Nat Struct Biol 2003; 10(1):13–18.
16. Bock JB et al. A genomic perspective on membrane compartment organization. Nature 2001; 409(6822):839–841.
17. Bennett MK, Calakos N, Scheller RH. Syntaxin: a synaptic protein implicated in docking of synaptic vesicles at presynaptic active zones. Science 1992; 257(5067):255–259.
18. Calakos N et al. Protein-protein interactions contributing to the specificity of intracellular vesicular trafficking. Science 1994; 263(5150):1146–1149.
19. Sollner T et al. A protein assembly-disassembly pathway in vitro that may correspond to sequential steps of synaptic vesicle docking, activation, and fusion. Cell 1993; 75(3): 409–418.
20. Schiavo G et al. Tetanus and botulinum neurotoxins are zinc proteases specific for components of the neuroexocytosis apparatus. Ann N Y Acad Sci 1994; 710:65–75.
21. Sollner TH. Intracellular and viral membrane fusion: a uniting mechanism. Curr Opin Cell Biol 2004; 16(4):429–435.
22. Calakos N, Scheller RH. Synaptic vesicle biogenesis, docking, and fusion: a molecular description. Physiol Rev 1996; 76(1):1–29.
23. Lin RC, Scheller RH. Mechanisms of synaptic vesicle exocytosis. Annu Rev Cell Dev Biol 2000; 16:19–49.
24. Schuette CG et al. Determinants of liposome fusion mediated by synaptic SNARE proteins. Proc Natl Acad Sci U S A 2004; 101(9):2858–2863.
25. Tucker WC, Weber T, Chapman ER. Reconstitution of Ca2+-regulated membrane fusion by synaptotagmin and SNAREs. Science 2004; 304(5669):435–438.
26. Sakaba T et al. Distinct kinetic changes in neurotransmitter release after SNARE protein cleavage. Science 2005; 309(5733):491–494.
27. Capogna M et al. Ca2+ or Sr2+ partially rescues synaptic transmission in hippocampal cultures treated with botulinum toxin A and C, but not tetanus toxin. J Neurosci 1997; 17(19):7190–7202.

28. Owe-Larsson B et al. Distinct effects of Clostridial toxins on activity-dependent modulation of autaptic responses in cultured hippocampal neurons. Eur J Neurosci 1997; 9(8): 1773–1777.
29. Lawrence GW, Foran P, Oliver Dolly J. Insights into a basis for incomplete inhibition by botulinum toxin A of Ca2+-evoked exocytosis from permeabilised chromaffin cells. Toxicology 2002; 181–182:249–253.
30. Verderio C et al. SNAP-25 modulation of calcium dynamics underlies differences in GABAergic and glutamatergic responsiveness to depolarization. Neuron 2004; 41(4):599–610.
31. Swaminathan S, Eswaramoorthy S. Structural analysis of the catalytic and binding sites of Clostridium botulinum neurotoxin B. Nat Struct Biol 2000; 7(8):693–699.
32. Breidenbach MA, Brunger AT. Substrate recognition strategy for botulinum neurotoxin serotype A. Nature 2004; 432(7019):925–929.
33. Lacy DB et al. Crystal structure of botulinum neurotoxin type A and implications for toxicity. Nat Struct Biol 1998; 5(10):898–902.
34. Breidenbach MA, Brunger AT. 2.3 A crystal structure of tetanus neurotoxin light chain. Biochemistry 2005; 44(20):7450–7457.
35. Umland TC et al. Structure of the receptor binding fragment HC of tetanus neurotoxin. Nat Struct Biol 1997; 4(10):788–792.
36. Pellizzari R et al. Structural determinants of the specificity for synaptic vesicle-associated membrane protein/synaptobrevin of tetanus and botulinum type B and G neurotoxins. J Biol Chem 1996; 271(34):20353–20358.
37. Rossetto O et al. SNARE motif and neurotoxins. Nature 1994; 372(6505):415–416.
38. Vaidyanathan VV et al. Proteolysis of SNAP-25 isoforms by botulinum neurotoxin types A, C, and E: domains and amino acid residues controlling the formation of enzyme-substrate complexes and cleavage. J Neurochem 1999; 72(1):327–337.
39. Washbourne P et al. Botulinum neurotoxin types A and E require the SNARE motif in SNAP-25 for proteolysis. FEBS Lett 1997; 418(1–2):1–5.
40. Breidenbach MA, Brunger AT. New insights into Clostridial neurotoxin-SNARE interactions. Trends Mol Med 2005; 11(8):377–381.
41. Greene PE, Fahn S. Use of botulinum toxin type F injections to treat torticollis in patients with immunity to botulinum toxin type A. Mov Disord 1993; 8(4):479–483.
42. Rosales RL, Bigalke H, Dressler D. Pharmacology of botulinum toxin: differences between type A preparations. Eur J Neurol 2006; 13(suppl 1):2–10.
43. Foran PG et al. Evaluation of the therapeutic usefulness of botulinum neurotoxin B, C1, E, and F compared with the long lasting type A. Basis for distinct durations of inhibition of exocytosis in central neurons. J Biol Chem 2003; 278(2):1363–1371.
44. Eleopra R et al. Different time courses of recovery after poisoning with botulinum neurotoxin serotypes A and E in humans. Neurosci Lett 1998; 256(3):135–138.
45. O'Sullivan GA et al. Rescue of exocytosis in botulinum toxin A-poisoned chromaffin cells by expression of cleavage-resistant SNAP-25. Identification of the minimal essential C-terminal residues. J Biol Chem 1999; 274(52):36897–36904.
46. Simpson LL et al. The role of exoproteases in governing intraneuronal metabolism of botulinum toxin. Protein J 2005; 24(3):155–165.
47. Fernandez-Salas E et al. Plasma membrane localization signals in the light chain of botulinum neurotoxin. Proc Natl Acad Sci USA 2004; 101(9):3208 3213.
48. Koticha DK, McCarthy EE, Baldini G. Plasma membrane targeting of SNAP-25 increases its local concentration and is necessary for SNARE complex formation and regulated exocytosis. J Cell Sci 2002; 115(Pt 16):3341–3351.
49. Ibanez C et al. Modulation of botulinum neurotoxin A catalytic domain stability by tyrosine phosphorylation. FEBS Lett 2004; 578(1–2):121–127.
50. Ferrer-Montiel AV et al. Tyrosine phosphorylation modulates the activity of Clostridial neurotoxins. J Biol Chem 1996; 271(31):18322–18325.
51. Keller JE, Neale EA. The role of the synaptic protein snap-25 in the potency of botulinum neurotoxin type A. J Biol Chem 2001; 276(16):13476–13482.

52. Sanes JR, Lichtman JW. Development of the vertebrate neuromuscular junction. Annu Rev Neurosci 1999; 22:389–442.
53. de Paiva A et al. Functional repair of motor endplates after botulinum neurotoxin type A poisoning: biphasic switch of synaptic activity between nerve sprouts and their parent terminals. Proc Natl Acad Sci USA 1999; 96(6):3200–3205.
54. Atassi MZ. Basic immunological aspects of botulinum toxin therapy. Mov Disord 2004; 19(suppl 8):S68–S84.
55. Atassi MZ, Dolimbek BZ. Mapping of the antibody-binding regions on the HN-domain (residues 449–859) of botulinum neurotoxin A with antitoxin antibodies from four host species. Full profile of the continuous antigenic regions of the H-chain of botulinum neurotoxin A. Protein J 2004; 23(1):39–52.
56. Atassi MZ et al. Mapping of the antibody-binding regions on botulinum neurotoxin H-chain domain 855–1296 with antitoxin antibodies from three host species. J Protein Chem 1996; 15(7):691–700.
57. Rosenberg JS, Middlebrook JL, Atassi MZ. Localization of the regions on the C-terminal domain of the heavy chain of botulinum A recognized by T lymphocytes and by antibodies after immunization of mice with pentavalent toxoid. Immunol Invest 1997; 26(4): 491–504.
58. Sharma SK, Singh BR. Immunological properties of Hn-33 purified from type A Clostridium botulinum. J Nat Toxins 2000; 9(4):357–362.
59. Singh BR et al. Gene probe-based detection of type E botulinum neurotoxin binding protein using polymerase chain reaction. Toxicon 1996; 34(7):737–742.
60. Aoki KR. Pharmacology and immunology of botulinum toxin serotypes. J Neurol 2001; 248(suppl 1):3–10.
61. Santos AF, Caroni P. Assembly, plasticity and selective vulnerability to disease of mouse neuromuscular junctions. J Neurocytol 2003; 32(5–8):849–862.
62. Stamatialis DF, Rolevink HH, Koops GH. Passive and iontophoretic controlled delivery of salmon calcitonin through artificial membranes. Curr Drug Deliv 2004; 1(2):137–143.
63. Cross SE, Roberts MS. Physical enhancement of transdermal drug application: is delivery technology keeping up with pharmaceutical development? Curr Drug Deliv 2004; 1(1): 81–92.
64. Chaddock JA et al. Inhibition of vesicular secretion in both neuronal and nonneuronal cells by a retargeted endopeptidase derivative of Clostridium botulinum neurotoxin type A. Infect Immun 2000; 68(5):2587–2593.
65. Chaddock JA et al. A conjugate composed of nerve growth factor coupled to a non-toxic derivative of Clostridium botulinum neurotoxin type A can inhibit neurotransmitter release in vitro. Growth Factors 2000; 18(2):147–155.
66. Gonelle-Gispert C et al. SNAP-25a and -25b isoforms are both expressed in insulin-secreting cells and can function in insulin secretion. Biochem J 1999; 339 (Pt 1):159–165.

# 23

# Botulinum Toxins in the Treatment of Dystonia

**Mark A. Stacy**
*Department of Medicine/Neurology, and Movement Disorders Center, Duke University Medical Center, Durham, North Carolina, U.S.A.*

## INTRODUCTION

In the 1820s, a German physician, Justinus Kerner, reported his clinical experience with 230 patients who developed weakness, gastrointestinal disturbances, dry eyes, and dry skin associated with the ingestion of contaminated meat. This condition, termed by Kerner as "sausage poison," was later named "botulism," from the Latin term *botulus* or sausage (1). A century later, Edward Schantz first cultured *Clostridium botulinum* and isolated the toxin. In 1973, Alan Scott first used botulinum toxin type A (BoTN-A) in monkey experiments, and in 1980 he was able to first test this drug in humans (2). This work led to therapeutic trials in dystonia by a number of investigators, culminating with U.S. approval of Oculinum®/Botox® for the treatment of strabismus, blepharospasm, and hemifacial spasm in December 1989. An indication for approval for treatment of cervical dystonia (CD) was given in 2000. Dysport®, another BoTN-A, developed in Europe received approvals outside the United States in a similar time frame. Myobloc™, a BoTN-B therapy, was approved in the United States for the treatment of CD in 2000; this agent is also approved for usage in Europe under the trade name Neurobloc® (Table 1) (3).

While the greatest factors for successful treatment of a dystonic muscle concern identifying the affected muscles, and appropriate intramuscular dosage injection, determining a BoTN dosage does play a role (4). This chapter will outline toxin selection strategies and compare the relative potencies and regulatory data of these agents in the treatment of dystonia.

## BOTULINUM TOXIN A

There are three types of BoTN-A: Botox, Dysport, and NT 301 (Xeomin®; available only in Germany). Given the differences in potencies for Dysport and Botox, it is important to clarify the toxin by the manufacturer when considering dosing issues. Each toxin is produced by the Gram-negative anaerobic bacterium *C. botulinum* and harvested from a culture medium, after fermentation of a toxin-producing

**Table 1** Dysport® and Botox® Indications Approved by Regulatory Agencies

| | Dysport | Botox |
|---|---|---|
| Blepharospasm[a] | Argentina, Australia, Brazil, Denmark, France, Germany, Greece, Ireland, Italy, Mexico, Netherlands, New Zealand, Spain, United Kingdom | Argentina, Australia, Brazil, Denmark, Finland, France, Germany, Greece, Iceland, Ireland, Italy, Mexico, Netherlands, New Zealand, Norway, Spain, Sweden, United Kingdom, United States |
| Hemifacial spasm | Argentina, Australia, Brazil, France, Germany, Ireland, Italy, Netherlands, Spain, United Kingdom | Argentina, Denmark, Finland, France, Germany, Greece, Iceland, Ireland, Italy, Mexico, Netherlands, Norway, Spain, Sweden, United Kingdom, United States |
| Torticollis/cervical dystonia (CD)[a] | Argentina, Australia, Brazil, Denmark, Finland, France, Germany, Greece, Iceland, Ireland, Italy, Mexico, Netherlands, New Zealand, Norway, Spain, Sweden, United Kingdom | Argentina, Australia, Brazil, Canada, Denmark, Finland, France, Germany, Greece, Iceland, Ireland, Italy, Mexico, Netherlands, New Zealand, Norway, Spain, Sweden, United Kingdom, United States |
| Spasticity | Argentina, Australia, Brazil, France, Greece, Iceland, Ireland, Italy, Mexico, New Zealand, Norway, Spain, Sweden | Argentina, Australia, Brazil, Canada, Denmark, Finland, France, Germany, Greece, Iceland, Ireland, Italy, Mexico, Netherlands, New Zealand, Norway, Spain, Sweden, United Kingdom, United States |
| Hyperhydrosis | Argentina, Brazil, Denmark, Iceland, New Zealand, Norway | Argentina, Australia, Brazil, Canada, Denmark, Finland, France, Germany, Greece, Iceland, Ireland, Italy, Mexico, Netherlands, New Zealand, Norway, Spain, Sweden, United Kingdom, United States |
| Cerebral palsy (pediatric) | Argentina, Australia, Brazil, Finland, France, Greece, Iceland, Ireland, Italy, Mexico, New Zealand, Norway, Spain, Sweden, United Kingdom | Argentina, Australia, Brazil, Canada, Denmark, Finland, France, Germany, Greece, Iceland, Ireland, Italy, Mexico, Netherlands, New Zealand, Norway, Spain, Sweden, United Kingdom, United States |

[a]Myobloc®/Neurobloc® is approved for treating CD in Austria, Canada, France, Germany, Ireland, Italy, Portugal, Spain, United Kingdom, and United States. Xeomin® is approved for use in blepharospasm and CD in Germany.

strain. The toxin is then extracted, precipitated, purified, and finally crystallized with ammonium sulfate. Because of different purification processes, packaged toxins differ with respect to size of the active molecule and additional, nonactive protein subcomponents. Botox (900 kD) and Xeomin (150 kD) differ with respect to toxin complex size, but not in amounts of accompanying protein subcomponents (5). The active toxin components in Dysport are measured at 500 kD, and the nonactive proteins appear to be higher (6).

The potency of BoTN is expressed as mouse units (U), with 1 U equivalent to the median lethal dose (LD 50) for mice. Botox and Xeomin are packaged in 100 U vials, while a vial of Dysport contains 500 U (5,6). The relative potencies of Botox units to Dysport units is approximately 1:4, but this may differ with patient and clinical setting. Botox and Xeomin appear to be of similar potencies in early comparator trials, but Xeomin has not been directly compared to Dysport (7–9). Botulinum toxin type A (BoTN-A) should be diluted with preservative-free saline and the preparation used within four hours of reconstitution. Conditions for stability of the toxin in solution include pH 4.2 to 6.8 and temperature less than 20°C (5,6). Most physicians dilute these products with 1 to 4 mL of saline, depending on the amount of toxin diffusion desired from an injection session.

## Botox®

Botox has been available in the United States for treating blepharospasm and cranial nerve VII disorder (hemifacial spasm) since 1990. Other neurological conditions include spasmodic torticollis (CD), limb dystonia, oromandibular dystonia, laryngeal dystonia, and limb spasticity (Table 1). This agent has also been shown to be effective in patients with tremor (10,11), headache (12,13), stuttering (14), sialorrhea (15), hyperhydrosis (16,17), pain (18), facial wrinkles (19), gastrointestinal dysmotility disorders (20,21), and bladder detruser hyperactivity (22). Subjects with dystonia receive amounts ranging from 1 to 400 U in a single injection session. Small muscles such as the vocal cords may receive as little as 0.75 U, whereas larger neck muscles may require 100 to 150 U and lower limb muscles may require 200 to 300 U to exert a desirable effect. In an early placebo-controlled study of BoTN-A in CD, 55 subjects were randomized to placebo or Botox therapy (23). The subjects receiving active drug demonstrated statistically significant improvement in the severity of torticollis, disability, pain, and degree of head turning. There were no serious side effects. Long-term treatment data using Botox suggest that this agent remains effective for many years. A multicenter, retrospective analysis of 172 subjects treated for a total of 1059 treatments over two years found toxin dosages remaining fairly stable and ranging from 241.80 to 254.07 units with a slight increase in dosing interval from 108.48 to 114.14 days (24). A single-center retrospective review of 2616 injections in 235 patients reported continued benefit in most patients for more than five years (25). Subjects with blepharospasm reported a 90% benefit, while hemifacial spasm (88%), CD (63%), jaw opening dystonia (100%), lower limb dystonia (100%), and writer's cramp (56%) also improved. Of the 28% of patients who discontinued, 9.1% had an insufficient initial response, 7.5% developed secondary resistance, and 1.3% reported unacceptable adverse events. Adverse events were most common in blepharospasm (22 of 36 patients), followed by hemifacial spasm (21 of 70 patients) and CD (17 of 106).

After injection of BoTN-A, a clinical response is usually seen within 24 to 72 hours, and maximal effect occurs after about 14 days; benefit may last for three to six months (5). In 1997, the U.S. agency approved a new bulk toxin source, with a

**Table 2** Dosing Range

| Indication | Dosage (U) | | | |
|---|---|---|---|---|
| | Botox® | Dysport® | Xeomin® | Myobloc® |
| Blepharospasm | 15–50 | 100–120 | 35 | 1,000–2,500 |
| Hemifacial spasm | 15–50 | 100–120 | – | 750–1,000 |
| Cervical dystonia | 40–360 | 50–1,000 | 70–300 | 2,500–10,000 |
| Spasmodic dysphonia | 0.5–10 | 2–40 | – | 50–150 |
| Limb dystonia | 40–300 | 100–500 | – | 2,000–10,000 |
| Spasticity | 50–540 | 500–1,500 | – | 2,000–10,000 |
| Cerebral palsy | 50–200 | 200–600 | – | 2,000–10,000 |

substantial improvement in toxin purity. This BoTN-A preparation has a lower neurotoxin complex protein load than the original BoTN-A preparation and may reduce antigenic potential. In a double-blind CD trial comparing these two preparations, 133 subjects were treated with original and current bulk toxin sources using a crossover design (26). There were no differences in the preparations regarding efficacy or adverse events (Table 2).

## Dysport®

Dysport has its origin and greatest usage in Europe but is also approved in countries in Asia, South America, and Canada. This toxin has been approved for the treatment of abnormal gait in ambulatory pediatric patients with cerebral palsy and adult spasmodic torticollis, blepharospasm, hemifacial spasm, and in some countries, cosmetic treatment (6) (Table 1) (27,28). This toxin is also used for treating symptoms of spasmodic dysphonia (29), hyperhydrosis (17), headache (30), tremor (31), and sialorrhea (32,33). Injections in monkeys are associated with an onset of response with a delay from two to three days, with maximum effects appearing at day 5 to 6 after the injection. The action duration, measured as a change in the eye alignment, and the muscle paralysis varied from two weeks to eight months (6). Dysport is also stored between 2°C and 8°C and should be used within eight hours after dilution.

Like Botox, injection dosages with Dysport are altered according to muscle size and other considerations (Table 3). Smaller muscles of the face require less toxin

**Table 3** Dosing Considerations

| Increase dosage | Decrease dosage |
|---|---|
| Large body size ( > 80 kg) | Small stature |
| Large muscle mass | Small muscle mass |
| Male gender | Female gender |
| Distant from risk of dysphagia | Injecting SCM, digastric, hypoglossus |
| | Less that 14 yr in age |
| Severe symptoms | Lower facial target |
| | Nerve injury or denervation surgery |
| | Muscle injury (obicularis oculi myectomy) |
| | Anticipate long duration of therapy |
| | Injecting multiple sites (neck and limb) |

than limb or cervical muscles. In a retrospective assessment of patients with hemifacial spasm, a dose range from 28 to 220 U with a mean dosage of 92 ± 29.4 U was reported (25). The average duration of benefit from 855 treatments was 3.4 months. The most common side effect was ptosis (22.1%). A number of studies have examined dosage response in the treatment of CD (34–37). An early dose-ranging study of 75 de novo subjects, randomly assigned to receive placebo or doses of 250, 500, and 1000 U Dysport, demonstrated that significant decreases in the modified Tsui score were at week 4 for the 500 and 1000 unit groups versus placebo ($p < 0.05$) (34). The time to benefit was eight days for all actively treated groups, with the 500 and 1000 U group demonstrating benefit at both four and eight weeks. Despite the improved efficacy at 1000 U, these authors suggest an initial starting dose of 500 U Dysport to avoid the significant increase in neck muscle weakness and voice changes seen at the higher dosage. In an earlier placebo-controlled study of 68 patients, Wissel et al. found that the subjects receiving 500 U demonstrated significant differences in terms of responder rate, pain, and head posture, when compared to placebo at four and eight weeks after the procedure (35). The results of a pivotal trial in the United States show similar benefit when 80 subjects were randomized to Dysport 500 U or placebo. In this 20-week trial, statistically significant benefit was seen at 4, 8, and 12 weeks, with similar incidence of adverse events (36). In a long-term analysis of 616 patients, 303 patients with CD demonstrated sustained benefit (37). The most common adverse event was dysphagia, occurring on average 9.7 days after injection and averaging 3.5 weeks. Secondary loss of response was seen in approximately 5% of patients with neutralizing serum antibodies in 2% (Table 2).

## BOTULINUM TOXIN B

In 2000, a botulinum toxin type B (BoTN-B) product (Myobloc$^{TM}$) was approved by the FDA in the United States for the treatment of CD (38) and, similar to BoTN-A, it is also used to treat blepharospasm, oromandibular dystonia, hemifacial spasm, tremor, tics (39), limb dystonia, spasticity (40), spasmodic dysphonia (41), sialorrhea (42), hyperhydrosis (43), facial lines (44,45), anal fissure (46), and bladder difficulties (47). This product also received marketing authorization from the European Union Committee for Proprietary Medicinal Products as Neurobloc. Myobloc Injectable Solution is a sterile liquid formulation of a purified neurotoxin, produced by fermentation of the bacterium *C. botulinum* type B, and is a clear, colorless, sterile solution in single-use vials containing 2500 U, 5000 U, or 10,000 U. The diluent also contains 0.05% human albumin, 0.01 M sodium succinate, and 0.1 M sodium chloride at approximately pH 5.6 and does not require reconstitution prior to injection (38).

Like BoTN-A, dosing should vary with muscle size and potential for side effects. Although no controlled trial data for blepharospasm or hemifacial spasm are available, Adler et al. have reported the effects of BoTN-B in the treatment of adductor spasmodic dysphonia in a single-site, open-label, dose-finding study in 13 patients (41). At the eight-week assessment, no benefit was seen in 3 subjects receiving 50 U, 1 of 3 patients receiving 100 U, and 8 of 10 patients receiving 200 U. Breathiness was the most common side effect.

An initial dose-ranging study in CD randomized 122 subjects to receive intramuscular injections of either BoTN-B (2500, 5000, or 10,000 U) or placebo (48). Concurrent trials comparing placebo to 5000 U or 10,000 U, or placebo to 10,000 U demonstrated significant benefit at week 4, which continued for both active treatment arms through the 12-week assessment period (49,50). Dry mouth and dysphagia were reported more frequently in the treated groups (51). A long-term efficacy and safety study of BoTN-B in the CD population, examining 10 repeated dosing sessions in 34 patients receiving doses from 10,000 to 25,000 U, demonstrated continued benefit in all subjects. Interestingly, the magnitude of response and dry mouth frequency decreased with each session, while flu-like symptoms and weakness increased (Table 2) (52).

## TOXIN DOSAGE SELECTION

When considering injection of facial muscles, dosage effects to these small muscles are more likely to produce targeted muscle weakness beyond a therapeutic intent, and added caution should be used (53). Weakness from injections of cervical and limb musculature is more likely to result from poorly targeted sites or from injection of unaffected muscles. However, diffusion also occurs, and in the neck, most seriously, will produce dysphagia or dysarthria. In rare, and serious, instances, a feeding tube may be required. Dysphagia has been reported more commonly with BoTN-B and may be a result of both weakness and decreased saliva production.

Prior to toxin injection, particularly at the initial procedure, it is important to provide the patient with expectations of the procedure, including the typical time of onset, time to peak effect, and duration of benefit. In some instances, a simple drawing of a dose–response curve is helpful to illustrate the desired response versus under- or overtreated response (Fig. 1). This approach allows a patient some understanding of the importance of dosage, and may allow for better dosage communication in future sessions.

Although each toxin should be dosed independently of other toxin response, there are some common features influencing dosage selection (Table 3). In general,

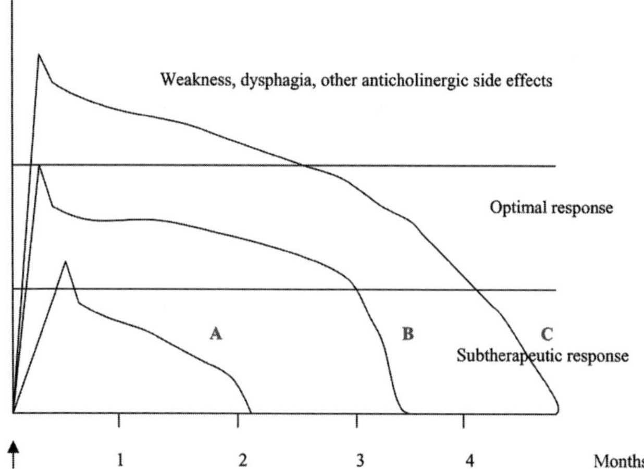


**Figure 1** *Curve A*: Dose too low. A delay in benefit for two weeks with less than two weeks benefit. Consider a 30% increase at the next scheduled injection session. *Note*: Injections prior to the scheduled three months increases the risk of the development of antibodies. *Curve B*: Ideal response. A kick-in at one week with a three-month benefit. No change in future dosing. *Curve C*: Dose too high. The patient would report a brisk response within one week, with weakness for three months, and response for more than four months. Consider at least 30% decrease after recovery from the prior treatment.

it is always better to initiate toxin therapy with a conservative dosing choice and increase the dosage to maximal benefit. Recording a time of onset, time to peak benefit (or best response), and duration of benefit is useful in determining whether a dose may be increased. In addition, a report of side effects, with both day of onset and duration of the symptom, will assist in determining the amount of decrease at the next dosage (Fig. 1). A typical, and desired response from any injection session would be an initial response within five to seven days (BoTN-A) or two to three days (BoTN-B), and a duration of benefit beyond 10 weeks. Increasing the dosage 10% to 20% may produce a benefit of two to four weeks' duration but may also produce adverse events. A 30% increase in dosage may be necessary if a duration of benefit is less than four weeks. Patients reporting weakness as an adverse event usually require dosage reduction. In patients reporting a complication beyond four weeks, a dosage reduction of at least 30% is recommended (Table 4).

## SIDE EFFECTS AND SAFETY

The most common side effect of BoTN injection is directly related to its action, muscle weakness. Given the intended action of the agent is to weaken a targeted muscle, clearly a dosage beyond the therapeutic range of benefit will produce weakness. In addition, diffusion of toxin to adjacent muscles will also lead to weakness, as well as injection of an unintended or, simply, wrongly identified muscle will produce this side effect. Patients with excessive weakness from amytrophic lateral sclerosis, neuromuscular junction disorders, or severe myopathy should not be treated with intramuscular BoTN. In addition, individuals being treated with aminoglycoside antibiotics, because of the effect on neuromuscular transmission, should not receive toxin injections (53).

**Table 4** Dosing Algorithm

| | | |
|---|---|---|
| Initial injection | | |
| Choose low end of dosing range for toxin and indication | | |
| Increase based on size of the patient and the muscle to be injected | | |
| Use increased caution: anterior neck > periorbitally > lower face > limb | | |
| Follow-up injection dosage determination | Increase | Decrease |
| Time to response | | |
| >2 wk | Mild | |
| >4 wk | Moderate | |
| Duration of response | | |
| <8 wk | Mild | |
| <4 wk | Moderate | |
| Side effect duration | | |
| Weakness | | |
| <1 wk | | Mild |
| >2 wk | | Moderate |
| Mild dysphagia | | |
| <1 wk | | Mild |
| >1 wk | | Moderate |
| No benefit | | |
| Consider technique, muscle selection. If prior response to injections, consider neutralizing antibodies | | |

Other side effects from toxin injections are similar to any procedure associated with needle puncture. These include pain, bleeding, soreness, or bruising (50). While anticoagulant therapy is not an absolute contraindication to therapeutic injections, added caution should be used. Patients treated with aspirin may be able to hold this agent for two days prior to the procedure—especially if undergoing treatment for blepharospasm. Care should be taken during the injection procedure to avoid needle insertion in an area of increased vascularity, edema, or inflammation. Changing to a 30-gauge needle, after drawing up the solution, and using care from the point of needle insertion to removal may reduce these unintended complications.

Some patients with CD may report pain beginning several days after the procedure; this may result from inflammation at the infusion site or, perhaps, from weakness or postural change associated with decreased muscle tone. This pain usually will respond to several days of treatment with anti-inflammatory medications.

Because BoTN is rapidly internalized at the neuromuscular junction, systemic side effects from toxin injections are exceedingly rare. Single fiber EMG has demonstrated subtle neuromuscular transmission alterations at sites remote from targeted muscles, but these are not clinically significant (54). BoTN-B, particularly at higher dosages, may have an increased capacity to influence autonomic cholinergic synapses and may produce more noticeable symptoms of dry mouth, blurred vision, and GI symptoms such as heartburn or constipation (55). Racette et al. have reported a subject who developed ptosis and blurred vision after treatment with BoTN-B for CD (56). While intramuscular injection of BoTN is not likely to produce remote side effects, unintended toxin infusion to local blood vessels or nerves would potentially produce harmful results. In addition, patients with hypersensitivity to any of the ingredients in a toxin vial should not receive these products (57). The fetal risk of BoTN in pregnancy is unknown, but successful and safe treatment with Botox has been reported (58). Long-term safety data with Botox, Dysport, and Myobloc are extensive, and more specific information may be found in the package inserts for each product (5,6,38).

## ANTIBODY FORMATION

The development of resistance to BoTN therapy is an area of concern when treating patients with these biological agents. In general, limiting treatment sessions to no more often than every three months and not exceeding dosage recommendations for each session will reduce the risk of treatment failure from antibodies to these agents. It is important to emphasize that not all treatment failures are from neutralizing antibody formation, and prior to serious consideration of this rare development, an injector should review other causes of treatment failure. Most often, these issues relate to the effective dosing of the intended muscles, either from selected dosage amounts or from the toxin not reaching the affected muscle (59). A retrospective analysis of 90 CD patients, 10 years beyond the initial BoTN-A treatment, found that 57 (63%) remained on toxin therapy, with loss of response in only three subjects (Table 4).

While neutralizing antibodies are rarely reported with all of the botulinum toxins, some suggest that antibodies may be a function of accompanying protein in each vial (53). Jankovic et al. have carefully compared the differences between the original and second-generation formulations of Botox (60). In this retrospective analysis, the authors found neutralizing antibodies in 4 of 42 (9.5%) subjects exposed only to the original Botox and none in the 119 subjects treated only with the current Botox ($p < 0.004$). These authors emphasized that the differences seen in the rate of antibody formation reflected the 25 ng protein in each of the original preparation as opposed to 5 ng of protein in the current formulation (61). This same group has analyzed longitudinal follow-up data on 45 patients receiving Botox treatments continuously for at least 12 years (62). While the duration and response to treatment did not change in this group, the dose per visit did significantly increase. In addition, 20 adverse events occurred in 16 of 45 (35.6%) patients after their initial visit and 11 adverse events in 10 of 45 (22.2%) patients at their most recent injection visit. Antibody testing was carried out in 22 patients due to nonresponsiveness, and antibodies were confirmed in 4 of 22 (18%) patients. Of the nonantibody subjects, 16 resumed responsiveness after dose adjustments, and 2 persisted as nonrespondents. Although none of the subjects followed in this clinic developed resistance to the new toxin preparation, one subject has been reported in another center (63). Rollnik et al. compared 6 antibody-positive with 12 antibody-negative CD patients treated with BoTN-A (Dysport) and found significant differences in cumulative dose ($5984 \pm 3151$ U for nonresponders vs. $3143 \pm 1294$ U for responders; $p < 0.05$) and age (mean age $= 41.3 \pm 5.9$ years for nonresponders vs. $56.8 \pm 15.3$ years for responders; $p < 0.05$) (64). Longitudinal experience with Myobloc is less than with these other products, but two patients have been reported to develop antibodies to this agent after an initial injection. These patients received 14,400 and 7200 U, but each had been treated with BoTN-A earlier (65).

## COMPARISON TRIALS

### Botox® Vs. Dysport®

A number of trials have compared the efficacies of Botox versus Dysport. While these trials serve to underscore the difficulties with conversion from one to another using a simple (Botox:Dysport or B:D) 1:3 or 1:4 U ratio, reports suggesting a 1:2 conversion factor seem to be somewhat low. In normal mouse *gastrocnemius* muscle, Wohlfarth et al. have reported a potency ratio of roughly 1:3 (66). Studies comparing these BoTN-A products in small muscles include conditions such as anal fissure (B:D = 1:3) (21), esophageal achalasia (1:2.5) (20), glabellar lines (1:2.5) (67), hemifacial spasm or blepharospasm (1:4) (68), and blepharospasm (1:4) (69,70). An early comparison of Dysport and Botox, using a 4:1 ratio, in the treatment of blepharospasm demonstrated statistically similar duration of response with but a difference in adverse event for Botox (17.0%) and Dysport (24.1%) subjects ($p < 0.05$) (68). In addition, a retrospective analysis of six European sites' published experience with blepharospasm ($n = 45$) and CD (69) patients receiving at least one treatment with each product found a dosing comparison ranging from 1:2 to 1:11. However, all but 13 of the subjects fell into ratios ranging from 1:3 to 1:6, and only 21% below the ratio of 1:4 (70). The mean conversion ratios for all five sites ranged from 1:3.60 to 1:4.88 B:D for both indications.

An early CD trial compared 73 patients randomized to Botox ($n = 35$) or Dysport (37) in approximately a 1:3 ratio (71). The Dysport group received a mean dose of 477 U (range 240–720), and the Botox group received a mean 152 U (range 70–240). Both groups showed substantial and statistically similar improvement with respect to change in Tsui scale with a peak effect at week 4. The duration of benefit was also similar and beyond 80 days for both groups. During the study,

58% of Dysport patients and 69% Botox patients reported adverse events. A later trial compared Botox to Dysport in both 1:3 and 1:4 ratios (72). There were no differences between these groups regarding the primary outcome variable, change in Tsui scale at four weeks. Secondary outcome comparisons suggest greater improvement in pain and duration of response with Dysport, while the frequency of adverse events was also higher with this agent. The most frequent adverse event was dysphagia, found in 3%, 15.6%, and 17.3% (Botox, Dysport 1:3 and 1:4, respectively) of the patients. The mean duration of action was 25 days longer for Dysport 1:4 than for Botox ($p = 0.02$). Published correspondence by Dresser emphasizes the uniqueness of each of these toxins: the potential for greater diffusion of Dysport as possible explanation for the increase in side effects and the 491-day duration of benefit range in the 1:4 group as a confounding factor for the increase in duration of benefit (73). The author response emphasized that this investigation was not designed to compare duration of action between the three preparations and agreed with the suggestion that diffusion rates may explain the differences between adverse events (Table 5) (74).

## Botox® Vs. Xeomin® (NT 201)

While extensive data regarding NT 201 are lacking, the initial studies with this agent suggest a 1:1 ratio with Botox. In normal human volunteers, 4 U of either product produced similar decline in the compound muscle action potential with maximum effect at 7 to 14 days and a continued 40% decline at 90 days postinjection (75). A comparison study in subjects with blepharospasm in 256 completers (304 enrolled) produced similar magnitude of benefit in all outcome measures with equivalent dosages of toxin (76). There were no significant differences in adverse events. In addition, a comparator trial in 463 CD subjects yielded similar (70–300 U) benefit and adverse events (Table 5) (77).

## Botox® Vs. Myobloc®/Neurobloc®

Sloop et al. have provided elegant data concerning dose–response curve for Botox and Myobloc (78). In this human muscle model, 10 healthy volunteers received a randomized dosage of either toxin to the Extensor Digitorum Brevis muscle. A 57-week follow-up demonstrated maximal paralysis two weeks postinjection with 320 to 480 U of BoTN-B was 50 to 75%, and 70 to 80% with 7.5 to 10 U of BoTN-A. BoTN-B–induced paralysis had improved by 66% with complete improvement by 11 weeks postinjection, and BoTN-A–induced paralysis had improved by 6% at 7 weeks, and by 22% at 57 weeks. Small muscle comparison trials for Botox:Myobloc® have been completed within cosmetic indications. Matarasso reports more rapid onset, but shorter duration of action, for the BoTN-B site in ten women randomly assigned to have 15 U BoTN-A injected into one set of lateral canthal rhytides and 750 U BoTN-B into the opposite side, using a 1:50 ratio (79). Lowe et al. compared two dosing ratios, B:M 1:50 or 1:100 U, in treating brow furrows (19). In this trial, BoTN-A doses at 20 U resulted in a 16-week benefit after onset at 3 to 7 days, while BoTN-B 1000 and 2000 U resulted in a 6- to 8-week or 10- to 12-week benefit, respectively, and a shorter time to onset at 2 to 3 days.

There have been two studies assessing Myobloc and Botox equivalencies. Blitzer treated 32 patients with adductor spasmodic dysphonia by starting with a 1:50 Botox:Myobloc conversion of 1 U of BoTN-A to 50 U of BoTN-B (80). After a

**Table 5** Comparative Clinical Trials

| Trial | Indication | Dosages (*n*) | Benefit | Side effects |
|---|---|---|---|---|
| Jost et al. (75) | Normal EDB | BT: 4 U<br>XM: 4 U | Max = 40%, duration = 90 days | None |
| Sloop et al. (78) | Normal EDB | BT: 10 U<br>MB: 480 U | Max 80%, D > 57 wk<br>Max 80%, D = 11 wk | None |
| Eleopra et al. (82) | APB | BT: 15 U<br>MB: 1500 U | No difference<br>1:100 ratio | None |
| Blitzer (80) | Spasmodic dysphonia | BT: 1<br>MB: 50 | O = 3.2 days D = 17 wk<br>O = 2.1 days D = 10.8 wk | MB—dry mouth |
| Nussgens and Roggenkamper (68) | Blepharospasm | BT: 45.4 ± 14.3 U<br>DP: 182.1 ± 55.1 U | No difference in benefit or duration | All AE DP > BT 0.05<br>Ptosis DP > BT 0.01 |
| Marchetti et al. (70) | Blepharospasm (*n* = 45) | BT: 28–40 U<br>DP: 88–111 U | 82% used ratio<br>BT:DP > 1:3 | Ptosis = 12, total = 5<br>Ptosis = 29, total = 42 |
| Marchetti et al. (70) | Cervical dystonia (*n* = 70) | BT: 106–156 U<br>DP: 399–817 U | BT:DP range by site: 1:3.6–4.9 | Dysphagia = 12, total = 16<br>Dysphagia = 19, total = 32 |
| Benecke et al. (77) | Cervical dystonia | BT:XM 1:1 | No difference | No difference |
| Ranoux et al. (72) | Cervical dystonia | BT:<br>DP: 1:3<br>DP: 1:4 | Benefit/pain<br>*p* = 0.02/.04<br>*p* = 0.01/.02 | Dysphagia 3%<br>Dysphagia 15.6%<br>Dysphagia 17.3% |
| Odergren et al. (71) | Cervical dystonia | BT: 152 ± 45 U,<br>DY: 477 ± 131 U | Peak 4 wk, duration > 80 days | No difference |
| Sampaio et al. (69) | Cervical dystonia | BT<br>DY = 4:1 | Duration = 11.2 wk; booster = 12%<br>Duration = 13.3 wk; booster = 23% | AE = 47%<br>AE = 50% |
| Comella et al. (81) | Cervical dystonia (*n*=122) | BT: 205 U<br>MB:8520 U | Duration 14.0w<br>Duration 12.1 w | MB > dysphagia drymouth |
| Matassaro et al. (79) | Canthal rhytids | BT: 15 U<br>MB: 750 U | No difference | None |
| Lowe et al. (67) | Brow furrows | BT: 20 U<br>MB: 1000 U<br>MB: 2000 U | 16 wk<br>6–8 wk<br>10–12 wk | None |

(*Continued*)

**Table 5** Comparative Clinical Trials (*Continued*)

| Trial | Indication | Dosages ($n$) | Benefit | Side effects |
|---|---|---|---|---|
| Lowe et al. (19) | Glabellar lines | BT: 20<br>DP: 50 | No difference | None |
| Anesse et al. (20) | Achalasia | BT: 100 U<br>DP: 250 U | No difference in 1-mo change or benefit duration | None |
| Brisinda et al. (21) | Anal fissure | BT: 50 U<br>DP: 150 U | 2-mo eval, similar benefit | Mild flatus incontinence |

*Abbreviations*: BT, Botox®; DP, Dysport®; MB, Myobloc™; XM, Xeomin®; EDB, extensor digitorum brevis; APB, abductor pollicis brevis; AE, adverse events.

one-year process of dosage adjustment, a conversion ratio was found to be 52.3:1 U. The onset of action of type B was more rapid [2.09 days vs. 3.2 days ($p = 0.028$)], with a shorter duration of benefit [10.8 weeks vs. 17 weeks ($P = 0.002$)]. The Dystonia Study Group compared BoTN-A (Botox) and BoTN-B (Myobloc) in the treatment of CD (81). Subjects were randomly assigned to treatment with BoTN-A (up to 250 units) or BoTN-B (up to 10,000 units). A total of 122 subjects (BoTN-A, $n = 63$; BoTN-B, $n = 59$) were enrolled in the study. The Toronto Western Spasmotic Torticollis Rating Scale (TWSTRS) did not differ at baseline [mean 42.7 (SD $\pm$9.7)], or at the time of maximal effect. BoTN-A (14 weeks) had a longer duration of clinical effect than BoTN-B (12.1 weeks, $p = 0.025$). Dysphagia and dry mouth were greater following BoTN-B ($p < 0.05$). Although the maximum dosage for each arm resulted in a B:M ratio of 1:40, the actual dosage ratio was slightly higher (81) with BoTN-A 205 U (range 75–250) and BoTN-B 8,520 U (range 1520–12,000). While the frequency and severity of adverse events were similar for most groups, the BoTN-B group did have greater frequency and severity of dysphagia and dry mouth (Table 5).

## CONCLUSION

Treating patients with dystonic and other motor disorders with BoTN may be extremely rewarding. While toxins differ in dosing units and response profiles, successful treatment remains dependent upon identifying the correct muscle or muscles producing the dystonic posture and reaching that muscle with a needle to infuse toxin. If these tasks are accomplished, toxin dosing may be determined by beginning with a conservative initial dosage and upwardly titrating to optimal response at scheduled three-month injection intervals. The goal for each injection session should then be simply: three-month resolution of dystonic muscle spasm with no toxin-related side effects.

The choice of toxin is often dependent upon external market forces, such as regulatory approval and patient insurance carrier approval, as well as injector preference. However, each of these preparations exhibits differences in molecular size, diffusion characteristics, antibody potential, and efficacy profile. Because of the relatively low prevalence of dystonia, and therefore fewer opportunities to try alternate toxin approaches, becoming highly familiar with the response of one toxin type may be advantageous to a physician with a small patient population.

## REFERENCES


1. Scott AB. Development of botulinum toxin therapy. Dermatol Clin 2004; 22:131–133.
2. Schantz EJ, Johnson EA. Preparation and characterization of Botulinum Toxin Type A for Human Treatment. In: Jankovic J, Hallett M, eds. Therapy with Botulinum Toxin. Marcel Dekker, Inc., 1994:41–50.
3. Jankovic J. Botulinum toxin in clinical practice. J Neurol Neurosurg Psychiatry 2004; 75(7):951–957.
4. Jankovic J, Brin MF. Therapeutic uses of botulinum toxin. N Engl J Med 1991; 324: 1186–1194.
5. Botox®. Package insert.
6. Dysport®. Package insert.
7. Jost WH. Other indications of botulinum toxin therapy. Eur J Neurol 2006; 13(suppl 1): 65–69.
8. Cheng CM, Chen JS, Patel RP. Unlabeled uses of botulinum toxins: a review, part 1. Am J Health Syst Pharm 2006; 63:145–152.
9. Cheng CM, Chen JS, Patel RP. Unlabeled uses of botulinum toxins: a review, part 2. Am J Health Syst Pharm 2006; 63:225–232.
10. Brin MF, Lyons KE, Doucette J, et al. A randomized, double masked, controlled trial of botulinum toxin type A in essential hand tremor. Neurology 2001; 56:1523–1528.
11. Jankovic J, Schwartz K, Clement W, Aswad A, Mordaunt J. A randomized, double-blind, placebo-controlled study to evaluate botulinum toxin type A in essential hand tremor. Mov Disord 1996; 11:250–256.
12. Dodick, DW, Mauskop A, Elkind AH, De Gryse R, Brin MF, Silberstein SD, Botox® Study Group. Botulinum toxin type a for the prophylaxis of chronic daily headache: subgroup analysis of patients not receiving other prophylactic medications: a randomized double-blind, placebo-controlled study. Headache 2005; 45:315–324.
13. Schulte-Mattler WJ, Martinez-Castrillo JC. Botulinum toxin therapy of migraine and tension-type headache: comparing different botulinum toxin preparations. Eur J Neurol 2006; 13(suppl 1):51–54.
14. Brin MF, Stewart, Blitzer, Diamond B. Laryngeal botulinum toxin injections for disabling stuttering in adults. Neurology 1994; 44:2262–2266.
15. Lagalla G, Millevolte M, Capecci M, Provinciali L, Ceravolo MG. Botulinum toxin type A for drooling in Parkinson's disease: a double-blind, randomized, placebo-controlled study. Mov Disord 2006; [Epub ahead of print].
16. Connor KM, Cook JL, Davidson JR. Botulinum toxin treatment of social anxiety disorder with hyperhidrosis: a placebo-controlled double-blind trial. J Clin Psychiatry 2006; 67:30–36.
17. Schlereth T, Mouka I, Eisenbarth G, Winterholler M, Birklein F. Botulinum toxin A (Botox®) and sweating-dose efficacy and comparison to other BoTN preparations. Auton Neurosci 2005; 117:120–126.
18. Lang AM. A preliminary comparison of the efficacy and tolerability of botulinum toxin serotypes A and B in the treatment of myofascial pain syndrome: a retrospective, open-label chart review. Clin Ther 2003; 25:2268–2278.
19. Lowe PL, Patnaik R, Lowe NJ. A comparison of two botulinum type a toxin preparations for the treatment of glabellar lines: double-blind, randomized, pilot study. Dermatol Surg 2005; 31:1651–1654.
20. Annese V, Bassotti G, Coccia G, et al. Comparison of two different formulations of botulinum toxin A for the treatment of oesophageal achalasia. The Gismad Achalasia Study Group. Aliment Pharmacol Ther 1999; 13:1347–1350.
21. Brisinda G, Albanese A, Cadeddu F, et al. Botulinum neurotoxin to treat chronic anal fissure: results of a randomized "Botox® vs. Dysport®" controlled trial. Ailment Pharmacol Ther 2004; 19:695–701.
22. Moore C, Rackley R, Goldman H. Urologic applications of botox. Curr Urol Rep 2005; 6:419–423.

23. Greene P, Kang U, Fahn S, Brin M, Moskowitz C, Flaster E. Double-blind, placebo-controlled trial of botulinum toxin injections for the treatment of spasmodic torticollis. Neurology 1990; 40:1213–1218.
24. Brashear A, Hogan P, Wooten-Watts M, Marchetti A, Maga R, Martin J. Longitudinal assessment of the dose consistency of botulinum toxin type A (BOTOX®) for cervical dystonia. Adv Ther 2005; 22:49–55.
25. Hsiung GY, Das SK, Ranawaya R, Lafontaine AL, Suchowersky O. Long-term efficacy of botulinum toxin A in treatment of various mov disord over a 10-year period. Mov Disord 2002; 17:1288–1293.
26. Naumann M, Yakovleff A, Durif F; Botox® Cervical Dystonia Prospective Study Group. A randomized, double-masked, crossover comparison of the efficacy and safety of botulinum toxin type A produced from the original bulk toxin source and current bulk toxin source for the treatment of cervical dystonia. J Neurol 2002; 249:57–63.
27. Jipimolmard S, Tiamkao S, Laopaiboon M. Long term results of botulinum toxin type A (Dysport®) in the treatment of hemifacial spasm: a report of 175 cases. J Neurol Neurosurg Psychiatry 1988; 64:751–757.
28. Ascher B, Azkine B, Kestemont P, Baspeyras M, Bougara A, Santini J. A multicenter, randomized, double-blind, placebo-controlled study of efficacy and safety of 3 doses of botulinum toxin A in the treatment of glabellar lines. J Am Acad Dermatol 2004; 51:223–233.
29. Galardi G, Guerriero R, Amadio S, et al. Sporadic failure of botulinum toxin treatment in usually responsive patients with adductor spasmodic dysphonia. Neurol Sci 2001; 22:303–306.
30. Rollnik JD, Dengler R. Botulinum toxin (DYSPORT®) in tension-type headaches. Acta Neurochir Suppl 2002; 79:123–126.
31. Wissel J, Masuhr, Schelosky L, Ebersbach G, Poewe W. Quantitative assessment of botulinum toxin treatment in 43 patients with head tremor. Mov Disord 1997; 12:722–726.
32. Mancini F, Zangaglia R, Cristina S, et al. Double-blind, placebo-controlled study to evaluate the efficacy and safety of botulinum toxin type A in the treatment of drooling in parkinsonism. Mov Disord 2003; 18:685–688.
33. Lipp A, Trottneberg T, Schink T, Kupsh A, Arnold G. A randomized trial of botulinum toxin A for treatment of drooling. Neurology 2003; 61:1279–1281.
34. Poewe W, Deuschl G, Nebe A, et al. What is the optimal dose of botulinum toxin A in the treatment of cervical dystonia? Results of a double blind, placebo controlled, dose ranging study using Dysport®. German Dystonia Study Group. J Neurol Neurosurg Psychiatry 1998; 64:13–17.
35. Wissel J, Kanovsky P, Ruzicka E, et al. Efficacy and safety of a standardised 500 unit dose of Dysport® (clostridium botulinum toxin type A haemaglutinin complex) in a heterogeneous cervical dystonia population: results of a prospective, multicentre, randomised, double-blind, placebo-controlled, parallel group study. J Neurol 2001; 248:1073–1078.
36. Truong D, Duane DD, Jankovic J, et al. Efficacy and safety of botulinum type A toxin (Dysport®) in cervical dystonia: results of the first US randomized, double-blind, placebo-controlled study. Mov Disord 2005; 20:783–791.
37. Kessler KR, Skuta M, Benecke R. Long-term treatment of cervical dystonia with botulinum toxin A: efficacy, safety, and antibody frequency. German Dystonia Study Group. J Neurol 1999; 246:265–274.
38. Myohloc™ Package insert.
39. Wan XH, Vuong KD, Jankovic J. Clinical application of botulinum toxin type B in movement disorders and autonomic symptoms. Chin Med Sci J 2005; 20:44–47.
40. Brashear A, McAfee AL, Kuhn ER, Fyffe J. Botulinum toxin type B in upper-limb poststroke spasticity: a double-blind, placebo-controlled trial. Arch Phys Med Rehabil 2004; 85:705–709.
41. Adler CH, Bansberg SF, Krein-Jones K, Hentz JG. Safety and efficacy of botulinum toxin type B (MyoblocÔ) in adductor spasmodic dysphonia. Mov Disord 2004; 19:1075–1079.
42. Ondo WG, Hunter C, Moore W. A double-blind placebo-controlled trial of botulinum toxin B for sialorrhea in Parkinson's disease. Neurology 2004; 62:37–40.

43. Baumann L, Slezinger A, Halem M, et al. Pilot study of the safety and efficacy of MyoblocÔ (botulinum toxin type B) for treatment of axillary hyperhidrosis. Int J Dermatol 2005; 44:418–424.
44. Baumann L, Slezinger A, Vujevich J, et al. A double-blinded, randomized, placebo-controlled pilot study of the safety and efficacy of Myobloc® (botulinum toxin type B)-purified neurotoxin complex for the treatment of crow's feet: a double-blinded, placebo-controlled trial. Dermatol Surg 2003; 29:508–515.
45. Sadick NS. Prospective open-label study of botulinum toxin type B (MyoblocÔ) at doses of 2,400 and 3,000 U for the treatment of glabellar wrinkles. Dermatol Surg 2003; 29: 501–507.
46. Jost WH. Botulinum toxin type B in the treatment of anal fissures: first preliminary results. Dis Colon Rectum 2001; 44:1721–1722.
47. Ghei M, Maraj BH, Miller R, et al. Effects of botulinum toxin B on refractory detrusor overactivity: a randomized, double-blind, placebo controlled, crossover trial. J Urol 2005; 174:1873–1877.
48. Lew MF, Adornato BT, Duane DD, et al. Botulinum toxin type B: a double-blind, placebo-controlled, safety and efficacy study in cervical dystonia. Neurology 1997; 49: 701–707.
49. Brashear A, Lew MF, Dykstra DD, et al. Safety and efficacy of Neurobloc® (botulinum toxin type B) in type A-responsive cervical dystonia. Neurology 1999; 53:1439–1446.
50. Brin MF, Lew MF, Adler CH, et al. Safety and efficacy of Neurobloc® (botulinum toxin type B) in type A-resistant cervical dystonia. Neurology 1999; 53:1431–1438.
51. Lew MF, Brashear A, Factor S. The safety and efficacy of botulinum toxin type B in the treatment of patients with cervical dystonia: summary of three controlled clinical trials. Neurology 2000; 12(suppl 5):S29–S35.
52. Factor SA, Molho ES, Evans S, Feustel PJ. Efficacy and safety of repeated doses of botulinum toxin type B in type A resistant and responsive cervical dystonia. Mov Disord 2005; 20:1152–1160.
53. Brin MF, Dressler D, Aoki RK. Pharmacology of Botulinum Toxin Therapy. In: Brin MF, Comella CL, Jankovic J, eds. Dystonia: Etiology, Clinical Features, and Treatment. Philadelphia: Lippincott Williams & Wilkins, 2004:93–112.
54. Girlanda P, Vita G, Nicolosi C, Milone S, Messina C. Botulinum toxin therapy: distant effects on neuromuscular transmission and autonomic nervous system. J Neurol Neurosurg Psychiatry 1992; 55:844–845.
55. Tintner R, Gross R, Winzer UF, Smalky KA, Jankovic J. Autonomic function after botulinum toxin type A or B: a double-blind, randomized trial. Neurology 2005; 65:765–767.
56. Racette BA, Lopate G, Good L, Sagitto S, Perlmutter JS. Ptosis as a remote effect of therapeutic botulinum toxin B injection. Neurology 2002; 59(9):1445–1447.
57. Li M, Goldberger BA, Hopkins C. Fatal case of BOTOX-related anaphylaxis? J Forensic Sci 2005; 50:169–172.
58. Newman WJ, Davis TL, Padaliya BB, et al. Botulinum toxin type A therapy during pregnancy. Mov Disord 2004; 19:1384–1385.
59. Haussermann P, Marczoch S, Klinger C, Landgrebe M, Conrak B, Ceballos-Baumann A. Long-term follow-up of cervical dystonia patients treated with botulinum toxin A. Mov Disord 2004; 19:303–308.
60. Jankovic J, Vuong KD, Ahsan J. Comparison of efficacy and immunogenicity of original versus current botulinum toxin in cervical dystonia. Neurology 2003; 60:1186–1188.
61. Mejia NI, Vuong KD, Jankovic J. Long-term botulinum toxin efficacy, safety, and immunogenicity. Mov Disord 2005; 20:592–597.
62. Racette BA, Stambuk M, Perlmutter JS. Secondary nonresponsiveness to new bulk botulinum toxin A (BCB2024). Mov Disord 2002; 17:1098–1100.
63. Goschel H, Wohlfarth K, Frevert J, Dengler R, Bigalke H. Botulinum A toxin therapy: neutralizing and nonneutralizing antibodies–therapeutic consequences. Exp Neurol 1997; 147:96–102.

64. Rollnik JD, Wohlfarth K, Dengler R, Bigalke H. Neutralizing botulinum toxin type a antibodies: clinical observations in patients with cervical dystonia. Neurol Clin Neurophysiol 2001; 2001:2–4.
65. Dressler D, Bigalke H, Benecke R. Botulinum toxin type B in antibody-induced botulinum toxin type a therapy failure. J Neurol 2003; 250:967–969.
66. Wohlfarth K, Kampe K, Bigalke H. Pharmacokinetic properties of different formulations of botulinum neurotoxin type A. Mov Disord 2004; 19(suppl 8):S65–67.
67. Lowe NJ, Yamauchi PS, Lasik GP, Patnaik R, Moore D. Botulinum toxins types A and B for brow furrows: preliminary experiences with type B toxin dosing. J Cosmet Laser Ther 2002; 4:15–18.
68. Nussgens Z, Roggenkamper P. Comparison of two botulinum-toxin preparations in the treatment of essential blepharospasm. Graefes Arch Clin Exp Ophthalmol 1997; 235:197–199.
69. Sampaio C, Ferreira JJ, Simoes F, et al. DYSBOT: a single-blind, randomized parallel study to determine whether any differences can be detected in the efficacy and tolerability of two formulations of botulinum toxin type A—Dysport® and Botox®–assuming a ratio of 4:1. Mov Disord 1997; 12:1013–1018.
70. Marchetti A, Magar R, Findley L, et al. Retrospective evaluation of the dose of Dysport® and BOTOX® in the management of cervical dystonia and blepharospasm: the REAL DOSE study. Mov Disord 2005; 20:937–944.
71. Odergren T, Hjaltason H, Kaakkola S, et al. A double blind, randomised, parallel group study to investigate the dose equivalence of Dysport® and Botox® in the treatment of cervical dystonia. J Neurol Neurosurg Psychiatry 1998; 64:6–12.
72. Ranoux D, Gury C, Fondarai J, Mas JL, Zuber M. Respective potencies of Botox® and Dysport®: a double blind, randomised, crossover study in cervical dystonia. J Neurol Neurosurg Psychiatry 2002; 72:459–462.
73. Dressler D. Correspondence: Dysport produces intrinsically more swallowing problems than Botox: unexpected results from a conversion factor study in cervical dystonia. J Neurol Neurosurg Psychiatry 2002; 73:604.
74. Ranoux D, Zuber M, Gury C. Author's reply: Dysport produces intrinsically more swallowing problems than Botox: unexpected results from a conversion factor study in cervical dystonia. J Neurol Neurosurg Psychiatry 2002; 73:604.
75. Jost WH, Kohl A, Brinkmann S, Comes G. Efficacy and tolerability of a botulinum toxin type A free of complexing proteins (NT 201) compared with commercially available botulinum toxin type A (BOTOX®) in healthy volunteers. J Neural Transm 2005; 112:905–913.
76. Roggenkamper P, Jost WH, Bihari K, Comes G. Efficacy and safety of a new botulinum toxin type A free of complexing proteins in the treatment of blepharospasm. J Neural Transm 2006; 113:303–312.
77. Benecke R, Jost WH, Kanovsky P, Ruzicka E, Comes G, Grafe S. A new botulinum toxin type A free of complexing proteins for treatment of cervical dystonia. Neurology 2005; 64:1949–1951.
78. Sloop RR, Cole BA, Escuitin RO. Human response to botulinum toxin injection: type B compared with type A. Neurology 1997; 49:189–194.
79. Matarasso SL. Comparison of botulinum toxin types A and B: a bilateral and double-blind randomized evaluation in the treatment of canthal rhytides. Dermatol Surg 2003; 29:7–13.J Neurol Neurosurg Psychiatry 2002; 73:604.
80. Blitzer A. Botulinum toxin A and B: a comparative dosing study for spasmodic dysphonia. Otolaryngol Head Neck Surg 2005; 133:836–838.
81. Comella CL, Jankovic J, Shannon KM, et al. Dystonia Study Group. Comparison of botulinum toxin serotypes A and B for the treatment of cervical dystonia. Neurology 2005; 65:1423–1429.
82. Eleopra R, Tugnoli V, Quatrale R, Rossetto O, Montecucco C. Different types of botulinum toxin in humans. Mov Disord 2004; 19(suppl 8):S53–S59.

# 24
# Phenol Injections in Dystonia

**Lauren C. Seeberger**
*Colorado Neurological Institute Movement Disorders Center, Englewood, and Department of Neurology, University of Colorado Health Sciences Center, Denver, Colorado, U.S.A.*

## INTRODUCTION

Phenol, carbolic acid, is one of the earliest known disinfectant substances, and is an extremely astringent antiseptic, capable of sterilizing to the point of cauterizing wounds. Shortly following Louis Pasteur's discovery that microorganisms caused infection, Joseph Lister (1827–1912) demonstrated that the use of carbolic acid to sterilize surgical instruments and dress wounds produced a state of asepsis that greatly reduced postoperative septic mortality. Even today, phenol remains the standard against which new disinfectants are tested.

Phenol kills microorganisms by denaturing proteins and dissolving cell membranes. This corrosive nature has been tamed by dilution to lower concentrations and harnessed for use as a therapeutic agent.

## HISTORICAL BACKGROUND IN THE THERAPEUTIC USE OF PHENOL

The use of intrathecal absolute alcohol in performing chemical rhizotomy to injure nerves and reduce lower body pain, especially cancer-related pain, was widespread in the 1930s and 1940s. This intervention subsequently lost favor because of erratic results and diffuse pathological damage induced by alcohol. It was later felt that phenol would be a superior compound for neurolysis because of certain properties, including greater ease of instillation due to higher viscosity, ability to combine with a radio-opaque material and an initial anesthetic response to guide placement. Thus, phenol has been used therapeutically since the mid-1950s when it was employed for treatment of pain. Maher (1) first administered the compound in a lipid solution into the thecal sac in end-stage cancer patients and found that there was good pain relief. Within four years, physicians were using phenol in the treatment of spasticity, theorizing improvement resulted from disruption of the hyperactive stretch reflex arc. Nathan (2) injected intrathecal phenol into a series of 25 patients with spastic paraplegia using techniques to maximize damage to the targeted nerves with "most satisfactory" results in pain and spasm reduction from the conversion of spastic paralysis to flaccid paralysis. The next several years brought studies in spasticity using lower concentrations of intrathecal phenol, 5% to 10%, with fine results (3,4) and no worsening of weakness (5). Interestingly, about that same time, the first use in movement disorders was reported (1960), when three patients with parkinsonism were noted to have significant improvement in lower extremity tone but no improvement in tremor after intrathecal phenol (6).

### Peripheral Neurolysis

Physicians began instilling phenol directly onto nerves in open surgical procedures or administering the solution percutaneously to peripheral nerves in an effort to expand treatment of spasticity to the upper extremities. Using dilute 2% or 3% aqueous phenol solutions, Khalili et al. reported two series of 39 and 126 blocks in which phenol was injected using nerve stimulation technique in severe spasticity patients (7,8). These interventions had minimal side effects and were felt to be safe and effective. Patients showed improved range of motion and ability to perform activities of daily living, as well as, improved movement, reduction in clonus, and reduced or eliminated need for therapeutic stretching.

### Motor Point Blocks

Muscle motor point block using phenol was undertaken in 1965. This innovation led the way for current use in dystonia. Halpern and Meelhuysen (9) rationalized that if given procaine, a local anesthetic, and alcohol produced a loss of muscle tone with motor point injection, phenol may also be utilized to provide safe, prolonged reduction in hypertonia. The total volume of solution ranged from 0.2 to 3 mL per muscle. There was a correlation between the dosage strength and the outcome with longer effects from 5% and 7% aqueous phenol solutions. The majority of their 39 patients treated had a "good" improvement in function or relaxation of tone and only three patients had a poor result from the intervention. Although predominantly used for spasticity, there have now been several reports of phenol motor point block and direct intramuscular injections in the treatment of dystonia (10–14). Methods are described in the technique section of this chapter.

## PROPERTIES/PREPARATION OF PHENOL

Phenol is a weak acid with bactericidal and fungicidal properties. It is the major oxidized metabolite of benzene. The name is derived from its benzene ring structure and there is an attached hydroxyl group. The –OH bond allows interactions with other phenolic compounds and water, and is highly soluble. Phenol has analgesic properties at low concentration and at higher concentrations can be used as a disinfectant or to destroy nerve tissue. There is a direct correlation between amount of nerve

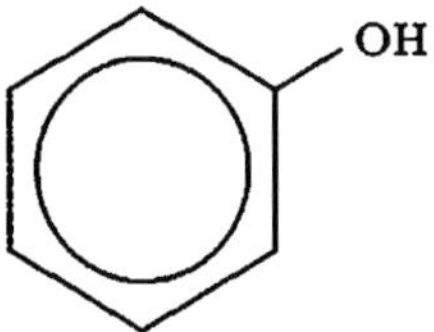

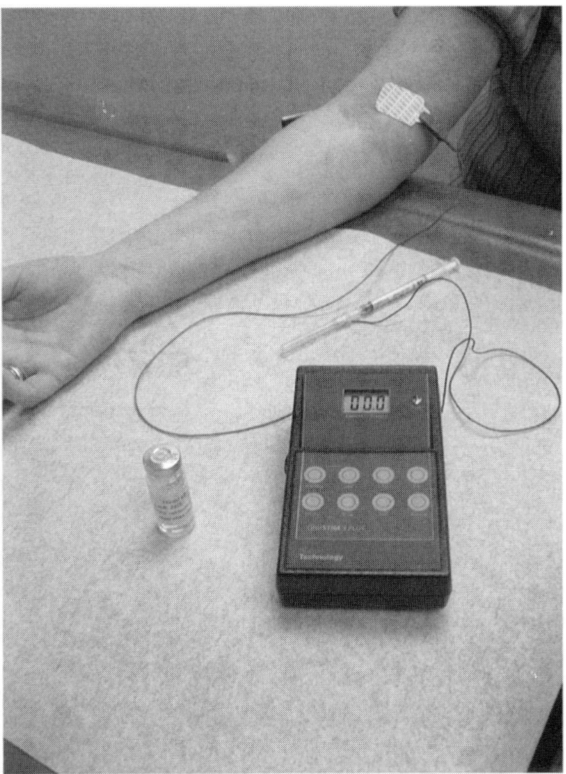

**Figure 1** Equipment setup for phenol block: teflon coated hollow-bore EMG needle, reference electrode with connector, nerve stimulator with rheostat and milliamp readout screen, freshly prepared phenol.

damage and concentration of the solution. Phenol crystals are dissolved in a solvent, usually sterile water or anhydrous glycerin, to achieve the desired concentration. Phenol in glycerin is less caustic than aqueous phenol solutions (15), with a 5% glycerin-based solution having a similar effect on nerves as a 0.1% aqueous solution (16). The most commonly used concentrations of phenol in clinical practice are 3% to 6% (17). Concentrations greater than 8% will show precipitation of solution at room temperature.

After dissolving the phenol crystals in solution, it is then sterilized by heating. Sterilization does not affect its activity. The solution should be clear and colorless without evidence of yellowing or precipitant. It should have a pungent, distinctive odor. Phenol is primarily excreted from the body by the kidney. Exposure to very high concentrations may cause central nervous system dysfunction with tremor, followed by seizures, cardiovascular collapse, and respiratory failure (18). The toxic dose for adult humans is 8 to 15 g.

## MECHANISM OF ACTION AND PATHOLOGICAL STUDIES

Phenol is known to have a high affinity for nervous and cardiovascular tissues. It was initially felt that phenol had activity only on the small-diameter nerve fibers; that its therapeutic activity came from selective involvement of muscle spindle innervation (gamma fibers) with relative preservation of large-diameter fibers serving motor function (7). Histopathological studies in man and cat, however, revealed that the damage from phenol was present irrespective of fiber size with relatively normal fibers lying beside those completely degenerated (19–21). Muscle study following phenol nerve block demonstrates severe neurogenic atrophy (22). Additionally, electromyographic assessment following phenol demonstrates active denervation that indicates destruction of alphamotor fibers (23).

The effect of phenol on nervous tissue is twofold. First, there is a short-term anesthetic effect primarily on small-diameter fibers, e.g., C-fibers, and then a long-term effect from a nonselective block of all fiber types (24). The long-term effect is from blocked neural transmission due to dose-dependent protein denaturation with severe demyelination and Wallerian degeneration in axons of all types. Phenol causes total destruction of some myelin sheaths with proliferation of Schwann cells. As expected, depth of degeneration into the nerve has been shown to be greatest at the injection site and is lessened distal from that point (25). Animal studies suggest peak nerve damage at two weeks with regeneration as early as seven weeks in nerves injected with 10% phenol solution (26–28) and correlates with the temporary benefit from this approach.

Phenol can also be used for blocking muscle motor points. Motor points are typically located at the entry point of the nerve into the muscle, usually near the muscle belly. Intramuscular neurolysis, or motor point block, causes neurogenic muscle atrophy with subsequent reinnervation and regeneration of muscle fibers. There is blockage of small mixed nerves. Diffusion of phenol into nearby muscle fibers also leads to atrophy and inflammatory changes in the muscle fibers themselves. Electron microscope studies confirm that phenol denatures tissue protein (27) including muscle. This damage to muscle fibers through neurogenic mechanisms as well as direct tissue injury weakens the power of contraction. The weakening of a specific muscle is useful to reduce inappropriate muscle tone in dystonia. Thus, motor point blocks and intramuscular phenol injections are used to weaken a specific muscle, such as in dystonia, whereas nerve blocks are used to reduce contractions in a group of muscles innervated by one nerve, e.g., in spasticity.

## CLINICAL APPLICATION OF PHENOL IN DYSTONIA

For those with focal or segmental dystonia, botulinum neurotoxin (BoNT) injections have become the treatment option of choice. Some patients, however, do not respond to BoNT injections. These patients may try medications for ease of their symptoms but many will not obtain optimal relief. In those with cervical or limb dystonia who are nonresponsive to BoNT and who fail medication treatment trials, phenol injections to relax involved muscles are a reasonable therapeutic option.

Massey (11) first reported the use of intramuscular phenol in torticollis. She described two patients, one nonresponsive to BoNT type A and one with intolerable side effects from BoNT type A in whom phenol injections were undertaken. Clinical examination and EMG recording from muscles involved in the abnormal posturing guided the injections. Both patients had considerable pain relief and improved control of head movements. Beneficial effects lasted approximately five to six months and side effects were limited to temporary pain and redness at the injected site. These results were not confirmed in another small series involving three torticollis patients. In this open trial, intramuscular phenol injection produced sustained benefit in one, partial response in one (three months) and a lack of benefit in the last (12) and in retrospect emphasizes that improvement may be highly dependent on technical proficiency with this relatively difficult procedure. Since that time, Massey (29) has reported a much larger series, 56 BoNT-resistant torticollis patients, again using EMG guidance for intramuscular placement. Patients were rated using the Toronto Western Spasmodic Torticollis Rating Scale severity score, physician and patient assessments of head control, and pain. By these three assessments, 45% of patients were moderately to markedly improved; 27% of patients had mild improvement; and 28% failed to improve but were not worse. Follow-up of the patients was from 6 to 46 months. Phenol solution was spread throughout the muscle with 0.5 to 4 mL injected per muscle depending on size. The concentration was 1% to 5% solution with 20 to 25 mL maximum total dose per session. Subsequent EMG testing of the injected muscles demonstrated fibrillations, positive waves, complex repetitive discharges, and abnormal motor unit potentials suggesting a direct muscle effect. Local swelling, erythema, and pain were found in most patients. Also common were temporary dysesthesias over the scalp, neck, and shoulder. Three patients had mild weakness in the arm or shoulder girdle with resolution by six months. Duration of benefit was from four to six months (Tables 1 and 2).

At this time, experience with phenol neurolysis in cervical dystonia using motor point block technique is limited. Takeuchi et al. (14) isolated motor points through surface electrodes then by percutaneous nerve stimulation (see section "Motor Point Blocks"). These authors used phenol blocks in 16 torticollis patients who had failed medication trials and physical rehabilitation (prior to the approval of BoNT in this country). A solution of 2% phenol was administered into one, two, or three active muscles as determined by clinical exam and surface electrode recordings. Volumes of 2.2 mL up to 6.6 mL were given. A blinded rater assessed the patients using the Tsui scale score before and two weeks postphenol injections. The Tsui scale score showed significant reduction following injections with better neck movement and head position. Four patients (25%) had dysesthesia of the anterior neck ipsilateral to the injected *sternocleidomastoid* (SCM) muscle felt secondary to involvement of the transverse cutaneous nerve. The authors suggest avoiding the mid-portion of the SCM to minimize this complication or using a local anesthetic first. An injection of a local anesthetic prior to injecting phenol solution may help gauge expected results from the motor point block.

A report of a single case of idiopathic foot dystonia treated with phenol motor point block expands the use of the agent into treatment of limb dystonia (13). A patient with gait-induced posturing of the left ankle, nonresponsive to BoNT injections, was successfully treated with phenol. The *peroneus longus* and *brevis muscles* were blocked using 5% aqueous phenol solution, 1.0 and 0.5 mL volume, respectively. Sustained gait improvement was reported at one year.

**Table 1** Phenol Use in Cervical Dystonia

| |
|---|
| Nonresponsive botulinum neurotoxin patients |
| 1–5% aqueous phenol solution |
| 0.5–4.0 cc phenol per muscle, dependent on muscle size |
| Maximum recommended dose 20–25 cc/day |
| Several series of injections may be needed to achieve results |
| Duration of benefit 4–6 mo |

**Table 2** Comparison of Botulinum Neurotoxin Vs. Phenol for Dystonia

| | Botulinum neurotoxin | Phenol |
|---|---|---|
| Cost | Expensive | Inexpensive |
| Properties | Neurotoxin | Disinfectant |
| Technique | Palpation or electromyography (EMG) guidance; given every 3 mo | EMG motor end-plate technique or nerve stimulation; given as often as tolerated |
| Side effects | Less common, temporary | Frequent, may be permanent |
| Mechanism of action | Prevents presynaptic acetylcholine release | Destroys myelin nerve sheath and muscle tissue |
| Benefit | Temporary | Mostly temporary |
| Ease of technique | Fairly easy with knowledge of muscle anatomy | Advanced level of nerve type and muscle anatomy; labor intensive, prolonged sessions |
| Safety | Large therapeutic window | Relatively large therapeutic window |
| Resistance | May develop in some patients | None |

## TECHNIQUE

The patient is prepared for the injection by cleansing the skin over the muscle to be targeted. For motor point block, isolation of the motor point insertion into the muscle can be done either by transcutaneous stimulation with a superficial electrode or by direct intramuscular stimulation. There is insulation of the stimulating/recording needle by a Teflon coating except at its beveled end. This limits stimulation or EMG recording to the very tip of the needle. The hollow bore in the needle allows direct injection of phenol from a syringe once placement is confirmed.

### Motor Point Blocks

For motor point blocks, the needle electrode is attached to a nerve stimulator with a manually operated rheostat. The nerve stimulator is capable of delivering 0.2 ms square wave monophasic pulses at repetitions of one every second. Output current is adjustable in 0.1 milliamp (mA) increments with a range from 0 to 6.0 mA. Anatomical knowledge of the approximate points of entry of the motor branches of the nerve into the muscle belly is needed. The needle electrode is then inserted near these points and is slowly advanced while continuously stimulating at 5.0 mA. Once muscle contractions are obtained, the current is reduced to see if the muscle contraction remains as strong at lower stimulation strength. The closer the needle electrode is to the nerve branch the easier it should be to achieve contraction of the muscle. Confirm that the muscle contracting is the target muscle and not multiple muscles supplied by a nearby peripheral nerve. The stimulating current is progressively reduced as the needle approaches the nerve. The motor point is reached when there is a minimal amount of current required to cause the maximum contraction of the muscle. The rheostat reading should be less than or equal to 1 mA while still causing a detectable motor response. This confirms that the needle electrode is in very close proximity to the nerve. After first aspirating to ensure that the needle tip is not intravascular, 0.2 to 0.5 mL of phenol solution are instilled. The patient may complain of a burning sensation for a few seconds after the injection. Within several seconds to a minute there should be a decrease in the contraction of the muscle. If muscle contractions continue with repeat stimulation, then 0.2 to 0.5 mL may be additionally given. At that point, there should be a definite decrease or cessation in the muscle contractions. If the muscle is not enough relaxed then the needle can be slightly redirected or reinserted. The technique is again repeated to block additional nerve fibers (usually three or four sites) in the same muscle until sufficient relaxation or until 3.0 to 4.0 mL has been injected. The effects of phenol are typically seen immediately because of the anesthetic properties, then as the secondary effects occur maximum relaxation is usually seen in the first 24 hours. Patients with contracture of the muscle will not benefit. The number of injections needed varies with the size and innervation of the muscle (30). Ranges of phenol used for a single motor point block are from 1 to 6 mL of a 2% to 6% solution. It is not recommended to inject more than 1 g in a single day (31). Electrical stimulation must be used to localize motor points. This is a lengthy procedure and can take over an hour to perform because of the tedious nature of motor point isolation. Two of the reports in dystonia describe use of this method (13,14).

### Intramuscular Injections in Cervical Dystonia

The patient is prepared by cleansing the skin overlying the muscles to be targeted. EMG guidance using standard electromyography equipment must be used for this procedure. The recording monopolar needle is used for accurate placement of the phenol near the motor end-plates according to methods described by DeLateur (32) and more recently by Massey (29). The hollow bore allows injection of the phenol solution through the recording needle/electrode. The Teflon-coated needle minimizes the recording area to the tip where the bevel is exposed. The injections should be in muscles that are actively assisting in the maintenance of the abnormal posture. Technically, a sharp rise of the motor unit potential without a positive deflection indicates close proximity to the end plate. These areas are sought out diligently throughout the muscle with small amounts of phenol instilled as they are located. Multiple sites are usually necessary to relax the muscle. Solutions of 1% to 5% phenol have been used with volumes from 0.5 up to 4 mL per muscle, dependent upon size, and a maximum total of 20 to 25 mL per injection session is recommended (29).

Massey champions the use of intramuscular phenol injections because of two technical problems with motor point injections of cervical muscles. First, the motor end plates are scattered through the length of the muscles and second, the nerves are not easily located, especially in the deeply situated neck rotators (29).

## RESULTS AND DURATION OF BENEFIT

The effectiveness of phenol motor point blocks vary depending on the concentration, type of solvent, volume used, physical tissues barriers, spread of solution, length of time of nerve exposure, and experience in placement of the agent. Sung et al. demonstrated that rabbits receiving perineural phenol injections had greater effect on the nerve with a significant reduction in compound muscle action potential (CMAP) amplitude related to the volume injected and there was a trend to the same reduction in CMAP amplitude with increasing phenol concentrations (25). In man, blocks with higher concentrations of phenol show longer-duration benefit and are less likely to need repeating. Certainly, the administration of phenol is more technically challenging than BoNT and results hinge on the experience of the clinician.

Duration of benefit for two to three months after motor point block for upper extremity spasticity in brain injury was described by Garland et al. (33); however, durations of six months or more are commonly reported (8,34–38). As well, intramuscular phenol injections for dystonia seem to have duration of benefit lasting about four to six months (11,29). Ultimately, the neurolytic and muscle effects are reversed by regeneration of neural and muscle tissue with a return of muscle overactivity.

## ADVERSE REACTIONS

With greater experience using phenol have come the realizations of its shortcomings. These include temporary results, nonspecific action on nerve fibers, and greater destruction of tissue at higher concentrations. There are both muscle and nerve destruction resulting from phenol injections (39). Pain and dysesthesia may occur from injury of the sensory component of mixed nerves. This usually involves a small area in the distribution of the blocked nerve. There can be sensitivity to touch in the affected region as well as burning pain lasting days to weeks. The incidence of paresthesias following nerve blocks is typically 20% to 30% (23,30) but ranges from 3% (40) to 36.4% (31).

Inflammatory reactions causing tender muscle nodules may be present from one to three weeks after the injections (30). Larger amounts of phenol are more likely to cause this reaction that may lead to fibrosis of the muscle. Fibrosis at the injection site can make future injections more difficult (41). Patients may also experience lethargy and nausea from systemic absorption. Rarely, there is necrosis of skin overlying the injection site.

In a large series of 521 phenol blocks, there was a severe complication with loss of an upper limb secondary to arterial thrombosis attributed to the phenol injections (42). Another report revealed thrombosis of the posterior spinal arteries with the cause "clearly thrombosis initiated by intrathecal phenol;" felt by the author to be compatible with necropsy descriptions of widespread tissue damage by phenol (43). It is now well established that phenol may cause thrombosis. Aspiration during the procedure should always be performed to avoid direct injection into a vessel.

No long-term significant adverse events have occurred in the dystonia patient groups reported. The most serious events thus far are the occurrence of temporary motor weakness in unintended muscle targets. The most common side effects are lightheadedness during injections, swelling with redness and pain at the injection sites and transient dysesthesias. Ice and nonsteroidal anti-inflammatory agents are recommended to help with local injection site pain and edema (29).

## CONCLUSIONS

Phenol has been used for over 50 years to treat neurological syndromes of muscle hypertonia. It is an inexpensive, neurolytic agent that can be used for intramuscular or motor point block in those with dystonia who are not able to afford or who are no longer responsive to BoNT. Phenol has the advantage of an immediate onset of action, fairly long duration of benefit, and it does not induce systemic resistance. Concentrations of phenol solution less than 3% will need frequent repeating, whereas those above 8% tend to spontaneously precipitate. For motor point block, the most effective and commonly used concentrations are 5% to 6% aqueous solution phenol.

For intramuscular injections in dystonia, concentrations ranging from 1% to 5% solution have been reported (11,29). Duration of benefit is variable and is affected by many factors. Technical expertise is invaluable for obtaining good results. The injections can be repeated as needed when symptoms return. Side effects of this caustic agent can include painful paresthesias, swelling, tissue necrosis, and inadvertent vascular thrombosis. Relatively, few significant adverse events have occurred in the dystonia patients reported. As with BoNT, phenol neurolysis should improve range of motion through muscle weakening leading to better performance of stretching maneuvers to maintain range and function. Intramuscular injections of phenol are an effective and viable treatment alternative in some patients with dystonia.

## REFERENCES


1. Maher RM. Relief of pain in incurable cancer. Lancet 1955; 268(6853):18–20.
2. Nathan PW. Intrathecal phenol to relieve spasticity in paraplegia. Lancet 1959; 2: 1099–1102.
3. Kelly RE, Gautier-Smith PC. Intrathecal phenol in the treatment of reflex spasms and spasticity. Lancet 1959; 2:1102–1105.
4. Koppang K. Intrathecal phenol in the treatment of spastic conditions. Acta Neurol Scand 1962; 38(Suppl 3):63–68.
5. Pedersen E, Juul-Jensen P. Intrathecal phenol in the treatment of spasticity. Acta Neurol Scand 1962; 38(Suppl 3):69–77.
6. Liversedge LA, Maher RM. Use of phenol in relief of spasticity. Br Med J 1960; 5191:31–33.
7. Khalili AA, Harmel MH, Forster S, Benton JG. Management of spasticity by selective peripheral nerve block with dilute phenol solutions in clinical rehabilitation. Arch Phys Med Rehabil 1964; 45:513–519.
8. Khalili AA, Betts HB. Peripheral nerve block with phenol in the management of spasticity. Indications and complications. JAMA 1967; 200(13):1155–1157.
9. Halpern D, Meelhuysen FE. Phenol motor point block in the management of muscular hypertonia. Arch Phys Med Rehabil 1966; 47(10):659–664.
10. Poemnyi FA, Barsukova MD, Gutorova Iu V. (Treatment of spastic torticollis with phenol-glycerin and alcohol-novocaine blockade). Zh Nevropatol Psikhiatr Im S S Korsakova 1976; 76(9):1326–1330.
11. Massey JM. Treatment of spasmodic torticollis with intramuscular phenol injection. J Neurol Neurosurg Psychiatr 1995; 58(2):258–259.
12. Garcia Ruiz PJ, Sanchez Bernardos V. Intramuscular phenol injection for severe cervical dystonia. J Neurol 2000; 247(2):146–147.
13. Kim JS, Lee KS, Ko YJ, Ko SB, Chung SW. Idiopathic foot dystonia treated with intramuscular phenol injection. Parkinsonism Relat Disord 2003; 9(6):355–359.
14. Takeuchi N, Chuma T, Mano Y. Phenol block for cervical dystonia: effects and side effects. Arch Phys Med Rehabil 2004; 85(7):1117–1120.
15. Cain HD. Subarachnoid phenol block in the treatment of pain and spasticity. Paraplegia 1965; 3(2):152–160.
16. Nathan PW, Sears TA. Effects of phenol on nervous conduction. J Physiol 1960; 150: 565–580.
17. Cullu E, Ozkan I, Culhaci N, Alparslan B. A comparison of the effect of doxorubicin and phenol on the skeletal muscle. May doxorubicin be a new alternative treatment agent for spasticity?. J Pediatr Orthop B 2005; 14(2):134–138.
18. Felsenthal G. Pharmacology of phenol in peripheral nerve blocks: a review. Arch Phys Med Rehabil 1974; 55(1):13–16.
19. Smith MC. Histological findings following intrathecal injections of phenol solutions for relief of pain. Br J Anaesth 1964; 36:387–406.

20. Nathan PW, Sears TA, Smith MC. Effects of phenol solutions on the nerve roots of the cat: an electrophysiological and histological study. J Neurol Sci 1965; 2(1):7–29.
21. Pedersen E, Reske-Nielsen E. Neuropathology of subarachnoid phenol-glycerin. Acta Neuropathol (Berl) 1965; 5(1):112–116.
22. Pedersen E, Juul-Jensen P. Treatment of spasticity by subarachnoid phenolglycerin. Neurology 1965; 15:256–262.
23. Brattstrom M, Moritz U, Svantesson G. Electromyographic studies of peripheral nerve block with phenol. Scand J Rehabil Med 1970; 2(1):17–22.
24. Gerbershagen HU. Neurolysis. Subarachnoid neurolytic blockade. Acta Anaesthesiol Belg 1981; 32(1):45–57.
25. Sung DH, Han TR, Park WH, et al. Phenol block of peripheral nerve conduction: titrating for optimum effect. Arch Phys Med Rehabil 2001; 82(5):671–676.
26. Lu L, Atchabahian A, Mackinnon SE, Hunter DA. Nerve injection injury with botulinum toxin. Plast Reconstr Surg 1998; 101(7):1875–1880.
27. Burkel WE, McPhee M. Effect of phenol injection into peripheral nerve of rat: electron microscope studies. Arch Phys Med Rehabil 1970; 51(7):391–397.
28. Mooney V, Frykman G, McLamb J. Current status of intraneural phenol injections. Clin Orthop Relat Res 1969; 63:122–131.
29. Massey JM. Electromyography-guided chemodenervation with phenol in cervical dystonia (spasmodic torticollis). In: Brin MF, Jankovic J, Hallett M, eds. Scientific and Therapeutic Aspects of Botulinum Toxin. Philadelphia: Lippincott, Williams & Wilkins, 2002: 459–462.
30. Easton JK, Ozel T, Halpern D. Intramuscular neurolysis for spasticity in children. Arch Phys Med Rehabil 1979; 60(4):155–158.
31. Wong AM, Chen CL, Chen CP, Chou SW, Chung CY, Chen MJ. Clinical effects of botulinum toxin A and phenol block on gait in children with cerebral palsy. Am J Phys Med Rehabil 2004; 83(4):284–291.
32. DeLateur BJ. A new technique of intramuscular phenol neurolysis. Arch Phys Med Rehabil 1972; 53(4):179–181.
33. Garland DE, Lilling M, Keenan MA. Percutaneous phenol blocks to motor points of spastic forearm muscles in head-injured adults. Arch Phys Med Rehabil 1984; 65(5): 243–245.
34. Caldwell C, Braun RM. Spasticity in the upper extremity. Clin Orthop Relat Res 1974(104):80–91.
35. Keenan MA, Todderud EP, Henderson R, Botte M. Management of intrinsic spasticity in the hand with phenol injection or neurectomy of the motor branch of the ulnar nerve. J Hand Surg (Am) 1987; 12(5 Pt 1):734–739.
36. Petrillo CR, Knoploch S. Phenol block of the tibial nerve for spasticity: a long-term follow-up study. Int Disabil Stud 1988; 10(3):97–100.
37. Yadav SL, Singh U, Dureja GP, Singh KK, Chaturvedi S. Phenol block in the management of spastic cerebral palsy. Indian J Pediatr 1994; 61(3):249–255.
38. Garland DE, Lucie RS, Waters RL. Current uses of open phenol nerve block for adult acquired spasticity. Clin Orthop Relat Res 1982(165):217–222.
39. Tilton AH. Injectable neuromuscular blockade in the treatment of spasticity and movement disorders. J Child Neurol 2003; 18(Suppl 1):S50–66.
40. Copp EP, Keenan J. Phenol nerve and motor point block in spasticity. Rheumatol Phys Med 1972; 11(6):287–292.
41. Esquenazi A, Mayer NH. Instrumented assessment of muscle overactivity and spasticity with dynamic polyelectromyographic and motion analysis for treatment planning. Am J Phys Med Rehabil 2004; 83(10 Suppl):S19–29.
42. Gibson II. Phenol block in the treatment of spasticity. Gerontology 1987; 33(5):327–330.
43. Hughes JT. Thrombosis of the posterior spinal arteries. A complication of an intrathecal injection of phenol. Neurology 1970; 20(7):659–664.

# 25
# Selective Denervation in Cervical Dystonia

**Carlos A. Arce**
*Department of Neurosurgery, University of Florida HSC, Jacksonville, Florida, U.S.A.*

## HISTORICAL PERSPECTIVE

Spasmodic torticollis is a condition that has held the attention of physicians since the 16th century, and the term torticollis has been attributed to the French physician, Francois Rabelais (1494–1553) (1). Physicians have been trying to help patients afflicted with this disabling condition by surgical means since the 17th century. The surgical procedures performed for torticollis can be divided into intracranial and extracranial procedures, with the latter emerging as the preferred method of treatment over several centuries. Finney and Hughson (2) first described bilateral peripheral denervations for torticollis in 1925, and also document a three-century history of surgical evolution from myotomy to tenotomy, and, finally, to nerve sectioning. In the 1600s, Isaac Minius reported open sectioning of the sternocleidomastoid, and Hendrick van Roonhuyze emphasized myotomies, and by 1812 Dupuytren attempted to treat torticollis by performing sternocleidomastoid tenotomy. The era of selective nerve sectioning began in 1866 when Campbell de Morgan (3) was credited with the first peripheral division of the accessory nerve, although Bujalski reported a similar technique in 1834. While Gross reemphasized multiple myotomies in 1873, nerve sectioning has emerged as the primary focus for extracranial surgical correction of spasmodic torticollis. Collier (4) proposed the quickly abandoned procedure of constricting the accessory nerve in the neck with a silver wire later that century. It was McKeen (5) who first described the division of the posterior divisions of the first three cervical nerves for torticollis in 1891 and, although this procedure became a procedure of choice for American and British surgeons, myotomy continued to be emphasized by German surgeons. In 1924, Mc Kenzie (1) reported a successful intracranial division of the accessory nerve and an intraspinal division of the roots of the first three cervical nerves, performed by Cushing that led to significant improvement in a patient with a rotational-type torticollis. A year later, Finney and Hughson (2) published a more extensive experience with bilateral peripheral denervations of the three first posterior divisions with excellent results (37% cured and 50% improved). However, this procedure never became widely used, probably because of the formidable incision and dissection. In 1930, Dandy (6) first described the bilateral intraspinal division of the roots of the first three cervical roots and the intracranial division of the spinal accessory nerve, with excellent results in five out of eight patients. Although initially he divided the anterior and posterior roots, he later modified this to sectioning of only the anterior roots. In 1955, McKenzie (7) advocated the peripheral sectioning of the accessory nerve to the sternocleidomastoid be added to the intraspinal procedure and the division of some rootlets of C4. Anterior rhizotomy, or the Dandy–McKenzie procedure, remained the procedure of choice until the late 1970s (8–10). In 1986, Colbassani and Wood (11), in a literature review of anterior rhizotomy series, warn of significant risks to this procedure, reporting an incidence of an unstable or weak neck (39%), dysphagia (30%), shoulder weakness (41%), and death (2%). Hemiparesis, subluxation requiring fusion (10) and quadriplegia (12,13) have also been reported with this operation. Because of the complications with anterior rhizotomies, the search for other procedures to treat this condition continued. Stereotactic procedures (14–16) were used in the 1970s, and electrical stimulation (17) and iontophoresis (18) were also tried without success. In 1978, Bertrand (19) reported the use of thalamotomy combined with selective denervation. Because of the significant complications with anterior rhizotomies and bilateral thalamotomies, he felt the combination of thalamotomy and peripheral denervation may lead to a safer and more successful treatment. After his initial experience, he returned to selective denervation without intracranial ablation, a more benign treatment for torticollis. Over the subsequent years he published his results and experience with this procedure (20–22). His descriptions of the use of a midline incision, innovative study of preoperative electromyographic (EMG) analysis, the identification of the muscles to be denervated for the different types of torticollis, as well as his low morbidity has led to the well-accepted surgery for spasmodic torticollis, appropriately termed Selective Peripheral Denervation (The Bertrand Procedure).

## SELECTIVE PERIPHERAL DENERVATION (THE BERTRAND PROCEDURE)

The principle behind selective denervation is that in cervical dystonia only a select group of muscles are involved, and the contractions of these muscles are going to determine the direction of the involuntary movement. By finding which muscles are involved, a peripheral or extraspinal selective denervation of only the muscles involved can be performed. The patient selection is of utmost importance. Not every patient with torticollis is a candidate for this procedure, and the operation requires careful tailoring to the particular muscle involvement and type of movement of the patient. The evaluation of the patient includes a complete physical exam and examination of the neck muscles. Neck examination should be done at rest and with active head movement to ensure the surgeon is aware of the specific muscles affected by dystonia. Determining the direction of the movement, and if the patient has a mixed movement or a unidirectional movement, is essential to make an informed surgical decision. Because patients have become accustomed to "fighting" the involuntary movement, especially when painful, an examiner must be convinced that the patient is fully relaxed before determining a surgical approach. Palpation of the neck musculature and observation of the involuntary movement at rest and with movements of the head in anterior–posterior, horizontal, and turning directions are equally important. This needs to be done both when the patient is at the maximum abnormal position and also when the patient is trying to bring the head in the opposite direction of the involuntary movement, especially in patients with forward flexion. Measurements of the angle of rotation, tilt, or extension of the head and the distance between the chin and the sternal notch are important to determine at baseline and for following the patient after the procedure. Preoperative and postoperative videotape of the patient should also be performed routinely. A four-channel EMG study to simultaneously assess agonist and antagonist neck muscle involvement is the third component of the presurgical evaluation. It is important that the surgeon and neurophysiologist be present during the exam. The recordings are done with the head in the abnormal position, trying to hold the head straight and turning or tilting in the opposite direction. Persistent and significant activity noted in involved muscles when the patient is trying to correct the torticollis is usually a good indication of muscle involvement and usually correlates well with a good outcome after denervation (Figs. 1 and 2). The muscles studied routinely during EMG study include the splenius capiti, semispinalis capiti, sternocleidomastoids, trapezii, and levator scapuli muscles, but depending on the movement and the exam other muscles may also be investigated.

## CANDIDATES FOR SELECTIVE DENERVATION

There are four types of torticollis that may be treated successfully with selective denervation: Rotational torticollis (Fig. 3), Lateral torticollis (Fig. 4), Retro-rotational torticollis (Fig. 5), and Retrocollis (Fig. 6). Patients with mixed movements can be treated but the success depends on the muscles involved and the type of associated movement. Patients with "rotational torticollis" often demonstrate involvement of the ipsilateral suboccipital group, ipsilateral splenius capitus, ipsilateral semispinalis capitis, and the contralateral sternocleidomastoid. The contralateral semispinalis may also be involved. In patients with a forward position of the ipsilateral shoulder, there is usual involvement of the ipsilateral levator scapulae, and less often, there may be activity of the contralateral trapezius or, rarely, the ipsilateral platysma. In the setting of "lateral torticollis," involvement of the ipsilateral suboccipital muscle group, ipsilateral splenius capitus, ipsilateral semispinalis capitus, ipsilateral levator scapulae, ipsilateral sternocleidomastoid, and in some cases the ipsilateral trapezius. "Retro-rotational torticollis" usually presents with

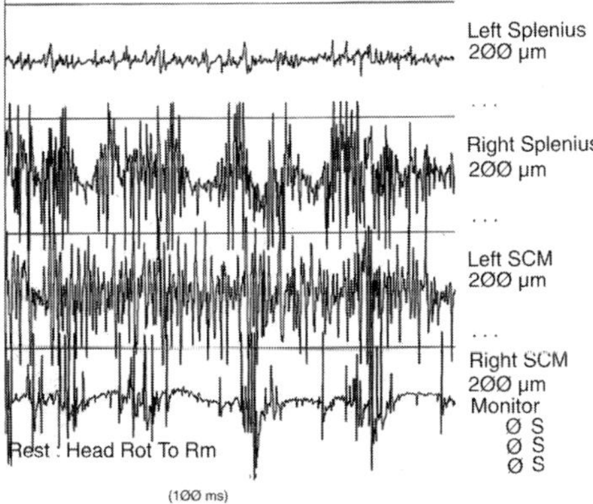


**Figure 1** Four-channel electromyographic recording in a patient with a rotational torticollis to the right. Channels 2 and 3 showed the activity in the right splenius capitis and left sternocleidomastoid. *Abbreviation*: SCM, sternocleidomastoid.

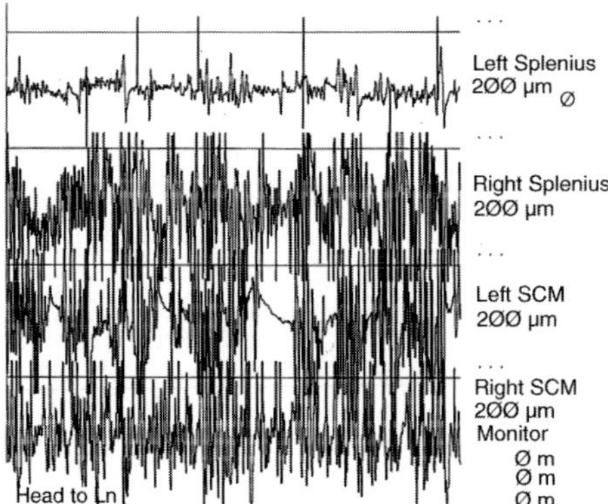


**Figure 2** Electromyographic recording of the same patient turning his head to the left. There is activity in the right SCM (channel 4) and the left splenius (channel 1) activity is increasing, but the right splenius capitis and the left sternocleidomastoid are not relaxing and continue to show significant activity, making it difficult for the patient to turn left. *Abbreviation*: SCM, sternocleidomastoid.

ipsilateral suboccipital muscle groups, ipsilateral splenius capitus, ipsilateral semispinalis capitus, contralateral sternocleidomastoid, and contralateral semispinalis involvement. Subjects with "retrocollis" demonstrate bilateral involvement of the suboccipital muscle groups, semispinalis capiti, and splenius capiti.

## FACTORS THAT AFFECT THE SUCCESS OF SELECTIVE DENERVATION

### Fixed Posture, Secondary to Soft-Tissue Fibrosis or Skeletal Changes

The most important problem encountered in patients who are being evaluated for selective denervation is the presence of a fixed, abnormal posture of the head and

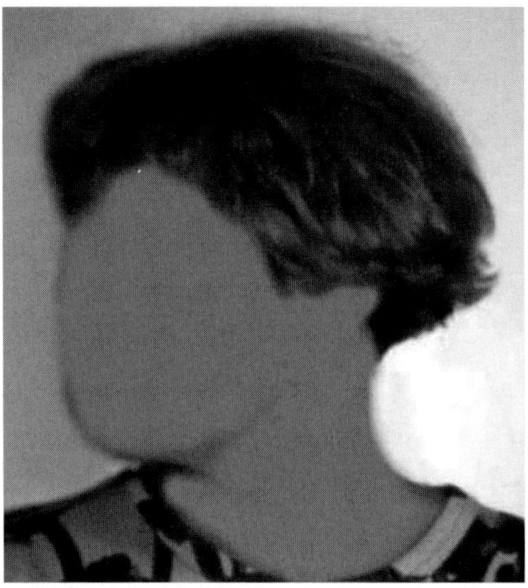

**Figure 3** Patient with rotational torticollis to the right.

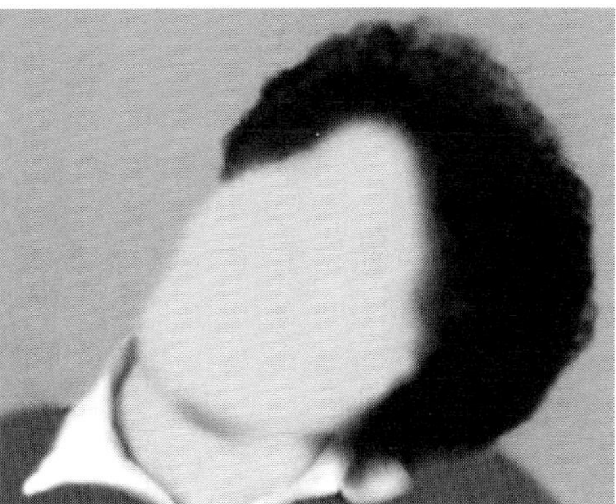

**Figure 4** Patient with laterocollis to the left.

neck, secondary to the years of torticollis, and the difficulty they have turning in the opposite direction of the movement. Fibrosis of muscles and joints from the constant abnormal position, coupled with atrophy of the antagonistic muscles, leads to the development of these fixed postures. In addition, subjects presenting with torticollis, because of the typical age of presentation, commonly the fourth or fifth decades, and long-term posture changes, often have degenerative changes of the spine. Commonly, severe degenerative changes with facet hypertrophy and fibrosis, usually occur on the side toward the head turn or tilt, leading to a fixed, abnormal posture. Chawda et al. (23) studied 34 patients with torticollis and found 14 with severe degenerative changes in the side of the direction of movement. Once a fixed, abnormal posture has developed, the potential for benefit from selective denervation decreases significantly. In a series of 45 consecutive patients evaluated for selective denervation (24), the position of the head and neck was studied under general anesthesia with full chemical paralysis. Only 18% of the patients had a normal range of movement and position of the head. The rest of the patients had significant restriction of movement and different degrees of fixed scoliosis, which was severe in 35% of the patients. Figure 7 shows a patient in her normal position with a rotational

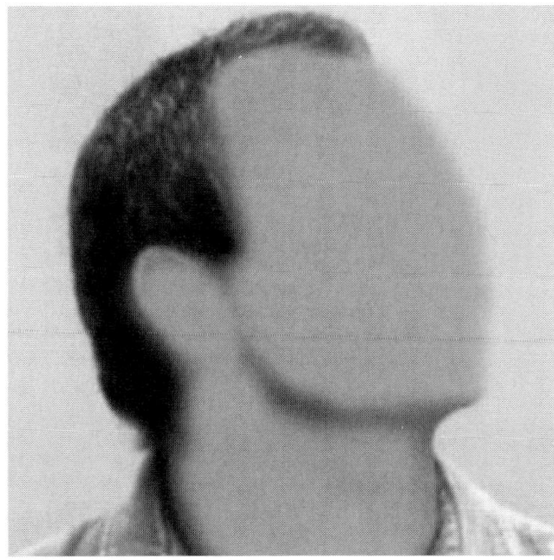

**Figure 5** Patient with retro-rotational torticollis to the left.

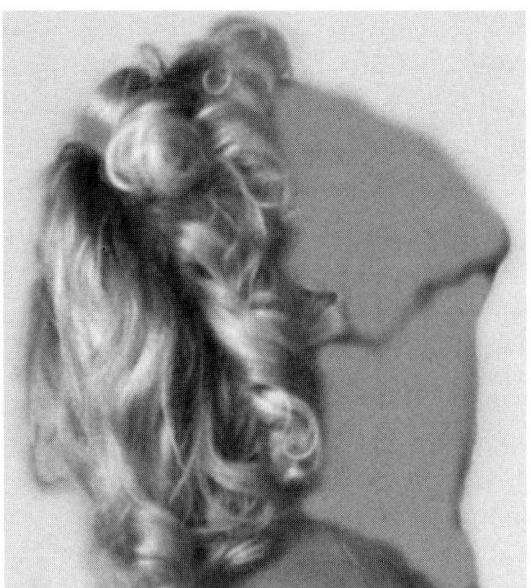

**Figure 6** Patient with retrocollis.

torticollis to the left. Figure 8 shows the same patient under anesthesia. Although fully paralyzed, the head of the patient is fixed and leaning to the left.

Because the development of a fixed posture, by either muscle or soft-tissue fibrosis or spinal column degeneration or hypertrophy will limit the potential for any therapeutic intervention, it is important that patients with torticollis be constantly monitored for the development of this problem. Patients over 40 years, patients who are noticing progressive difficulty bringing the head to the midline or turning in the opposite direction of the abnormal movement, and patients who in addition to the difficulty turning, start having increased pain, should be evaluated for the development of a fixed, abnormal posture. A short exam under anesthesia with the patient fully paralyzed may assist in determining whether a fixed posture

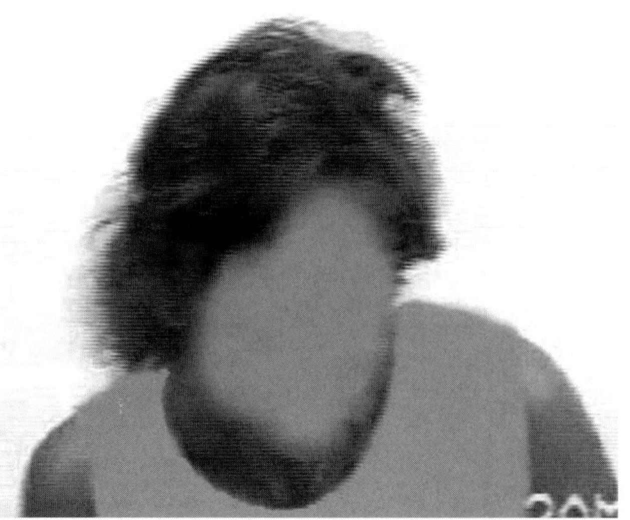

**Figure 7** Patient with rotational torticollis to the left, awake, in her normal position.

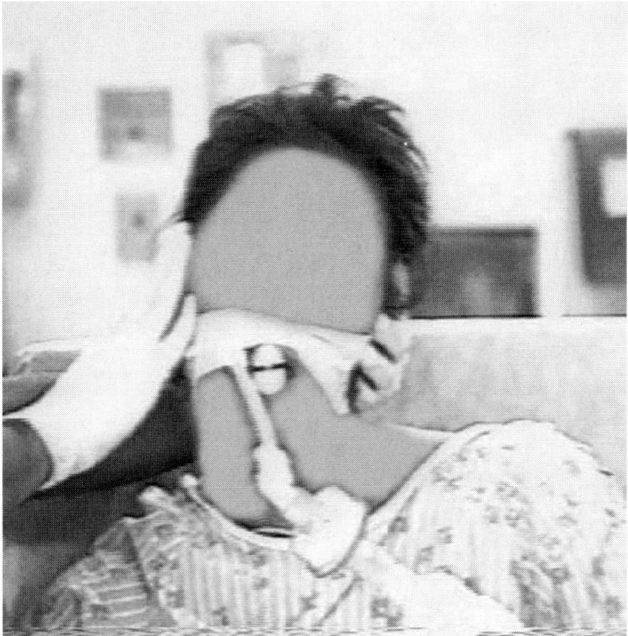

**Figure 8** Same patient under general anesthesia and fully paralyzed. Instead of her head being relaxed and moveable, it is rigid and fixed, tilted left.

is the cause for poor therapeutic response. While not proven, some clinicians support active physical therapy in patients with severe or long-time spasmodic torticollis to prevent this problem.

## Multiple Areas of Dystonia

Other factors or conditions that limit the success of selective denervation are the presence of a more than one primary movement (e.g., torticollis and lateral torticollis), especially the presence of anterior torticollis. A mixed movement is not a contraindication for selective denervation, but the success would depend on the types of movement and muscles involved.

## Presence of Dystonic Muscle Contractions in Other Areas

The presence of oromandibular dystonia does not seem to affect the success of selective denervation; however, the presence of brachial or axial dystonia would decrease the success. In these patients, as well as in patients with generalized dystonia, selective denervation could be performed, but only with the goal of decreasing the number of muscles involved trying to improve the result with other treatments, such as botulinum toxin.

## Involvement of the Trapezius Muscle

The denervation of the trapezius muscle, although a simple surgical procedure can be very disabling, not only because of the shoulder weakness, but also because of the shoulder pain that many patients have afterwards. This muscle can be treated with botulinum toxin very easily. For this reason, in patients with this problem it is very important that selective denervation be performed before they developed resistance to botulinum toxin.

### Resistance to Botulinum Toxin

Historically, torticollis patients with poor response to botulinum toxin also do not respond well to selective denervation procedures. Conversely, complementary toxin injection after successful selective denervation in certain cases may offer these patients a greater improvement of their symptoms.

### Posttraumatic Dystonia

Patients with this type of dystonia behave differently than patients with idiopathic cervical dystonia, and often have involvement of the trapezius muscle. Assessment is also difficult because EMG findings are often unexpected. At minimum, this group of patients should be reevaluated several times before proceeding with selective denervation. The best results are obtained in patients with EMG findings that clearly correlate with the type of movement. In some cases, the abnormal movement is brought on only by certain activities. In these cases, it is prudent to perform several evaluations before deciding to proceed with selective denervation.

## SURGICAL PROCEDURE

The selective denervation procedure for spasmodic torticollis is performed in the sitting position. Although, theoretically, there is a small risk of air embolism, this has not been reported in more than 1000 patients undergoing this surgery. In a study of 100 selective denervation patients (25) there was only one minor episode detected by cardiac Doppler, without clinical significance. Although adequate and careful hemostasis and vigilance is important, bleeding has not been a problem in most series. However, Taira (26) has proposed an intradural sectioning of C1 and C2 to decrease the risk of bleeding from the venous plexus that usually surrounds these nerves, but, this approach has not produced additional benefit, and adds the risk of an intraspinal procedure. Figure 9 shows the different incisions that have been used to perform selective denervation.

Over the last three years, an increasing preference for a lateral muscle-splitting approach (27) has been endorsed, and allows easier access to the superior posterior cervical rami (of C1 to C5). The main advantage of this approach is that the trapezius and cervical muscle attachments to the midline are not touched, and muscles, such as the semispinalis capitis, may be split instead of divided. This technique appears to be associated with significant decrease in the postoperative pain and a faster recovery. The branches of the posterior rami are found using unipolar stimulation (usually 3v) and then followed proximally until the main branch is identified. The C1 and C2 anterior branches are usually preserved. Successful sectioning of C3 and C4 is highly dependent on locating the lateral branches, given that the procedural result is compromised if these branches remain intact. Denervation of the levator requires identification of the anterior fascicles of C3 and C4 with every precaution to identify and avoid sectioning of the branches innervating the trapezius and diaphragm. Complete denervation of this muscle is difficult to achieve, and

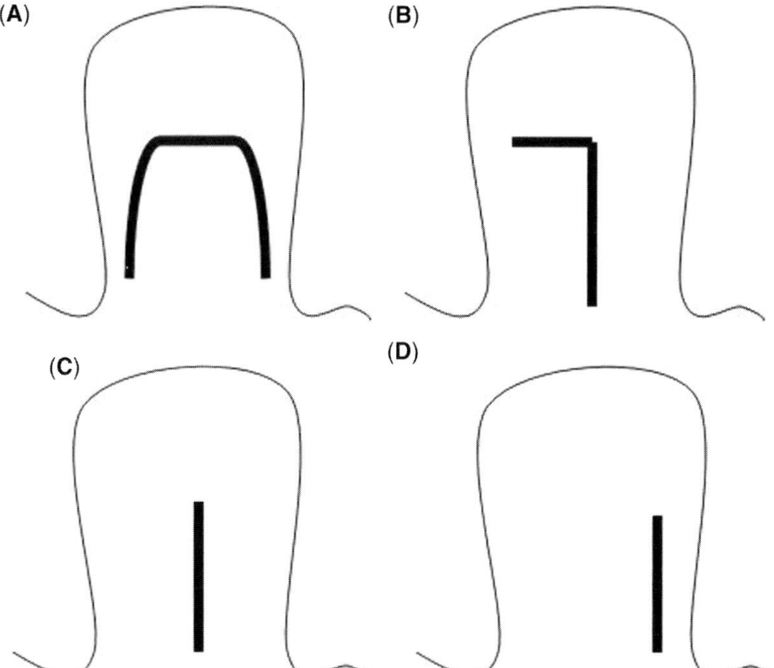


**Figure 9** These drawings show the incisions advocated by Finney Hughson (**A**), Bertrand (**B**), Richter (**C**), and Arce (**D**).

additional myotomy is recommended. The nerves are clipped proximal to the branches and divided and avulsed. Denervation of the sternocleidomastoid muscle is performed through an incision in the lateral aspect of the neck, starting below the lobe of the ear and extended to the supraclavicular area. The branch to the trapezius is identified with stimulation and followed proximally, where the branches to the sternocleidomastoid are divided with care to preserve the main trunk to the trapezius.

In most patients with rotational, lateral torticollis, and retrocollis the procedure can be performed in one stage. However, when there is bilateral posterior involvement, such as in some patients with rotational torticollis or in patients with retro-rotation, a two-stage procedure is recommended. When bilateral posterior denervations and denervation of the sternocleidomastoid are performed in one stage, there is increased risk of dysphagia. This problem is avoided if the surgery is performed in stages six months apart. A more recently developed lateral approach to the denervation of the posterior group has decreased significantly the postoperative recovery and the postoperative pain. Most of the patients are discharged within 24 hours, and require only oral medication for pain control. After surgery it is very important that patients do posture exercises to regain a sense of midline, and to improve the range of movement.

## RESULTS

In Bertrand's series of 260 patients (28), 89% of the patients had excellent or very good results. In a more recent series of 145 patients undergoing the Bertrand approach, 85%

of the patients had the same type of results (29). A modification of this procedure, using a lateral muscle-splitting approach yields very similar results (27). Chen (30), in his series of 361 patients on whom he performed selective denervation and myectomies, reports that 88% of his patients obtained these types of results. Braun and Richter (31) report excellent-to-moderate benefit in 75% of 155 patients, while Cohen-Gadol et al. (32) notes excellent-to-moderate benefit in 70% of 130 patients. Munchau et al. (33), using the Toronto Western Spasmodic Torticollis Rating Scale (TWSTRS), reported a significant improvement in 68% of 40 patients who underwent selective denervation. In more than 1000 published cases, only one mortality has been reported. This patient was also diagnosed with an underlying myopathy, and suffered respiratory compromise the day after surgery (32). No major morbidity has been associated with this surgery. Numbness associated with C2 sectioning has not been a significant problem, but some subjects have reported dysesthesia. Bertrand (34) and other authors have also described cases in which the dystonic process in other areas of the body worsened temporarily. Other complications reported less often include temporary weakness of the trapezius muscle and dysphagia. However, swallowing difficulties are much less common when only a unilateral posterior ramisectomy is performed. The recurrence of spasmodic torticollis postoperatively is approximately 10%. Possible etiologies are an incomplete denervation, involvement of other muscles, or progression of the condition. Reoperation can be helpful if other muscles are involved; however, if there is incomplete denervation, reoperation is less successful due to scarring.

## SUMMARY

Selective Peripheral Denervation, or the Bertrand Procedure, is a safe and effective surgical treatment for patients with cervical dystonia. Careful preoperative evaluation is essential to benefit from this procedure, and every patient with torticollis needs to be treated on an individual basis. Patients with the same direction of movement do not necessarily have the same muscles involved. For example, patients who turn right have involvement of the right posterior group and left sternocleidomastoid, but some of them have involvement of the ipsilateral levator, or the contralateral semispinalis; some of them have involvement of the ipsilateral platysma (35) or the contralateral trapezius. It is for these reasons that the preoperative evaluation, including a careful observation of the movement, palpation of the musculature, study of the videotape, and a complete EMG evaluation are needed to determine the direction of movement and the muscles involved. Once this has been determined, the surgery needs to be tailored to that particular patient. It is important that patients with cervical dystonia be monitored very closely for the development of a fixed, abnormal posture, and permanent loss of range of movement. Once this happens, the success of any treatment would be decreased. Although botulinum toxin is a standard and successful treatment, every patient should be individualized, and surgery should not be used only as a last resort or only when the patient is resistant to botulinum toxin. Selective denervation has proved to be a safe procedure that helps a significant number of patients. The use of botulinum toxin after the denervation, if needed, could significantly enhance the results of the surgery in some cases, and this needs to be considered in determining the best time for the patient to have the surgery. Our increased understanding of the muscles involved in cervical dystonia, the development of the lateral muscle-splitting approach which allows a fast recovery, the decrease in side effects by staging the procedure, and the good success rate of the procedure, with only minor side effects, makes selective denervation a safe alternative for patients with cervical dystonia.

## REFERENCES

1. McKenzie KG. Intrameningeal division of the spinal accessory and roots of the upper cervical nerves for the treatment of spasmodic torticollis. Surg Gynecol Obstet 1924; 39:5–10.
2. Finney JMT, Hughson W. Spasmodic Torticollis. Ann Surg 1925; 81:255–269.
3. DeMorgan C. A case in which severe spasmodic contraction of cervical muscle is produced by movement. Lancet 1867; 2:180.
4. Collier M. Spasmodic torticollis treated by nerve ligature. Lancet 1890; 1:1354–1355.
5. McKeen WW. A new operation for spasmodic wry neck. Namely, division or exsection of the nerves supplying the posterior rotator muscles of the head. Ann Surg 1891; 13:44–47.
6. Dandy WE. An operation for the treatment of spasmodic torticollis. Arch Surg 1930; 20:1021–1032.
7. McKenzie KG. The surgical treatment of spasmodic torticollis. Clin Neurosurg 1955; 2:37–43.
8. Sorensen BF, Hamby WB. Spasmodic torticollis: Results in 71 surgically treated patients. JAMA 1965; 194:706–708.
9. Hamby WB, Schiffer S. Spasmodic torticollis: Results after cervical rhizotomy in 50 cases. J Neurosurg 1969; 31:323–326.
10. Tasker RR. The treatment of spasmodic torticollis by peripheral denervation: the McKenzie operation. In: Morley TP, ed. Current Controversies in Neurosurgery. Philadelphia: WB Saunders, 1976:448–454.
11. Colbassani HJ, Wood JH. Management of spasmodic torticollis. Surg Neurol 1986; 25:153–158.
12. Scoville WB, Bettis DB. Motor tics of the head and neck: Surgical approaches and their complications. Acta Neurochir 1979; 48:47–66.
13. Adams CBT. Vascular catastrophy following the Dandy-McKenzie operation for spasmodic torticollis. J Neurol Neurosurg Psychiatry 1984; 47:990–994.
14. Hassler R, Dieckmann G. Stereotactic treatment of different kinds of spasmodic torticollis. Confin Neurol 1970; 32:135–143.
15. Mundinger F, Riechert T, Disselhoff J. Long term results of stereotactic treatment of spasmodic Torticollis. Confin Neurol 1972; 34:41–46.
16. Bertrand C. The treatment of spasmodic torticollis with particular reference to thalamotomy. In: Morley TP, ed. Current Controversies in Neurosurgery. Philadelphia: WB Saunders, 1976:455–459.
17. Gildenberg PL. Treatment of spasmodic torticollis with dorsal column stimulation. Applied Neurophysiol 1978; 27:899–900.
18. Svein HJ, Cody DTR. Treatment of spasmodic torticollis by suppression of labyrinthine activity: Report of a case. Mayo Clin Proc 1969; 44:825–827.
19. Bertrand C, Molina-Negro P, Martinez SN. Combined stereotactic and peripheral surgical approach for spasmodic torticollis. Appl Neurophysiol 1977; 41:122–133.
20. Bertrand C, Molina-Negro P, Martinez SN. Technical aspects of selective peripheral denervation for spasmodic torticollis. Appl Neurophysiol 1982; 45:326–330.
21. Bertrand C, Molina-Negro P. Selective peripheral denervation in 111 cases of spasmodic torticollis: rationale and results. In: Fahn S, Marsden C, Calne D, eds. Dystonia 2. Advances in Neurology. New York: Raven Press, 1988:637–643.
22. Bertrand C, Molina-Negro P, Bouvier G, et al. Observations and analysis of results in 131 cases of spasmodic torticollis after selective denervation. Appl Neurophysiol 1987; 50:319–323.
23. Chawda SJ, Munchau A, Johnson D, et al. Pattern of premature degenerative changes of the cervical spine in patients with spasmodic torticollis and the impact on the outcome of selective denervation. J Neurol Neurosurg Psychiatry 2000; 68:465–471.

24. Arce C. Permanent abnormal postures in cervical dystonia (spasmodic torticollis). Mov Disord 1998; 13(2):33.
25. Lobato EB, Black S, DeSoto H. Venous air embolism and selective denervation for torticollis. Anesth Analg 1977; 84(3):551–553.
26. Taira T, Hori T. Peripheral neurotomy for torticollis: a new approach. Stereotact Funct Neurosurg 2001; 77:40–43.
27. Arce C. A new muscle-splitting approach for selective denervation for cervical dystonia: Experience in 36 cases. Mov Disord 2005; 20(10):160.
28. Bertrand C. Selective peripheral denervation for spasmodic torticollis: Surgical technique, results and obdervations in 260 cases. Surg Neurol 1993; 40:96–103.
29. Arce C. Selective Peripheral denervation–Analysis and results in 145 patients. Mov Disord 1995; 10(5):98.
30. Chen X, Ma A, Liang J, et al. Selective denervation and resection of cervical muscles in the treatment of spasmodic torticollis: long term follow-up results in 207 cases. Stereotact Funct Neurosurg 2000; 75:96–102.
31. Braun V, Richter HP. Selective peripheral denervation for spasmodic torticollis: 13 year experience with 155 patients. J Neurosurg 2002; 97:207–212.
32. Cohen-Gadol AA, Ahlskog JE, Matsumoto J, et al. Selective peripheral denervation for the treatment of intractable spasmodic torticollis: experience with 168 patients at Mayo Clinic. J Neurosurg 2003; 98:1247–1254.
33. Munchau A, Palmer JD, Dressler D, et al. Prospective study of selective peripheral denervation for botulinum-toxin resistant patients with cervical dystonia. Brain 2001; 124: 769–783.
34. Bertrand C, Benabou R. Surgical treatment of spasmodic torticollis: Selective peripheral denervation revisited. In: Germano IM, ed. Neurosurgical Treatment of Movement Disorders. Illinois: AANS Publications, 1998:239–254.
35. Arce C. Role of the platysma muscle in cervical dystonia and experience with surgical denervation/resection of this muscle. Mov Disord 2002; 17(5):297–298.

# 26
# Brain Surgery for Dystonia

**William J. Marks, Jr.**
*Department of Neurology, University of California, San Francisco, California, U.S.A.*

## INTRODUCTION

Surgical treatments have been used for decades to treat a variety of movement disorders including tremor disorders, Parkinson's disease, and dystonia. Beneficial effects of serendipitous lesions in corticospinal, thalamic, and basal ganglia regions resulted in the deliberate use of ablative techniques directed at various components of pyramidal and extrapyramidal pathways. As the pathophysiology underlying movement disorders came to be appreciated, surgical intervention with a rational anatomicophysiological basis emerged. Procedures initially entailed destructive lesioning of nuclei exhibiting aberrant neurophysiological activity—thalamotomy and pallidotomy. More recently, the advent of deep brain stimulation (DBS) has provided a means of reversibly modulating activity in thalamic and basal ganglia nuclei in a manner that is nondestructive, adjustable, and safer for bilateral use using an implantable device.

Initial treatment of dystonia is pharmacological in nature. Oral medications, used for all types of dystonia, include dopaminergic drugs, anticholinergic medications, baclofen, benzodiazepines, and dopamine-depleting drugs. Chemodenervation treatment with botulinum toxin (type A or B) is highly effective for focal and regional use in many patients. More widespread dystonia may respond to intrathecal baclofen, which can be chronically delivered using an implantable pump system.

These treatments have limitations, though. Oral pharmacotherapy is often only modestly effective in suppressing dystonic symptoms, and the neurological and systemic adverse effects of these agents commonly impose a dose ceiling for their tolerable use. Chemodenervation may provide a robust effect initially, but this can wane over time, and some patients never achieve an adequate level of symptom control with this strategy. Furthermore, chemodenervation is impractical for patients with widespread involvement of their dystonia. Intrathecal baclofen, while often impressive in treating spasticity, seems to be less helpful for dystonia. For patients with dystonia in whom symptoms are inadequately controlled with pharmacological measures, the use of surgical treatments, particularly DBS, can provide improved symptom control and enhanced functional capacity.

## ABLATIVE PROCEDURES FOR DYSTONIA

### Overview

Thalamotomy and pallidotomy are ablative procedures in which tissue within the target is precisely destroyed, usually using radiofrequency thermocoagulation (1). These procedures involve the use of stereotactic neurosurgical methods, whereby a frame with coordinate markings affixed to the patient's head or fiducial markers embedded in the outer portion of the skull, in conjunction with a brain image obtained by computed tomography or magnetic resonance imaging, are used to calculate the location of the brain target to be operated upon. Although lesioning can be accomplished via noninvasive radiosurgery, there are several disadvantages to such an approach (2); hence, an invasive procedure is usually performed. A small burr hole in the skull allows the surgeon to pass a recording electrode and then lesioning probe to the intended target. Precise targeting of these small structures deep in the brain is achieved using imaging and intraoperative recordings of brain activity. The procedures are typically performed using local analgesia in an awake patient to allow neurological examination and questioning of the patient, important in confirming surgical targeting during the course of the procedure. Modern stereotactic neurosurgical techniques allow ablative surgery to be relatively safe. In a review of 1116 patients who underwent microelectrode-guided pallidotomy for Parkinson's disease, symptomatic intracerebral hemorrhage occurred in 1.5% of patients (3). Encroachment of the surgical lesion into neighboring neural structures can also produce permanent neurological sequelae, such as hemiparesis, dysarthria, dysphagia, and visual field deficits. The incidence of such complications in the modern surgical era ranges from 3% to 16% and is higher with bilateral procedures (3,4). The irreversible, destructive, and nonadjustable nature of ablative procedures has resulted in these procedures being used much less commonly once the technique of DBS became available.

### Outcomes

The use of thalamotomy and pallidotomy to treat dystonia has a rich history. Much of the outcome data predates the modern era of functional stereotactic neurosurgical techniques, making its interpretation and current applicability challenging. In addition, the absence of standardized rating scales with which to assess patient outcomes makes evaluation of the clinical results difficult. The extensive experience of Cooper in the use of thalamic ablation to treat generalized dystonia showed that the majority of patients experienced moderate-to-excellent improvement at long-term evaluation (5). These patients typically underwent more than one operation, often receiving multiple lesions directed at the ventrolateral thalamus, centromedian nucleus of the thalamus, and pallidal and cerebellar afferents to the thalamus. Other relatively early reports described a range of outcomes. Only a quarter of generalized dystonia patients (of mixed etiology) showed considerable benefit in a series of 16 patients treated with thalamotomy, although nearly two-thirds of patients with cervical dystonia in that series were "much improved" (6). Another report indicated that "all" patients with cervical dystonia (mainly torticollis) improved after unilateral thalamotomy (7). More recent reports include a series of 54 patients with primary and secondary dystonia, in which 59% of patients exhibited at least a 25% improvement and another 23% showed slight improvement following ventral thalamotomy (8), and a series of 17 patients with mean improvements in dystonia severity of 43% and 50% in patients with primary and secondary dystonia, respectively (9). A variety of case reports suggest efficacy of thalamotomy in focal dystonia, tardive dystonia, and pantothenate kinase-associated neurodegeneration (PKAN) (10–12). While operative mortality in these series is low, a consistent finding is a relatively high rate of persistent dysarthria (15% in the Cooper series), particularly following bilateral thalamotomy.

Pallidotomy, although occasionally used for dystonia in the early era of functional neurosurgical treatment, has been explored in more depth during the modern era, particularly with its resurgence to treat Parkinson's disease. Several reports document the efficacy of bilateral pallidotomy for generalized dystonia (13–16). Improvements in the Burke—Fahn–Marsden Dystonia Rating Scale (BFMDRS) movement scores ranged from 58% to 79% at relatively short-term follow-up. Benefits tended to lag the operative procedure and continued to accrue over the course of three to six postoperative months. Patients with dystonia, particularly children, appear to tolerate bilateral treatment with few persistent adverse effects (17). Patients with secondary generalized dystonia appear to receive less benefit than those with primary disorders. One report noted that only 8 of 18 patients derived benefit (18), while another noted an overall improvement of 13% in the BFMDRS movement score and 9% in the disability score (19,20). Cases of beneficial outcomes following pallidotomy have been reported for individual patients with dystonia due to PKAN, glutaric aciduria, Huntington's disease, perinatal hypoxia, and neuroleptic exposure (20–25).

In a nonrandomized comparative study, patients with primary dystonia realized significantly more improvement following pallidotomy compared with those who had undergone thalamotomy (26). Patients with secondary dystonia had similarly modest levels of improvement with either procedure.

## DEEP BRAIN STIMULATION FOR DYSTONIA

### Overview

Benabid and colleagues pioneered the use of high-frequency electrical stimulation of deep brain nuclei via implanted electrodes in 1987 to treat essential tremor and Parkinson's disease (27). Chronic DBS is a nondestructive and reversible means of disrupting the abnormal function of thalamic and basal ganglia nuclei that occurs in a variety of movement disorders. DBS mimics the effect of a lesion in the target structure that is stimulated, although the exact mechanism by which this occurs remains unclear and is likely to be more complex than that of a lesion. The DBS system consists of a four-contact lead placed into the brain that is connected to a programmable neurostimulator (also called an implantable pulse generator), implanted in the subclavicular region, via a wire tunneled under the scalp down to the chest (Fig. 1). Stimulation parameters can be programmed noninvasively to deliver the appropriate level of stimulation to the optimal anatomic region to maximize symptomatic benefit and minimize adverse effects. The benefits of DBS compared to ablative surgery include its nondestructive nature, reversibility, and adjustability. In addition, when used bilaterally the technique does not typically produce the permanent speech, swallowing, or cognitive complications sometimes seen with ablative procedures; thus, DBS is safer for bilateral use. DBS implantation is safe, with serious surgical complications relatively uncommon. Intracerebral hemorrhage producing persistent symptoms occurs in about 0.6% of patients (28). Infection, most commonly occurring in the region of the neurostimulator, occurs in about 4% of patients and usually requires device explantation and treatment with intravenous

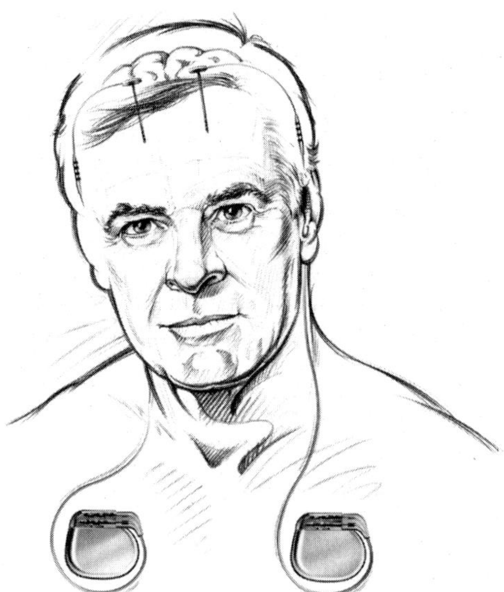

**Figure 1** Illustration of the deep brain stimulation system, which consists of brain leads, extensions, and neurostimulators. *Source*: courtesy of Medtronic Neurological.

antibiotics (29). Complications related to unintended stimulation of adjacent structures (e.g., visual phenomena from optic tract or tonic motor contraction from internal capsule) are readily reversible by altering stimulation parameters.

## Technical Issues

DBS therapy uses a device with three implantable components: a quadripolar brain lead, a neurostimulator, and an extension that connects the two. The DBS lead, containing an array of four electrodes on its distal end, is implanted into the deep brain target using stereotactic neurosurgical techniques. Such procedures typically use image-based targeting and intraoperative physiological confirmation to accurately implant the DBS lead into the appropriate target, generally the motor subterritory of the globus pallidus internus (GPi) when treating dystonia (30). DBS lead implantation is often performed using local anesthesia in the awake patient to optimize the recording of physiological data during the mapping procedure, as well as to elicit the patient's report of stimulation-induced adverse effects during intraoperative test stimulation of the lead. For young patients or those with extreme dystonic postures or spasms, the procedure can be performed under general anesthesia.

Following lead implantation on one side of the brain for contralateral hemidystonia or both sides for other syndromes, the neurostimulator is implanted under general anesthesia. The neurostimulator is typically placed in the subclavicular region, although it can be located elsewhere. Bilateral stimulation necessitates the implantation of two single-channel neurostimulators or one dual-channel neurostimulator. Extension wires, tunneled under the skin, connect the brain leads to the neurostimulator(s).

## Postoperative Management

Days to weeks after device implantation, stimulation is activated. Using the DBS programmer, the clinician can select which electrodes on the DBS lead to use to deliver stimulation, as well as the stimulation parameters themselves (including amplitude, pulse width, and frequency of stimulation). Usually, the one or two electrodes within, or closest to, the sensorimotor region of the target nucleus are activated. Typical stimulation parameters include amplitude of 2.0 to 4.0 V, pulse width of 90 to 450 $\mu$sec, and frequency of 130 to 185 Hz (30). Some investigators cite benefit at lower frequencies (e.g., 60 Hz), as well (31). Because beneficial effects commonly take weeks or months to become evident, stimulation settings initially are guided by tolerability, rather than by efficacy. Following activation of stimulation, some patients may experience a transient worsening in dystonic spasm that necessitates a reduction in stimulation intensity. As acclimatization to stimulation occurs, stimulation parameters can then gradually be increased. The time course for response varies among patients; some exhibit rapid improvement in dystonic signs, but in most patients there is a lag of weeks to months after initiation of stimulation until improvement is seen, with full accrual of benefit taking many months. In one study in which extent of dystonia was scored repeatedly over time, 95% of maximal long-term improvement had been reached six months after activation of stimulation (32).

## Outcomes

DBS has only recently been used to treat dystonia, and thus efficacy and outcome data are relatively limited and continue to evolve. The majority of patients worldwide have been treated with DBS directed at the GPi, although thalamic stimulation has been used in a limited number of patients (33–37). Additionally, recent interest in the use of the subthalamic nucleus target has emerged (38,39). Because the vast majority of outcome data are currently in patients treated with pallidal stimulation, the discussion that follows pertains to that target.

### *Primary Generalized Dystonia*

The use of DBS to treat dystonia was first reported in a seven-year-old girl with severe and rapidly progressive primary generalized dystonia (40). This child, who required general anesthesia and assisted ventilation due to the severity of her dystonia, had failed exhaustive attempts at pharmacological management. Following implantation of bilateral DBS leads into the globus pallidus (GP) and activation of stimulation, the patient experienced rapid and dramatic improvement in her dystonic signs and associated disability. This finding lead to the use of DBS in additional patients with disabling dystonia.

Indeed, primary generalized dystonia syndromes appear to be the most robustly responsive dystonic disorders to treatment with DBS. In an open-label, uncontrolled series of 31 subjects, a mean improvement of 79% in the BFMDRS movement score and 65% in the disability score was reported at two-year follow-up evaluation (41). In this study, patients were evaluated following stimulation at 3, 6, 12, and 24 months. Robust improvement was typically evident by three months but continued to gradually improve over time. Significant improvement occurred in children and in adults; movement scores tended to be somewhat more improved in children, although disability scores improved to a similar extent. In this series, no significant difference in mean response was found between those patients positive for the *DYT1* mutation and those without that genotype. The only adverse event observed in the group of 31 patients was an infection at the neurostimulator site in one patient.

A prospective, controlled, multicenter study in 22 patients with primary generalized dystonia documented mean improvements in the 12-month postoperative

BFMDRS movement and disability scores of 54% and 44%, respectively (42). All but 2 of the 15 patients without the *DYT1* mutation experienced benefit, and all of those with the *DYT1* mutation realized improvement. Benefits were obvious at the three-month evaluation period and persisted at 12 months. Significant improvements in the general health and physical functioning domains of the Short-Form General Health Survey (SF-36), a health-related quality-of-life instrument, also occurred. Five adverse events in three patients occurred, all of which resolved rapidly and without permanent sequelae.

A number of additional reports consistently document the excellent degree of motoric and functional response realized by patients with primary generalized dystonia treated with pallidal deep brain stimulation (30,32,43–53). Mean improvement in dystonia scores in these series ranges from 47% to 74%. Importantly, while it was common for the majority of patients in these reports to exhibit a substantial improvement in their dystonia status, a subgroup of patients in virtually all series realized a more modest response or, rarely, no meaningful benefit. The basis for this diminished improvement is currently unclear, and therefore it is difficult to predict in advance which patients will or will not achieve a significant response. Suboptimal DBS lead location may explain some, but certainly not all, of these instances of underwhelming response. Perhaps some variants of primary generalized dystonia unassociated with the *DYT1* mutation have underlying pathophysiological changes that fail to be modulated by existing stimulation techniques. As the pathophysiology of dystonia and mechanism of action of DBS become better understood, the ability to predict outcomes and counsel patients preoperatively will likely increase. Until then, pallidal DBS remains the most effective treatment for primary generalized dystonia, and clinicians can advise patients and their families that the majority of patients will appreciate a meaningful benefit from this therapy.

### *Idiopathic Cervical Dystonia*

Because a sizeable number of patients with idiopathic cervical dystonia fail to achieve long-term, sustained benefit from chemodenervation therapy (54), the availability of other treatment options is important. Accumulating evidence supports the efficacy of pallidal DBS for cervical dystonia. Most reports thus far consist of individual case reports or series with small numbers of patients (30–32,43–45,47,52,55–62), although a prospective, multicenter trial with blinded evaluators is underway (63). The vast majority of patients have been treated with bilateral pallidal stimulation, however two reports suggest efficacy with unilateral stimulation (one ipsilateral to the affected sternocleidomastoid muscle, the other contralateral to the involved muscle) (61,62). Reported mean postoperative improvement in the Toronto Western Spasmodic Torticollis Rating Scale (TWSTRS) severity score ranges from 48% to 76%. Mean improvements in TWSTRS disability and pain scores range from 60% to 75% and 38% to 100%, respectively. Despite these favorable overall improvements, some patients fail to exhibit benefit (30). Some patients with modest motor improvement nevertheless report marked and sustained improvement in the pain associated with their cervical dystonia (60).

### *Other Primary Dystonia Syndromes*

The use of DBS for other primary dystonia syndromes is somewhat limited, but outcome data are beginning to emerge. Several reports document significant improvement of craniofacial dystonia and dystonia involving craniofacial and axial regions (64–67). Prompt resolution or substantial improvement of blepharospasm and oromandibular dystonia occurred after stimulation was initiated. Pallidal DBS has also been reported to improve both the dystonic and the myoclonic components of the myoclonus–dystonia syndrome (68,69).

*Tardive Dystonia*

Several published reports suggest that tardive dystonic syndromes are responsive to pallidal DBS (30),(37),(70–72). Significant improvements in dystonic and choreiform components have been seen. The largest series of tardive patients treated with DBS of the GP showed rapid and sustained improvement in all five patients (72). Other reports describe some tardive dystonia patients as not deriving significant benefit from DBS (30,52).

*Other Secondary Dystonias*

DBS has been applied to treat a variety of secondary dystonic disorders. Benefits have generally been less robust than those seen in primary dystonia syndromes (43), yet clinically meaningful improvements in dystonia scores and in patient function have been observed in some patients.

In a large series of dystonia patients treated with pallidal DBS at the same center, the mean improvement in the BFMDRS movement score was 31% for those patients with secondary dystonia syndromes versus 73% for patients with primary disorders (46). Of note, the 21 patients with secondary dystonia in that report had severe, medically intractable dystonia due to a variety of etiologies, including perinatal anoxia, postanoxic encephalopathies, mitochondrial cytopathies, and PKAN. Those with PKAN seem to represent a particularly responsive subset of secondary dystonia patients, with studies consistently documenting sustained excellent benefit (75–80% improvement in movement scores) from pallidal DBS (30,52,73,74).

Limited cases of posttraumatic dystonia treated with DBS have been reported, with symptom improvement described in some patients (30,48,61,75), but not in others (45,52). The few reported outcomes in patients with postanoxic dystonia, poststroke dystonia, and postencephalitic dystonia treated with DBS have been variable but generally modest or disappointing (30,43,46,51,52).

## Mechanism of Action

Significant gaps currently exist in understanding the mechanism of action by which electrical stimulation of basal ganglia nuclei improves movement disorders in general and dystonia in particular. The pathophysiology of dystonia itself is also poorly understood.

In dystonia, abnormalities at the level of basal ganglia nuclei have been documented, with intraoperative recordings of single unit neuronal activity in GPi demonstrating reduced discharge rates, increased oscillatory activity, and increased bursting activity compared to normal nonhuman primates (76). This abnormal pallidal activity may lead to uncontrolled synchrony throughout the subcortical–cortical network, disruption in cortical and brainstem output, and the resultant disordered movement seen in dystonia (77). Indeed, functional imaging studies demonstrate abnormalities at the cortical level, with $H_2{}^{15}O$ positron emission tomography (PET) blood flow data suggesting inappropriate overactivity in motor executive areas (78).

DBS, which delivers regularly patterned, high-frequency stimulation, may convert the aberrant neuronal activity in the GPi from a pattern disruptive to motor information processing to a pattern that has less deleterious impact on cortical regions (79). PET studies in patients with dystonia show that DBS of GPi reverses abnormal overactivity in cortical motor regions (80,81). This modulation of pathological network activity appears to underlie the basis for clinical improvement, although many details remain to be established.

## DYSTONIA PATIENT CANDIDACY FOR SURGICAL TREATMENT

In selecting dystonia patients for surgical treatment, the heterogeneous nature of dystonia requires an approach that is individualized to each patient. For each patient, a number of factors, summarized in Table 1, need to be considered. These include the type of their dystonia and its associated natural history; level of disability, functional impairment, pain, and associated musculoskeletal deformity produced by their dystonia; extent to which other appropriate treatments, administered in an optimal manner, have been undertaken and have failed to produce sufficient benefit; willingness of the patient to accept the potential risks of surgery and the potential for no meaningful benefit or incomplete control of symptoms. When treatment with DBS is being considered, the patient and their family must understand key issues related to use of that treatment for dystonia, including the need for repeated follow-up visits to adjust the stimulation, the probable lag time until benefit occurs, and device-related issues.

Patients with childhood or adolescent-onset primary generalized dystonia associated with documented *DYT1* mutation are the most straightforward candidates in whom to recommend surgical treatment, particularly DBS. The known natural history of the disorder is one of progressive and often severe disability, this type of dystonia generally is refractory to pharmacological therapy, and the syndrome usually responds dramatically to DBS of the GP. Indeed, whenever possible for these patients,

**Table 1** Dystonia Patient Candidacy for Surgical Treatment: Issues to Consider

| Factor | Comments |
|---|---|
| Dystonia type and its likelihood of responding to surgical intervention | Primary dystonia syndromes tend to be more responsive than most secondary disorders; tardive dystonia and dystonia associated with pantothenate kinase-associated neurodegeneration can be responsive |
| Natural history of the dystonia syndrome | Surgical intervention may be considered before maximum disability ensues for those syndromes known to typically progress and lead to significant disability |
| Level of disability produced by the dystonia | Is the severity of dystonia sufficient to justify the potential risks of surgery; relevant issues include functional limitations, musculoskeletal deformity, and pain |
| Extent to which the dystonia has failed treatment with pharmacological measures | Appropriate oral medications and, where indicated, chemodenervation treatment should be tried prior to surgery |
| Patient and family expectations | The patient should understand the potential risks of surgery and conclude that these risks are acceptable to them in light of their level of disability and impaired quality of life. They should understand and accept the range of potential benefits, the lag time that may occur before full benefit is realized, and the therapy requirements (e.g., adjustment of deep brain stimulation settings) |

intervention at the onset of troubling symptoms—rather than after severe disability and associated physical and psychosocial sequelae have ensued—seems prudent.

Patients with other primary dystonias can exhibit very favorable responses to surgical treatment, but their less consistent and sometimes less robust response must be factored into the decision-making process. Certainly, patients with idiopathic cervical dystonia and other focal or regional dystonias potentially amenable to treatment with chemodenervation should be treated optimally with botulinum toxin before referral for brain surgery. If chemodenervation and oral pharmacotherapy fail to provide sufficient benefit, then surgical intervention should be entertained. Patients with tardive dystonias, owing to their often favorable response to DBS therapy, should also be considered for surgical treatment when pharmacological measures fall short.

Because of the less consistent and less dramatic response commonly encountered in patients with most nontardive, secondary dystonia syndromes, weighing of the risk/benefit ratio and confirmation of realistic expectations is particularly important in counseling such patients and their families. Even when modest improvements occur in this group of patients, the results can be clinically meaningful.

## CONCLUSIONS

The limited capacity of current pharmacological measures to adequately treat dystonia makes the availability of surgical treatments important in the management of patients with these disorders. In particular, the ability to modulate aberrant motor systems activity using DBS offers an attractive option in the treatment of many patients with pharmacoresistant dystonia. Neuromodulation strategies will undoubtedly continue to evolve as the pathophysiology of dystonia becomes better understood, surgical techniques become even more refined, and technological improvements in neuromodulation therapies occur. In the meantime, using current procedures in appropriately selected patients, surgical intervention can provide dramatic suppression of dystonic symptoms and significant improvement in function.

## REFERENCES

1. Starr PA, Vitek JL, Bakay RA. Ablative surgery and deep brain stimulation for Parkinson's disease. Neurosurgery 1998; 43(5):989–1013; discussion 1013–1015.
2. Okun MS, Stover NP, Subramanian T, et al. Complications of gamma knife surgery for Parkinson disease. Arch Neurol 2001; 58(12):1995–2002.
3. Hua Z, Guodong G, Qinchuan L, et al. Analysis of complications of radiofrequency pallidotomy. Neurosurgery 2003; 52(1):89–99; discussion 99–101.
4. Akbostanci MC, Slavin KV, Burchiel KJ. Stereotactic ventral intermedial thalamotomy for the treatment of essential tremor: results of a series of 37 patients. Stereotact Funct Neurosurg 1999; 72(2–4):174–177.
5. Cooper IS. 20-year follow-up study of the neurosurgical treatment of dystonia musculorum deformans. Adv Neurol 1976; 14:423–452.
6. Andrew J, Fowler CJ, Harrison MJ. Stereotaxic thalamotomy in 55 cases of dystonia. Brain 1983; 106(Pt 4):981–1000.
7. von Essen C, Augustinsson LE, Lindqvist G. VOI thalamotomy in spasmodic torticollis. Appl Neurophysiol 1980; 43(3–5):159–163.

8. Yamashiro K, Tasker RR. Stereotactic thalamotomy for dystonic patients. Stereotact Funct Neurosurg 1993; 60(1–3):81–85.
9. Cardoso F, Jankovic J, Grossman RG, et al. Outcome after stereotactic thalamotomy for dystonia and hemiballismus. Neurosurgery 1995; 36(3):501–507; discussion 507–508.
10. Mempel E, Kucinski L, Witkiewicz B. (Writer's cramp syndrome treated successfully by thalamotomy).
11. Hillier CE, Wiles CM, Simpson BA. Thalamotomy for severe antipsychotic induced tardive dyskinesia and dystonia. J Neurol Neurosurg Psychiatr 1999; 66(2):250–251.
12. Tsukamoto H, Inui K, Taniike M, et al. A case of Hallervorden-Spatz disease: progressive and intractable dystonia controlled by bilateral thalamotomy. Brain Dev 1992; 14(4):269–272.
13. Teive HA, Sa DS, Grande CV, et al. Bilateral pallidotomy for generalized dystonia. Arq Neuropsiquiatr 2001; 59(2–B):353–357.
14. Vitek JL, Bakay RAE, Hashimoto T, et al. Microelectrode-guided pallidotomy: technical approach and application for medically intractable Parkinson's disease. J Neurosurg 1998; 88:1027–1043.
15. Ondo WG, Desaloms JM, Jankovic J, et al. Pallidotomy for generalized dystonia. Mov Disord 1998; 13(4):693–698.
16. Lozano AM, Kumar R, Gross RE, et al. Globus pallidus internus pallidotomy for generalized dystonia. Mov Disord 1997; 12(6):865–870.
17. Krack P, Vercueil L. Review of the functional surgical treatment of dystonia. Eur J Neurol 2001; 8(5):389–399.
18. Lin JJ, Lin SZ, Chang, DC. Pallidotomy and generalized dystonia. Mov Disord 1999; 14(6):1057–1059.
19. Lin JJ, Lin SZ, Lin GY, et al. Treatment of intractable generalized dystonia by bilateral posteroventral pallidotomy—one-year results. Zhonghua Yi Xue Za Zhi (Taipei) 2001; 64(4):231–238.
20. Justesen CR, Penn RD, Kroin JS, et al. Stereotactic pallidotomy in a child with Hallervorden-Spatz disease. Case report. J Neurosurg 1999; 90(3):551–554.
21. Kyriagis M, Grattan-Smith P, Scheinberg A, et al. Status dystonicus and Hallervorden-Spatz disease: treatment with intrathecal baclofen and pallidotomy. J Paediatr Child Health 2004; 40(5–6):322–325.
22. Rakocevic G, Lyons KE, Wilkinson SB, et al. Bilateral pallidotomy for severe dystonia in an 18-month-old child with glutaric aciduria. Stereotact Funct Neurosurg 2004; 82(2–3): 80–83.
23. Cubo E, Shannon KM, Penn RD, et al. Internal globus pallidotomy in dystonia secondary to Huntington's disease. Mov Disord 2000; 15(6):1248–1251.
24. Lin JJ, Lin GY, Shih C, et al. Benefit of bilateral pallidotomy in the treatment of generalized dystonia. Case report. J Neurosurg 1999; 90(5):974–976.
25. Weetman J, Anderson IM, Gregory RP, et al. Bilateral posteroventral pallidotomy for severe antipsychotic induced tardive dyskinesia and dystonia. J Neurol Neurosurg Psychiatr 1997; 63(4):554–556.
26. Yoshor D, Hamilton WJ, Ondo W, et al. Comparison of thalamotomy and pallidotomy for the treatment of dystonia. Neurosurgery 2001; 48(4):818–824; discussion 824.
27. Benabid AL, Pollak P, Louveau A, et al. Combined (thalamotomy and stimulation) stereotactic surgery of the VIM thalamic nucleus for bilateral Parkinson disease. Appl Neurophysiol 1987; 50(1–6):344–346.
28. Binder DK, Rau GM, Starr PA. Risk factors for hemorrhage during microelectrode-guided deep brain stimulator implantation for movement disorders. Neurosurgery 2005; 56(4):722–732; discussion 722–732.
29. Umemura A, Jaggi JL, Hurtig HI, et al. Deep brain stimulation for movement disorders: morbidity and mortality in 109 patients. J Neurosurg 2003; 98(4):779–784.
30. Starr PA, Turner RS, Rau G, et al. Microelectrode-guided implantation of deep brain stimulators into the globus pallidus internus for dystonia: techniques, electrode locations, and outcomes. Neurosurg Focus 2004; 17(1):E4.

31. Goto S, Mita S, Ushio Y. Bilateral pallidal stimulation for cervical dystonia. An optimal paradigm from our experiences. Stereotact Funct Neurosurg 2002; 79(3–4):221–227.
32. Bittar RG, Yianni J, Wang S, et al. Deep brain stimulation for generalised dystonia and spasmodic torticollis. J Clin Neurosci 2005; 12(1):12–16.
33. Sellal F, Hirsch E, Barth P, et al. A case of symptomatic hemidystonia improved by ventroposterolateral thalamic electrostimulation. Mov Disord 1993; 8(4):515–518.
34. Mundinger F. [New stereotactic treatment of spasmodic torticollis with a brain stimulation system (author's transl)].
35. Andy OJ. Thalamic stimulation for control of movement disorders. Appl Neurophysiol 1983; 46(1–4):107–111.
36. Vercueil L, Krack P, Pollak P. Results of deep brain stimulation for dystonia: a critical reappraisal. Mov Disord 2002; 17(Suppl 3):S89–S93.
37. Trottenberg T, Paul G, Meissner W, et al. Pallidal and thalamic neurostimulation in severe tardive dystonia. J Neurol Neurosurg Psychiatr 2001; 70(4):557–559.
38. Benabid AL, Koudsie A, Benazzouz A, et al. Deep brain stimulation of the corpus luysi (subthalamic nucleus) and other targets in Parkinson's disease. Extension to new indications such as dystonia and epilepsy. J Neurol 2001; 248(Suppl 3):III37–III47.
39. Chou KL, Hurtig HI, Jaggi JL, et al. Bilateral subthalamic nucleus deep brain stimulation in a patient with cervical dystonia and essential tremor. Mov Disord 2005; 20(3):377–380.
40. Coubes P, Humbertclaude V, Bauchet L, et al. Bilateral chronic electrical stimulation of the internal globus pallidus as a treatment of idiopathic dystonia in musculorum deformans: case report. Stereotact Funct Neurosurg 1997; 67:70.
41. Coubes P, Cif L, El Fertit H, et al. Electrical stimulation of the globus pallidus internus in patients with primary generalized dystonia: long-term results. J Neurosurg 2004; 101(2): 189–194.
42. Vidailhet M, Vercueil L, Houeto JL, et al. Bilateral deep-brain stimulation of the globus pallidus in primary generalized dystonia. N Engl J Med 2005; 352(5):459–467.
43. Eltahawy HA, Saint-Cyr J, Giladi N, et al. Primary dystonia is more responsive than secondary dystonia to pallidal interventions: outcome after pallidotomy or pallidal deep brain stimulation. Neurosurgery 2004; 54(3):613–619; discussion 619–621.
44. Yianni J, Bain PG, Gregory RP, et al. Post-operative progress of dystonia patients following globus pallidus internus deep brain stimulation. Eur J Neurol 2003; 10(3): 239–247.
45. Yianni J, Bain P, Giladi N, et al. Globus pallidus internus deep brain stimulation for dystonic conditions: a prospective audit. Mov Disord 2003; 18(4):436–442.
46. Cif L, El Fertit H, Vayssiere N, et al. Treatment of dystonic syndromes by chronic electrical stimulation of the internal globus pallidus. J Neurosurg Sci 2003; 47(1):52–55.
47. Bereznai B, Steude U, Seelos K, et al. Chronic high-frequency globus pallidus internus stimulation in different types of dystonia: a clinical, video, and MRI report of six patients presenting with segmental, cervical, and generalized dystonia. Mov Disord 2002; 17(1): 138–144.
48. Vercueil L, Pollak P, Fraix V, et al. Deep brain stimulation in the treatment of severe dystonia. J Neurol 2001; 248(8):695–700.
49. Tronnier VM, Fogel W. Pallidal stimulation for generalized dystonia. Report of three cases. J Neurosurg 2000; 92(3):453–456.
50. Krauss JK, Loher TJ, Weigel R, et al. Chronic stimulation of the globus pallidus internus for treatment of non-dYT1 generalized dystonia and choreoathetosis: 2-year follow up. J Neurosurg 2003; 98(4):785–792.
51. Zorzi G, Marras C, Nardocci N, et al. Stimulation of the globus pallidus internus for childhood-onset dystonia. Mov Disord 2005; 20(9):1194–1200.
52. Krause M, Fogel W, Kloss M, et al. Pallidal stimulation for dystonia. Neurosurgery 2004; 55(6):1361–1368; discussion 1368–1370.
53. Kupsch A, Klaffke S, Kuhn AA, et al. The effects of frequency in pallidal deep brain stimulation for primary dystonia. J Neurol 2003; 250(10):1201–1205.

54. Hsiung GY, Das SK, Ranawaya R, et al. Long-term efficacy of botulinum toxin A in treatment of various movement disorders over a 10-year period. Mov Disord 2002; 17(6):1288–1293.
55. Krauss JK, Loher TJ, Pohle T, et al. Pallidal deep brain stimulation in patients with cervical dystonia and severe cervical dyskinesias with cervical myelopathy. J Neurol Neurosurg Psychiatr 2002; 72(2):249–256.
56. Andaluz N, Taha JM, Dalvi A. Bilateral pallidal deep brain stimulation for cervical and truncal dystonia. Neurology 2001; 57(3):557–558.
57. Parkin S, Aziz T, Gregory R, et al. Bilateral internal globus pallidus stimulation for the treatment of spasmodic torticollis. Mov Disord 2001; 16(3):489–493.
58. Krauss JK, Pohle T, Weber S, et al. Bilateral stimulation of globus pallidus internus for treatment of cervical dystonia. Lancet 1999; 354(9181):837–838.
59. Eltahawy HA, Saint-Cyr J, Poon YY, et al. Pallidal deep brain stimulation in cervical dystonia: clinical outcome in four cases. Can J Neurol Sci 2004; 31(3):328–332.
60. Kulisevsky J, Lleo A, Gironell A, et al. Bilateral pallidal stimulation for cervical dystonia: dissociated pain and motor improvement. Neurology 2000; 55(11):1754–1755.
61. Chang JW, Choi JY, Lee BW, et al. Unilateral globus pallidus internus stimulation improves delayed onset post-traumatic cervical dystonia with an ipsilateral focal basal ganglia lesion. J Neurol Neurosurg Psychiatr 2002; 73(5):588–590.
62. Escamilla-Sevilla F, Minguez-Castellanos A, Arjona-Moron V, et al. Unilateral pallidal stimulation for segmental cervical and truncal dystonia: which side? Mov Disord 2002; 17(6):1383–1385.
63. Kiss ZH, Doig K, Eliasziw M, et al. The Canadian multicenter trial of pallidal deep brain stimulation for cervical dystonia: preliminary results in three patients. Neurosurg Focus 2004; 17(1):E5.
64. Foote KD, Sanchez JC, Okun MS. Staged deep brain stimulation for refractory craniofacial dystonia with blepharospasm: case report and physiology. Neurosurgery 2005; 56(2):E415; discussion E415.
65. Capelle HH, Weigel R, Krauss JK. Bilateral pallidal stimulation for blepharospasm-oromandibular dystonia (Meige syndrome). Neurology 2003; 60(12):2017–2018.
66. Houser M, Waltz T. Meige syndrome and pallidal deep brain stimulation. Mov Disord 2005; 20(9):1203–1205.
67. Muta D, Goto S, Nishikawa S, et al. Bilateral pallidal stimulation for idiopathic segmental axial dystonia advanced from Meige syndrome refractory to bilateral thalamotomy. Mov Disord 2001; 16(4):774–777.
68. Cif L, Valente EM, Hemm S, et al. Deep brain stimulation in myoclonus-dystonia syndrome. Mov Disord 2004; 19(6):724–727.
69. Magarinos-Ascone CM, Regidor I, Martinez-Castrillo JC, et al. Pallidal stimulation relieves myoclonus-dystonia syndrome. J Neurol Neurosurg Psychiatr 2005; 76(7):989–991.
70. Eltahawy HA, Feinstein A, Khan F, et al. Bilateral globus pallidus internus deep brain stimulation in tardive dyskinesia: a case report. Mov Disord 2004; 19(8):969–972.
71. Franzini A, Marras C, Ferroli P, et al. Long-term high-frequency bilateral pallidal stimulation for neuroleptic-induced tardive dystonia. Report of two cases. J Neurosurg 2005; 102(4):721–725.
72. Trottenberg T, Volkmann J, Deuschl G, et al. Treatment of severe tardive dystonia with pallidal deep brain stimulation. Neurology 2005; 64(2):344–346.
73. Umemura A, Jaggi JL, Dolinskas CA, et al. Pallidal deep brain stimulation for longstanding severe generalized dystonia in Hallervorden-Spatz syndrome. Case report. J Neurosurg 2004; 100(4):706–709.
74. Castelnau P, Cif L, Valente EM, et al. Pallidal stimulation improves pantothenate kinase-associated neurodegeneration. Ann Neurol 2005; 57(5):738–741.
75. Loher TJ, Hasdemir MG, Burgunder JM, et al. Long-term follow-up study of chronic globus pallidus internus stimulation for posttraumatic hemidystonia. J Neurosurg 2000; 92(3):457–460.

76. Starr PA, Rau GM, Davis V, et al. Spontaneous pallidal neuronal activity in human dystonia: comparison with Parkinson's disease and normal macaque. J Neurophysiol 2005; 93(6):3165–3176.
77. Vitek JL. Pathophysiology of dystonia: a neuronal model. Mov Disord 2002; 17(Suppl 3): S49–62.
78. Ceballos-Baumann AO, Boecker H, Bartenstein P, et al. A positron emission tomographic study of subthalamic nucleus stimulation in Parkinson's disease: enhanced movement-related activity of motor-association cortex and decreased motor cortex resting activity. Arch Neurol 1999; 56:997–1003.
79. Montgomery EB Jr. Deep brain stimulation for hyperkinetic disorders. Neurosurg Focus 2004; 17(1):E1.
80. Kumar R, Dagher A, Hutchison WD, et al. Globus pallidus deep brain stimulation for generalized dystonia: clinical and PET investigation. Neurology 1999; 53(4):871–874.
81. Detante O, Vercueil L, Thobois S, et al. Globus pallidus internus stimulation in primary generalized dystonia: a H215O PET study. Brain 2004; 127(Pt 8):1899–1908.

# Index